A Clinician's Guide to Tuberculosis

A Clinician's Guide to Tuberculosis

Michael D. Iseman, M.D.
Girard and Madeline Beno Chair in Mycobacterial Diseases
National Jewish Medical and Research Center, and
Professor of Medicine
University of Colorado School of Medicine
Denver, Colorado

LIPPINCOTT WILLIAMS & WILKINS
A **Wolters Kluwer** Company
Philadelphia • Baltimore • New York • London
Buenos Aires • Hong Kong • Sydney • Tokyo

Acquisitions Editor: Jonathan W. Pine, Jr.
Developmental Editor: Kathleen Courtney Millet
Production Editor: Robin E. Cook
Manufacturing Manager: Tim Reynolds
Cover Designer: Tik Chuaviriya
Compositor: Maryland Composition
Printer: Edwards Brothers

Printed in the USA

Library of Congress Cataloging-in-Publication Data

Iseman, Michael D.
A clinician's guide to tuberculosis / Michael D. Iseman.
p. cm.
Includes bibliographical references and index.
ISBN 0-7817-1749-3
1. Tuberculosis. I. Title.
[DNLM: 1. Tuberculosis. WF 200 178c 2000]
RC311.I74 2000
616.9′ 95—dc21
DNLM/DLC
for Library of Congress

99-40515
CIP

Care has been taken to confirm the accuracy of the information presented and to describe generally accepted practices. However, the authors, editors, and publisher are not responsible for errors or omissions or for any consequences from application of the information in this book and make no warranty, expressed or implied, with respect to the currency, completeness, or accuracy of the contents of the publication. Application of this information in a particular situation remains the professional responsibility of the practitioner.

The authors, editors, and publisher have exerted every effort to ensure that drug selection and dosage set forth in this text are in accordance with current recommendations and practice at the time of publication. However, in view of ongoing research, changes in government regulations, and the constant flow of information relating to drug therapy and drug reactions, the reader is urged to check the package insert for each drug for any change in indications and dosage and for added warnings and precautions. This is particularly important when the recommended agent is a new or infrequently employed drug.

Some drugs and medical devices presented in this publication have Food and Drug Administration (FDA) clearance for limited use in restricted research settings. It is the responsibility of the health care provider to ascertain the FDA status of each drug or device planned for use in their clinical practice.

10 9 8 7 6 5 4

To my mother, the nurse, Eileen Croghan Iseman, R.N. who, in ministering to my childhood maladies, first taught me tender loving care—the essence of medicine. To my wife Joan, and sons, Tom and Matt, who have brought joy and meaning that sustained me through the times of doubt and discouragement. And, finally, to those patients in whose care I have had the privilege to participate. The many and varied manifestations of their illnesses have instructed me about the disease; and their dignity, forbearance, and bravery in the face of devastating sickness and arduous treatment have informed me of the best aspects of humanity.

Contents

Preface

Mycobacterium tuberculosis is the most pervasive, morbid, and lethal microbial pathogen of humans. From the equator to the polar circles, on all seven continents, males and females, young and old of all races are at risk from this debilitating, disabling, and potentially fatal infection.

Tuberculosis has no intermediate vector like the mosquito of malaria; it is transmitted solely by direct human-to-human spread. It has no reservoir in nature like the polluted water of cholera; its only vessel for transport through time and across space is a person infected with the bacillus.

Tuberculosis primarily attacks the lungs, but the microbe has been noted to invade virtually every organ system from the skin to the bowel, from the brain to the bones.

The tubercle bacillus' primary habitat within the human body is the mononuclear phagocyte or macrophage. Paradoxically, this cell is the body's primary mode of defense against tuberculosis. The scientific unraveling of this puzzling duality offers exciting insights into the subtle, fragile balance between the host and this biologically clever parasite.

Unlike viral epidemic illnesses such as polio and smallpox that have been amenable to vaccine control, tuberculosis had defied the efforts of twentieth-century scientists to create a vaccine which is epidemiologically effective—that is, one which interrupts the cycle of transmission of infection.

The one truly successful battle that humans have waged against the tubercle bacillus has been the development of effective antimicrobial drugs. After millennia of desperate searches for a remedy, medications which proffered nearly universal cures have been discovered in the latter half of this century. Perversely, however, curative treatment requires extended periods of administration, taxing both the tolerance of the individual patient and the assets of society. Sadly, we have witnessed the widespread squandering of this precious legacy as inadequate treatment programs have generated escalating levels of resistance to these medicines among strains of *M. tuberculosis* around the globe.

In addition to breaching our biological defenses, tuberculosis has shown a striking propensity for attacking through social frailties such as poverty, overcrowding, and malnutrition. This phenomenon was poignantly delineated by René and Jean Dubos in *The White Plague* (1952):

> Tuberculosis is a social disease, and presents problems that transcend the traditional medical approach. . . . Its understanding demands that the impact of social and economic factors on the individual be considered as much as the mechanisms by which the tubercle bacilli cause damage to the human body. . . . It is the consequence of gross defects in social organization, and of errors in individual behavior.

As predicted by the Duboses, the concept of a scientific conquest of tuberculosis has proven hubristic. The extensive social problems of the developing nations have proven to be a substantial but anticipated barrier to tuberculosis control. Somewhat surprisingly, though, there remain extensive groups in the more prosperous, industrialized nations whose socioeconomic circumstances have proven to be major impediments to the prevention and cure of tuberculosis in the last decade of this century.

In retrospect, one of the great ironies of twentieth-century medical science has been the widely held perception that the advent of chemotherapy meant the death knell for the disease. Indeed, despite the immense global morbidity and mortality of tuberculosis, there has been a shameful paucity of research related to the disease over the last four decades.

But, the most ominous recent element in the ongoing duel between humankind and the tubercle bacillus has been the appearance and explosive spread of the human immunodeficiency virus (HIV). This virus abets tuberculosis in both the biological and demographic arenas. By attacking and disabling the T-lymphocytes, HIV progressively vitiates the cellular immune mechanisms which control tubercle bacilli within the body. Thus, HIV-infected persons are at greatly increased risk of endogenous reactivation of latent tuberculosis infection and probably are at heightened jeopardy of acquiring new infection. Demographically, tuberculosis and HIV infection have tended to congregate in the same populations. Following the explosion of HIV in sub-Saharan Africa, tuberculosis case rates have soared there. In large areas of the United States, HIV has proven a powerful facilitator of surging tuberculosis case rates. Having established beachheads in large cities in Latin America, Asia and the Indian subcontinent, HIV appears poised to spread throughout these regions with potentially immense implications for the epidemiology of tuberculosis. Indeed, because of its impact on host defenses and its predilection for groups and regions in which tuberculosis infections are highly prevalent, HIV may be expected to unleash immense morbidity and mortality from tuberculosis over the next two decades, no matter what advances are made in the near future regarding the diagnosis, treatment, or prevention of either of these infections.

Acknowledgments

We are all the products of our academic culture, an intellectual lineage. Sir Isaac Newton once said that if he had seen further, it was because he was "standing on the shoulders of Giants." The father of the Bellevue Hospital tuberculosis program and chest service was J. Burns Amberson whose teaching and clinical skills spawned several generations of pulmonary academic leaders. Among his followers at Bellevue was Julia Jones, M.D., whose unassuming manner, immense decency, and warmth became a beacon and inspiration for many of my generation. Gently, she taught us at the weekly case conferences about the enormous complexity and subtlety of tuberculosis. Dr. Jones arranged my participation in a research project in the laboratory of Gladys Hobby, Ph.D., in East Orange, New Jersey. Dr. Hobby was a stern and demanding mentor, and her respect for the sanctity of data was absolute and memorable.

Gerald Bertram Webb came to Manitou Springs, Colorado from foggy England, seeking the sunshine and fresh-air cure for his wife Jenny's consumption. Having interrupted his studies at Guy's Hospital in London because of his wife's sickness, he completed his medical degree in Denver and helped set in motion the scientific fascination with tuberculosis that has been a dominant theme of medicine in Colorado throughout this century. Among the patients treated by Dr. Webb was James J. Waring, who contracted tuberculosis while a medical student at Johns Hopkins. After he was cured, Waring went on to become the chief of medicine at the fledgling University of Colorado School of Medicine. He, in turn, recruited Roger Mitchell to head up the newly formed Webb-Waring Institute for the cure and prevention of tuberculosis. Dr. Mitchell, whose training in neurology at the Massachusetts General Hospital had been interrupted by tuberculosis, went on to study consumption while recovering at the famous Trudeau Sanatorium in Saranac Lake, New York. Professor Mitchell continued to attend our tuberculosis conferences well into his eighties, sharing his invaluable wisdom.

In the early part of the twentieth century, when tuberculosis was rampant, thousands flocked every year to Colorado, desperately seeking "the mountain cure." Many of them were without any resources. In response to their great needs, the Jewish community of Denver raised a modest amount of money and opened a small facility for their care. Thus, was born the National Jewish Hospital, which over the years recruited a distinguished faculty, most recently Drs. Paul Davidson and Marian Goble, two wonderful clinicians. Sustaining its tuberculosis programs when others in North America boarded up or turned to trendier diseases, National Jewish has proven a unique repository for clinical and basic science related to this ancient scourge.

Finally, I owe immense gratitude to two persons. Dr. Charles Ragan was my chief of medicine at both Bellevue and Harlem Hospitals in New York. He was a quiet but strong man who patiently instructed and nurtured his residents, inspiring many of us to consider careers in academic medicine. After I moved to Colorado in 1972 to take a position at Denver General Hospital, I had the good fortune to work with a boundlessly enthusiastic teacher and student of tuberculosis, John Sbarbaro. A counselor, mentor, and special friend, John facilitated my involvement with tuberculosis at both the local and national level, promoting my opportunities in a most generous way.

Medical Knowledge

An Historical Process

"The truth" in medical science is the goal of all clinicians. As students we study avidly—in varying priority—to pass exams, shine (or, at least, spare ourselves from embarrassment) on rounds, prepare for boards, and equip ourselves to establish diagnoses and treat patients. At that stage of our experience, we are prone to chuckle smugly at the gross misunderstandings or naivete of prior generations and to feel comfortably reassured that we—bolstered by "vastly superior" scientific methods—enjoy true understanding. We tell ourselves: "If only I can master this material I will be equipped for a long and distinguished career."

However, within a few years of graduation, many of our verities have gone by the wayside, replaced by "newer truth." Indeed, it is apparent that the process is like peeling an infinite onion: layer-by-layer we futilely seek the core of knowledge. Try as we might, perfect understanding eludes us. Like quicksilver, our conceptions and models refuse to remain in place; perturbed by new research or observations, the data jiggle about until they are reorganized into new paradigms for future generations to embrace as the ultimate revelation.

Having witnessed, reluctantly, this process for over three decades, I have attempted to write my version of tuberculosis from a historical perspective, to frame my analyses or recommendations as imperfect iterations of contemporary understanding. While I am sure that Professor Eric Goldman, for whom I wrote my collegiate senior thesis (on radical agrarian political movements during the Great Depression) would have been critical of my awkward efforts to think and write as a historian, I hope that he would have approved of my efforts to honor his teachings.

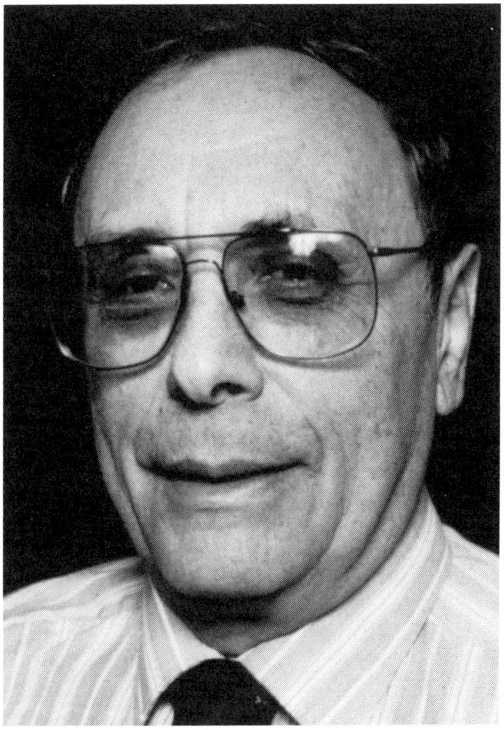

Dr. Leonid Heifits

Dr. Leonid Heifits immigrated to the United States from the Soviet Union in 1978. Coming to Colorado as a research associate, he rapidly rose to prominence as perhaps the most visionary clinical laboratorian of this era. Recognizing the critical importance of prompt and accurate diagnostic services, Leonid pioneered in rapid culture techniques and quantitative in vitro susceptibility methods. He has also been a persuasive advocate for centralized, sophisticated laboratory services in both industrialized and developing nations.

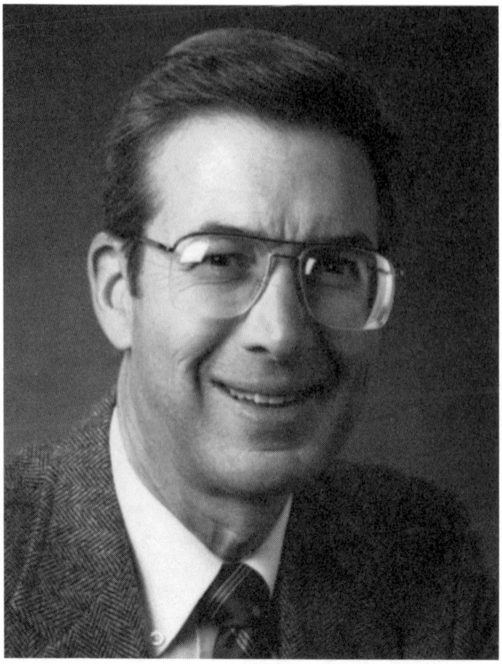

Dr. John Sbarbaro

Dr. John Sbarbaro was probably the first person in the United States to fully comprehend the implications and challenges of patients' noncompliance with chemotherapy. Utilizing the seminal work of the BMRC on twice weekly therapy, he developed programs of supervised intermittent chemotherapy in Denver, first for individuals of proven refractoriness, then as a community norm. Underlying his philosophy was a singular insight into the public health implications of this disease: the mandate that the community be protected against preventable transmission.

Drs. Wallace Fox and *Denis Mitchison* led a remarkable group of clinicians, epidemiologists, and bacteriologists at the British Medical Research Council to conduct a series of elegant chemotherapy trials which essentially defined the modern chemotherapy for tuberculosis. The trials were done largely in cooperation with investigations in Madras, India, East Africa, Hong Kong, and Singapore. They were brilliantly conceived to ask and answer vital questions about the roles of the individual drugs, requisite duration of ther-

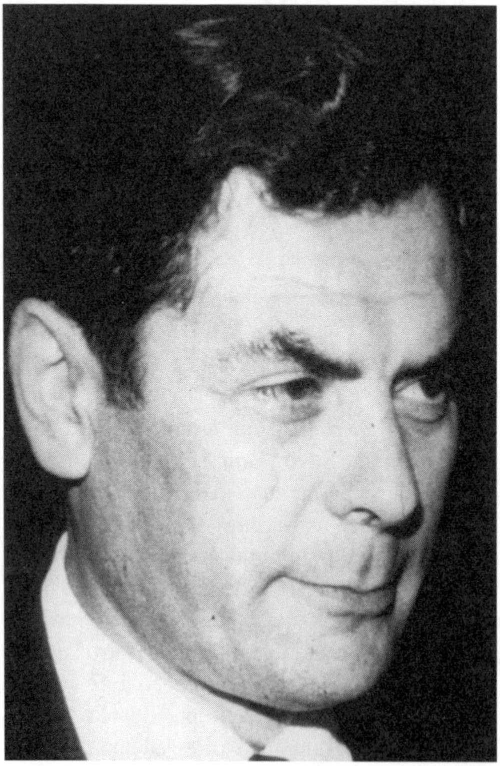

Dr. Wallace Fox

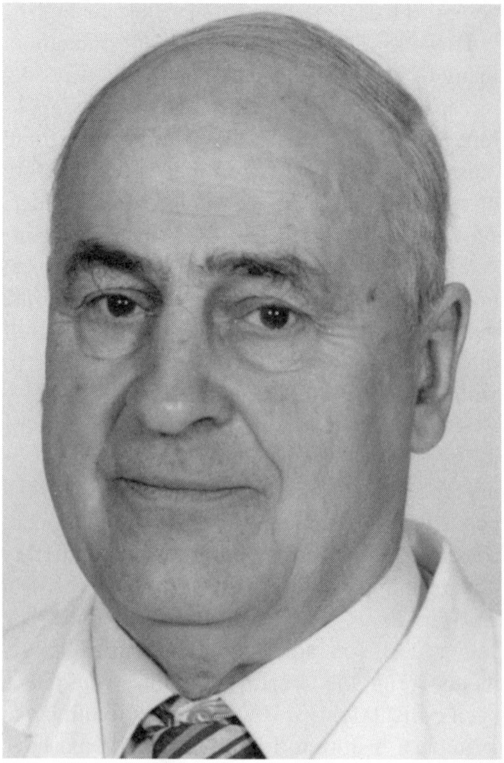

Dr. Denis Mitchison

apy, and convenient rhythms to facilitate directly-observed treatment. Indeed, their names have become synonymous with "short-course" treatment, and—given the critical efficiency of this model—they must be recognized as two of the most important figures of global medicine in the latter half of the twentieth century.

Dr. George Comstock is a wonderfully kind, thoughtful, and humble scholar whose keen insights into the epidemiology of tuberculosis helped shape highly successful public-health policies in the United States over the past forty years. He insisted with typical modesty that great credit be given as well to two of his mentors and collaborators, Shirley Ferbee Woolpert and Carroll Palmer. The recognition by this trio of the dominant contribution of reactivation tuberculosis morbidity led to the adoption of preventive chemotherapy (rather than vaccination) as the basic mode of prevention for the U.S. Public Health Service. Dr. Comstock's careful manuscripts and lucid lectures helped generations of young students to grasp the intricacies of a very complx disease.

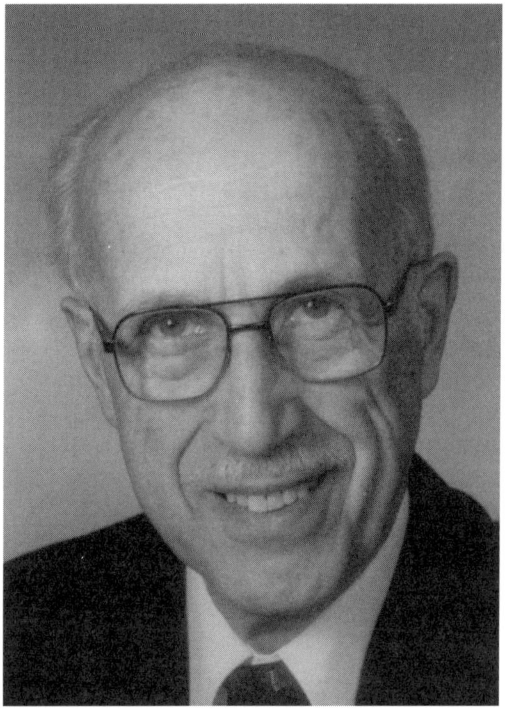

Dr. George Comstock

1

Tuberculosis Down Through the Centuries

The history of tuberculosis is rich with insight and enlightenment. While a temporal perspective is desirable for any field of study, it is particularly compelling in this singular infection. Among the immense intellectual capital to be derived from revisiting this disease are the often bizarre explanations for the causes of this malady, the desperate searching for remedies that so often resulted in mischief and misery rather than benefit, and the plodding advancement toward recognition of the etiological agent and effective treatment of this disease. This is a story marked by some of humankind's most heroic scientific advancements, as well as its most arrogant charlatanism.

Much of the information in this chapter has been derived from the following selected sources: an article by H.J. Corper, "Founders of Our Knowledge of Tuberculosis," published in 1929 (1); a monograph, *Tuberculosis,* by Gerald B. Webb, which was part of the Clio Medica Series on medical history published in 1936 (2); R.Y. Keers's marvelous 1978 book, *Pulmonary Tuberculosis: A Journey Down the Centuries* (3); Rene and Jean Dubos's moving tale of tuberculosis, man, and society, *The White Plague,* published in 1952 (4); Thomas D. Brock's biography, *Robert Koch: A Life in Medicine and Bacteriology,* published in 1988 (5); and *The Forgotten Plague,* Frank Ryan's recounting of the heroic struggles leading to the discovery in the twentieth century of streptomycin, para-amino-salicylate, and isoniazid (6).

TUBERCULOSIS IN REMOTE CIVILIZATIONS

Egyptian culture probably arose around 4,000 B.C. The fragmentary writings of the period related to medicine do not clearly document illness mindful of tuberculosis. However, Keers pointed out two clear lines of evidence documenting the presence of tuberculosis among the Egyptian people: graphic representations of individuals with dorsal spine deformities, which authorities deem classic for the gibbus deformity of tuberculosis, and examination of mummified human remains (3). He noted evidence of osseous tuberculosis dating back to the early dynastic period (circa 3,400 B.C.) and cited a case of spinal tuberculosis with an associated psoas abscess found in the mummified remains of a Twenty-First Dynasty priest, Nesperahan (7).

Other historical allusions to pulmonary and nonpulmonary diseases that very likely included tuberculosis were noted in Chinese writings as remote as 2,698 B.C. (8). Also, references were made to probable pulmonary tuberculosis in writings of the Indo-Aryan Hindu civilization (circa 1,500 B.C.) (2).

TUBERCULOSIS AND EARLY GREECE

The most detailed and thoughtful references to tuberculosis occurred with the burgeoning civilization of ancient Greece. Keers noted the evolution of Greek medicine in three phases: (a) myths, legends, and demigods such as Aesculapius, who was allegedly taught healing by

Apollo, only to be slain through the machinations of Pluto; (b) the early philosophers, such as Pythagoras, who fostered reason and inquiry; and (c) the golden era of Hippocrates (circa 460–375 b.c.), whom many regard as the intellectual fountainhead for medical science and practice (3). In the Hippocratic Collection are the first references to *phthisis* (pronounced *tisis* or *taisis*), which meant literally, "I am wasting." Indeed, the various stages and forms of tuberculosis are described in this collection, although the Greeks—as did many who came later—failed to recognize the common source of these pleomorphic disorders. From these and other writings, Webb surmised that tuberculosis "was raging in Greece" during this era (2).

HISTORICAL PERSPECTIVE ON THE TUBERCULOSIS BACILLUS

From these sources, one may conclude that disease caused by a microbe, presumably identical or very similar to the currently recognized pathogen, *Mycobacterium tuberculosis,* has been extant in diverse human populations for many thousands of years. Indeed, by using a variety of sophisticated molecular biological indicators, Kapur et al. (9) recently estimated that the tubercle bacillus is approximately 15,000 years old (see Chapter 2 for more on the evolution and taxonomy of *M. tuberculosis*). Current evidence indicates clearly that *M. tuberculosis* is spread exclusively by human-to-human transmission without significant animal or environmental reservoirs. Webb speculated that the tubercle bacillus may have been introduced to humans when cattle were first domesticated. Given the evidence of the close genetic relatedness of *M. tuberculosis* and *Mycobacterium bovis* (an endemic pathogen of wild cattle and other animals), it is attractive to conjecture that the human tubercle bacillus was derived from the zoonotic pathogen *M. bovis* and underwent subtle mutations that are responsible for its current distinct reservoirs, transmission patterns, and pathogenicity (see Chapter 2). There has been epidemic waxing and waning of tuberculosis because of various biological and socioeconomic factors, but most evidence indicates that no major population in modern times has been entirely free of the disease. This information is of much more than historical import. We must conclude that the microorganism has been engaged in an ongoing, adaptive relationship with human defenses over these thousands of years. During this time, the tubercle bacillus has, in a distinctly darwinian manner, been under selective pressure for those attributes which have facilitated survival of its species. Consider the following factors: (a) Although only 10% to 15% of most populations infected with *M. tuberculosis* go on to develop overt illness, those who come down with disease do so over years and decades; this ensures that diverse populations, staggered in time, are exposed and newly infected. In this manner, endemicity of this infection is ensured (see Chapter 5). (b) The tubercle bacillus has adapted itself handsomely to the intracellular milieu of the host. While most infected persons are able to restrain the mycobacteria from ungoverned replication, the bacilli are capable of surviving for extended periods, emerging when events result in attenuation of the host's immune capabilities. (c) In the pathogenesis of tuberculosis, the microbes subvert an important component of the immune response, delayed-type hypersensitivity, to their ends. By causing liquefaction-cavitation of pulmonary lesions (see Chapter 4), this phenomenon results in massive replication of the bacilli, facilitating infectious aerosol generation and propagation of the infection of new human hosts. (d) In stark contrast to the great preponderance of infectious conditions, exposure to and subclinical infection with *M. tuberculosis* does not confer substantial protection against the microbe in the future. Indeed, the great majority of cases in the Western world occur as a result of endogenous reactivation of old, latent foci (see Chapters 4 and 5). This not only has implications in the epidemiologic arena, but it also informs us of the extreme difficulties that can be anticipated in pursuing an effective vaccine.

FOUNDERS OF OUR MODERN UNDERSTANDING OF TUBERCULOSIS

The study of the evolution of our intellectual, scientific appreciation of tuberculosis is a journey through the elite firmament of medicine; surely no other disease has enjoyed the impassioned attention given to this malady by the most distinguished minds of nearly every era. We may occasionally smile at some of the formulations, which, in retrospect, seem unimaginably ill-founded or bizarre, or we may be awestruck by the brilliant insights garnered by scholars who had only the scantiest of "hard data," relying instead on remarkable powers of observation and deduction. The matter should inform, inspire, and amuse us. Also, it should alert us to the clinical tragedies and impediments to scientific advancements that can result from the misguided dogma of influential, prideful physicians.

Greek Era

As noted above, the first systematic description of the clinical manifestations and epidemiologic features of phthisis was recorded in the Hippocratic Collection, compiled around 400–350 B.C. In these writings the tuberculous process in the lungs was called a "phyma," and Hippocrates observed that "those patients in whose lungs phymata are formed expectorate blood 40 days after the onset of the malady, and—if they survive—they practically always become phthisical" (2). While he evinced no clear understanding of the infectious nature of the disease, Hippocrates described with remarkable vision the pathogenetic sequence of pulmonary tuberculosis, including the evolution of cavitary lesions and distinguished tuberculous distortion of the spine—the gibbous deformity—from other spinal disorders (2). Notable in their insights into tuberculosis, the Hippocratic school did not benefit from autopsies. It was not until the development of the Alexandrian (Egypt) school hundreds of years later that postmortem studies were performed regularly.

During the post-Hippocratic centuries of the Greek hegemony, little more understanding of phthisis was engendered. However, Aristotle (354–322 B.C.)—not a physician, but a philosopher and biologist—did discern a pattern that suggested the disease was contagious:

> Why when one comes near consumptives. . . does one contract their disease, while one does not contract dropsy, apoplexy. . .? With the consumption, the reason is that the breath is bad and heavy. . .in approaching the consumptive, one breathes this pernicious air. One takes the disease because there is in this air something disease-producing (2).

Roman Empire

The Roman Empire emerged to supplant Greece, and medical science became a low priority. In fact, medicine was regarded by the Romans as a secondary profession, left commonly to foreigners or slaves. Thus it was that two Greek physicians working under the Romans provided the next significant recorded delineations of tuberculosis. Aretaeus, the Cappodocian (circa A.D. 150) described in careful detail the terminal illness of the consumptive, including notations of clubbing, diarrhea, lassitude, nocturnal fever, and sweats (3); he also distinguished phthisis from empyema (2). Aretaeus was overshadowed, however, by another Greek physician of that era, Galen, the Pergamite (A.D. 131–201), who studied medicine at the Alexandrian school before returning to his home in Asia Minor. Galen, a physiologist, anatomist, and prolific writer, was the last flare of the medical candle before the Dark Ages. His approach to the care of tuberculosis (which he deemed contagious) was based on early recognition, rest, a rich diet, and gentle cough suppression. This should be contrasted to some of the barbaric, obviously hurtful remedies practiced 1,500 years later in Europe and North America.

With the fall of the Roman Empire in the sixth century, the lights of open inquiry flickered out and medical science went into a 1,000-year eclipse. If analysis had been undertaken in this period, it could not be reported, lest it appear to be heterodoxy of any sort, for the Church and its minions were major providers of care. It was during this period, also, that the royal healing of tuberculosis commenced, with Clovis the Franc (circa A.D. 500) laying on hands to cure scrofula.

Early Renaissance: Anatomy and Pathology

Keers described the emergence of Western civilization from this medieval blight in most elegant terms:

> It required the wonderful phenomenon of the Renaissance to enable men to throw off the tyranny of scholastic dogmatism, to break the stranglehold of the Church and to restore to learning and the pursuit of knowledge the position of honor and prestige with which they had been endowed in the civilizations of Greece and Rome (3).

With the new-found freedom of the Renaissance, Andreas Vesalius from the school of Padua (1514–1564) took advantage of the lifting of the ban of dissection to reawaken interest in anatomy through his treatise, *De Humani Corporis Fabrica,* which was published in 1543 and established him as the founder of modern anatomical science. A contemporary scholar, Antonio Benivieni, used dissection for a different purpose, the study of disease; thus he launched the modern discipline of pathological anatomy. Among his observations were cases of tuberculosis of the lymph nodes, mesentery, hip, and hilar lymph nodes (2).

Frascatorius and Contagion

The next truly significant insight related to tuberculosis came from Girolamus Frascatorius (1483–1553), who in 1546 systematically described three major modes of transmitting infection in his book *De Contagioni:* (a) spread by direct contact, (b) spread by intermediary (e.g., fomites), and (c) infection at a distance. The last concept entailed his postulation of minute infectious particles which he called "seminaria." The conceptualization of Frascatorious was truly prescient: "It may be considered that the force of the disease lies in these seeds since they have the power to propagate and reproduce their own kind" (2). He also, in describing tubercular patients, used the term "tabes," which translated to "decline." This term, "decline," became the favored euphemism of the nineteenth century to describe gradual death from tuberculosis.

Tubercle and Phthisis: Sylvius, Willis, and Morton

As physicians began to perceive phthisis more clearly as a contagious disease, anxiety arose about the hazards of necropsy. Among the seventeenth-century medical luminaries who chose not to risk contagion were Valsalva, Morgagni, and Richard Morton, about whom we will hear more later. By contrast, one who learned an immense amount from the postmortem examination of consumptive patients was a professor of anatomical medicine at Leyden, Franciscus de la Boe, or Sylvius (1614–1672). Examining the tissues of phthisical patients, he was struck by the profusion of various-sized nodulations which he, in the Greek tradition, referred to as "tubercles." Sylvius theorized that these nodular lesions tended to enlarge and soften, eventually forming cavities. He erred, however, in believing them to be lymph glands that were, he deduced wrongly, part of the predisposition to phthisis. Nonetheless, he believed the disease to be contagious: ". . .the air expired by consumptives . . .is drawn in. . .irritating emanations are carried from the affected party to others, especially relatives. . .they also fall into phthisis" (10).

Thomas Willis (1621–1675), a student of medicine at Leyden, went on to develop a more unified conceptualization of phthisis, recognizing it as a systemic illness with wasting that typically, but not universally, resulted in gross lung destruction. His work entailed clinicopathological correlations that found fuller expression subsequently in the writings of Morton, Bayle, and Läennec (vide infra).

Richard Morton (1637–1698) contributed another step forward in the understanding of tuberculosis with his work, *Phthisiologia,* published in 1689. His writings correlated clinical manifestations with necropsy findings, including fever and wasting associated with progression from a solid tubercle to cavitation. Among his memorable contributions to the lore of tuberculosis are these two pithy observations:

- On considering the extraordinary number of patients whom he saw with phthisis: ". . .I cannot sufficiently admire that anyone, at least after he comes to the flower of his youth, can die without a touch of consumption (11)."
- On the effects of age on phthisis: "The consumption of young men that are in the flower of their age, when the heat of blood is yet brisk, and therefore more disposed to a fever-

ish fermentation, is for the most part acute. But, in old men, where the natural heat is decayed, it is more chronical (11)."

Overall, a clear transition in the perception of tuberculosis occurred with the contributions of Sylvius, Willis, and Morton. They were able to tease out tuberculosis from other wasting illnesses, associating it with the specific tissue finding, the tubercle. Sylvius's contention that tubercles represented enlargement of lymph glands was challenged later by Pierre Desult (1675–1737), a French physician who contended that tubercles were new structures that evolved as a consequence of phthisis, not lymph nodes that marked a predisposition. In addition, Desult maintained that the illness was contagious with the transmitting principal being the sputum, but his analysis lay neglected for 50 years (3).

Benjamin Marten's Remarkable Vision

Another scholar whose extraordinary insights into tuberculosis were to be roundly ignored was Benjamin Marten (1704–1782), a precocious student of medicine who, before his 20th birthday, published a book, *A New Theory of Consumptions More Especially of a Phthisis or Consumption of the Lungs,* which, in the words of a 20th century medical historian, ". . .anticipated, in thoughts, the deeds of Pasteur, Villemin, and Robert Koch" (12). With preternatural clarity, Marten foresaw much of that which was to be proven about the microbial etiology, epidemiology, and transmission of tuberculosis 150 years later:

> The original and essential cause may possibly be some certain species of animalculae or wonderfully minute living creatures that, by their peculiar shape or disagreeable parts, are inimical to our natures; but, however, capable of subsisting in our juices and vessels (13).

Rather than serving as a beacon to inspire other investigators to test (and confirm) his theories, Marten was ridiculed and his work dismissed by the medical poohbahs of his time. Thus it was that clinicians of the eighteenth and nineteenth centuries continued to focus on heredity, various predispositions, and other noninfectious mechanisms to explain consumption, which was wreaking unimaginable havoc on the populations of Europe.

Unlike Marten's schema of the nature of phthisis, which he apparently derived largely by intuition, two other physicians of the later 18th century obtained their understanding of the disease the traditional way: they earned it by performing careful necropsies on consumptives. William Stark (1741–1770) and Matthew Baillie (1761–1823) made primary contributions to the delineation of the disease process by recognizing that tubercles were simply the reaction of the tissues to the phthistical process, that the various-sized tubercles represented different stages of that process, and that cavities ("vomicae") arose from the confluence and progression of these tubercles.

Clinicopathological Correlation and Physical Examination: Bayle and Läennec

The next sentinel strides in tuberculosis were to occur in the first 25 years of the nineteenth century in Paris, where two brilliant young men synergistically worked to unravel further the mysteries of consumption before dying themselves of the disease. Gaspard Laurent Bayle (1774–1816) and Rene Theophile Hyacinthe Läennec (1781– 1826) worked at the Hopital de la Charite in the department of Jean Nicholas Corvisart (1775– 1821), who was Professor of Medicine at the College de France and subsequently Napoleon's personal physician.

Corvisart's principal contribution to the foment lay with his uncovering and translating into French in 1797 an obscure treatise penned 36 years earlier by an Austrian physician, Leopold Auenbrugger (1722–1809). Auenbrugger had performed a seven-year study on a substantially new concept: deriving understanding of intrathoracic pathology by physical examination, namely, percussion of the chest. Corvisart saw the utility of the technique and, in so doing, initiated a movement toward physical examination that resulted in Läennec's momentous innovation, the stethoscope, for auscultation of the chest.

Bayle performed a prodigious number of autopsies on phthistic patients, 900 such studies being the subject of his 1810 report, "Recherches sur la Phthisis Pulmonair." Notably, the necropsies were accompanied by detailed antemortem histories of the illness, enabling physicians to make heretofore impossible clinicopathological correlations. Läennec, with whom Bayle shared a rich personal friendship during their brilliant but short careers, described Bayle as being:

> . . .gifted with wondrous powers of concentration and perseverance; nothing could tire or dishearten him, indeed application seemed to be so inherent in his habits that none of his friends and fellow workers ever saw him, through lassitude, discouragement or neglect, omit to do that which was to be done (12).

However, in his writings, Bayle seemed unable to make the leap of understanding that would have incorporated the various manifestations within the lungs and other organs into one nosological category. That distinction was to fall to Läennec, who was to survive 10 years after Bayle's death from consumption, only to fall to the same disease at the age of 45.

Läennec's autopsy studies, detailed in his opus, *Traite de L'Auscultation Mediate et des Maladies des Poumons et du Couer* (1821), indicated to him that the diverse forms of tubercles all fit under the rubric of a single disorder, thus echoing and reinforcing the partially formed impressions of prior scholars such as Morton, Stark, and Baillie. For the clinician, Läennec's work meant substantial improvement in the antemortem diagnosis of tuberculosis, an observation of great import to the art of prognostication, something which clinicians of that era performed much better than therapy.

Läennec came from a family riddled with phthisis, and he obviously suffered with chronic consumption throughout his entire adult life. Indeed, he became so debilitated while working in Paris that he, on several occasions, sought respite in his family's home in coastal Brittany. Enjoying remarkable improvement with the visits and noticing less phthisis among the Bretons, Läennec inferred some salutary effect of seaweed and, on return to his hospital in Paris, had seaweed strewn about the wards.

In addition to this therapeutic naivete, Läennec failed to concede the contagious quality of consumption, despite his family pattern of disease, his close observation of the epidemic raging through Paris, and his personal experience of several direct inoculation infections of his hands ("prosector's warts") incurred while performing autopsies of tuberculous patients.

The French successor to Bayle and Läennec was Pierre Charles Alexander Louis (1787–1872), a physician whose own series of necropsies on consumptives, published in 1825, reaffirmed Läennec's unitary theory. In particular, Louis noted the significance of cavitary disease in the clinical manifestations and prognosis of the disease. Anticipating current views of pathogenesis, he averred that, "after the age of fifteen, one could not have tubercle in any organ of the body without at the same time having tubercle in the lungs," an aphorism that became known as Louis's law (2). Also notable, Louis found evidence of latent tuberculosis in the lungs of patients dying of other causes; this was a potentially momentous finding, for it was latency following tuberculosis exposure/infection that did more to dissuade clinicians of the contagious nature of the disorder than any other factor.

Microscopy, Histopathology, and Microbiology

The clinicopathological aspects of tuberculosis having been sequentially refined by the abovementioned scholars, the next challenge before medical scientists was the identification of an etiological principle for the disease. Here, for the first time, the microscope came into play. Developed by Anthony Van Leeuwenhoek and used by him to describe protozoa (1674) and bacteria (1676), the instrument was not engaged meaningfully in the study of tuberculosis until more than 150 years later. Microscopy made two fundamental contributions to the understanding of tuberculosis: the histopathology of tissue lesions to identify characteristic cellular responses and, later, recognition of the microbe itself in the tissues. The latter had to await the genius of Koch in 1882; the former was fodder for disputation throughout the mid-nineteenth century.

Hermann Lebert, in an 1843 addendum to P.C.A. Louis's writings, commented that, based on his microscopic studies, tubercles were not simple pus, the previously held notion of most anatomical pathologists. Rokitansky first described in 1855 the giant cell that remains a characteristic feature of tubercles; Langhans in 1868 embellished the histological characterization of these cells, earning for himself eponymic association with them. Rudolf Virchow (1821–1902), who was the preeminent figure in German medicine until eclipsed by Koch, identified two other cellular constituents of the tubercle, lymphocytes, and epitheloid monocytes. However, he disputed that tubercles were unique to a specific disease, phthisis, setting himself retrospectively athwart Läennec's unitary thesis. Prospectively, this set the stage for Koch's confrontation with Virchow, the *Geheimrat* (dominant academic leader) in March 1882.

Until the middle of the nineteenth century, all investigators had been restricted to theoretical or inferential means of establishing an infectious etiology for a disease. However, inspired by the work of Louis Pasteur (including his proof in 1857 of the microbial origins of fermentation), scientists began direct investigations to demonstrate contagiousness and to search for the specific agent. The first documentation of a transmissible infectious disease was the work of Casimir Joseph Davaine in 1863 with anthrax (14).

Also in France, Jean Antoine Villemin, a physician in the military service, began a series of experiments in 1865 that laid substantial groundwork for Koch's later scientific blitzkrieg. Taking material from tuberculous human tissue, Villemin inoculated a series of six rabbits and was able to demonstrate disseminated tubercles in all; he used controls in each experiment, which remained disease free (12). Results in hand, Villemin presented them to the Academy of Medicine in December 1865; to his apparent dismay, his data were greeted locally with a mixture of skepticism and lukewarm interest. However, the report caught the attention of interested parties in Great Britain, and a Dr. Burdon-Saunderson was sent to France to study and attempt to replicate Villemin's findings. The Englishman observed tuberculosis lesions in 50 of 53 rabbits he so inoculated. On the brink of a major breakthrough in the understanding of tuberculosis, however, Burdon-Saunderson conceived of a different control method to test the validity of the inoculation model. He placed unbleached, sterile cotton (instead of tuberculous matter) in the shoulders of two guinea pigs, analogous to the rabbit experiments. Sadly, one of the guinea pigs experienced a fatal disseminated infection of unknown etiology, presumably attributable to contaminated surgery. This was interpreted by the British group as refutation of Villemin's theory of specific transmission of "tuberculosis," thus slowing scientific appreciation of this concept for many years. Undaunted, however, Villemin went on to analyze the epidemiology of tuberculosis and to perform numerous in vivo inoculation experiments. In 1868, he published a book, *Etudes sur la Tuberculose,* in which he accurately characterized some of the epidemiologic features of tuberculosis that supported its contagious nature. In the final chapters of his book, Villemin reported a series of inoculation experiments, human to animal and animal to animal, that irrefutably demonstrated the transmissibility of the disease, including the infectiousness of the bronchial secretions of diseased animals! Notably, however, Villemin's work did not include microscopic identification or in vitro isolation of the putative infectious agent; thus he was to be denied the fame and adulation that came to Koch 14 years later.

Reinforcing Villemin's transmission model, Julius Cohnheim performed an inoculation study in 1877 in which tuberculous material was introduced into the anterior chambers of rabbits' eyes, resulting in the formation of characteristic tubercles (1).

Koch: The Brilliant Coalescence

In many respects, the extended saga of phthisis from Hippocrates to 1882 seemed like a mammoth wagnerian opera filled with drama, suffering, pathos, and uncertainty. Then, in the final act, an unassuming 39-year-old tenor walked on stage and enunciated a brief, unembellished coda that resolved centuries of confusion, fear, and contentiousness. And, ironically, it was reported that the audience was so stunned by the import of his performance that they neglected to applaud.

Robert Koch had previously performed a laudable but relatively minor operetta: from 1874 to 1876 he had, through the ingenious and innovative uses of microscopy and culture techniques, characterized *Bacillus anthracis,* the etiological agent of the zoonosis, anthrax (15).

Following this feat, Koch spent the next 5 years refining his basic laboratory skills. Obvious genius, coupled with immense tenacity, allowed Koch, from 1876 to 1878, to improve substantially upon photomicroscopy (working largely on his own) and plain microscopy (working in concert with Ernst Abbe at the Carl Zeiss factory to develop the first oil-immersion lens) (5). His next major contribution to the discipline of bacteriology/microbiology was delineation of a method for isolation of pure cultures. Louis Pasteur's liquid medium methods relied on randomness and good fortune (5). Joseph Lister had published a report in 1878 of a pure culture technique, also employing liquid medium. This system was used not to study an infectious agent, but to determine the cause of souring milk (16). Working in his laboratory in Berlin in 1880–1881, Koch modified the methods of Schroeter to create "nutrient gelatin" plates, which revolutionized the science of bacteriology (5).

These honed laboratory skills were to prove vital to Koch in his assault on the mysteries of tuberculosis. Koch commenced work on August 18, 1881; he presented his research findings, which were deemed ". . .one of the great scientific discoveries of the age" (17), only 217 days later, on March 24, 1882. Noteworthy is the fact that he presented his findings to the Berlin Physiological Society, not the more appropriate Pathological Society. This probably reflects the antipathy of Virchow—Dean of German Pathology at this time—to Koch's message, which ran contrary to the views which had been espoused by Virchow over the previous 20 years.

As indicated above, there was considerable experimental evidence and inferential data that tuberculosis was an infectious disease caused by a specific microorganism. As stated by another medical historian, ". . .it was no longer a question of was there a tubercle bacillus but rather who would find it first (3)." Koch moved resolutely to overcome the barriers to recognition which had kept the tubercle bacillus shrouded in mystery well into the bacteriological era. One of the truly ingenious aspects of his research was his method for staining the bacilli. He employed, among various agents, Ehrlich's methylene blue, with which he saw very tiny, thin rods in tuberculous material. In an effort to obtain photomicrographs, Koch counterstained his preparation with Bismarck brown (vesuvin), then photographed these slides with blue light. As recorded in the recollections of his colleague Loeffler, Koch found that the brown counterstain absorbed the blue light, while the blue-stained rods remained bright and transparent (18). This technique proved very sensitive in demonstrating the bacilli in many and varied sources. However, when Koch attempted to employ a new batch of methylene blue, he could not identify the bacilli. While others were baffled by this turn, Koch reasoned that the prior batch, which had been standing in the laboratory for a considerable period, must have absorbed something from the atmosphere that altered its chemical characteristics. He deduced that the most probable candidate for this was ammonia, which acted as an alkali. Koch then added ammonia or other bases such as potassium or sodium hydroxide to the second batch of methylene blue and restored its tinctorial affinity for the bacillus. In another instance of happenstance, Koch noted that accidental heating of a slide increased the uptake of the dye by the bacilli. Serendipity and the prepared mind! Koch's first report stated:

> It seems likely that the tubercle bacillus is surrounded with a special wall of unusual properties, and that the penetration of a dye through this wall can only occur when alkali, aniline, or similar substance is present (19).

Employing this staining system, Koch proceeded to examine multiple specimens from tuberculous patients of the Charite Hospital, which was located near his laboratory in Berlin. He reported in his March 1882 presentation that:

> . . .in all tissues in which the tuberculosis process has recently developed and is progressing most rapidly, these bacilli can be found in large

> numbers, especially at the edge of large, cheesy masses. The bacilli occur almost exclusively in large numbers free of the tissue cells. . .on the basis of my extensive observations, I consider it as proved that in all tuberculous conditions of man and animals there exists a characteristic bacterium which I have designated as the tubercle bacillus, which has specific properties which allow it to be distinguished from all other microorganisms.

The next major component of Koch's initial investigations took the form of proving a causal relationship between these stainable objects and the disease tuberculosis. Essentially, this work took the form that had been taught to him by his mentor Jakob Henle, but that became known as Koch's Postulates:

> In order to prove that tuberculosis is brought about by the tubercle bacillus. . .the bacilli must be isolated from the body. . .cultured so long in pure culture that they are freed from any diseased production of the animal organism which may still be adhering to the bacilli. . .the isolated bacilli must bring about the transfer of the disease to other animals. . . .(19)

Koch, indeed, did exactly this. The culture plate technique that he had perfected over the previous years did not suffice. However, after many trials he succeeded by employing the coagulated blood serum techniques of Tyndall, modified in part by allowing the serum to gel when the test tubes were slanted, thus creating a larger surface area for cultivation. Recovery of the microbes by this system, however, was not easy. Microbiologists of this era had been working with bacteria such as streptococci or staphylococci that grew up in a matter of hours on media; Koch, though, watched patiently and carefully as microscopic colonies began to appear in the second week on his blood serum media.

The next component of the process entailed introduction of the cultured microbes into animals to see if they induced tuberculosis. As he reported:

> . . .the substance to be tested for its virulence was inoculated each time into 4 to 6 guinea pigs. The result was uniform throughout. . . without exception, animals injected with bacilliferous material had far-advanced tuberculosis, four weeks after inoculation (19).

On the surface, this sounds rather straightforward, but, in truth, Koch was rigorous and critical in establishing his theory. He actually reported 13 separate experiments using a variety of animal models (guinea pigs, mice, hamsters, rabbits, rats, cats, and dogs) and routes of inoculation (subcutaneous, intraocular, intraperitonial, and intravenous), all of which confirmed his hypothesis.

In his concluding comments of this original paper, Koch included an assortment of observations that testify to his broad understanding of tuberculosis. In summary, he noted the following:

- The life cycle of tubercle bacilli entailed human-to-human transmission without external, natural reservoirs: that the microbes "are true and not occasional parasites."
- The portal of entry was the lungs, and the source of the microbes was patients with cavitary disease who expectorate immense numbers of bacilli (he had found the bacilli in the sputum of most patients with tuberculosis and in none of the sputa from patients without the disease).
- Because of their slow rate of replication, the tubercle bacilli "cannot infect the body through every little wound, as do the fast-growing anthrax bacilli; if one wishes to render an animal tuberculous with certainty, the infectious material must be brought into a place where the bacilli have the opportunity to propagate in a protected position and where they can focalize."
- "Tuberculosis has so far been habitually considered to be a manifestation of social misery, and it has been hoped that an improvement in the latter would reduce the disease."

Certainly, Koch's saga was not without significant errors that, because of his immense status, had significant detrimental impact on medicine and society. Among the missteps were the following: (a) Probably influenced by his experience with anthrax, Koch thought the tubercle bacilli could exist outside the body in a pathogenic spore-form; this gave rise to the practice of regarding objects handled by or in contact with tuberculous patients as fomites.

The expensive, stigmatizing, and unnecessary practices of disposable plates, utensils, gowns, and the like persisted in many hospitals long into the twentieth century. (b) There was confusion between the human tubercle bacillus, *M. tuberculosis,* and the pathogen of cattle, *M. bovis.* At first, Koch regarded them as identical; then, once distinguishing them, Koch erroneously inferred that, since *M. tuberculosis* was not very pathogenic for cattle, *M. bovis* was not a significant threat for human disease. His attitude substantially delayed the practices of screening dairy herds for mycobacterial infection and pasteurizing milk in much of Europe, presumably resulting in considerable morbidity from *M. bovis* infections. These programs were implemented in 1917 in the United States through the influence of Theobald Smith; Germany and France began their national programs to eliminate tuberculosis in cattle in 1952 and 1955, respectively (20). (c) The most profound miscalculation to be made by Koch occurred in 1890 when he announced, based on his research with guinea pigs, an agent for the cure and prevention of tuberculosis. Clouded in secrecy for complex personal and governmental reasons, the substance was a glycerine extract of tubercle bacilli that we now call old tuberculin. Tragically for many patients and Koch, therapeutic application of the agent resulted in immense morbidity and even mortality through an immune reaction that became known as "Koch's phenomenon" (see Chapter 4). The discredit that came to Koch for this misadventure no doubt delayed his receipt of the obviously merited Nobel Prize until 1905, the fourth year of this award.

However, we should not allow these blemishes to diminish our appreciation of this extraordinary man and scientist. In addition to the aforementioned identification of the causative agents of anthrax and tuberculosis, Koch identified the etiologic agent of cholera in 1883, merely a year after his triumph in tuberculosis. In addition, research associates in his Berlin laboratories made a number of momentous discoveries with other infectious diseases in the 1880s: Gaffky isolated the causal organism, salmonella, of typhoid fever; Loeffler identified the causal agent of diphtheria, *Corynebacterium diphtheriae;* and von Behring and Kitasato developed diphtheria antitoxin, a sentinel event unto itself, but doubly important as an immunological model.

The sojourn through the millennia toward a modern understanding of the cause and nature of tuberculosis ended in Berlin in 1882 with the exposition by Koch. The illumination that resulted from Koch's research may be compared to a stellar nova, light from which still travels through our scientific universe. Koch stated that "my studies have been done in the interest of public health, and I hope that this will derive the largest profit from them (19)." Indeed so!

HISTORY OF THE TREATMENT OF PHTHISIS

No recounting of the history of tuberculosis would be complete without examination of the manifold treatments attempted over the centuries. As Webb (2) stated, "The human desire to help the sick prompted the most fantastic remedies for tuberculosis."

Two Thousand Years of Futility

The first detailed notations of therapy arose in Greece, and—because of the enduring impact of the Greek perceptions and treatment of disease—they are worth considering in broad outline. Early Greek scholars believed nature to consist of four basic elements: air, fire, water, and earth. In turn, they believed the human body to be composed of four humors: blood (produced by the heart), phlegm (produced by the brain), yellow bile (produced by the liver), and black bile (produced by the spleen). Illness was associated with perturbations of the humoral balance, and therapy was believed to redress these disturbances. At its essence, Greek medicine believed diseases to be natural phenomena and sought remedies from earthly sources. Dietary enrichments of various forms were popular, including milk from various sources. This is in sharp distinction to the theories of other cultures before and after the Greek era.

Primitive observers of human suffering were predisposed to attribute the misfortunes to the displeasure of deities or other supernatural events. Consequences of these belief systems included attempted remedy by religious ritual, exorcism, fasting, and—when it was believed that a fellow member of the community was responsible—expulsion or execution. Because of the supernatural component, members of the religious hierarchy or the royalty [who were empowered by god(s)] became important healers, typically to the detriment of the patient but to the benefit of their institutional coffers.

Physician-generated remedies were often noxious. Early therapists of the Greco-Roman schools tended to use plants or other natural products to restore humoral balance. However, these remedies gave way to more dramatic treatments such as bleeding, purging, emetics, or other interventions that were morbid at best and mortal in the extreme.

Sanatoria

Most benign, and possibly even efficacious, rest was employed among diverse schools of healing in the care of consumptives, appearing first in the hippocratic aphorism, "If the patient is treated early, before the hemorrhage is excessive and the body too emaciated, one can cure him by rest in bed (2)." It reappeared in the writings and practices of healers from the Roman era to the early 20th century (2). Rest literally included recumbency in bed, as well as curtailment of disruptive emotions such as fear, anger, or melancholy.

Manipulation of climatological variables has been employed in the treatment of many illnesses including tuberculosis, throughout history. Webb (2) found allusions to it in the ancient Hindu vedas: ". . .the consumptive should go and live in elevated regions." Hippocrates and Galen advocated mountainous retreats for their phthisical patients. Sea voyages became popular therapy during the Roman era; this modality reappeared during the eras of the Renaissance and the Enlightenment. Percy Bysshe Shelley drowned when, during a therapeutic voyage, his sailboat capsized during a sudden squall. A variant of climate therapy was the issue of the type of air to which the patient should be exposed. Common practice in 16th to 18th century European medicine was the confinement of consumptive patients to closed spaces; whether this was for the perceived benefit of the patient or society is not clear. But, early in the 19th century, George Bodington, a British physician, advocated fresh air: "To live in and breathe freely, the open air is one important and essential remedy in arresting its progress (2)." Bodington also employed rest and a nutritious diet, anticipating the elements noted by a later observer to be "the triad on which all sanatorium treatment is based (1)."

The sanatorium movement evolved from sentiments similar to those of Bodington. However, the individual credited with introduction of formal sanatorium treatment was Hermann Brehmer, who in 1859 opened a "Kurhaus" for tubercular patients. The notion of sanatorium care gradually grew in popularity over the next 40 years. Peter Dettweiler, a consumptive physician who was treated and "cured" by Brehmer, opened a sanatorium in 1870 with emphasis on the economically disadvantaged patient.

Edward Livingston Trudeau had just graduated from the Columbia College of Physicians and Surgeons in 1871 and set up his practice in New York City when he began to experience recurrent fevers. In his autobiography, Trudeau described the scene in the office of the famous Dr. Janeway, to whom he had been referred:

> He received me cordially and began the examination at once. When this was concluded he said nothing. So I ventured, "Well, Dr. Janeway, you can find nothing the matter?" He looked grave and said, "Yes, the upper two-thirds of the left lung is involved in an active tuberculous process." I think I know something of the feelings of the man at the bar who is told he is to be hanged on a given date, for in those days pulmonary consumption was considered as absolutely fatal (21)."

After a trial of the therapy then in vogue, regular exercise and horseback riding, Trudeau deteriorated with increasing fever and debility. In despondency, he surrendered to the tuberculosis:

> . . .it drove me, in spite of all the urgent protests of my friends and physicians, to bury myself in the Adirondacks—then an unbroken wilder-

> ness, and considered a most dangerous climate for a chest invalid—in order to live an open-air life in the great forest, alone with Nature. . .. (21)"

Trudeau's health improved in the mountains, and he returned to New York City, only to experience a relapse within the year. Thus, by 1874 he had returned to Saranac Lake for permanent residency. Inspired by Brehmer's sanatorium report and Koch's discovery of the tubercle bacillus, Trudeau in 1882 initiated his plan for a center for the care of consumptives. In February 1885, the first two patients were admitted to the now-famous Little Red Cottage. Driven by Trudeau's zeal, the treatment facilities expanded dramatically, and a research laboratory was founded as well. The institution became a global source for expertise and the training ground for generations of leaders in tuberculosis who spread Trudeau's message widely across North America.

Trudeau died in 1915, living far beyond his initial expectations in Dr. Janeway's office and ascribing his longevity to the salutary effects of his Adirondacks retreat. In the absence of the randomized, controlled trials that have become our gold standard for assessing efficacy of a form of treatment, it is difficult to determine the extent to which sanatorium/rest therapy was efficacious. Certainly, this form of care had much more to recommend it than some of the dangerous, miserable remedies that antedated it. And, surely for the patients, it was far more preferable than passively surrendering to the disease; in the sanatoria, they were surrounded by caregivers with missionary zeal and enjoyed the company of fellow consumptives with whom they could rejoice or mourn. While it is without scientific basis and perhaps naive, I believe that there probably was significant merit in this approach and that future advances in the field of mind-body interaction will identify the means by which improvement was effected.

An interesting sidelight to this system of care lies in the field of heliotherapy or sunshine treatment. Niels R. Finsen, a Danish physician, reported in 1893 that arc-light treatment of cutaneous tuberculosis, lupus vulgaris, was beneficial (1). Finsen himself died prematurely of consumption, but a Swiss doctor, A. Rollier, commenced in 1903 to use heliotherapy for various forms of extrapulmonary tuberculosis (1). Corper, on reviewing the issue in 1929, noted that: "light alone is not a specific agent for the treatment of any form of tuberculosis, but it must be. . .an adjunct in treatment to. . .fresh air, rest, and nutritious food (1)."

In a related vein, milk and cod-liver oil were among the most prominently noted nutritional supplements used in the sanatoria. Given what has subsequently been learned about the role of vitamin D as a potential enhancer of tuberculoimmunity (see Chapter 4), it is fascinating to consider that the physicians of this era may have stumbled onto early, valid forms of immunomodulation.

The contributions of the sanatorium movement may be seen in the light of public health and welfare, rather than from the perspective of the tuberculous patient. Again, it is impossible to quantify the impact on tuberculosis epidemiology that resulted from sanatorium care. It is very likely that the declining incidence of tuberculosis throughout the first 50 years of the twentieth century has a multifactorial explanation. However, it is counter-intuitive to believe that removal of tens of thousands of patients from homes, schools, and workplaces did not curtail, somewhat, the transmission of the infection, ultimately reducing the prevalence of tuberculosis in this country. The number of sanatorium beds rose from 11,953 in 1908 to 30,000 in 1915, 80,054 in 1931, and 97,720 in 1942 (National Tuberculosis Association: *Tuberculosis Hospital and Sanatorium Directory,* New York, 1942).

Before leaving the subject of sanatorium care, it is worth considering the words of Trudeau as he reflected upon his experiences:

> As I look back on my life, ever since that day in 1886 when my brother came to me sick at Newport [Trudeau nursed him through his terminal months of consumption], tuberculosis looms up as an ever-present and relentless foe. It robbed me of my dear ones, and brought me the first two great sorrows of my life; it shattered my health when I was young and strong, and relegated me to a remote region, where ever since I have witnessed its withering blight

laid upon those about me, and stood at the death-beds of many of its victims whom I had learned to love. Of late it has condemned me to years of chronic invalidism, helplessness and physical misery and suffering (21)."

Collapse Therapy

Arising in the same era as sanatorium/rest care, "collapse therapy" was the last major thrust of clinicians to cure tuberculosis before the modern era of chemotherapy. Keers noted that the first distinct reference to collapsing the lung to control tuberculosis was made by M. Bourru in 1770 in an introduction to another book on consumption (3). He then traces the parentage of this concept to James Carson, a Scottish physician, who reasoned that if the elastic lung were allowed to contract down to an uninflated state, it would be more likely to heal. Carson did induce artificial pneumothorax in rabbits and actually attempted the procedure in 1822 on two patients with consumption. However, because of pleural adhesions, neither patient's lung collapsed, and Carson abandoned the practice.

For the next 60 years there was a smattering of reports suggesting that some consumptive patients who experienced spontaneous pneumothorax enjoyed improvements of their respiratory or constitutional symptoms. In 1885, Pierre Carl Edouard Potain, a physician at the Neckar and Charite Hospitals, introduced air into the chests of three consumptives, two of whom "recovered." The procedure, however, did not catch hold in France. Rather, it appeared next in Italy under the sponsorship of Carlo Forlanini. An avid student of consumption, Forlanini reasoned that collapsing the lung would reduce "the phthisiogenic process of the lung (3)." Over 11 years, Forlanini refined his technique, finally publishing in 1906 a series of 25 patients and claiming invention rights for the procedure in a German journal (22).

A rival of Forlanini for precedence with the procedure was an American surgeon, John B. Murphy, who reported on a case so managed in 1898 (1). Murphy's associate, A.E. Lemke, reported on 53 cases treated with intrapleural nitrogen installation in 1899. However, this focus of interest in America came to an end when Lemke succumbed to tuberculosis in 1906, and Murphy returned to formal thoracic surgery.

Pneumothorax therapy advanced gradually in the first 20 years of this century, undergoing subtle modifications, including the recognition by Saugman that measuring intrapleural pressure by manometry could reduce the risk of gas embolization (3) and the observation that partial, not total, collapse of the lung was sufficient. With the advent of the partial-collapse strategy, some practitioners actually conducted bilateral pneumothorax therapy.

Among the major barriers to pneumothorax were pleural adhesions, which prevented sufficient collapse. Hans Christian Jacobeus, a Swedish clinician, developed a technique for lysis of these adhesions via an endoscope (23). This procedure, the predecessor of contemporary thoracoscopic procedures, became known as closed intrapleural pneumolysis and was an essential component of the technique of pneumothorax therapy.

For some tuberculous patients, however, pneumothorax was not feasible because of the extent of the pleural fibrosis. For such patients, Ludolph Brauer developed a technique that entailed collapsing the bony thorax itself down against the mediastinum (1). This procedure, known as thorocoplasty, was refined and popularized by Wilms and Sauerbruch (3).

Efforts to collapse the lung to promote healing of tuberculous cavities or to halt hemoptysis took other diverse forms. For patients with dense apical adhesions, extrapleural pneumolysis—stripping the parietal pleura away from the chest wall—followed by plombage (instillation of paraffin wax, dense sponges, or, later, Lucite balls) enjoyed some popularity.

Unilateral interruption of the phrenic nerve was reported by Stuertz in 1911; the procedure, known as phreniclasis, entailed blunt compression of the phrenic nerve as it coursed along the neck. In this manner, the theory went, the axon would be disrupted, but the perineural sheath left intact. Thus, the diaphragm on the side of the cavity would become flaccid, putting the lung at rest. Eventually—after the cavity had healed—the axon would grow back within the sheath, restoring diaphragmatic function.

By the 1940s, pneumoperitoneum had become a popular modality of collapse. In this technique, air or nitrogen was regularly instilled into the peritoneal cavity to pneumatically elevate the diaphragm; it was sometimes employed with abdominal wraps or phreniclasis to exaggerate the diaphragm elevation (24). Happily, all of these measures were phased out of use within the first decade of effective drug treatment (see Chapter 10).

Looking back from 40 years of the chemotherapy era on these dangerous, deforming, and desperate efforts to arrest tuberculosis, it is easy to deride some of the unfortunate misadventures that resulted. However, it is appropriate that we reconsider the words with which Webb ended his chapter on the history of consumption:

> We think our fathers fools. . .so wise we grow:
> Our wiser sons, no doubt, will think us so (2)."

The Holy Grail: Curative Chemotherapy

The choice of the most significant medical advance of the twentieth century clearly is subjective and arbitrary. However, a compelling case can be made for the discovery of three drugs which, taken collectively, transformed tuberculosis from being an overwhelmingly lethal killer of millions to a predictably curable infection. It is difficult to construct a suitable analogy in contemporary medicine. Acquired immunodeficiency syndrome (AIDS) comes to mind, but—while there is a great tragedy in the deaths of so many young persons—the current scale of morbidity and mortality cannot begin to compare with that of consumption 50 years ago. Numerically, curative treatment for tuberculosis might be compared best to cancer today. Neoplastic diseases in the aggregate have approximately a 50% five-year survival—a rate comparable to pulmonary tuberculosis in 1944. Thus, if one wishes to conjure the drama associated with the discovery of the medications that cured tuberculosis, one should try to imagine the excitement that would greet a generic, assured remedy for cancer today.

Frank Ryan has written one of the finest medical books of the recent era in his tale of the scientists who struggled to find drugs to combat the tubercle bacillus, *The Forgotten Plague: How the Battle Against Tuberculosis Was Won—and Lost.* Originally titled *The Greatest Story Never Told,* the book was to be a celebration of the conquest of tuberculosis. However, the author subsequently recognized that the careless administration of drugs, failure to develop adequate control programs, and human immunodeficiency virus (HIV) infection had allowed drug resistance and burgeoning case rates to unravel the tenuous hold that had been established over the disease. Rewritten to include these elements, the book remains a stirring tale of the heroic efforts of Waksman and Schatz, Lehmann, and Domagk.

Curiously, these scientists were working with very little awareness of the efforts of the others, following substantially different pathways, intellectually, to their discoveries.

Lehmann's Vision: Para-Aminosalicylate

Born in Denmark in 1898, Jorgen Lehmann was recognized throughout his life for his creative, if unconventional, intellect. He studied medicine at the University of Lund in Sweden, writing his thesis in 1929 on the chemistry of enzymes. Later, he worked at Rockefeller University in New York, studying nerve conduction. One of his young colleagues on the faculty there was Rene Dubos.

Lehmann returned to Europe, first becoming a professor of biochemistry at Aarhus, Denmark, and later moving to Gothenburg, Sweden, where he was affiliated with the school of medicine. Among his early accomplishments were delineation of the pathogenesis of pellagra and elucidation of the clotting-anticoagulant effects of vitamin K and coumarin, studies which led to the production of the antithrombotic agent dicoumarol.

However, his focus was to shift to tuberculosis because of receipt of a reprint of an article from *Science* from an American acquaintance, Fredrick Bernheim, working at Duke University (Chapel Hill, NC). Bernheim had shown that salicylate greatly augmented oxygen uptake by tubercle bacilli in vitro; searching for an analogue to produce competitive inhibition of this pathway, Bernheim had come upon 2,3,5, triiodobenzoate. This was the report that he sent to Lehmann in 1941.

Because of his work on dicoumarol, Lehmann did not become active in tuberculosis research until 1943. By a leap of logic that was a mix of intuition and extraordinary intellect, he reasoned that the para-amino salt of salicylate would be the most effective antituberculosis compound in this system. He approached Ferrosan, a Swedish pharmaceutical firm, to enlist their aid in developing this compound. However, synthesis of para-aminosalicylate (PAS) proved very elusive. Karl-Gustave Nordahl, a Ferrosan chemist, developed a method to produce the compound, albeit in miniscule quantities. Working with meager amounts of PAS, Lehmann showed that the compound was a potent in vitro inhibitor of *M. bovis* BCG (Bacillus of Calmette and Guerin) and later demonstrated protection in vivo for guinea pigs infected with virulent tubercle bacilli.

After the safety of the drug was tested upon Lehmann himself, PAS was given to two children with osseous and soft tissue tuberculosis in March 1944. Encouraged by these results, Gylfe Vallentin next treated a series of patients with tuberculous empyema, again with impressive results. Then, one month before a young woman with pulmonary tuberculosis was treated with streptomycin in Minnesota, Sigrid, a young woman with rapidly progressive tuberculous pneumonia, was treated with PAS. She received the drug orally from October 1944 to the end of March 1945, at which time her sputum smears were negative and she underwent resection of a cavity in the right lobe of her lung. The age of tuberculosis chemotherapy had begun.

Waksman, Schatz, and Streptomycin

Selman Waksman was born in the Ukraine in 1888 and emigrated to the United States in 1910. Aided by family, he enrolled at Rutgers University in New Brunswick, New Jersey, graduating in 1915 with a bachelor of science degree in agricultural studies and acquiring a master's degree one year later. Possessed by a singular fascination with the microbes of soil, he obtained a doctorate from the University of California at Berkeley, where he focused on the mechanisms by which fungal enzymes acted. He returned to Rutgers, where he rose rapidly through the academic ranks, and in 1927 he wrote a definitive textbook, *Principles of Soil Microbiology.*

Among the many students who came to work with Waksman was a young Frenchman, Rene Dubos. Dubos participated in research pursuing "antibiotics" produced by soil microbes, but he never found an agent of clinical utility. Tragically, he was to eventually lose his first wife to tuberculosis and subsequently write (with his second wife) a book that captured much of the cultural and biological intrigue of tuberculosis, *The White Plague.*

The most significant young scientist who came to work with Waksman at Rutgers was Albert Schatz. The son of Russian immigrants, he also had a passion for microbiology and came to New Jersey in 1943 to begin working on an antibiotic research program in Waksman's laboratories.

Based on an earlier observation in his laboratory that he was unable to reproduce, Waksman believed there was a microbe in the soil that produced a compound lethal to the tubercle bacillus. Schatz's interest gravitated to the actinomyces, taking an immense variety of these organisms and streaking them on agar plates that contained other microbes, testing whether the actinomycetes produced inhibition of the various bacteria. Working with phenomenal energy, Schatz happened upon a species that appeared to have highly powerful antimicrobial properties. Originally referred to as *Actinomyces griseus,* the organism had only recently been renamed as a streptomyces. On October 19, 1943, Schatz took to Waksman the plate in which a streaked growth of *Streptomyces griseus* had produced wide zones of inhibition for routine pathogens. As the laboratory mobilized its energies to study this finding, it was Schatz who set out to determine whether the product of this streptomyces would inhibit the tubercle bacillus as well. To his gathering excitement, the material isolated from the cultures of *S. griseus*—named, by then, "streptomycin"—totally inhibited the growth of an avirulent laboratory strain of tubercle bacilli on Lowenstein-Jensen slants!

By coincidence, William Feldman, a doctor of veterinary medicine from the Mayo Clinic, visited Waksman's laboratories in November 1943, looking for new leads in the treatment of tuberculosis. Feldman was working in Minnesota in collaboration with Corwin Hinshaw. They had previously studied the effects of a sulfa-derived agent called promin, which had modestly favorable but toxicity-limited effects against pulmonary tuberculosis. Feldman and Hinshaw had developed plans for the systematic testing of antituberculosis therapy in patients in mental institutions, but were seeking new and more promising agents.

From the meeting of Feldman, Waksman, and Schatz, arrangements were made for Feldman to send a virulent strain of *M. tuberculosis* H37-Rv to Rutgers for screening potential compounds. Streptomycin was highly active in vitro against H37-Rv, so Schatz laboriously prepared 10 g of streptomycin, which was sent to Feldman to use in vivo to treat four guinea pigs infected with tubercle bacilli. It worked! All four survived the predictably lethal infection. Eagerly, the group attempted to press ahead with streptomycin research. But it required the assistance of a pharmaceutical manufacturer to produce sufficient streptomycin for meaningful studies. Merck & Company, located nearby in Rahway, New Jersey, was, at that time, intensely committed to producing penicillin for the war effort. But George Merck saw the potential implication of this new drug and committed his company to the endeavor.

Further studies in large numbers of mice persuaded Feldman and Hinshaw not only that streptomycin was highly effective, but also that it was strikingly benign in terms of drug toxicity. Encouraged by these results, Hinshaw and colleagues commenced treatment in humans. Their first patient was a man with acute miliary disease associated with genitourinary tuberculosis; after an initially favorable response, the patient died abruptly. The postmortem indicated that his death was due to pulmonary embolism, but the tuberculosis had undergone involution. Encouraged by these findings, they next set out to treat a young woman, Patricia, who was dying of consumption. With gradually increasing doses, she was treated with streptomycin from November 1944 to the end of April 1945, enjoying a clinical remission (although her sputum remained positive for tubercle bacilli). She went on to discharge from the sanatorium, marriage, and three children. Across the world, with neither group aware of the other, the second blow against tuberculosis had been delivered.

Domagk Undaunted: Isoniazid

Gerhard Domagk was born in 1895 in the province of Brandenburg, Germany. His education was interrupted by service in World War I, where he eventually became a medical assistant. Working with the wounded soldiers, he was indelibly impressed by the havoc wrought by uncontrolled wound infections.

Returning home to a country grimly depressed by Germany's loss in the war, Domagk plunged resolutely into his medical studies at Kiel. His postgraduate studies were focused on infection and immunity, with Domagk helping to originally characterize the reticuloendothelial system. In 1927, at age 31, he was recruited to the Bayer Laboratories of Farben Industries. There, he was immersed in the intellectual lineage of Paul Ehrlich, Robert Koch's contemporary and colleague. Based on the affinity of bacteria for various types of dyes or stains, Ehrlich had hypothesized that dyes or similar compounds could be modified and made toxic or lethal for the microbes. One of his followers had joined Bayer and initiated a project to search for anti-infective chemotherapy agents.

Domagk tested numerous compounds synthesized by an associate, Josef Klarer, for their ability to protect mice from a particularly virulent strain of streptococci. Despite an extended run of failures, Domagk persisted with this line of study. Finally, at Christmas of 1931, his tenacity was rewarded. A red dye compound designated K1-730, which had no activity in vitro against streptococci, was wholly protective in the mouse against these same microbes.

Domagk and colleagues spent the next 18 months producing, characterizing, and testing this compound—named Prontosil rubrum—against various microbes. In 1933, the drug was given to the first patient, a young girl with streptococcal abscesses of the pharynx complicated by septic phlebitis; this apparently saved her life. Prontosil cured a variety of infections over the next few years, gradually overcoming the skepticism of a profession and the public that had hopes dashed too many times by spurious claims of "wonder drugs." However, the study was to be complicated further: French scientists showed that it was not the entire Bayer molecule that was active, but only the sulfanilamide side chain. Prontosil rubrum was not active in vitro because it required cleavage by the host to release the active compound!

Domagk and others tested sulfanilamide for activity against the tubercle bacillus. Although there was some in vitro inhibition and slight protection in animal models, the amounts required would be highly toxic in humans. In the midst of his studies in 1939, Domagk experienced the heights and depths, almost simultaneously. He was awarded the Nobel Prize for his discovery of Prontosil. But Germany was immersed in World War II, and he was arrested by the Gestapo rather than allowed to travel to receive his prize. Domagk returned to the laboratories in Elberfeld.

During the war, Domagk was simultaneously driven by concerns for wound infections and for the tuberculosis epidemic that he knew would follow the conflict. To his gratification, German military surgeons eventually conceded the utility of the sulfa drugs against such dreaded conditions as gas gangrene and sepsis. And, remarkably, his directors at Bayer chose to continue to support his search for an effective antituberculosis compound, despite the distractions and demands of the war.

Robert Behnisch, a clever young chemist, was assigned to work with Domagk. Behnisch noted that the only sulfonamide compounds with in vitro activity against tuberculosis involved a thiazole side chain. Focusing on this moiety, he synthesized a variety of cleavages and side chains. Soon, it became apparent that the active principle lay in a structure, thiosemicarbazone. Excited by this finding, Domagk struggled to keep his research proceeding, despite repeated bombings by the Allies, dwindling staff, shrinking financial support, and sorely limited supplies. Through 1942 and 1943 he remained steadfast in his working discipline, despite unimaginable stress. Threats existed not only from the bombs raining down from the sky, but also for the safety of his Jewish wife, Flora, who was eventually wrested from him in 1944 and sent to a concentration camp. [She was one of the survivors, returning to her family following Germany's surrender.]

Following the war, Benisch and Domagk reassembled a team in Elberfeld to resume work with the thiosemicarbazone. They distilled their list down to three compounds, the best of which was thioacetazone, also know as TB-1 or Conteben. In 1946, this drug was first given to a woman with a long history of deforming lupus vulgaris, tuberculosis of the skin. She responded well to such therapy, and other cases of cutaneous tuberculosis were also treated. Bolstered by these successes, Domagk traveled about northern Germany, enlisting colleagues to collaborate in testing his new drug.

Thioacetazone was not to be a major first-line antituberculosis medication. Nonetheless, it was a foundation upon which the German scientists and others could build. As part of the treaty ending the war, the Allies were empowered to exact reparations by sending scientists into the laboratories of the vanquished. American researchers who visited Germany carried back with them information regarding the structure and function of the thiosemicarbazone compounds. Among the data brought back to North America were the observations of two distinguished visitors—Corwin Hinshaw and Walsh McDermott—that Conteben appeared to have activity comparable to that of PAS.

From 1948 to 1951, chemists in Europe and North America created numerous variations of this pleomorphic molecule, looking for the ultimate weapon against tuberculosis. And, in a remarkable event that must have been more than coincidence, three different scientists came to identify a singularly potent compound, isonicotinic acid hydrazide, as the apex of this family of drugs: Gerhard Domagk of Bayer, Herbert Fox of LaRoche, and Jack Bernstein of Squibb Pharmaceuticals.

Thus, in early 1952, the world welcomed the final element of a millennial search. Within two years, it was recognized that combining isoniazid, streptomycin, and PAS afforded nearly universal, lifetime cures of a scourge that had ravaged humankind like no other.

Bittersweet Postscripts to the Miracle

Ideally, accomplishments such as those described above—heroic feats that stemmed from brilliant intellect, inspired intuition, and exceptional perseverance—would be rewarded with acclaim, recompense, and personal satisfaction. Sadly, many of the major figures in this saga experienced far less. True, Selman Waksman received the Nobel Prize for Medicine in 1952. However, his young associate Albert Schatz was ignored by both the Nobel committee and Dr. Waksman; the latter scarcely mentioned Schatz's role in the discovery and development of streptomycin during the Nobel acceptance speech or subsequent public comments, leaving the young man embittered and frustrated. Schatz also felt deceived by Waksman regarding the patent and royalties, eventually bringing a successful suit against Waksman and Rutgers. Belatedly, Schatz received the Rutgers University Award in 1994, 50 years after his momentous finding. Similarly, Corwin Hinshaw and William Feldman (who developed life-threatening disease from his laboratory research with virulent tubercle bacilli) felt ignored in the Nobel award, and suspected an associate at the Mayo Clinic of sabotaging their candidacy.

Jorgen Lehmann, whose wife—feeling neglected by his fanatical commitment to the research—had left him in the midst of his quest for PAS, felt betrayed at his omission from this award. Despite the fact that Lehmann's drug had been used to treat and arrest tuberculosis before Waksman's agent was employed, the report of this event was delayed by judgments of persons around Lehmann. And, it was rumored that personal antagonism by a member of the Nobel Committee had poisoned Lehmann's chances.

Gerhard Domagk received a Nobel Prize in 1939, not for his work that led ultimately to isoniazid, but for his discovery of Prontosil. However, he had been incarcerated by the Nazis rather than allowed to travel to Stockholm. He eventually visited Sweden in 1947 to receive his award; but Domagk—who had labored under the most adverse circumstances of all, the Allied bombing, the disintegration of his country, and the immense threat to himself and his family—had to feel acrid resentment when his intellectual property was pilfered, allowing others simultaneously to reach the pinnacle of the line of investigation which clearly was the product of his labors.

Financially, patent rights and royalties—modest by today's standards—flowed to Waksman, Rutgers, and Merck & Company for streptomycin. However, because of prior, nonmedical synthesis and description of both PAS and isoniazid, no patent rights could be obtained for either of these drugs.

REFERENCES

1. Corper HJ. Founders of our knowledge of tuberculosis. *Hygeia* 1929;October-November:1–13.
2. Webb GB. Tuberculosis. In (ed), Clio Series 1936.
3. Keers RY. *Pulmonary tuberculosis: a journey down the centuries.* London: Cassell Ltd., 1978.
4. Dubos R, Dubos J. *The White Plague: tuberculosis, man, and society.* Boston: Little, Brown and Company, 1952.
5. Brock TD, Koch R. *A life in medicine and bacteriology.* Madison, WI: Science Tech Publishers, 1988.
6. Ryan F. *The forgotten plague.* Boston: Little, Brown and Company, 1992.
7. Cave AJE. The evidence for the incidence of tuberculosis in ancient Egypt. *Br J Tuberc* 1939;33:142.
8. Meachen GN. *A short history of tuberculosis.* London: John Bale & Sons.
9. Kapur V, Whittam TS, Musser JM. Is *Mycobacterium tuberculosis* 15,000 years old? *J Infect Dis* 1994;170: 1348–1349.
10. Flick LF. *Development of our knowledge of tuberculosis.* Philadelphia: 1925.
11. Morton R. *Phthisiologica,* 2nd ed. Publisher unknown, 1689.
12. Cummins SL. *Tuberculosis in history: from the 17th century to our own times.* Baltimore: Williams & Wilkins, 1949.
13. Marten B. *A new theory on consumptions more especially of a phthisis or consumption of the lungs.* London: Knaplock, 1720.
14. Davaine CJ. Recherches sur las infusoires du sang dons la maladie connue sur le nome de sang de rate. *Comptes Rendu Acad Sci Paris* 1863;LV II:??.
15. Koch R. Die aetiologie der Mitzbrandkrankenheit, be-

grundet auf die entwicklungsgeschicte des Bacillus anthracis. *Beitr Biol Pflanzen* 1876;2:277–310.
16. Lister J. On the lactic fermentation and its bearing on pathology. *Trans Pathol Soc Lond* 1878;29:425–469.
17. *New York Times.* May 3, 1882.
18. Loeffler F. Zum 25 jahrigen gedenletage der entdeckung des tuberkalbacillus. *Deutsche Med* 1907;33:449–451.
19. Koch R. Die aetiologie der tuberculose. *Berl Klinische Wochenschr* 1882;19:221–230.
20. Woodward TE. Epidemiologic classics of Carter, Maxcy, Trudeau, and Smith. *J Infect Dis* 1992;165: 235–244.
21. Trudeau EL. *An autobiography.* New York: Doubleday & Company, 1951.
22. Forlanini C. Zur behandlung der lungenschwindsucht durch kunstlich erzengten pneumothorax. *Deutsche Med Wochenschr* 1906;32:1401.
23. Jacobeus HC. The cauterization of adhesions in artificial pneumothorax treatment of pulmonary tuberculosis under thoracoscopic control. *Proc R Soc Med* 1922;45.
24. Mitchell RS, Hiatt JS, McCain PP, Easom HF, Thomas CD. Pneumoperitoneum in the treatment of pulmonary tuberculosis. *Am Rev Tuberc* 1947;44:306–331.

2

Biology and Laboratory Diagnosis of Tuberculosis

WHAT IS TUBERCULOSIS?

"Tuberculosis" is an old term, referring generically to the small, potatolike ("tuber"), indurated anatomical lesions found throughout tissues involved by this disease. The formal naming of the disease "tuberculosis" is attributed to Johann Lukas Schoenlein in 1839 (1). However, considerable confusion still reigns over this terminology. Considering only the anatomical-histological findings, there are numerous infections, pneumoconioses, and idiopathic diseases such as sarcoidosis which can result in the formation of tuberclelike lesions in human tissues; these disorders, though, have generally been referred to as "granulomatous." Greater controversy still lies with the distinction between diseases caused by the various pathogens of the genus *Mycobacterium.* Many authors still refer to all of these assorted infections as "tuberculosis," later identifying the species involved [e.g., "Human Tuberculosis due to *Mycobacterium bovis:* Report of 10 Cases" (2)]. This usage is confusing to professional and lay persons and should be abandoned. Because of the unique implications for transmission patterns and public health practices, I suggest that the term "tuberculosis" should be reserved exclusively for disease caused by *Mycobacterium tuberculosis.* A more precise way to refer to the other mycobacterial diseases might employ a phrase such as "mycobacteriosis, due to *Mycobacterium* "*x*". In support of this logic is the manner in which we refer to Hansen's disease: we do *not* say "tuberculosis due to *Mycobacterium leprae.*"

The taxonomic grouping of mycobacteria *M. tuberculosis, M. bovis, M. microti,* and *M. africanum* as "tuberculosis complex" may cause further confusion. However, given the rarity with which these organisms cause human disease and the vastly differing public health implications for infection by these microbes, I even would argue against referring to them as causes of "tuberculosis."

TAXONOMY

Etymologically, "mycobacterium" is derived from the Greek for fungus *(myces)* and small rod *(bakterion).* The "fungus" component of the name derives from the tendency of these microorganisms to spread diffusely over the surface of liquid medium in a moldlike growth pattern. Most consistently, the mycobacteria have been identified by their unique tinctorial properties, specifically, their "acid-fastness." The mycobacteria resist staining with conventional bacterial stains; clinical specimens examined with Gram stain technique typically appear "neutral" or as unstained ghost-forms. This resistance to standard dyes and the avidity with which the mycobacteria retain certain dyes, once impregnated, are both due to the high lipid content of their cell walls. Generally, gram-positive bacteria have about 5% lipid or wax content in their cell walls, gram-negative organisms around 20%, and the mycobacteria roughly 60%. The mycobacteria are all acid-fast on staining (see below for detailed description of staining and microbial structure/chemistry); however, not all acid-fast microbes are mycobacteria. Most nocardia and rhodococci, some actinomyces and corynebacteria, and one species of legionella are weakly acid-fast.

Several of the microbes that share this tinctorial property are phylogenetically closely related to the mycobacteria (Fig. 2.1). While many of the Actinomycetaceae are environmental, nonpathogenic organisms, a few of the *Nocardia* and *Actinomyces* species are significant sources of human disease. And, mindful of internecine human conflict, the *Streptomyces* species have provided several of the most potent antituberculosis drugs, notably, the aminoglycoside antibiotics including streptomycin and the rifamycin agents.

Among the mycobacteria there are various criteria employed to distinguish species. For the purposes of laboratory identification, numerous morphological, biochemical, and growth characteristics previously have been employed (3), but these have largely been supplanted in modern laboratories by more rapid and accurate methodologies that employ radiometric cultivation and/or molecular biology techniques (see below).

However, the newer methodologies generally identify only *M. tuberculosis* complex and do not distinguish among the species/subspecies within that grouping. There is such a high degree of genetic relatedness among these "species" that they are grouped as a "complex" (3). Very likely, they have evolved from a common source (4). Nonetheless, the criteria cited above, as well as various epidemiological and biological properties, argue, I believe, for continued species distinction.

MORPHOLOGY OF THE ORGANISMS

M. tuberculosis is typically a slightly curved or straight rod-shaped microbe. Its typical size when cultivated in vitro is 1 to 4 mm in length and 0.3 to 0.6 mm in diameter, making it smaller than most bacterial pathogens. However, the tubercle bacilli in the tissues of diseased hosts may assume different characteristics (5). When *M. tuberculosis* was cultivated in human cell cultures, it was observed that the bacilli assumed longer, more curved forms and tended to accept stains in an irregular fashion with more prominent beading (5).

CELL-WALL STRUCTURE AND BIOCHEMISTRY

Delineation of the chemical constituents and architecture of the cell wall of *M. tuberculosis* (and other mycobacterial pathogens) very well may lead to enhanced understanding of such critical issues as pathogenesis, immunity, vaccine development, and rational drug design. Brennan and his colleagues at Colorado State

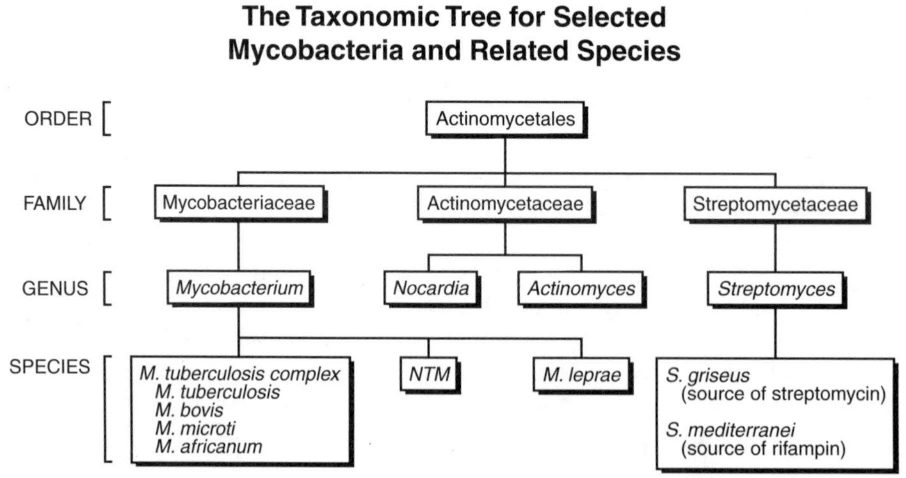

FIG. 2.1. The taxonomic tree for selected mycobacteria and related species. NTM, nontuberculous mycobacteria.

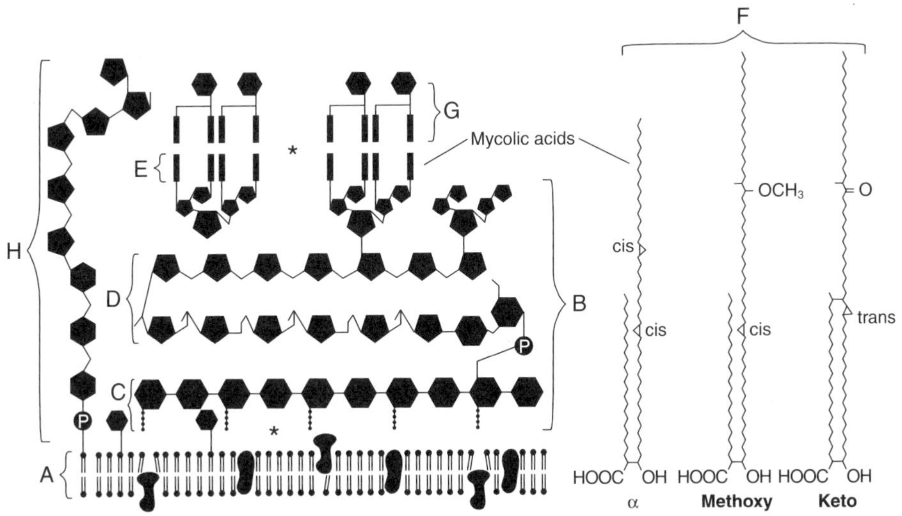

FIG. 2.2. This schematic view of the cell wall of the tubercle bacillus has been developed largely through the research of Patrick Brennan and colleagues at Colorado State University, Fort Collins, Colorado. The components include (A) plasma membrane and (B) complex polymer that is associated with the plasma membrane. The plasma membrane is composed of (C) peptidoglycans, (D) arabinogalactan, and (E) mycolic acids, which for Mycobacterium tuberculosis include (F) methoxy, and keto types. (G) Glycolipid surface molecules associate with the mycolic acids to form a second bilayer. (H) Lipoarabinomannan (LAM) units traverse the entire depth of the cell wall; the terminal components of these LAM units may be important determinants of pathogenicity (see text). Phosphodiester bonds (I) link the complex polymer units and LAM moieties to the cell membrane. * Various proteins are interspersed within the plasma membrane, between the plasma membrane and the peptidoglycan layer, and along the peripheral cell wall.

University have recently conducted a series of elegant studies on these topics; this material comprises major elements of this section (6).

Historically, ultrastructural research has suggested that mycobacterial cell walls consist of a number of layers. There is an electron-dense region abutting or intercalated with the outer leaf of the plasma membrane. The next outward layer is electron transparent. It and the inner electron-dense layer appear common to all of the mycobacterial species thus far analyzed. Peripheral to these layers are variable strata that also contain electron-dense materials and appear to be distinctive for different species.

Biochemical studies have indicated that the major building blocks of the mycobacterial cell wall skeletons consist of three macromolecules: peptidoglycans, arabinogalactans, and mycolic acids (see Fig. 2.2). The peptidoglycans are common to other bacteria. Mycolic acids are found almost exclusively among the mycobacteria and, as fatty acids, are believed to be essential to, but not the sole source of, the unique staining properties (acid-fastness) of the mycobacteria. The least well characterized component of the cell wall has been the arabinogalactans. However, substantial advances have been made recently in the delineation of the biochemical and architectural features of the arabinogalactans and their coelements in the cell wall.

Among the most significant aspects of this structural model is the potential pathogenic role in the mycobacterial diseases of two lipopolysaccharides, lipoarabinomannan (LAM) and lipomannan (6). Based on the role of LAM in directing macrophage function (7,8), its capacity to inhibit the processing of mycobacterial peptides/proteins by antigen-presenting cells (9), and its induction of tumor necrosis factor production (10,11), this compound is currently considered by some authorities to be a mycobacterial virulence factor (8). Indeed, a recent analysis by Brennan's group identified biochemical differences in the terminal structures of the LAM moieties of classically virulent and avirulent strains of *M. tuberculosis,* Erdmann and H37Ra, respectively (12).

GROWTH CHARACTERISTICS

M. tuberculosis is a slow-growing microbe with generation times ranging from 12 to 24 hours depending on environmental and microbial variables. One characteristic but not distinctive property of *M. tuberculosis* is the tendency to form "cords" or dense clusters of bacilli in parallel alignment, like a cord of wood. This quality was noted by Koch in his initial report on the etiological agent of tuberculosis. The biochemical source of this phenomenon was identified by Bloch in 1950 and titled "cord factor" (13). Originally deemed to be associated with a virulence principle of *M. tuberculosis,* cording was subsequently observed to occur among other mycobacterial species of lesser or no observed virulence (14). Cord factor, later identified as a highly unusual biological compound, trehalose 6,6'-dimycolate (15–18), was observed to cause highly morbid, often lethal consequences when injected serially into animal models (15). However, the role of this compound in the pathogenesis of tuberculosis is unresolved. Arguing against a central role in virulence, the compound is found in other nonpathogenic mycobacteria; however, their avirulence could be due to unrelated factors. Evidence in support of a virulence role of cording factor was developed by Kato (19,20), who showed that mice immunized against the compound (that was rendered antigenic by complexing it with bovine serum albumin) were less susceptible to challenge with virulent tubercle bacilli. However, the same investigator also demonstrated that mice immunized with a strain of bacille Calmette-Guérin (BCG) that was positive for cord factor were partially protected, despite the absence of antibodies to this compound (20).

PHYSIOLOGY

Considerable investigation of the physiologic properties of *M. tuberculosis* has been conducted in this century. Consistent features of the bacillus include the following attributes.

Aerobic

The growth of mycobacteria in vitro and in vivo appears closely linked to the availability of oxygen. Grown in liquid medium without agitation or detergent, the bacilli tend to form a thin pellicle on the surface; this is presumed to be due to the proliferation at the air (oxygen) interface, as well as their hydrophobic, waxy coats. The bacilli that sink to the bottom of the liquid remain viable but do not replicate. Wayne (21) suggested that such microbes may assume an analogous state in chronic lesions within the human body, and he demonstrated that such bacilli assume replication soon after reexposure to oxygen.

Non–Spore Forming

Because of their waxy coats, which limit fluid loss across the cell membrane, mycobacteria remain viable much longer than most other bacteria in an airborne or exposed state. However, this is not a true sporulation.

Growth Variation In Vivo

There are several vital issues in the pathogenesis and natural history of tuberculosis that relate to the physiology of the mycobacterial life cycles. In the subsequent sections, we examine two states, cell-wall–deficient, non–acid-fast forms and organ tropism, that may be of great biological significance in clinical tuberculosis.

Cell-Wall–Deficient, Non–Acid-Fast Forms

In 1908, Much (22) claimed to detect minute, granular variants of tubercle bacilli that did not stain acid-fast with Ziehl's stain. Much's granules, as these forms became known, have remained controversial among students of mycobacterial diseases ever since. Mattman and colleagues described "L-forms" of mycobacteria in a series of reports from 1960 to 1970 (23–25). Subsequently, Ratnam and Chandrasekhar published two studies on this topic far apart in time. In 1976, they reported that cell-wall–deficient forms (spheroplasts) of *M. tuberculosis* persisted in a viable state after injection into guinea pigs but did not produce overt disease or consistent tuberculin reactivity over a 5-week period (26). However, animals observed for 10 or 16 weeks manifested substantial rates of tuberculin reactivity, autopsy-demonstrated tuberculosis, or premature death from tuberculosis. The authors showed that spheroplasts reverted back to conventional forms of *M. tuberculosis,* and that this phenomenon was associated with the morbidity in their guinea pigs. They speculated that reactivation-type tuberculosis might involve persistence in tissue of spheroplast forms. Sixteen years later, they reported on their ongoing studies of these cell-wall–deficient, non–acid-fast (CWD/NAF) forms (27). In their second report, the authors described an improved method for derivation of these CWD/NAF variants in vitro (a technique that reduced contamination with normal bacillary forms) and reported that, while the CWD/NAF forms did not produce overt infection or tuberculin conversion in normal guinea pigs, among immunodeficient animals they did produce skin test reactivity and the eventual recovery of normal forms of *M. tuberculosis.* Of considerable interest, the CWD/NAF form found in tissue had a granular character mindful of Much's original description. Chandrasekhar and Ratnam noted that macrophages from competent hosts were able to denude tubercle bacilli of their cell walls as one means of creating these variant forms. They also noted that a cell-wall antibiotic, cycloserine, was useful in creating CWD/NAF forms. Crowle et al. (28) also observed the formation of CWD/NAF forms when tubercle bacilli within macrophages were exposed to ethambutol, another cell-wall–active agent.

The real clinical significance of these findings may well relate to two puzzling problems: (a) the phenomenon of "persistence" whereby tubercle bacilli continue to survive in tissue despite microbicidal concentrations of antibiotics and (b) reactivation of tuberculosis years or decades after the initial infection (29). Khomenko's report (30) of "ultrafine" forms of *M. tuberculosis* that were invisible on conventional staining techniques may be consistent with the CWD/NAF phenomena described above. In the walls of cavitary pulmonary lesions, he found filterable forms which on electron microscopy had no cell walls; the number of these ultrafine forms rose during the introduction of chemotherapy. These "invisible" forms were said to be able to revert to typical bacterial forms on careful recultivation. These CWD/NAF and ultrafine forms may possibly be related to the phenomena of persistence and recrudescence of tuberculosis.

Virulence and Organ Tropism

Bacteriology is replete with examples of microbes that undergo adaptation for survival or virulence utility. Segal and Bloch (31) showed that a strain of *M. tuberculosis* grown in vitro had significantly different properties than organisms of the same strain that were passed through a murine host; among the distinctions noted by these investigators were enhanced virulence and reduced immunogenicity for the tubercle bacilli passed through the mouse (32,33). Probably related to such adaptations were the observations made by Collins and Montalbine (34) that organisms that had been recovered from the lungs of animals, after extended residency there, tended to selectively collect in the lungs of subsequent animals when injected intravenously. Subsequently, it was found that cultures grown longer in vitro developed similar tropism for the lungs (35). Based on variations of staining properties of the bacilli grown in vivo, it was speculated that there may have been alterations in the sulfolipids of the mycobacteria, which potentially could have been responsible for the changes in virulence and organ tropism noted above (36). While these laboratory observations may appear to be abstract or academic, they may be relevant to some of the peculiarities of transmission and virulence that have puzzled epidemiologists for decades. Based on these and other like observations, a plausible case may be made that strains of *M. tuberculosis* that have passed through certain hosts could have become more transmissible (likely to establish infection in exposed individuals) or more virulent (likely to produce clinically active disease in those infected); see Chapter 3 for a more thorough discussion.

CLINICAL LABORATORY AND TUBERCULOSIS

Laboratories serve major roles in the diagnosis and management of tuberculosis. In this section, sputum processing, microscopic identification of mycobacteria in secretions or tissues, cultivation techniques, drug susceptibility testing, serological testing, and novel molecular biological methods including polymerase chain reaction (PCR) and restriction fragment length polymorphism (RFLP) are reviewed.

Two trends have combined to create a new pattern in laboratory services: (a) the technology has become more sophisticated and expensive and (b) the prevalence in the industrialized nations of mycobacterial diseases, especially tuberculosis, has diminished. Because of these considerations, a three-tiered program is evolving. Level I laboratories collect and ship specimens; if adequate safety standards are met, they may also perform smears and acid-fast stains. Level II laboratories perform level I services plus culture and identify isolates as *M. tuberculosis;* nontuberculous mycobacterial isolates are sent on to Level III facilities. Level II facilities may perform in vitro susceptibility testing for *M. tuberculosis* or may refer them elsewhere. Level III laboratories perform all of the services of Levels I and II, as well as conducting species identification and drug susceptibility testing. For a comprehensive and masterful review of laboratory organization, standard procedures, and new techniques, see *Clinical Mycobacteriology,* edited by Heifets (37).

Sputum Processing

Sputum is the most common sample submitted to the laboratory for study. To obtain the best microscopic and cultivation results, such specimens should be handled carefully. Important elements in sputum study include how to obtain the specimen and transport it to the laboratory for homogenization/digestion, decontamination, and concentration. This process is shown schematically in Fig. 2.3. These methods are described in detail in several recent reviews (38–40).

Collection of a Good Specimen

For patients with a deep cough that is readily productive of lower respiratory tract secretions, such material may be collected at any time [note: because coughing may generate highly infectious aerosols, health care workers should be extremely careful that cough-inducing procedures are performed in a well-ventilated and/or ultraviolet (UV)-irradiated area]. For patients with less productive cough, early-morning specimens that take advantage of overnight accumulations are preferred. Unlike sputum cultures for nonmycobacterial pneumonias, specimens that represent an admixture of sputum and upper airway secretions are acceptable (although not ideal) for tuberculosis diagnosis. Other methods for obtaining lower respiratory secretions include formal sputum induction (typically by heated saline nebulization), bronchoscopy, or gastric aspiration (see Chapter 6 for techniques and indications). Sputum or similar specimens should be collected in screw-capped centrifuge tubes or cups.

Transport to Laboratory

For the purposes of both early reporting and optimal bacteriology, specimens should be taken promptly to the laboratory. If this cannot be accomplished, refrigeration of the specimen will serve to reduce the risk of overgrowth by nonmycobacterial organisms. Microbial inhibitors such as cetylpyridium chloride may be added to retard bacterial growth.

Homogenization and Decontamination

Respiratory secretions typically include a thick, proteinaceous matrix. To disrupt this dense material, a mucolytic agent such as N-acetyl cysteine may be added to the sputum. Also, to diminish the risk of overgrowth by other

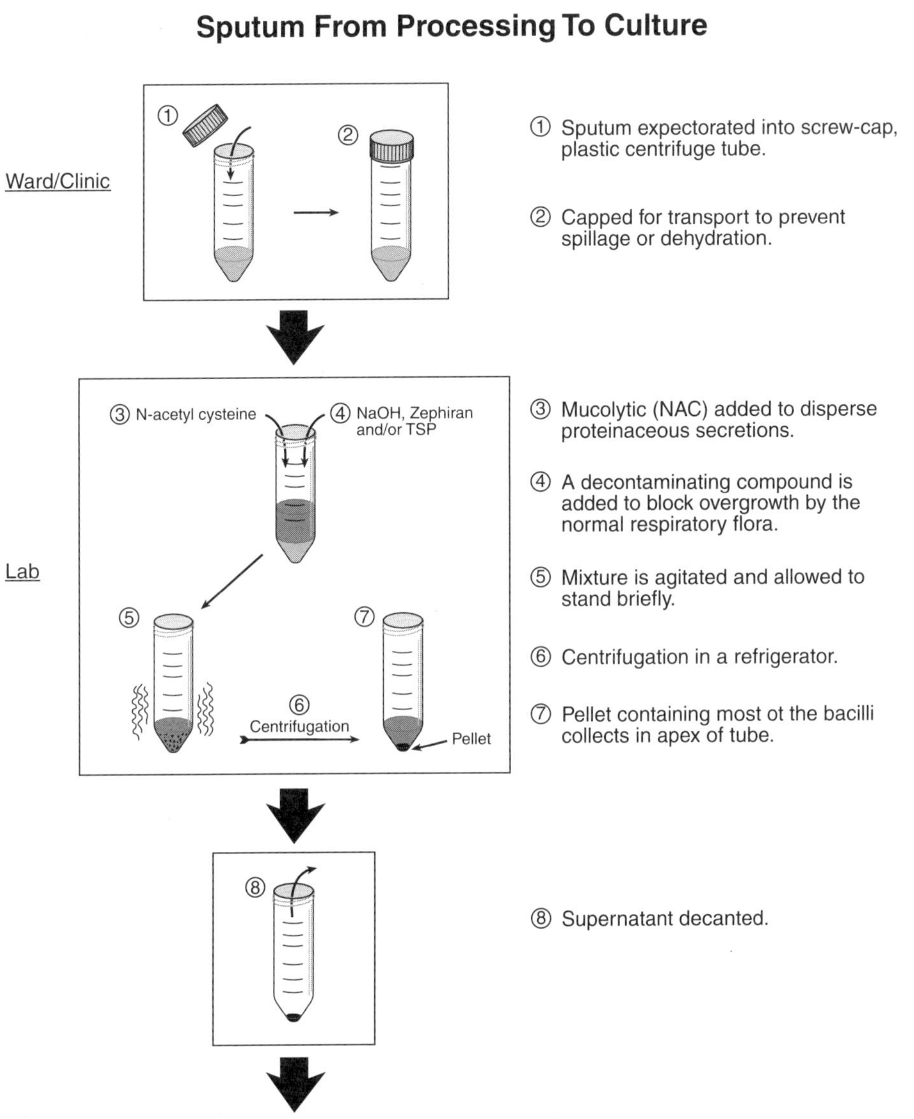
Sputum From Processing To Culture
Ward/Clinic
①
②
① Sputum expectorated into screw-cap, plastic centrifuge tube.
② Capped for transport to prevent spillage or dehydration.
Lab
③ N-acetyl cysteine
④ NaOH, Zephiran and/or TSP
⑤
⑥ Centrifugation
⑦
Pellet
③ Mucolytic (NAC) added to disperse proteinaceous secretions.
④ A decontaminating compound is added to block overgrowth by the normal respiratory flora.
⑤ Mixture is agitated and allowed to stand briefly.
⑥ Centrifugation in a refrigerator.
⑦ Pellet containing most ot the bacilli collects in apex of tube.
⑧
⑧ Supernatant decanted.

A

FIG. 2.3. Sputum from processing to culture. *Ward/Clinic:* 1, Sputum expectorated into screw-cap, plastic centrifuge tube; 2, Capped for transport to prevent spillage or dehydration. *Lab:* 3, Mucolytic (NAC) added to disperse proteinaceous secretion; 4, A decontaminating compound is added to block overgrowth by the normal respiratory flora; 5, Mixture is agitated and allowed to stand briefly; 6, Centrifugation in a refrigerator; 7, Pellet containing most of the bacilli collects in apex of tube; 8, Supernatent decanted. *Microscopy:* 9, Pellet sampled into loop and; 10, smeared on glass slide for fixation, staining and; 11, microscopic examination. *Culture*: 12, Bovine serum albumin added to pellet; 13, Pellet suspended in BSA by agitation; 14, BACTEC liquid 7H-12 medium; 15, 7H-11 (nonselective); 16, 7H-11S (selective); 17, L-J (nonselective).

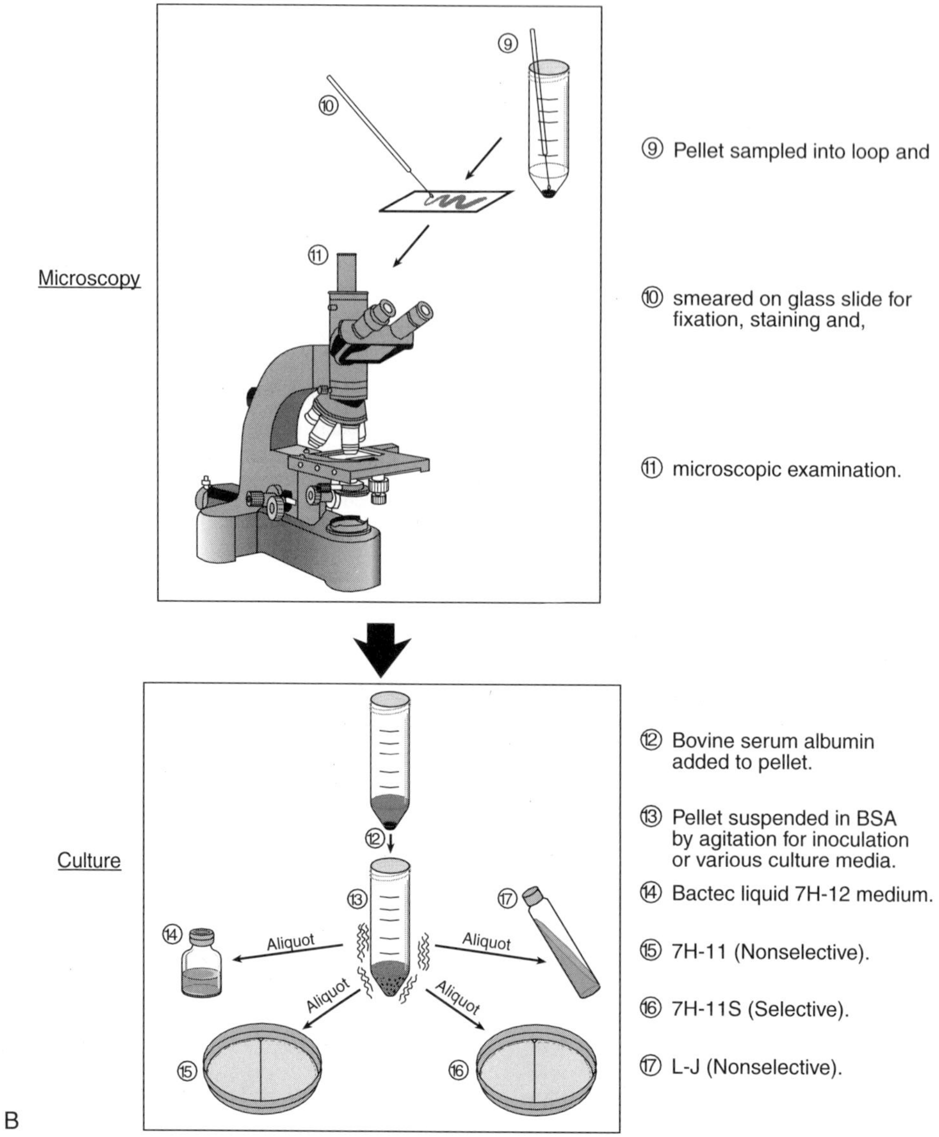
Microscopy
⑨ Pellet sampled into loop and
⑩ smeared on glass slide for fixation, staining and,
⑪ microscopic examination.
Culture
Aliquot
Aliquot
Aliquot
Aliquot
⑫ Bovine serum albumin added to pellet.
⑬ Pellet suspended in BSA by agitation for inoculation or various culture media.
⑭ Bactec liquid 7H-12 medium.
⑮ 7H-11 (Nonselective).
⑯ 7H-11S (Selective).
⑰ L-J (Nonselective).
B

FIG. 2.3. *Continued*

bacteria, decontamination with dilute sodium hydroxide, benzalkonium chloride, or trisodium phosphate should be employed. However, care must be taken not to injure the mycobacteria by overexposure to the basic solutions.

Concentration

After the sputum has undergone homogenization/digestion and decontamination, the specimen should be promptly spun down in a refrigerated centrifuge (to prevent heat injury to the mycobacteria), and the supernatant decanted. The pellet should then be sampled for smear and microscopy; because of the concentration effect, this specimen is far more sensitive to the presence of mycobacteria than is the raw sputum. To culture this material, the pellet must be resuspended in bovine serum albumin and agitated to uniformly distribute mycobacteria.

Microscopy

Because of the unique tinctorial properties of the mycobacteria, sputum (and other diagnostic specimens) should be examined with care by the microscopic techniques described below. The two major limitations of microscopy are its relative insensitivity and lack of specificity (see below for details); however, until novel techniques (noted below in "Molecular Biology Techniques") are more fully developed, microscopy remains the first line of diagnosis in tuberculosis.

Koch fortuitously came upon a dye that was capable of staining the cell wall in 1881–1882: the methylene blue he employed had absorbed enough ammonia from the laboratory atmosphere to become sufficiently alkaline to penetrate the waxy mycobacterial coat (see Chapter 1). However, within two decades, improved stains had been developed, techniques that are still employed today—the carbol-fuchsin methods of Ziehl-Neelsen or Kinyoun. The fundamental principles of these methods relate to the avidity of the waxy, lipid-rich mycobacterial cell wall for the carbol-fuchsin dye. The mycobacterial cell walls are encouraged to take up the red carbol-fuchsin by alkalinity (and heat, with the Ziehl-Neelsen method); once the cells are so impregnated, they resist decolorization even with a potent hydrochloric acid-ethanol solution (acid-alcohol). So, when the slide is counterstained with methylene blue (Ziehl-Neelsen) or malachite green (Kinyoun), the mycobacteria appear as red rods against a uniform counterstain. This property is responsible for the familiar appellation, "red snappers," employed by generations of health care workers.

While generally reliable, these "acid-fast" carbol-fuchsin techniques are visually problematic: the red bacilli do not contrast well with the blue and white background. Therefore, material stained in this manner must be viewed under oil immersion, which is arduous and time-consuming. Since 1989, fluorescence microscopy has largely supplanted the older, acid-fast methods in modern laboratories. Fundamentally, this technology relies on the same lipid-related avidity for dyes, but the stain in this case is auramine-rhodamine. The mycobacteria absorb this agent and resist decolorization with acid-alcohol; however, the auramine-rhodamine–stained bacilli fluoresce when excited with UV or other specially filtered light frequencies. The mycobacteria appear as bright yellow rods against an inky black background in the UV system. Because of the physiology of human retina, this is much easier to perceive than the red-blue contrast of the carbol-fuchsin stain. Therefore, microscopy smears can be examined under a 25× or 40× objective, allowing for much faster reading of specimens, 1 to 2 minutes per slide in contrast to the 15 minutes given traditionally for the Ziehl-Neelsen technique. Also, the yellow-black contrast eliminates the potential problem of red-blue color-blindness among male microscopists.

Regardless of the technique employed, microscopy is modestly less sensitive than culture in detecting mycobacteria in sputum. Most patients with cavitary lung disease have abundantly positive sputum smears (41). However, for patients with less extensive, noncavitary disease, there is a substantial probability that a sputum smear (or several sputa) will be negative, despite the presence of viable bacilli in the specimens. For example, among a group of 1,710 patients in Hong Kong who, by suspect chest radiographs, were thought likely to have "active" tuberculosis but who had had four or more negative sputum smears, 592 (35%) had one or more positive cultures (42). In one rigorous study, which entailed reading 100 oil-immersion fields, smears became negative when culture counts fell below 7,800 bacilli per milliliter of sputum (43); a previous study had indicated the cut-off point to be 9,500 bacilli per milliliter (44).

Another major shortcoming of microscopy lies with the nonspecificity of the finding: are the microbes on the smear *M. tuberculosis* or other mycobacteria? Although experienced technologists may form impressions about the etiological agents from microscopic morphology (e.g., ". . .*M. kansasii* tends to appear longer, more slender or filamentous, and more beaded. . ." or ". . .*M. avium-intracellulare* tends to be smaller, more curved, or cocco-bacillary in shape. . ."), they are quick to point out that such visual impressions are insufficiently reliable to formulate management plans. Certainly, in an area of very high tuberculosis prevalence, such as a developing nation in Africa or Asia, positive sputum smears have a very high prior probability of representing disease attributable to *M. tuberculosis* (45). However, in western Europe, Canada, Japan, or the United States, where mycobacterial disease attributable to *M. avium* complex, *M. kansasii,* or *M. fortuitum-chelonae* constitutes an increasing portion of the total mycobacterial morbidity, a positive sputum smear alone generally is not adequate grounds for the diagnosis of tuberculosis. A recent report from San Francisco indicated that a sputum microscopy result had a positive predictive value of more than 90% for pulmonary tuberculosis (46). However, in other communities, in which *M. avium* is relatively more prevalent, the test would not perform so well. Nonetheless, among patients whose epidemiological profile puts them at significant risk of tuberculosis, a positive sputum smear for mycobacteria must be presumed tuberculosis until cultures or other techniques prove contrary.

Cultivation and Susceptibility Testing

Cultivation in vitro of the etiological agent has been essential for species identification, drug susceptibility testing, and monitoring response to therapy. The slow growth rate of *M. tuberculosis* (and most other mycobacterial pathogens) has been a puzzling and frustrating phenomenon for clinicians, technologists, and public health authorities. In Koch's original report in 1882, he noted that microcolonies appear on the medium gradually during the third week of incubation; *110 years later,* remarkably, most of the laboratories around the United States and the world still employ cultivation techniques that require 3 to 6 weeks to achieve growth. In substantial measure, this reflects the slow generation time inherent in the tubercle bacillus; but, sadly, it also reflects premature abandonment of tuberculosis research programs.

Material prepared from sputum or other diagnostic specimens ideally should be inoculated on/into a variety of media to maximize the probability of recovery of *M. tuberculosis* or other potentially pathogenic mycobacteria. Because of other microbes in the specimen or peculiar growth requirements of diverse strains of *M. tuberculosis* or other mycobacteria, each of the cultivation media may be expected to yield certain advantages in isolating mycobacteria.

Rapid Culture Techniques

The rapid radiometric system employing 7H-12 liquid medium offers considerable advantage in time-to-growth identification over conventional solid media (Table 2.1) (46). (Incidentally, the radiometric system was largely devel-

TABLE 2.1. *Characteristics of various culture media for tuberculosis*

Medium	Time to positivity (*Mycobacterium tuberculosis*)	Comments
7H-12 BACTEC liquid	5–10 days, m = 8.7	Rapid; advantages for recovery of nontuberculosis mycobacteria and fragile strains of drug-resistant *M. tuberculosis.* Requires CO_2 incubator.
7H-11 Agar	18–28 days, m = 21	Faster than 7H-10; more supportive for growth of INH-resistant strains of *M.* tuberculosis. Requires CO_2 incubator.
7H-11 Selective agar	21–28 days	Inhibits overgrowth by other bacteria that survive decontamination. Requires CO_2 incubator.
Löwenstein-Jensen inspissated egg	21–42 days, m = ?	Favorable for strains multiresistant or partially inhibited (by treatment). Grows slowly, but does not require CO_2 incubator.

INH, isoniazid.

7H-12 BACTEC®, Becton-Dickinson, Baltimore, MD.

oped through the efforts of Gardner Middlebrook, himself a victim of tuberculosis early in his medical career.) For facilitation of treatment, it—or other rapid systems—should be used more widely today (37,47,48). The basic principles of the radiometric system are displayed in Fig. 2.4. In most sputum specimens that are positive for *M. tuberculosis,* the radiometric system gives evidence of the presence of mycobacteria within 4 to 8 days, depending on inoculum size and vitality. Once there is evidence of logarithmic-phase growth, prompt steps may be taken to (a) identify the species and (b) assess drug susceptibility.

Species identification may be performed by two methods. The BACTEC system provides a vial containing a substance [para-nitro-alpha-acatylamine-hydroxypropiophenone (NAP*)], which selectively suppresses the growth of *M. tuberculosis* complex species; if a subculture from the initial vial fails to demonstrate growth in the NAP, that is presumptive evidence for a species within *M. tuberculosis* complex. Performed serially, this process requires about 14 to 18 days to cultivate and establish species for smear-positive specimens under usual laboratory conditions. The second method to identify species is somewhat faster and has gained preference in most centers. When there is evidence of rapid growth in the first vial, a sample is taken and tested with a variety of commercial genetic probes which, by nucleic acid amplification techniques, may identify species or groups (49). These tests take less than one day, thereby reducing the time for isolation and speciation for smear-positive specimens to the range of 7 to 12 days. While none of these methods can distinguish *M. tuberculosis* from the other species of the complex, *M. bovis, M. africanum,* and *M. microti* are not associated with significant morbidity in North America; thus, a positive finding is tantamount to species identification of *M. tuberculosis.* Others, in this setting, have used high-performance liquid chromatography to identify species based on their constituent mycolic acids (50).

The radiometric system facilitates rapid drug susceptibility testing. The method entails comparing the inhibitory effects of different concentrations of antimicrobials with control vials; depending on the inoculum size, clear data regarding susceptibility may be obtained in 4 to 8 days. Thus, on average, initial isolation, species determination, and in vitro susceptibility may be obtained with the rapid radiometric system in 14 to 21 days (37).

A high degree of concordance has been documented between susceptibility data from the BACTEC system and those obtained by the conventional solid-media methods (37). In fact, the rapid radiometric system offers a substantially more quantitative approach to the determination of susceptibility than other methods (37). By testing with serial concentrations of the drugs, it is possible to determine a minimum inhibitory concentration (MIC) or minimum bactericidal concentration (MBC) against the specific strain in question. These values are of particular importance in the management of patients with multidrug-resistant tuberculosis, since many of the medications employed in such cases have not had well-established, effective critical concentrations determined on solid media (see Chapter 10).

One of the major advantages of the rapid radiometric system also is the unique ability to characterize in vitro susceptibility resistance for the drug pyrazinamide (PZA). PZA has become one of the major agents in modern, short-course regimens. However, the drug is not active at the "normal" pH range (7.0–7.4), at which other agents are tested in vitro; PZA is active only in the pH range of 5.0 to 6.0. Most strains of *M. tuberculosis* will not grow in vitro at these pH values. Heifets and Lindholm-Levy (51) have developed a method which relies on their observation that most strains of *M. tuberculosis* inoculated into the BACTEC system will not initiate growth at pH 5.5, but if a strain is allowed to commence replication at pH 7.0 until logarithmic growth is achieved, the pH then can be lowered to 5.5 or 6.0 without impeding continued generation. Hence, this methodology entails observing a culture until the system indicates robust growth; then, phosphoric acid is added to lower the pH to 6.0 in two vials. In one of the vials PZA is added, and the continued growth in the two vials is compared to determine the inhibitory effect of PZA.

The Principles of Rapid Radiometric Culture (Bactec®)

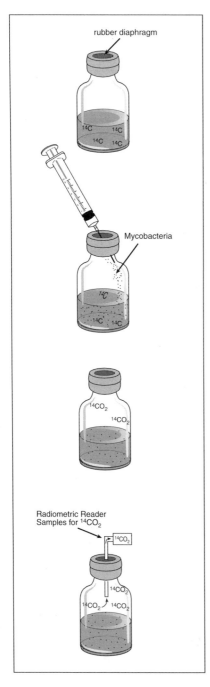

① 7H-12 liquid medium in a sealed vial with a rubber diaphragm across the top; the medium contains several broad spectrum antimicrobials that supress the growth of contaminants.

② The only source of carbohydrates in the liquid medium is palmitate that has been prepared with carbon ^{14}C tagging.

③ The processed specimen is injected into the vial across the diaphram.

④ Mycobacteria, if present and viable in the specimen, become metabolically active, consuming the tagged palmitate.

⑤ As the mycobacteria consume the palmitate, they elaborate carbon dioxide (CO_2) that is labelled with ^{14}C, $^{14}CO_2$.

⑥ This tagged ^{14}C appears in the gas mixture within the vial.

⑦ Periodically the automated needle probe punctures the diaphgram and samples the gas within the vial. As more mycobacteria proliferate, the concentration of ^{14}C rises. This is read as a "growth-index" (see sample reading of typical culture).

Because of regulatory issues surrounding the disposal of the radioactive materials involved with original methodology, the manufacturer has recently developed an alternative model that uses a novel fluorescent marker. In addition to avoiding radionuclide waste, the fluorescence can be read without elaborate instrumentation. This facilitates use of this system both in high-volume and smaller laboratories. The system, Mycobacterial Growth Indicator Tube (MGIT; Becton-Dickinson, Baltimore, MD), performed quite well in a comparative study versus the BACTEC radiometric system and conventional Lowenstein-Jensen (LJ) medium (52). In this study, which mostly involved patients with extensive pulmonary tuberculosis, the average times to recovery of tubercle bacilli from smear-positive sputum for the MGIT system, BACTEC radiometric method, and LJ medium were 9, 7, and 24 days, respectively. The MGIT system also performed well in a study from the Philippines; compared to LJ cultures, the MGIT detected *M. tuberculosis* in a much shorter time, 15.7 versus 29.9 days (53).

For a discussion of drug susceptibility testing performed by means of PCR or other nucleic acid amplification techniques, *not* by cultivation methods, see "Genomic Analysis for Drug Susceptibility Testing."

Conventional Culture Media

Although the radiometric systems or other rapid methods may offer advantages, optimal use of standard culture media may yield prompt growth and accurate species and susceptibility determination. At our institution, we have found that use of Middlebrook 7H-11 agar allows us to obtain susceptibility results in 18 to 21 days in most cases of smear-positive disease. In this method, when a new specimen is smear positive, some of the resuspended pellet is inoculated directly onto medium containing the drugs to be tested *simultaneously* with the initial plating (Fig. 2.5). The 7H-11 medium supports growth of most strains of tuberculosis very well, and in 85% of specimens there is sufficient growth for reading of susceptibility results in 18 to 21 days. This system employs the "proportionality" method in which the number of colony-forming units (CFU) on the drug quadrants are compared with the number on the control quadrant. Although there obviously are some significant operator-dependent variables in such a system, this technology—in well-supervised laboratories—yields consistent, highly useful data.

Molecular Biological Techniques

Recent molecular techniques have been employed in tuberculosis in several areas. These methods and their current and future applications in the diagnosis, drug susceptibility testing, and epidemiology of tuberculosis are reviewed in this section. To clarify the appropriate uses and limitations of these diagnostic methods, the Centers for Disease Control and Prevention (54) and American Thoracic Society (49) have both issued statements regarding their use.

Nucleic Acid Amplification for Diagnosis

The United States Food and Drug Administration has recently approved two new tests for the diagnosis of tuberculosis. Other commercial and institutional techniques that are similar have been developed, but because of their lack of availability, they are not discussed in detail in this chapter.

FIG. 2.4. The principles of rapid radiometric culture (BACTEC). 1, 7H-12 liquid medium in a sealed vial with a rubber diaphragm across top; the medium contains several broad spectrum antimicrobials that suppress the growth of contaminants. 2, The only source of carbohydrates in the liquid medium is palmitate that has been prepared with carbon ^{14}C tagging. 3, The processed specimen is injected into the vial across the diaphragm. 4, Mycobacteria, if present and viable in the specimen, become metabolically active, consuming the tagged palmitate. 5, As the mycobacteria consume the palmitate, they elaborate carbon dioxide (CO_2) that is labelled with ^{14}C, $^{14}CO_2$. 6, This tagged ^{14}C appears in the gas mixture within the vial. 7, Periodically, the automated needle probe punctures the diaphragm and samples the gas within the vial. As more mycobacteria proliferate, the concentration of ^{14}C rises. This is read as a "growth-index" (see sample reading of typical culture).

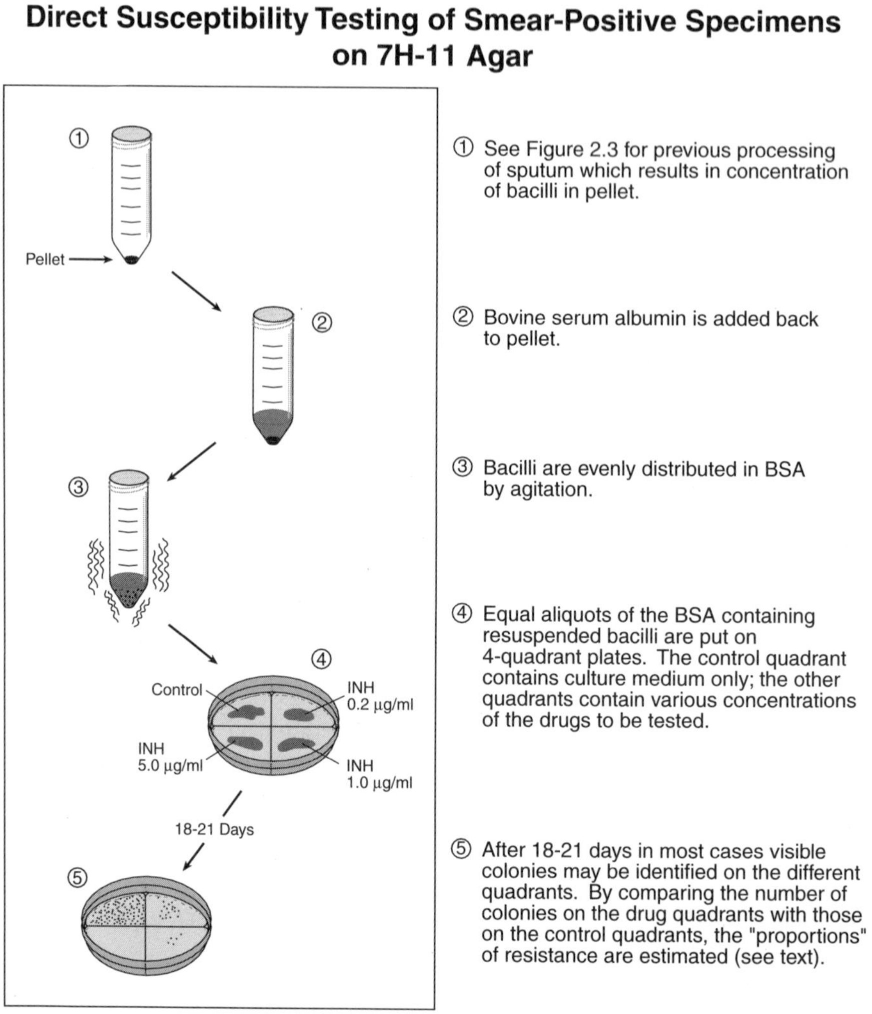
Direct Susceptibility Testing of Smear-Positive Specimens on 7H-11 Agar
①
Pellet
②
③
④
Control
INH 0.2 µg/ml
INH 5.0 µg/ml
INH 1.0 µg/ml
18-21 Days
⑤
① See Figure 2.3 for previous processing of sputum which results in concentration of bacilli in pellet.
② Bovine serum albumin is added back to pellet.
③ Bacilli are evenly distributed in BSA by agitation.
④ Equal aliquots of the BSA containing resuspended bacilli are put on 4-quadrant plates. The control quadrant contains culture medium only; the other quadrants contain various concentrations of the drugs to be tested.
⑤ After 18-21 days in most cases visible colonies may be identified on the different quadrants. By comparing the number of colonies on the drug quadrants with those on the control quadrants, the "proportions" of resistance are estimated (see text).

FIG. 2.5. Direct susceptibility testing of smear-positive specimens on 7H-11 agar. 1, See Figure 2.3 for previous processing of sputum which results in concentration of bacilli pellet. 2, Bovine serum albumin is added back to pellet. 3, Bacilli are evenly distributed in BSA by agitation. 4, Equal aliquots of the BSA containing resuspended bacilli are put on 4-quadrant plates. The control quadrant contains culture medium only; the other quadrants contain various concentrations of the drugs to be tested. 5, After 18-21 days in most cases, visible colonies may be identified on the different quadrants. By comparing the number of colonies on the drug quadrants with those on the control quadrants, the "proportions" of resistance are estimated (see text).

Ribotyping

The methodology of ribotyping (amplified *Mycobacterium tuberculosis* direct test [MTD], Gen-Probe [Gen-Probe Inc., San Diego, CA]) employs probes that recognize fragments of ribosomal RNA that are typically present in multiple copies and are characteristic for *M. tuberculosis* complex; they are amplified by transcription-mediation. Commercially available kits for this purpose are used to establish the species (or complex) of cultured material. The original methodology was entitled Accuprobe; it has been succeeded by a more rapid system, MTD (49). To date, the MTD system has been approved only for use in sputum specimens that are smear positive on microscopic examination. While it is clearly helpful for a clinician to know whether the organisms in the sputum belong to the tuberculosis complex, this approach may be inappropriately restrictive. If the test *were* capable of detecting tubercle bacilli in specimens that are smear negative—as it appears to be—judicious use in selected, high-risk cases may be of considerable clinical utility. For limited comparisons of the performance of the MTD, the AMPLICOR (Roche) method, and other nucleic acid amplification techniques, see Tables 2.2 and 2.3).

Polymerase Chain Reaction

Polymerase chain reaction entails amplification of characteristic fragments of bacillary DNA that is found in diagnostic specimens (49). The test that is currently approved for use in the United States is the AMPLICOR system. (Roche Diagnostic Systems, Inc., Branchberg, NJ). It is to be used for sputum specimens that are smear positive or to identify species that are growing in culture medium. For a thoughtful perspective on this technique, as well as the ribotyping method noted above, see the comments of Charache (55) in a 1996 editorial.

The advantages and shortcomings of molecular diagnostic techniques were highlighted in a recent study that compared two major commercial techniques—the MDT and the Amplicor—and an in-house, noncommercial test, IS6110 PCR (56). The authors described 98 specimens as being "clinically positive" for tuberculosis, an amalgam of 91 culture-positive and 7 culture-negative specimens from patients deemed to have active tuberculosis. Of these specimens, only 49 (50%) were smear positive by the fluorochrome technique. Overall, culture was positive in 93%, MTD in 84%, AMPLICOR in 80%, and IS-6110 in 83%. From smear-negative specimens, the sensitivity diminished with the positivity for MTD being 64%; AMPLICOR, 57%; and IS-6110, 68%. These techniques also were useful in distinguishing *M. tuberculosis* from nontuberculous mycobacteria; in 31 smear-positive NTM cases, MTD yielded three false-positive results; AMPLICOR, two false-positive results; and IS-6110, only one false-positive result. The performance of these tests in this series of *specimens* is represented in Table 2.3. Categorized by performance for the 27 *patients* in this series with culture-proven pulmonary tuberculosis, 17 of 23 (63%) had one or more positive smears, 27 of 27 (100%) had one or more culture-positive results; 23 of 27 (85%) had one or more MTD-positive

TABLE 2.2. *Performance of Gen-Probe Mycobacterium tuberculosis Direct Test and Roche AMPLICOR Mycobacterium tuberculosis test direct in acid-fast bacillus smear-positive versus smear-negative patients (data reviewed by FDA)*

	Overall (%)	Smear-positive (%)	Smear-negative (%)
Sensitivity	77/80[a]	95/96[a]	48/53[a]
Specificity	96/99[a]	100[b]	96/99[a]
PPV	57/85[a]	100[b]	24/58[a]
NPV	99[b]	86/90[a]	99[b]

[a] For some results, the Gen-Probe assay had the higher value; for others, the Roche assay was higher. Table 2.2 does not identify which values are associated with either assay. The wide differences shown for positive predictive value in the overall and smear-negative columns cannot be used to infer that one of the tests was superior, both because the two tests were studied on different samples and because the confidence intervals for the results would overlap. If one manufacturer sought to claim superior performance for its test, that claim would have to be based on results from a controlled, head-to-head clinical trial.

[b] Single values indicate that the two assays had the same value.

FDA, U.S. Food and Drug Administration; PPV, positive predictive value; NPV, negative predictive value.

From ref. 49, with permission.

Pooled data analyzed at the ATS workshop indicated that the two methods considered, Gen-Probe *Mycobacterium tuberculosis* direct test (MTD) and Roche AMPLICOR, performed reasonably well in sputum smear-positive cases. As noted, the data did not allow direct comparisons of the two systems. Of potentially important clinical utility, the combination of negative sputum smears and a negative result on direct amplification test (DAT) offered a strong negative predictive value for tuberculosis (see Table 2.4 for the schema by which workshop attendees recommended use of these new diagnostic methods; by contrast, see schema in Table 2.5).

TABLE 2.3. *Results of smear and nucleic acid amplification techniques (using culture as the standard) for 388 respiratory specimens from patients who were not treated or who received antimycobacterial therapy for less than 7 days*

Direct smear	Culture report	NAAT: No. of specimens positive by AMPLICOR (%)	NAAT: No. of specimens positive by MDT (%)	NAAT: No. of specimens positive by IS6110-PCR (%)
Positive (n = 65)	No. of specimens positive for MTB (n = 28)	25 (89)	26 (93)	25 (89)
	No. of specimens positive for nontuberculous mycobacteria (n = 32)	3 (9)	4 (12)	2 (6)
	No. of negative specimens (n = 5)	0 (0)	0 (0)	0 (0)
Negative (n = 323)	No. of specimens positive for MTB (n = 28)	16 (57)	18 (64)	19 (68)
	No. of specimens positive for nontuberculous mycobacteria (n = 84)	4 (5)	1 (1)	1 (1)
	No. of negative specimens (n = 211)	8 (4)	3 (1)	0 (0)
Total no. of specimens (n = 388)	No. of specimens positive for MTB (n = 56)	41 (73)	44 (79)	44 (79)
	No. of specimens positive for nontuberculous mycobacteria (n = 116)	7 (6)	5 (4)	3 (3)
	No. of negative specimens (n = 216)	8 (4)	3 (1)	0 (0)

	Smear	AMPLICOR	MDT	IS6110-PCR
Sensitivity[a] (%)	50	73	79	79
Specificity[a] (%)	89	96	98	99
Positive predictive value[a] (%)	43	73	85	94
Negative predictive value[a] (%)	91	96	96	97

[a] Parameters were calculated on culture as the gold standard.

NAAT, nucleic acid amplification techniques; MDT, Gen-Probe amplified MTB direct test; PCR, polymerase chain reaction; AMPLICOR, Roche AMPLICOR PCR; MTB, *Mycobacterium tuberculosis*.

From ref. 56, with permission.

A mixture of patients from a private hospital and a public facility were studied prospectively to determine the comparative utility of three molecular diagnostic tests in comparison with fluorochrome-technique smears and BACTEC plus conventional culture media. Table 2.3 refers only to patients with culture-proven tuberculosis. Overall, the three tests performed reasonably well. However, for patients with smear-negative/culture-positive tuberculosis, the AMPLICOR test had a substantial number of false-positive results, which resulted in a positive predictive value in this group of only 57% (56). Thus, these tests have been approved to date only for patients with smear-positive disease (see Tables 2.4 and 2.5 for recommended usage of the Gen-Probe *Mycobacterium tuberculosis* direct test (MTD) and Roche AMPLICOR tests).

results; 21 of 27 (78%) had one or more AMPLICOR-positive results; and 23 of 27 (85%) had one or more IS-6110-positive results. These findings are comparable to data from other series in which the sensitivity of MTD (84% in this study) ranged from 65% to 98% (57–61). The sensitivity of AMPLICOR (80% in this study) ranged in other studies from 58% to 100% (62–64).

The ATS Workshop (San Diego, CA, 1996) offered recommendations regarding actions to be taken on the basis of the direct amplification tests (DATs) (Table 2.4) (49). However, Barnes

TABLE 2.4. *Potential action while waiting for culture result (ATS Workshop)*

		High clinical suspicion of tuberculosis				Low clinical suspicion of tuberculosis			
		Positive AFB smear		Negative AFB smear		Positive AFB smear		Negative AFB smear	
Potential action	DAT results	Action without DAT results	Action with DAT results	Action without DAT results	Action with DAT results	Action without DAT results	Action with DAT results	Action without DAT results	Action with DAT results
Treat	+	Yes	Yes	Yes	Yes	Yes	Yes	No	**?**
Isolate	+	Yes	Yes	Yes	Yes	Yes	Yes	No	**?**
Begin contact investigation	+	Yes	Yes	**No**	**Yes**	Yes	Yes	No	No
Treat	−	**Yes**	**?**	**Yes**	**?**	**Yes**	**No**	No	No
Isolate	−	**Yes**	**?**	**Yes**	**No**	**Yes**	**No**	No	No
Begin contact investigation	−	**Yes**	**No**	No	No	**Yes**	**No**	No	No

AFB, acid-fast bacilli; DAT, direct amplification test; +, positive; −, negative; ?, divided opinion among attendees; bold typeface, different actions with and without knowledge of DAT results.

From ref. 49, with permission.

Based on results of the clinical probability of tuberculosis, routine sputum smear results, and the direct amplification tests (DATs), attendees at the ATS workshop recommended clinical responses shown. As noted, for patients deemed of "high clinical suspicion," a positive DAT result did not alter the recommendation to treat presumptively for tuberculosis. But, a negative DAT result raised questions in this regard. My choice in this case would be to initiate therapy with an empirical regimen that would provide reasonable coverage against both tuberculosis and a nontuberculous mycobacterial infection such as *M. avium* complex (e.g., rifampin, ethambutol, ciprofloxacin, and amikacin). Obviously, these DATs cannot supplant the need to obtain cultures; only by cultures can species be fully identified, mixed infections be detected, and full drug susceptibility testing be performed.

TABLE 2.5. *Effect on clinical decisions of rapid diagnostic test results for tuberculosis*

Acid-fast smear	+	+	+	+	−	−	−	−
Clinical suspicion of tuberculosis	Int	Int	Low	Low	High	High	Int	Int
Rapid diagnostic test result	+	−	+	−	+	−	+	−
Antituberculosis therapy[a]	Yes	?	Yes	No	Yes	Yes	Yes	?
Further diagnostic tests[a]	No	Yes	No	Yes	No	Yes	No	Yes

[a] General guidelines only. Specific clinical circumstances must be considered to optimize decisions regarding antituberculosis therapy and further diagnostic evaluation.

Int, intermediate; +, positive; −, negative.

From ref. 65, with permission.

Barnes (65) recommended employing the amplified *Mycobacterium tuberculosis* direct test (MTD) (Gen-Probe) or the AMPLICOR polymerase chain reaction (PCR) test (Roche Diagnostics) in this manner. Obviously, considerable clinical judgement is employed, including risk classification of patients, chest radiographic findings, and the need or suitability of empirical therapy. Of note, he does not advocate use of the direct amplification tests (DATs) in patients who are at high risk for tuberculosis and who have positive sputum smears; they should all receive empirical therapy.

(65), in an editorial accompanying the workshop report, offered a set of modified recommendations which I believe are of greater clinical utility (Table 2.5). Another approach, which has the advantage of taking into account inhibiting substances, is represented in Fig. 2.6 (66).

Ribotyping and Polymerase Chain Reaction for Specimens Other Than Sputum

Numerous articles have reported on the utility of various PCR methods on miscellaneous materials other than sputum, including bronchial lavage or aspirate, pleural effusions, cere-

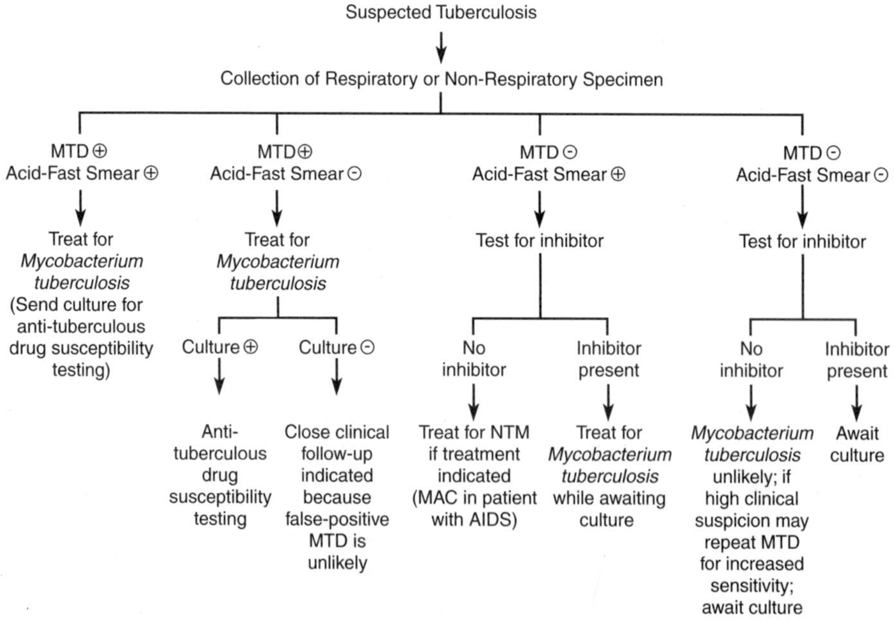

FIG. 2.6. A clinical algorithm applying acid-fast staining, MTD testing, and culture for the immunocompromised patient with suspected mycobacterial disease. The algorithm applies to respiratory tract and nonrespiratory specimens.

brospinal fluid, urine, gastric aspirates, lymph nodes, bone marrow, and blood.

In general, these studies largely employed PCR methods, although two reports involved the MTD techniques (61,67). Overall, they indicated significant promise for such methods, although there was considerable variability in results (68–75). In most series, the nucleic acid amplification techniques were more sensitive than microscopy. False-positive results, as defined by comparison with culture, were reported to occur, although it is possible that the technique truly was more sensitive than cultivation. Substances that interfered with PCR techniques were noted often, and these methods were typically time-consuming, laborious, and technically challenging. None of the techniques have been approved for use on specimens other than respiratory secretions in the United States, but we may anticipate that refined methods will be available for the diagnosis of extrapulmonary tuberculosis in the near future. Of rare, but possibly very helpful consequence, PCR has been shown to be effective in tissues already fixed in formalin and embedded in paraffin (76).

One particularly interesting use of such methodologies would be a "blood test" for tuberculosis. Theoretically, circulating polymorphonuclear leukocytes or monocytes that have traversed a site of active tuberculosis might carry with them enough mycobacterial RNA or DNA to give a positive signal on analysis of the buffy-coat of peripheral blood. In a brief report from New York City, PCR tests of a leukocyte concentrate of peripheral blood was positive in eight of eight patients with pulmonary tuberculosis (77); six of the eight patients had human immunodeficiency virus infection. However, a group from the Netherlands reported positive PCR results in only 1 of 11 persons with pulmonary or extrapulmonary tuberculosis, none of whom were HIV positive (78), and a group from Spain found blood to be PCR positive in only 8 of 19 patients (42%), a mixed population with 6 HIV-positive patients (79).

Genomic Analysis for Drug Susceptibility Testing

Recently, the genetic loci of resistance mutations for isoniazid, rifampin (RIF), PZA, ethambutol, streptomycin, and the fluoroquinolones have been identified (see Chapter 11 for details). Based on this type of methodology, developing molecular biology techniques to rapidly identify the susceptibility profile of a clinical strain appears feasible. Various methods have been employed to achieve this end, including PCR, RNA/RNA mismatch, direct gene sequencing, heteroduplex, and RFLP (80–84).

At present, the most attractive target for such testing is RIF. Two features make RIF an attractive agent for which to test: (a) a great preponderance of rifampin resistance mutations occurs within the RNA-polymerase β-subunit locus, *rpoB,* and (b) RIF resistance is a critical marker for multidrug-resistant tuberculosis, a situation which fundamentally alters the initial approach to therapy. The recent reports cited above have indicated the effectiveness of this approach in research laboratories (80–83). While not yet ready for widespread or commercial deployment, we may hope that within 5 years systems will be available to probe a clinical specimen and indicate "tuberculosis, yes or no?" and "RIF, susceptible or resistant?" Also of potential interest is a rapid method to detect resistance to isoniazid (INH) (84).

Restriction Fragment Length Polymorphism

Restriction fragment length polymorphism is a laboratory technique that can be employed for various purposes. As noted above, there is some interest in usage for rapid drug susceptibility testing. However, its most prominent role to date is as a method to "fingerprint" strains of *M. tuberculosis* to track patterns of transmission. In addition, RFLP has proven helpful in identifying false-positive cultures attributable to intralaboratory specimen contamination.

Molecular Epidemiology

Previous methods for distinguishing between strains of *M. tuberculosis* have relied primarily upon viral mycobacteriophage typing (85). However, this method was limited in its sensitivity and was technically difficult to perform. In 1986, two groups reported on the utility of RFLP in differentiating strains of *M. tuberculosis* (86,87). Basically, these techniques entail using restriction endonucleases to cleave the bacterial chromosomal DNA into fragments of varying lengths. These endonucleases cut only certain points in the DNA, and these points appear to vary widely among strains according to the locations of labile insertion elements. Because of great variability of the sites of these insertion elements among strains of *M. tuberculosis,* this technology has proven a sensitive and potentially very useful tool for "molecular epidemiology." One particular insertion sequence has proven most useful in this process, IS 6110. The great majority of strains of *M. tuberculosis* tested thus far have multiple copies of the genetic sequence, and there is great heterogeneity of the locations of IS 6110 in the mycobacterial DNA sequence. Hence, endonuclease cleavage at sites of this insertion sequence results in disparate and distinctive DNA fragment lengths among various strains of *M. tuberculosis,* or "restriction fragment length polymorphism." The discriminating power of this technique is greatest when there are many copies of IS 6110. If there are three or fewer, probing for an additional insertion sequence may help distinguish truly related strains; the TBN12 insertion sequence was shown to complement IS 6110 in two reports (88,89).

Examples of the utility of RFLP epidemiology include an analysis of new cases of tuberculosis occurring in San Francisco in 1990–1992 (90), a similar survey of cases in the Bronx, New York (91), and several other series in which RFLP analyses were central to recognition of patterns of community or institutional transmission (92–97). Currently, this technique is experimental; it is technically demanding and very labor intensive. The above series have largely employed analysis of insertion sequence 6110 as the critical marker; we may anticipate that combined analysis of other strain markers and IS 6110 will refine and enhance the specificity of this methodology, albeit making the method more costly and complicated. Overall, RFLP analysis has immense potential as a tool to study transmission patterns and the natural histories of primary and reinfection tuberculosis.

Detection of Laboratory Errors

Modern laboratories typically process large numbers of specimens daily, creating increased potential for cross-contamination of specimens. A false diagnosis of tuberculosis has many potential adverse consequences, including emotional distress, needless exposure to medications, delay in "true" diagnosis, and considerable financial outlays. Several recent reports have documented false-positive culture reports in 3 to 4% of culture positive cases (88, 89, 98, 99). These false-positive results were identified by RFLP testing of culture strains that were temporally grouped in the laboratory. These results reaffirm the importance of scrupulous laboratory techniques and remind clinicians to retain a reasonable skepticism for test results, even for a gold standard such as culture.

Luciferase Reporter Phages and Rapid Drug Susceptibility Testing

Jacobs et al. (100) have pursued a novel means of performing in vitro drug susceptibility tests, employing firefly luciferase. The system is based on the property of firefly luciferase to cause light emission when mixed with substrate luciferin and adenosine triphosphate (ATP). The group used viral phages to insert luciferase within the mycobacteria. Luciferin, when added to culture medium, was spontaneously taken up and internalized by the mycobacteria. Thus, all that was needed to produce light was mycobacterial ATP, a substance normally in abundance in a viable, metabolically active bacillus. Having set such a process in motion in vitro, antituberculosis agents were then added to the system. If the strain of mycobacteria were susceptible to the drug, the light emission was rapidly (within hours) extinguished. However, if the bacilli were resistant to the drug, light persisted. Using sensitive light-detecting systems, this phenomenon could be measured in terms of temporal evolution of drug effect and in a semiquantitative manner.

The clinical utility of such a system is not yet clear. Because it requires a substantial growth of the mycobacterial population (currently about 10^6 bacilli), the luciferase system would theoretically not be as rapid as nucleic acid amplification analysis directed against the bacilli in an initial sputum specimen. Yet, the potential of such methodology is intriguing, perhaps playing a role in industrial screening of large numbers of compounds for antimycobacterial activity (101).

Serological Methods for Diagnosis

A serological test for tuberculosis has been pursued throughout the twentieth century. Particular interest has been focused on patients with extrapulmonary forms of tuberculosis, since they generally do not have readily accessible diagnostic targets such as chest radiography or sputum. However, unlike many infectious diseases for which serodiagnosis has proven a highly valuable tool, tuberculosis has largely defied efforts at developing a methodology that is sensitive, specific, and practical for clinical use.

The major problem with the specificity issue lies with distinguishing between the *infected* versus the *diseased* state; also problematic is the serological reaction to prior BCG vaccination. This is particularly relevant in the developing nations where a simple test like serological examination would be of greatest utility: in such countries, approximately 40% of the population have latent tuberculosis infection, and substantial numbers have been vaccinated with *M. bovis* BCG, a member of the tuberculosis complex.

A lesser but still significant problem lies with distinguishing infection attributable to *M. tuberculosis* from the mycobacteria other than tuberculosis; this is more of a problem in the industrialized nations where the prevalences of tuberculosis disease and infection are relatively lower and the prevalence of mycobacteria, other than tuberculosis (MOTT) disease, is relatively higher.

Analysis of the many and varied studies of the serodiagnosis of tuberculosis indicates that there is a diversity of antigens potentially involved, that there is a wide array of immune responses associated with different forms of tuberculosis disease (cavitary pulmonary, noncavitary pulmonary, and extrapulmonary), and that Beyesian operator curves greatly influence the utility of tests among diversified populations. Specific seroantigens and techniques are reviewed below.

Antigen of 38 Kilodaltons

One promising system appears to be a 38-kd tuberculosis antigen that was found to be positive in 73% of extrapulmonary and 70% of smear-negative pulmonary cases with a chosen specificity of 98% (102). A second study employing this and other antigens was performed among patients with pulmonary tuberculosis (103). The 38-kd antigen performed well among patients with smear-positive pulmonary disease, with 80% sensitivity and 100% specificity. However, among the main target population for the serological test—the smear-negative cases—the 38-kd antigen alone yielded only 15% sensitivity. Combining the 38-kd with two other antigens raised the sensitivity to 64% with 95% specificity; however, the complexity and expense of this approach make it substantially less attractive and practical for widespread application.

Antigen 5

Multiple studies have examined the role of antigen 5 of *M. tuberculosis* in the serodiagnosis of tuberculosis. In general, these investigations have demonstrated marginal sensitivity of the technique. Daniel et al. (104) in 1985 calculated the receiver operating characteristics of the enzyme-linked immunosorbent assay (ELISA) they employed: for a population with a 15% prevalence of tuberculosis—a highly favorable scenario for the test—the sensitivity ranged between 45.8% and 63.4% with a specificity range of 98.3% to 91.5% depending on titer cut-off points of 1:80 or 1:40. In another study (105), antigen 5 ELISA serodiagnosis was found to be positive in only 42 of 61 Bolivian patients with active pulmonary tuberculosis, for a 69% sensitivity; it also was falsely positive in 14 of 113 patients who did not have tuberculosis, for a specificity of 88%. Subsequently, a decision analysis of the potential role for serodiagnosis in a setting like that in Bolivia was conducted (106). The study considered five possible diagnostic options: (a) direct sputum smear alone, (b) simultaneous sputum smear and chest x-ray, (c) sputum smear followed by chest x-ray *if* smear result is negative, (d) sputum smear followed by ELISA *if* smear is negative, and (5) ELISA alone. Options b and c had the highest probability of yielding the correct diagnosis—95% each—with ELISA alone being the lowest—81%. ELISA would not add to the diagnosis when sputum smear was available for diagnosis; however, it would roughly replace it at comparable costs if microscopy were not available. Nonetheless, another study (107) of serodiagnosis of tuberculosis with antigen 5 and hemagglutination assays of glycolipid antigens yielded very discouraging results. Among adult patients with smear-positive pulmonary disease, the various antigens were positive in 30% to 52%; among smear-negative cases, only 16% to 22% were positive. A more favorable study with antigen 5 was performed among children in Argentina (108). In this study, 21 patients aged 1 to 14 years with bacteriologically proven tuberculosis were compared with 19 control subjects, all of whom had received BCG vaccine. The authors calculated that in a population such as theirs, in which the prevalence of disease was 52.5% (21 of 40), the method had a sensitivity of 85.7%, a specificity of 100%, an accuracy of 92.5%, a positive predictive value of 100%, and a negative predictive value of 86.4%.

The authors also chose to examine carefully the power of antigen 5 *negative* results to *exclude* the presence of tuberculosis; they calculated a relationship between the prevalence of tuberculosis in a population and the accuracy of a negative prediction. As noted, a negative or low titer on this test would ostensibly have high utility in "ruling out" tuberculosis at prevalence rates seen even in developing countries.

Antigen A60

The main thermostable component of tuberculin [old tuberculin or purified protein derivative (PPD)] is referred to as antigen A60 (109). Notably, this antigen is found in *Nocardia* and *Corynebacterium* as well as *Mycobacterium* species. It has been employed, primarily in Europe, for the serodiagnosis of tuberculosis. Studies have been conducted examining ELISA assays for both immunoglobulin M (IgM) and immunoglobulin G (IgG) levels against A60. Among 83 hospitalized patients suspected of having pulmonary tuberculosis but with negative sputum smears, the sensitivity, specificity, and positive predictive value for IgM were 76%, 98%, and 95%, respectively, while for IgG the values were 48%, 71%, and 50%, respectively (110). Combining the IgM and IgG results yielded sensitivity of 68%, specificity of 100%, and positive predictive value of 100%. In this report, tuberculosis was confirmed by positive sputum cultures. The control subjects in this report were not well characterized; specifically missing were data regarding A60 levels in patients with other mycobacterial infections, a group of increasing size and significance in industrialized nations. The authors believed that IgM levels, which reflected more recent immunological experience, were more useful than IgG assays, which were more likely to represent remote infection.

Subsequently, a large-scale study in China of A60 among 560 patients with pulmonary and extrapulmonary tuberculosis and 734 "uninfected" control subjects was reported (111). Positive results for the following groups were recorded: (a) active primary tuberculosis: IgM, 80%; IgG, 36%; (b) active postprimary tuberculosis: IgM, 31%; IgG, 88.5%; (c) inactive tuberculosis: IgM, 0%; IgG, 41%; (d) active extrapulmonary tuberculosis [variable according to sites]: IgM, 30% to 61%; IgG, 69% to 86%. Among 529 healthy persons, most of whom had allegedly been vaccinated and 287 of whom were tuberculin reactors, there was less than 1% false-positive results. Incidentally, among patients with tuberculous meningitis, higher concentrations of anti-A60 IgG were found in the cerebrospinal fluid than serum, suggesting the potential utility of this assay for the diagnosis of tuberculous meningitis. Noteworthy is that none of the tuberculosis patients in this series were known to be HIV infected. Another study of A60 from Taiwan indicated sensitivity and specificity to be 80.8% and 88.4% with negative and positive predictive values of 93% and 71%, respectively; A60 performed better than the 38-kd and Kp90 antigens that were testing simultaneously (112). Combining the antigens offered no advantage, and the authors concluded that 80% sensitivity and specificity was the best this antigen could perform, making it a poor confirmatory test.

Antigen of 88 Kilodaltons

Laal et al. (113) have recently identified a new group of antigens which they believe have potential for serological diagnosis. They reasoned that the search for diagnostic antigens had been hindered by cross-reactivity with conserved regions from ubiquitous prokaryotes, and attempted to reduce this confusing process by preadsorption with *Escherichia coli* lysates. Using this process, they found that the secreted proteins contained the antigens against which humoral responses were most commonly and predictably directed during infection with *M. tuberculosis*. In particular, they identified an 88-kd antigen that elicited a strong antibody response in a high proportion of patients with pulmonary tuberculosis. Of novel interest, in a separate report, they noted that level of antibodies to this 88-kd antigen in the serum collected serially from HIV-infected persons predicted the clinical appearance of tuberculosis (114). These antibodies were present in the serum of 74% of the HIV-infected patients from 1.5 to 6.0 years before the clinical manifestations of tuberculosis; curiously, however, the antibodies were present in only 66% of the patients at the time tuberculosis was diagnosed. This suggests that the capacity to produce antibodies may be impaired at the time of active tuberculosis, diminishing the utility of serodiagnosis. The authors implied that screening HIV-infected persons with this 88-kd serological test may be useful to identify high-risk candidates for INH-preventive chemotherapy; yet, they have no data to assess its performance in comparison with the current standard, the tuberculin skin test. However, in a generally similar study from Italy, serum antibodies to two antigens, namely, anti-PPD and anti-diacyltrehalose, were present one year before the diagnosis of tuberculosis in 11 of 16 (69%) HIV-infected persons when only 4 of 16 (25%) had reactive PPD skin tests (115).

Multiantigen Analysis

In 1993, a group from the Netherlands (116) reported the results of an elaborate serodiagnosis study; in the trial, 91 newly diagnosed tuberculosis patients were compared with 17 tuberculosis patients under treatment and 220 control subjects. Control subjects included persons from areas endemic for tuberculosis, patients with sarcoidosis and Crohn's disease, and 100 healthy Dutch patients. The authors employed six different purified tuberculosis antigens with molecular weights of 10,000; 16,000; 24,000; 30,000; 38,000; and 70,000 kd, for which ELISA testing was performed. Also, monoclonal antibody TB 72 was tested by competitive ELISA. While the specificity of positive results for the individual antigens was high, ranging from 95% to 98%, the sensitivity ranges were low (29%–51%). The optimal results combining the tests came with the 16,000-kd antigen and the TB 72 monoclonal assay, yielding 65% sensitivity and 96% specificity. The positive predictive value (PPV) of the serological tests was, as typical of any similar modality, ultimately related to the prevalence of the disease in the studied population. If used in a group of patients who had a 30% prevalence of tuberculosis, the PPVs for various antigens ranged from 81% to 91%, but if used to screen a low-prevalence group (e.g., 1% disease), the PPV was useless. Notably, in this study, there were no patients with mycobacterioses other than tuberculosis in the control group, and among persons with HIV infection and active tuberculosis, the serological titers were substantially reduced.

Lipoarabinomannan

A unique LAM antigen (an important constituent of mycobacterial cell walls, possibly related to virulence) was employed in two studies of tuberculosis patients in Mexico (117,118). In the initial report, IgG antibodies against LAM were measured in 66 patients with pulmonary, pleural, and lymphatic tuberculosis and compared with a control group consisting of healthy persons, persons with histoplasmosis, and patients with nonmycobacterial lung diseases. In the authors' analysis, the test had a sensitivity of 73% and a specificity of 92%; curiously, the lowest sensitivity was seen in patients with pleural tuberculosis (43%), possibly indicating recently acquired infection and lower titers.

In the follow-up study, efforts were directed toward detecting LAM in the serum of patients with active tuberculosis. Strictly speaking, this is not a serological test because it does not measure the patients' responses to antigens. Rather, it employs rabbit antisera to LAM and a co-agglutination technique. The method yielded sensitivities of 88% in patients with smear-positive tuberculosis, 67% in those with smear-negative/culture-positive tuberculosis, and only 57% in persons with acquired immunodeficiency syndrome (AIDS) and tuberculosis. Using persons with other unspecified pulmonary diseases and healthy controls for comparison, the LAM assay had a specificity of 100%.

The authors speculated that the LAM they measured in this assay was mostly circulating as an antigen-antibody complex [and that they measured the antibodies in their first report (117)]. Regarding the lower levels of LAM found in their AIDS/tuberculosis patients, they conjectured that LAM is released as tubercle bacilli are degraded by macrophages and that, because of impaired host defenses, there was less of this carbohydrate antigen released into circulation.

Cord Factor

Cord factor, trehalose-6,6'-dimycolate, is produced by tubercle bacilli, as well as a small number of other mycobacteria that are generally nonpathogenic (see above, "Cell Wall Structure and Biochemistry," for discussion). A Japanese group (119) recently reported on their experience employing an ELISA for IgG antibodies against cord factor (CF) among 65 patients with active tuberculosis, 58 with inactive tuberculosis, 36 patients with other diseases, and 66 healthy adults (119). Among the 65 cases of tuberculosis, 53 of which were new, active, and untreated and 12 of which were chronic cases in patients on treatment regimens for a year but still smear positive, the anti-CF titers were significantly higher than the other groups. However, the sensitivity of the test among the 53 new cases was only 81%, with 43 of 53 reacting; the specificity of the test was 96%, with 4 of 102 control subjects reacting.

Notable aspects of this report included the following: (a) the anti-CF titers were higher among patients with more extensive disease; (b) there were no patients with extrapulmonary tuberculosis in this series, a group for whom serological diagnosis is of particular value; (c) there were no patients with known HIV infection in the study; and (d) titers of anti-CF fell during effective chemotherapy.

Antigen-Antibody Complex Assays

In addition to the classic serological tests noted above, other studies have focused on identification of circulating immune complexes as markers of active disease (120). While the method described indicated significant differences in immune-complex levels among patients with both smear-positive and smear-negative tuberculosis and control subjects, because of its technical complexity, this test is unlikely to be employed as a diagnostic system in high-prevalence, resource-poor countries. However, analysis of circulating immune complexes may offer significant insight into the pathogenesis and spectrum of various forms of tuberculosis (121).

Overview of Serological Testing

Although very attractive from a clinical perspective (a simple blood test to diagnose tuberculosis), serological testing with currently available technology offers neither sufficient sensitivity nor sufficient specificity to allow it to function as a primary, first-line screening test for the detection of active cases of tuberculosis. Most discouraging is the fact that most tests perform reasonably well for patients with sputum smear-positive pulmonary disease, but do significantly less well for smear-negative cases. Thus, they do little to enhance the diagnostic yield above the current, very economical standard diagnostic tool, microscopy. Furthermore, among HIV-infected persons, a group more likely to have smear-negative pulmonary disease, antibody production appears attenuated, making serological tests less sensitive. Conceivably, serological tests might be used not to prove but *to disprove* the presence of active tuberculosis. If one or more of the above tests were employed and interpreted in a manner that maximized their sensitivity, "clearly negative" results might effectively "rule out" tuberculosis in given patients. This could prove to be of considerable clinical and public health utility.

TUBERCULOSIS BIOLOGY: PAST, PRESENT, AND FUTURE

Two remarkable feats of virtuoso molecular biology must provoke us to consider the history and future horizons of the tubercle bacillus. First, the survey of strains from around the world by Musser and colleagues (4) in Texas suggested that *M. tuberculosis* has evolved into three large "groups." These are, to some extent, regionalized but—much as the "races" of *Homo sapiens*—the mycobacteria, transported by restless humans, are widely intermingled.

Second, an extraordinary multinational team (122) has just completed sequencing the entire genome of the H37Rv strain of *M. tuberculosis.* Composed of 4,411,529 base pairs, which form an estimated 4,000 genes, the inner workings of the microbe have been exposed to avid minds of current and future scientists and scholars. As noted by Young (123) in an editorial heralding this report, these data afford new opportunities to design antimicrobial agents, vaccines, and other elements to protectively modulate the immunopathogenesis of this devastating pathogen.

REFERENCES

1. Keers RY. *Pulmonary tuberculosis: a journey down the centuries.* London: Cassell Ltd., 1978.
2. Sauret J, Jolis R, Ausina V, Castro E, Cornudella R. Human tuberculosis due to *Mycobacterium bovis:* report of 10 cases. *Tuberc Lung Dis* 1992;73:388–391.
3. Shinnick TM, Good RC. Mycobacterial taxonomy. *Eur J Clin Microbiol Infect Dis* 1994;13:884–901.
4. Sreevatsan S, Pan X, Stockbauer KE, et al. Restricted structural gene polymorphism in the *Mycobacterium tuberculosis* complex indicates evolutionarily recent global dissemination. *Proc Natl Acad Sci U S A* 1997; 94:9869–9874.
5. Youmans GP. Tuberculosis. In: *The morphology and metabolism of mycobacteria.* Philadelphia: WB Saunders, 1979.
6. McNeil MR, Brennan PJ. Structure, function, and biogenesis of the cell envelope of mycobacteria in relation to bacterial physicology, pathogenesis and drug resistance: some thoughts and possibilities arising from recent structural information. *Res Microbiol* 1991;142: 451–463.
7. Sibley LD, Adams LB, Krahenbuhl JL. Inhibition of interferon-gamma–mediated activation in mouse macrophages treated with lipoarabinomannan. *Clin Exp Immunol* 1990;80:141–148.
8. Chan J, Fan X, Hunter SW, Brennan PJ, Bloom BR. Lipoarabinomannan: a possible virulence factor involved in persistence of *Mycobacterium tuberculosis* within macrophages. *Infect Immun* 1991;59:1755–1761.
9. Moreno C, Mehlert A, Lamb J. The inhibitory effects of mycobacterial lipoarabinomannan and polysaccharides upon polyclonal and monoclonal human T-cell proliferation. *Clin Exp Immunol* 1988;74:206–210.
10. Moreno C, Taverne J, Mehlert A, et al. Lipoarabinomannan from *Mycobacterium tuberculosis* induces the production of tumour necrosis factor from human and murine macrophages. *Clin Exp Immunol* 1989;76:240–245.
11. Barnes P, Fong S, Brennan P, Twomey P, Mazumder A, Modlin R. Local production of tumor necrosis factor and IFN-γ in tuberculous pleuritis. *J Immunol* 1990;145:149–154.
12. Chatterjee D, Lowell K, Rivoire B, McNeil M, Brennan P. Lipoarabinomannan of *Mycobacterium tuberculosis:* capping mannosyl residues in some strains. *J Biol Chem* 1992;267:6234–6239.
13. Bloch H. Studies on the virulence of tubercle bacilli: isolation and biological properties of a constituent of virulent organism. *J Exp Med* 1950;91:197–218.
14. Krasnow I, Wayne L, Salkin D. A microcolonial test for the recognition of virulent mycobacteria. *Am Rev Tuberc* 1955;71:361–370.
15. Bloch H, Sorkin E, Erlenmeyer H. A toxic lipid component of the tubercle bacillus ("cord factor"), II: isolation from petroleum ether extracts of young bacterial cultures. *Am Rev Tuberc* 1953;67:629–643.
16. Noll H, Bloch H. A toxic lipid component of the tubercle bacillus ("cord factor"), II: occurrence in chloroform extracts of young and older bacterial cultures. *Am Rev Tuberc* 1953;67:828–851.
17. Asselineau J, Bloch H, Lederer E. A toxic lipid component of the tubercle bacillus ("cord factor"), III: occurrence and distribution in various bacterial extracts. *Am Rev Tuberc* 1953;67:853–858.
18. Noll H, Bloch H, Asselineau J, Lederer E. The chemical structure of the cord factor of *Mycobacterium tuberculosis. Biochem Biophys Acta* 1956;20:299–317.
19. Kato M. Antibody formation to trehalose-6,6'-dimycolate (cord factor) of *Mycobacterium tuberculosis. Infect Immun* 1972;5:203–212.
20. Kato M. Effect of anti–cord factor antibody on experimental tuberculosis in mice. *Infect Immun* 1973;7:14–21.
21. Wayne LG. Dynamics of submerged growth of *M. tuberculosis* under aerobic and microaerophilic conditions. *Am Rev Respir Dis* 1976;114:807–811.

22. Much H. Die Nach Ziehl Nicht Darstellbaren Formen de Tuberkelbacillus. *Berl Klin Wochenschr* 1908; 45:691–694.
23. Mattman LH, Tunstall LH, Mathews WW, Gordon DL. L-variation in mycobacteria. *Am Rev Respir Dis* 1960;82:202–211.
24. Mattman LH. L-forms isolated from infections. In: Guze LB, ed. *Microbial protoplasts, spheroplasts and L-forms.* Baltimore: Williams & Wilkins, 1968:472.
25. Mattman LH. Cell wall deficient forms of mycobacteria. *Ann N Y Acad Sci* 1970;174:852–861.
26. Ratnam S, Chandrasekhar S. The pathogenicity of spheroplasts of *Mycobacterium tuberculosis. Am Rev Respir Dis* 1976;114:549–554.
27. Chandrasekhar S, Ratnam S. Studies on cell-wall deficient non-acid fast variants of *M. tuberculosis. Tuberc Lung Dis* 1992;73:273–279.
28. Crowle AJ, Sbarbaro JA, Judson FN, May MH. The effect of ethambutol on tubercle bacilli within cultured human macrophages. *Am Rev Respir Dis* 1985;132: 742–745.
29. Grange JM. The mystery of the mycobacterial "persistor." *Tuberc Lung Dis* 1992;73:249–251.
30. Khomenko AG. The variability of *Mycobacterium tuberculosis* in patients with cavitary pulmonary tuberculosis in the course of chemotherapy. *Tubercle* 1987; 68:243–253.
31. Segal W, Bloch H. Biochemical differentiation of *M. tuberculosis* grown *in vivo* and *in vitro. J Bacteriol* 1956;72:132–141.
32. Segal W. Comparative study of *in vivo* and *in vitro* grown *Mycobacterium tuberculosis,* IV: immunogenic differentiation. *Proc Soc Exp Biol Med* 1965;118:214–218.
33. Segal W, Bloch H. Pathogenic and immunogenic differentiation of *Mycobacterium tuberculosis* grown *in vitro* and *in vivo. Am Rev Tuberc* 1957;75:495–500.
34. Collins FM, Montalbine V. Distribution of mycobacteria grown *in vivo* in the organs of intravenously infected mice. *Am Rev Respir Dis* 1976;113:281–286.
35. Collins FM, Wayne LG, Montalbine V. The effect of cultural conditions on the distribution of *Mycobacterium tuberculosis* in the spleen and lungs of pathogen-free mice. *Am Rev Respir Dis* 1974;110: 147–156.
36. Segal W. Comparative study of mycobacterium grown *in vivo* and *in vitro,* V: differences in staining properties. *Am Rev Respir Dis* 1965;91:285–287.
37. Heifets LB. *Clinical mycobacteriology.* Philadelphia: WB Saunders, 1996.
38. Kiehn TE. The diagnostic mycobacteriology laboratory of the 1990s. *Clin Infect Dis* 1993;17:S447–S454.
39. Wolinsky E. Tuberculosis commentary. *Clin Infect Dis* 1994;19:396–401.
40. Salfinger M, Pfyffer GE. The new diagnostic mycobacteriology laboratory. *Eur J Clin Microbiol Infect Dis* 1994;13:961–979.
41. Kim TC, Blackman RS, Heatwole KM, Kim T, Rochester DF. Acid-fast bacilli in sputum smears of patients with pulmonary tuberculosis: prevalence and significance of negative smears pretreatment and positive smears post-treatment. *Am Rev Respir Dis* 1984; 129:264–268.
42. Hong Kong Chest Service/Tuberculosis Research Centre MBMRC. A controlled trial of 3-month, 4-month, and 6-month regimens of chemotherapy for sputum-smear negative pulmonary tuberculosis: results at 5 years. *Am Rev Respir Dis* 1989;139:871–876.
43. Hobby GL, Holman AP, Iseman MD, Jones J. Enumeration of tubercle bacilli in sputum of patients with pulmonary tuberculosis. *Antimicrob Agents Chemother* 1973;4:94–104.
44. Yeager HJ, Lacy J, Smith LR, LeMaistre C. Quantitative studies on mycobacterial populations in sputum and saliva. *Am Rev Respir Dis* 1967;95:998–1004.
45. Levy H, Feldman C, Sacho H, van der Meulen H, Kallenbach J, Koornhof H. A reevaluation of sputum microscopy and culture in the diagnosis of pulmonary tuberculosis. *Chest* 1989;95:1193–1197.
46. Siddiqi SH, Hwangbo CC, Silcox V, Good RC, Snider DE Jr, Middlebrook G. Rapid radiometric methods to detect and differentiate *Mycobacterium tuberculosis/M. bovis* from other mycobacterial species. *Am Rev Respir Dis* 1984;130:634–640.
47. Luquin M, Gamboa F, Barceló MG, et al. Comparison of a biphasic non-radiometric system with Löwenstein-Jensen and Bactec-460 system for recovery of mycobacteria from clinical specimens. *Tubercle Lung Dis* 1996;77:449–453.
48. Drowart A, Cambiaso CL, Huygen K, Serruys E, Yernault J-C, Van Vooren J-P. Detection of mycobacterial antigens present in short-term culture media using particle counting immunoassay. *Am Rev Respir Dis* 1993; 147:1401–1406.
49. American Thoracic Society. Rapid diagnostic tests for tuberculosis: what is the appropriate use? *Am J Respir Crit Care Med* 1997;155:1804–1814.
50. Butler WR, Kilburn JO. Identification of major slowly growing pathogenic mycobacteria and *Mycobacterium gordonae* by high-performance liquid chromatography of their mycolic acids. *J Clin Microbiol* 1988;26:50– 53.
51. Heifets L, Lindholm-Levy P. Pyrazinamide sterilizing activity in vitro against semidormant *Mycobacterium tuberculosis* bacterial populations. *Am Rev Respir Dis* 1992;145:1223–1225.
52. Casal M, Gutierrez J, Vaquero M. Comparative evaluation of the mycobacteria growth indicator tube with the BACTEC 460 TB system and Löwenstein-Jensen medium for isolation of mycobacteria from clinical specimens. *Int J Tuberc Lung Dis* 1997;1:81–84.
53. Rivera AB, Tupasi TE, Grimaldo ER, Cardano RC, Co VM. Rapid and improved recovery rate of *Mycobacterium tuberculosis* in mycobacteria growth indicator tube combined with solid Löwenstein Jensen medium. *Int J Tuberc Lung Dis* 1997;1:454–459.
54. Centers for Disease Control and Prevention. Nucleic acid amplification tests for tuberculosis. *MMWR* 1996;950–952.
55. Charache P. Editorial response: comparison of the amplified *Mycobacterium tuberculosis* (MTB) Direct Test, Amplicor MTB PCR, and IS6110-PCR for detection of MTB in respiratory specimens. *Clin Infect Dis* 1996;23:1107–1108.
56. Dalovisio JR, Montenegro-James S, Kemmerly SA, et al. Comparison of the amplified *Mycobacterium tuberculosis* (MTB) Direct Test, Amplicor MTB PCR, and IS6110-PCR for detection of MTB in respiratory specimens. *Clin Infect Dis* 1996;23:1099–1106.
57. Jonas V, Alden MJ, Curry JI, et al. Detection and identification of *Mycobacterium tuberculosis* directly from sputum sediments by amplification of rRNA. *J Clin Microbiol* 1993;31:2410–2416.

58. La Rocco MT, Wanger A, Ocera H, Macias E. Evaluation of a commercial rRNA amplification assay for direct detection of *Mycobacterium tuberculosis* in processed sputum. *Eur J Clin Microbiol Infect Dis* 1994;13:726–731.
59. Vlaspolder F, Singer P, Roggeveen C. Diagnostic value of an amplification method (Gen-Probe) compared with that of culture for diagnosis of tuberculosis. *J Clin Microbiol* 1995;33:2699–2703.
60. Bradley SP, Reed SL, Catanzaro A. Clinical efficacy of the amplified *Mycobacterium tuberculosis* direct test for the diagnosis of pulmonary tuberculosis. *Am J Respir Crit Care Med* 1996;153:1606–1610.
61. Gamboa F, Manterola JM, Lonca J, et al. Rapid detection of *Mycobacterium tuberculosis* in respiratory specimens, blood and other non-respiratory specimens by amplification of rRNA. *Int J Tuberc Lung Dis* 1997;1:542–555.
62. Chin DP, Yajko DM, Hadley WK. Clinical utility of a commercial test based on the polymerase chain reaction for detecting *Mycobacterium tuberculosis* in respiratory specimens. *Am J Respir Crit Care Med* 1995;151:1872–1877.
63. Ichiyama S, Iinuma Y, Tawada Y, et al. Evaluation of Gen-Probe amplified *Mycobacterium tuberculosis* direct test and Roche PCR-microwell plate hybridization method (AMPLICOR MYCOBACTERIUM) for direct detection of mycobacteria. *J Clin Microbiol* 1996;34:130–133.
64. Cohen RA, Muzaffar S, Schwartz D, et al. Diagnosis of pulmonary tuberculosis using PCR assays on sputum collected within 24 hours of hospital admission. *Am J Respir Crit Care Med* 1998;157:156–161.
65. Barnes PF. Rapid diagnostic tests for tuberculosis: progress but no gold standard. *Am J Respir Crit Care Med* 1997;155:1497–1498.
66. Gladwin MT, Plorde JJ, Martin TR. Clinical application of the *Mycobacterium tuberculosis* direct test: case report, literature review, and proposed clinical algorithm. *Chest* 1998;114:317–323.
67. Pfyffer GE, Kissling P, Jahn EMI, Welscher H-M, Salfinger M, Weber R. Diagnostic performance of amplified *Mycobacterium tuberculosis* direct test with cerebrospinal fluid, other nonrespiratory, and respiratory specimens. *J Clin Microbiol* 1996;34:834–841.
68. Shankar P, Manjunath N, Mohan K, et al. Rapid diagnosis of tuberculous meningitis by polymerase chain reaction. *Lancet* 1991;337:5–7.
69. deLassence A, Lecassier D, Pieere C, Cadrenel J, Sttern M, Hance AJ. Detection of mycobacterial DNA in pleural fluid from patients with tuberculous pleurisy by means of polymerase chain reaction: comparison of two protocols. *Thorax* 1992;47:265–269.
70. Querol JM, Mínguez J, García-Sánchez E, Farga MA, Gimeno C, García-de-Lomas J. Rapid diagnosis of pleural tuberculosis by polymerase chain reaction. *Am J Respir Crit Care Med* 1995;152:1977–1981.
71. Villena V. Polymerase chain reaction for the diagnosis of pleural tuberculosis in immunocompromised and immunocompetent patients. *Clin Infect Dis* 1998;26: 212–214.
72. Shah S, Miller A, Mastellone A, et al. Rapid diagnosis of tuberculosis in various biopsy and body fluid specimens by the AMPLICOR *Mycobacterium tuberculosis* polymerase chain reaction test. *Chest* 1998;113:1190–1194.
73. Folgueira L, Delgado R, Palenque E, Noriega AR. Detection of *Mycobacterium tuberculosis* DNA in clinical samples by using a simple lysis method and polymerase chain reaction. *J Clin Microbiol* 1993;31: 1019–1021.
74. Lombard EH, Victor T, Jordaan A, van Helden PD. The detection of *Mycobacterium tuberculosis* in bone marrow aspirate using the polymerase chain reaction. *Tuberc Lung Dis* 1994;75:65–69.
75. Pierre C, Olivier C, Lecossier D, Boussougant Y, Yeni P, Hance AJ. Diagnosis of primary tuberculosis in children by amplificatin and detection of mycobacterial DNA. *Am Rev Respir Dis* 1993;147:420–424.
76. Rish JA, Eisenach KD, Cave MD, Reddy MV, Gangadharam PRJ, Bates JH. Polymerase chain reaction detection of *Mycobacterium tuberculosis* in formalin-fixed tissue. *Am J Respir Crit Care Med* 1996;153: 1419–1423.
77. Schluger NW, Condos R, Lewis S, Rom WN. Amplification of DNA of *Mycobacterium tuberculosis* from peripheral blood of patients with pulmonary tuberculosis. *Lancet* 1994;344:232–233.
78. Kolk AHJ, Kox LFF, Kuijper S, Richter C. Detection of Mycobacterium tuberculosis in peripheral blood [letter]. *Lancet* 1994;344:694.
79. Aguado JM, Rebollo MJ, Palenque E, Folgueria L. Blood-based PCR assay to detect pulmonary tuberculosis. *Lancet* 1996;347:1836–1837.
80. Nash KA, Gaytan A, Inderlied CB. Detection of rifampin resistance in *Mycobacterium tuberculosis* by use of a rapid, simple, and specific RNA/RNA mismatch assay. *J Infect Dis* 1997;176:533–536.
81. Nachamkin I, Kang C, Weinstein MP. Detection of resistance to isoniazid, rifampin, and streptomycin in clinical isolates of *Mycobacterium tuberculosis* by molecular methods. *Clin Infect Dis* 1997;24:894–900.
82. Ohno H, Koga H, Kuroita T, et al. Rapid prediction of rifampin susceptibility of *Mycobacterium tuberculosis. Am J Respir Crit Care Med* 1997;155:2057–2063.
83. Williams DL, Spring L, Gillis TP, Salfinger M, Persing DH. Evaluation of a polymerase chain reaction-based universal heteroduplex generator assay for direct detection of rifampin susceptibility of *Mycobacterium tuberculosis* from sputum specimens. *Clin Infect Dis* 1998;26:446–450.
84. Dobner P, Rüsch-Gerdes S, Bretzel G, et al. Usefulness of *Mycobacterium tuberculosis* genomic mutations in the genes *katG* and *inhA* for the prediction of isoniazid resistance. *Int J Tuberc Lung Dis* 1997;1:365–369.
85. Snider DE, Jones WD Jr, Good RC. The usefulness of phage typing *Mycobacterium tuberculosis* isolates. *Am Rev Respir Dis* 1984;130:1095–1099.
86. Shoemaker SA, Fisher JH, Jones WE Jr, Scoggin CH. Restriction fragment analysis of chromosomal DNA defines different strains of *Mycobacterium tuberculosis* complex: analysis of restriction fragment heterogenicity using cloned DNA probes. *Am Rev Respir Dis* 1986;133:1065–1068.
87. Eisenach KD, Crawford JT, Bates JH. Genetic relatedness among strains of the *Mycobacterium tuberculosis* complex: analysis of restriction fragment heterogeneity using cloned DNA probes. *Am Rev Respir Dis* 1986;133:1065–1068.
88. Burman WJ, Stone BL, Reves RR, et al. The incidence of false-positive cultures for *Mycobacterium tuberculosis. Am J Respir Crit Care Med* 1997;155:321–326.

89. Braden CR, Templeton GL, Stead WW, Bates JH, Cave MD, Valway SE. Retrospective detection of laboratory cross-contamination of *Mycobacterium tuberculosis* cultures with use of DNA fingerprint analysis. *Clin Infect Dis* 1997;24:35–40.
90. Small PM, Hopewell PC, Singh SP, et al. The epidemiology of tuberculosis in San Francisco: a population-based study using conventional and molecular methods. *N Engl J Med* 1994;330:1703–1709.
91. Alland D, Kalkut GE, Moss AR, et al. Transmission of tuberculosis in New York City: an analysis by DNA fingerprinting and conventional epidemiologic methods. *N Engl J Med* 1994;330:1710–1716.
92. Genewein A, Telenti A, Bernasconi C, et al. Molecular approach to identifying route of transmission of tuberculosis in the community. *Lancet* 1993;342:841–844.
93. Coronado VG, Beck-Sague CM, Hutton MD, et al. Transmission of multidrug-resistant *Mycobacterium tuberculosis* among persons with human immunodeficiency virus infection in an urban hospital: epidemiologic and restriction fragment length polymorphism analysis. *J Infect Dis* 1993;168:1052–1055.
94. Jereb JA, Burwen DR, Dooley SW, et al. Nosocomial outbreak of tuberculosis in a renal transplant unit: application of a new technique for restriction fragment length polymorphism analysis of *Mycobacterium tuberculosis* isolates. *J Infect Dis* 1993;168:1219–1224.
95. Tabet SR, Goldbaum GM, Hooton TM, Eisenach KD, Cave MD, Nolan CM. Restriction fragment length polymorphism analysis detecting a community-based tuberculosis outbreak among persons infected with human immunodeficiency virus. *J Infect Dis* 1994;169: 189–192.
96. Sepkowitz KA, Friedman CR, Hafner A, et al. Tuberculosis among urban health care workers: a study using restriction fragment length polymorphism typing. *Clin Infect Dis* 1995;21:1098–1102.
97. Barnes PF, Yang Z, Preston-Martin S, et al. Patterns of tuberculosis transmission in central Los Angeles. *JAMA* 1997;278:1159–1163.
98. Frieden TR, Woodley CL, Crawford JT, Lew D, Dooley SM. The molecular epidemiology of tuberculosis in New York City: the importance of nosocomial transmission and laboratory error. *Tuberc Lung Dis* 1996;77:407–413.
99. Dunlap NE, Harris RH, Benjamin WH Jr, Harden JW, Hafner D. Laboratory contamination of *Mycobacterium tuberculosis* cultures. *Am J Respir Crit Care Med* 1995;152:1702–1704.
100. Jacobs WR, Barletta RG, Udani R, et al. Rapid assessment of drug susceptibilities of *Mycobacterium tuberculosis* by means of luciferase reporter phages. *Science* 1993;260:819–822.
101. Dubow MS. Antituberculosis drug screening [commentary]. *Lancet* 1993;342:448–449.
102. Wilkins EGL, Ivanyi J. Potential value of serology for diagnosis of extrapulmonary tuberculosis. *Lancet* 1990;336:641–644.
103. Bothamley GH, Rudd R, Festenstein F, Ivanyi J. Clinical value of the measurement of *Mycobacterium tuberculosis* specific antibody and pulmonary tuberculosis. *Thorax* 1992;47:270–275.
104. Daniel T, Debanne S, Van der Kuyp F. Enzyme-linked immunosorbent assay using *Mycobacterium tuberculosis* antigen 5 and PPD for the serodiagnosis of tuberculosis. *Chest* 1985;88:388–392.
105. Daniel TM, deMurillo GL, Sawyer JA, et al. Field evaluation of enzyme-linked immunosorbent assay for the serodiagnosis of tuberculosis. *Am Rev Respir Dis* 1988;134:662–665.
106. Steele B, Daniel TM. Evaluation of the potential role of serodiagnosis of tuberculosis in a clinic in Bolivia by decision analysis. *Am Rev Respir Dis* 1991;143:713– 716.
107. Chan SL, Reggiardo Z, Daniel TM, Girling DJ, Mitchison DA. Serodiagnosis of tuberculosis using an ELISA with antigen 5 and a hemagglutination assay with glycolipid antigens. *Am Rev Respir Dis* 1990;142:385–390.
108. Alde S, Pinasio H, Pelosi F, Budani H, Palma-Beltran O, Gonzalez-Montanez L. Evaluation of an enzyme-linked immunosorbent assay (ELISA) using an IgG antibody to *Mycobacterium tuberculosis* in the diagnosis of active tuberculosis in children. *Am Rev Respir Dis* 1989;139:748–751.
109. Cocito CG. Properties of the mycobacterial antigen complex A60 and its applications to the diagnosis and prognosis of tuberculosis. *Chest* 1991;100:1687–1693.
110. Charpin D, Herbault H, Gevaudan J, et al. Value of ELISA using A60 antigen in the diagnosis of active pulmonary tuberculosis. *Am Rev Respir Dis* 1990;142: 380–384.
111. Zou YL, Zhang JD, Chen MH, Shi GQ, Prignot J, Cocito C. Serological analysis of pulmonary and extrapulmonary tuberculosis with enzyme-linked immunosorbent assays for anti-A60 immunoglobulins. *Clin Infect Dis* 1994;19:1084–1091.
112. Chiang I-H, Suo J, Bai K-J, et al. Serodiagnosis of tuberculosis: a study comparing three specific mycobacterial antigens. *Am J Respir Crit Care Med* 1997;156: 906–911.
113. Laal S, Samanich KM, Sonnenberg MG, Zolla-Pazner S, Phadtare JM, Belisle JT. Human humoral responses to antigens of *Mycobacterium tuberculosis:* immunodominance of high-molecular-mass antigens. *Clin Diagn Lab Immunol* 1997;4:49–56.
114. Laal S, Samanich KM, Sonnenberg MG, et al. Surrogate marker of preclinical tuberculosis in human immunodeficiency virus infection: antibodies to an 88-kDa secreted antigen of *Mycobacterium tuberculosis. J Infect Dis* 1997;176:133–143.
115. Amicosante M, Richeldi L, Monno L, et al. Serological markers predicting tuberculosis in human immunodeficiency virus-infected patients. *Int J Tuberc Lung Dis* 1997;1:435–440.
116. Verbon A, Weverling GJ, Kuijper S, Speelman P, Jansen HM, Kolk AHJ. Evaluation of different tests for the serodiagnosis of tuberculosis and the use of likelihood ratios in serology. *Am Rev Respir Dis* 1993;148: 378–384.
117. Sada E, Brennan PJ, Herrera T, Torres M. Evaluation of lipoarabinomannan for the serological diagnosis of tuberculosis. *J Clin Microbiol* 1990;28:2587–2590.
118. Sada E, Aguilar D, Torres M, Herrera T. Detection of lipoarabinomannan as a diagnostic test for tuberculosis. *J Clin Microbiol* 1992;30:2415–2418.
119. Maekura R, Nakagawa M, Nakamura Y, et al. Clinical evaluation of rapid serodiagnosis of pulmonary tuberculosis by ELISA with cord factor (trehalose-6,6'-dimycolate) as antigen purified from Mycobacterium tuberculosis. *Am Rev Respir Dis* 1993;148:997–1001.
120. Bhattacharya A, Ranadive SN, Kale M, Bhattacharya S. Antibody-based enzyme-linked immunosorbent as-

say for determination of immune complexes in clinical tuberculosis. *Am Rev Respir Dis* 1986;134: 205–209.
121. Daniel TM. Circulating immune complexes in tuberculosis [editorial]. *Am Rev Respir Dis* 1986;134:199–200.
122. Cole ST, Brosch R, Parkhill J, et al. Deciphering the biology of *Mycobacterium tuberculosis* from the complete genome sequence. *Nature* 1998;393:537–544.
123. Young DB. Blueprint for the white plague. *Nature* 1998;393:515–516.

3
How Is Tuberculosis Transmitted?

In this chapter, current conceptions of the transmission of infection attributable to *Mycobacterium tuberculosis* are reviewed. Chapter 4 follows the fate of the tubercle bacilli in the newly infected host, focusing, in particular, on the newly infected individual's development of immunological responses and the roles they play in the pathogenesis of the disease known as tuberculosis.

PRINCIPLES AND VARIABLES OF TRANSMISSION

. . .the finest particles become part of the air itself [J. Burns Amberson (1)]

Physical Characteristics of Infectious Particles

As noted in Chapter 1, observers were very slow to accept that "consumption" was an airborne infection. Although many had speculated that it might be so, proof was elusive. Even when a dramatic outbreak persuaded observers that there was aerogenic spread, confusion reigned about the nature of the process. Generally, the dominant theme from ancient times to the 18th century was that the air itself was corrupted or "miasmatic," not that infectious particles were being transmitted. With the evolution of the experimental model in science, arising in the second half of the nineteenth century, scientists struggled to elucidate the means by which tuberculosis was spread. Fortified by Koch's discoveries and guided by the observation that the lungs appeared to be the portal of primary entry, efforts were made to assess the infectiousness of the air expired by consumptives. However, these projects yielded negative results, and the prevalent opinion from 1882 to the early twentieth century was that particles generated from dried sputum or contaminated articles were the main vehicles of transmission—a vestige of Koch's original 1882 treatise.

Flugge proposed in 1907 that it was fine droplets of respiratory secretions which bore bacilli to new hosts, and he performed limited studies showing infection of guinea pigs via inhalation of exhaled droplets from consumptives (2). However, definite proof of this was to wait another half-century for the work of Wells and Riley. William Firth Wells was the intellectual parent of the modern view of airborne transmission of infection. As detailed by Amberson in his introduction to Riley and O'Grady's book, *Airborne Infection,* Wells theorized that "most droplets atomized into air evaporate almost instantly, leaving disease germs drifting like cigarette smoke in the droplet nuclei (1)."

From this vision arose a series of arduous but elegant studies that still provide the clearest understanding of human-to-human transmission of tuberculosis. The results of these investigations are recounted in *Airborne Infection,* as well as in a series of original reports and reviews. Essential elements of this theory were a quantitative approach to the probability of infection based on the *concentration of the infectious particles* (not the total number of bacilli, but rather, those held within particles suitable for alveolar deposition) in relationship to the *volume of air* inhaled by the subjects. This infectious unit was designated a "quantum" by the investigators. Based on the period of time required during the era before chemotherapy for student nurses to convert their tuberculin skin tests (i.e., to be newly infected with tuberculosis), Wells had theorized about the concentration of these infectious particles in the ambient air of the wards. To test the validity of the "droplet-nucleus" concept and to quantify the risk of infection, Riley et al. (3) created a pilot ward at the Veterans Administration Hospital (VAH) in Baltimore, Maryland. The components of the droplet-nucleus theory and the results of their observations at the VAH are delineated below (see "Baltimore Veterans Administration Pilot Ward Experience").

The fundamental premise of the researchers was that tuberculosis was transmitted by liberating bacilli into the air in a physical form that could be inhaled deeply into the airways by a person sharing that air. The number of bacilli would be influenced (a) by a form of the disease that resulted in enhanced multiplication of the mycobacteria (typically, cavitary pulmonary disease) and (b) by events that promoted aerosolization of respiratory secretions. Their investigations primarily focused on the latter element.

During this era, Duguid had investigated the potential for various respiratory maneuvers to produce bacteria-containing aerosols. His studies measuring elaboration of small droplets (100 μm or less in diameter) yielded remarkable results (4):

- Speaking: 0 to 210 particles.
- Coughing: 0 to 3,500 particles.
- Sneezing: 4,500 to 1,000,000 particles.

The size of the particles was also critical in the droplet nucleus conceptualization of Wells. As noted by Riley and O'Grady (1):

> The size droplets swept by an air current from the surface of a liquid is determined primarily by the velocity of the air and the surface tension of the liquid. As the air velocity increases, the size of the droplets decreases until above 100m per second the diameter of the water droplets approaches a minimum of 10 microns. In sneezing and coughing, the peak air flow in the bronchi approaches 300m per second, and consequently the droplets ejected should be about 10 microns in diameter.

In fact, Duguid (5) measured droplets after sneezing and calculated the mean diameter to be 6 μm. Later, Wells (6) estimated this value to be 18 μm. These measurements closely approximated the predicted value of 10 μm! The significance of these observations related to the fate of various-sized particles: as Well had calculated, the large droplets and the mucoid matter rapidly fell to the ground where they became trapped in a matrix of dust forming large, complex structures. These particles—even if made airborne again by agitation—were highly unlikely to traverse the airways when inhaled. By contrast, the smaller particles would undergo rapid evaporation to produce the droplet nuclei which Wells had posited to be the conveyance for tuberculosis infection:

- Droplets less than 100 μm in diameter fall less than 2 feet in normal atmosphere before dehydration results in formation of droplet nuclei with diameters of 1 to 10 μm.
- Droplet nuclei settle at a rate of 0.2 mm per second; even the gentlest of air currents will keep them airborne for long periods.
- Small inhaled particles are far more likely to reach the periphery of the lung where tubercle bacilli can be implanted. Based on studies on the deposition of inorganic dusts in the lungs of animal models, it was determined that less than 10% of 8-μm particles reached the alveoli, but that roughly 40% of 2- 3-μm particles would do so (1). And Riley and O'Grady (1) calculated that, given their settling velocity of 0.2 mm per second, roughly 50% of droplet nuclei that reached the alveolar duct (diameter, 0.4 mm) or alveolus (diameter 0.1 mm) would be deposited there.
- Wells et al. (7) had previously shown dramatically increased implantation of tubercle bacilli in the lungs of rabbits exposed to a given number of organisms in a *fine* aerosol contrasted with implantations while exposed to an equal number of bacilli in a *coarse* aerosol.

Baltimore Veterans Administration Hospital Pilot Ward Experience

Several studies were conducted between 1956 and 1961 on a special facility at the Baltimore, Maryland, Veterans Administration Hospital (VAH). Essentially, the ward consisted of six rooms under balanced negative pressure with the entire effluent air being passed through a series of cages located in a "penthouse" over the patients' area (8). In these cages were kept 150 to 240 guinea pigs. Before placement in the cages, the guinea pigs were quarantined for 30 days and had tuberculin skin tests (TSTs) to verify that they did not harbor latent mycobacterial infection. The animals had TSTs monthly during the study period, and those found to be reactors were sacrificed and underwent autopsy. After an initial study period, the system was revised in the following manner: (a) The effluent air was split into two equal columns, each serving a different population of 120 guinea pigs; however, one column underwent ultraviolet (UV) irradiation before delivery to the animal area. (b) By drug susceptibility profiles and temporal patterns of exposure, the guinea pig infections were assigned to specific patients. Salient findings of these studies included the following:

- The air in the penthouse cages was equally infectious as air from the patients' room.
- The average time to infect one guinea pig among the whole population was 10 days.
- Based on the exposure time and the calculated volume of air inspired by each guinea pig (8 cubic feet per day), the authors calculated that there was one infectious dose (quantum) in every 11,000–12,500 cubic feet of air.
- Extraordinary heterogeneity of infectiousness among the patients was seen in the second phase of the study, as follows:
  - One patient with tuberculous laryngitis was responsible for 14 of the total of 63 infected animals (this person was calculated to produce one infectious particle for every 200 cubic feet of air, a density equal to measles cases).
  - Of the 130 patients who occupied the ward, 8 patients (including the laryngitis case, whose time on the ward constituted only 1% of the total patient days during the second phase) generated 46% of the total number of guinea pig infections.
  - Untreated patients with drug-susceptible disease were substantially more infectious than those being treated: 29 of 30 infections with drug-susceptible bacilli were caused by the untreated group (time of exposure: untreated, 7% of total; treated, 15%). This translated to a 10- to 50-fold increased risk of infection before treatment.
  - Patients with drug-susceptible disease were significantly more infectious than those with drug-resistant disease, the risk ranging from fourfold to eightfold higher.
  - Among most of the newly infected guinea pigs there was only one solitary pulmonary tubercle per animal found at autopsy. Although many of the animals had hilar lymphadenopathy and splenic involvement, this single pulmonary focus suggested that the infection and disease had resulted from the inhalation of a single "quantum" that probably contained only one or a few bacilli. Notable as well, some of the animals that converted their TSTs and on autopsy had evidence of tuberculosis had no demonstrable primary lesions in their lungs, suggesting invasion and bacteremia without significant pulmonary inflammation.
  - There were *no infections* among the guinea pigs exposed to the air that had been UV irradiated. This finding both reinforced the notion of airborne transmission and testified to the potency of UV irradiation in reducing tuberculosis communicability (see Chapter 14 for contemporary issues regarding UV irradiation in tuberculosis control).

The authors concluded that the Flugge-Wells theory of droplet-generated tuberculosis transmission had been validated: ". . .it is inferred that the droplet-nucleus mechanism alone is adequate to account for the spread of tuberculosis." Issues that were not fully addressed by this group include the transmissibility and virulence of different strains of *M. tuberculosis* and the frequency of cough among the different patients; these are reviewed later in this chapter.

Other Epidemics and Transmission

Subsequent to the observations made on the pilot ward at the VAH, there were two epidemics of tuberculosis wherein the patterns of transmission supported the concept of droplet-nucleus transmission.

Arkansas Industrial School

The first epidemic occurred in an industrial school in Arkansas (9). Two young male residents were found to have active, sputum smear-positive pulmonary disease. By studying dormitory, classroom, and extracurricular patterns, the observers noted significantly higher probability of transmitted infection (". . .at the 1 per cent level") among those who sang in the choir with one of the residents who had the disease than among other residents, including dormitory mates. The authors inferred that the vigorous exhalation associated with singing, abetted perhaps by the rapidly vibrating vocal cords, was a highly effective means of generating droplet nuclei.

U.S.S. Richard E. Byrd Study

The second epidemic occurred on a U.S. Navy ship, the U.S.S. *Richard E. Byrd.* This outbreak was well described in two classic articles in 1968 (10,11). Because there had been six other recent epidemics of tuberculosis among U.S. Navy ships, when the outbreak on the *Richard E. Byrd* was detected, an extraordinarily thorough investigation of the personnel and the physical characteristics of the ship was undertaken. Studies of the sailors included serial TSTs, chest radiographs (including whole-lung tomography for those whose x-rays were deemed suspect), and sputum-induced sputum/gastric aspirates for mycobacterial smear and culture. Sleeping quarters, work areas, and recreational patterns for all sailors were noted. Ventilation systems and their cross-connections were studied in detail. Important findings of the *Richard E. Byrd* study were as follows:

- In September 1966, the initial case was noted; the patient had been symptomatic, including having chronic cough, for 6 months. His chest radiograph revealed a 5-cm cavity, and his sputum smear revealed numerous bacilli.
- Of the 308 enlisted crew members at risk, 139 (45%) had converted their TSTs at the initial screen. Seven other crew members (2.2%) were found to have clinical-radiographic evidence of active disease.
- Six of the seven other active cases were found in individuals in the compartment in which the person with the index case slept. In this compartment (compartment 1), 47 of the other 59 sailors converted their TSTs. Overall, 53 of 66 individuals at risk (80%) had tuberculous morbidity.
- In another compartment (compartment 2), which shared ventilation with compartment 1, 43 (53%) of the 81 sailors at risk converted their TSTs. Of particular interest, most of these TST converters slept near inlets where air from compartment 1 entered. Sailors who slept *elsewhere* had significantly lower rates of new infections than the men in compartments 1 and 2. Of note, these other sleeping areas did *not* share ventilation with compartment 1.
- However, in one of the other compartments there was an unexplained clustering of TST reactors. The intensive medical evaluation to which all men were subjected revealed that one of the sailors whose bunk was in this area had strongly *positive sputum cultures,* despite *normal plain chest radiographs* and whole-lung tomograms. Perhaps coincidentally, his pastime was playing the guitar and singing songs to his compartment mates. As the authors stated, whimsically, "Besides the pleasure of his singing, they may also have acquired tuberculosis infection during these musical interludes."

The authors concluded that the evidence strongly supported the airborne droplet-nucleus mode of transmission with apparent dilutional effect associated with spatial gradients in the intensity of transmission. In view of the appearance of some unexpected late TST conversions, they discussed the possibility of dust-fomite infections, but speculated as well about the role of newly infected contacts with normal chest radiographs shedding enough bacilli in their respiratory secretions to infect others (see above).

Fennelly's Cough Box

After all of the inferential data, Fennelly and Martyny (12) provided direct observations on the generation of fine particles containing tubercle bacilli by a patient with respiratory tract tuberculosis. Interested in the size and configuration of the putative infectious particles, Fennelly and Martyny—working at the National Jewish Medical and Research Center in Denver, Colorado—devised a method to sample expired air. Fennelly's earlier efforts to assay room air with high-volume samplers had been thwarted by overgrowth with *Aspergillus* species; therefore, the researchers created a Plexiglas box with a volume of approximately one cubic foot. Patients were induced to cough through tubing into this box; the air within this box was then sampled with a sophisticated six-stage device that allowed estimation of the size of the bacilli-containing particles.

One of the first patients to be studied was a diabetic woman with multidrug-resistant tuberculosis with bilateral cavities and laryngeal disease. Before effective therapy was initiated, she generated 637 CFUs of *M. tuberculosis* with 10 minutes of coughing. By comparison, of nine other sputum-smear positive and culture-positive patients, only one generated cultivatable particles, but only 3 CFUs. Notably, the first patient had been, as determined by contact tracing, a highly effective transmitter of tuberculous infection, including transmission to two health care workers (HCWs) who had visited her home *while wearing personal respiratory tract protection devices.* Based on calculations from the air-sampling device, Fennelly and Martyny estimated that 49% of the particles containing bacilli were in the range of 1.1–2.1 μm range, but that a considerable number of particles smaller than one μm had been generated by this patient's cough. The authors have suggested that perhaps the bacilli, when traveling rapidly through the air, actually aligned themselves in a linear manner, behaving like a fiber; if this were so, such particles would require very-high-efficiency filtration for exclusion.

Sputum Status and Transmission Risk

Overall, there is abundant experimental and epidemiological evidence that the immense preponderance of tuberculosis transmission occurs through the vehicle of the airborne droplet nucleus. Most instances of transmission involve patients with extensive pulmonary disease including cavitary lesions and positive sputum smears. Data from contact investigations show a clear, consistent association between positive sputum microscopy and the prevalence of infection and disease among contacts (13,14). An analysis by Rouillon et al. (15), published in 1976, helped quantify this phenomenon (Tables 3.1–3.3; Fig. 3.1). These findings were subsequently confirmed by two other studies, which correlated risk with sputum-smear status. A study from Alabama found this gradient of skin-test reactivity of contacts: household contacts (HHCs) to smear-positive cases, 46%; non-HHCs to smear-positive cases, 34%; HHCs to smear-negative, culture-positive cases, 28%; and non-HHCs to smear-negative, culture-posi-

TABLE 3.1. *Risk of transmitting tuberculosis in relation to the index case's sputum smear status: three reports of household contacts 0 to 14 years of age*

	England, 1954[a]	Canada, 1954[b]	Netherlands, 1967–1969[c]
Index case	709 contacts	1876 contacts	148 contacts
Sputum status		Percentage of positive TST results	
Smear +/culture +	65%	45%	5%
Smear −/culture +	27%	26%	5%
	(22%)[d]	(2.5%)[d]	(1%)[d]

[a] From ref. 34.
[b] From ref. 35.
[c] From ref. 36.
[d] Estimate of prevalence of TST reactivity in general or similar population.
+, positive; −, negative.

Three studies describe substantially higher rates of tuberculin reactivity among contacts to index cases when sputum is both smear and culture positive than in cases whose sputa are culture positive but smear negative. Inference from the data are discussed more fully in the text.

TABLE 3.2. *Risk of tuberculosis transmission in relation to index cases' sputum smear status and closeness of contact: Netherlands, 1963–1964 (all ages of contacts)*

	Contact status	
	Household	Casual
Index case status	858 contacts	4,207 contacts
Smear +/culture +	20.2% Infected	3.7% Infected
Smear −/culture +	1.1% Infected	0.2% infected

+, positive; −, negative.
From ref. 18.

As in the Canadian Survey (Fig 3.1), these data from the Netherlands demonstrate clear gradients for risk of transmission/infection on the bases of index case smear status and intimacy of exposure.

tive cases, 24% (13). Also, a recent report from Finland documented the risk of disease, not infection, by index-case smear positivity (16); over 2 years of observation, all four cases of disease among contacts occurred among those exposed to patients with strongly positive smears.

It has been long recognized that not all cavitary, smear-positive cases are equally infectious (17). Certainly, some of the variables in aerosol generation noted previously come into play in this instance. Interestingly, one logical candidate for variance—the frequency of cough—was studied and found to be less powerful than chest radiograph or sputum microscopy in predicting case infectivity (18). However, the study did document a rapid reduction in cough frequency with commencement of chemotherapy, a factor that may contribute to the diminished risk of transmission seen with treatment.

Virulence, Infectivity, and Transmission

A theoretical factor in discrepant transmissibility of tuberculosis would be potential differences in the "virulence" or "infectivity" of various strains of *M. tuberculosis*. Because of ambiguities in the usage of these terms, it is appropriate to clarify their application in this discussion.

Virulence, I believe, should be reserved for description of the capacity of a strain to produce progressive disease. Quantitative variables in virulence might include the number of bacilli within organs, the severity of tissue reaction/damage within the organ(s), or the number of organs involved (e.g., the tendency to cause disseminated disease). There are reasonable animal-model observations to support these features as strain-dependent variables (see below).

By contrast, **infectivity** should be limited to demonstrate differences in the propensity to cause infection upon exposure to an aerosol of that strain. This is harder to document, in large measure because of imperfections in the way we measure "exposure" (we can only infer that animals or humans inhale a certain number of bacilli in a given laboratory or clinical situation) and "infection" (the TST is the usual marker in animal studies, such as the Baltimore VAH study cited above, or in human contact investi-

TABLE 3.3. *Likelihood of developing active tuberculosis in relation to sputum smear status of index case: Canada*

	Active disease among contacts			
Index case	Close	Casual	Close	Casual
	Ages: 0 to 14 y		Ages: 15 to 29 y	
Smear +/culture +	38%	24%	11%	6%
Smear −/Culture +	18%	18%	1%	3%

From ref. 22.

Among infected contacts to patients with positive sputum smears, subsequent rates of clinically active tuberculosis were modestly higher than disease rates among infected contacts of smear-negative, culture-positive cases. This was most pronounced among close contacts in both age groups. The most obvious explanation relates to inoculum size, but other phenomena should be considered (see text).

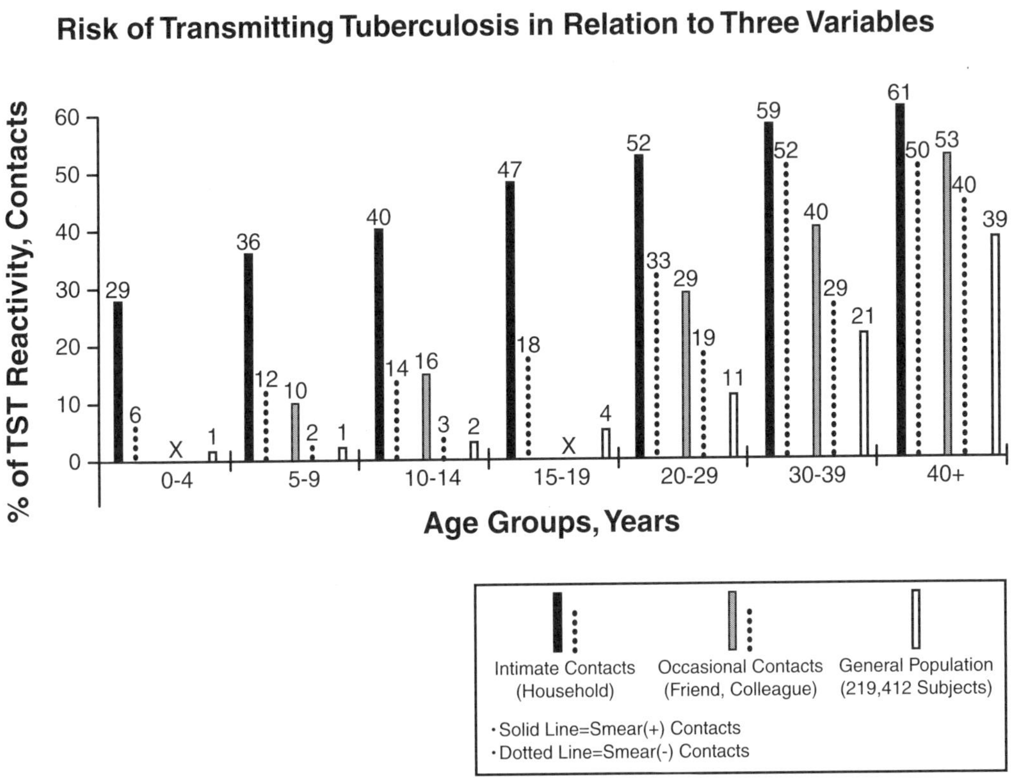

FIG. 3.1. The risk of transmitting tuberculosis in relation to three variables: index-case smear status, age of contacts, and intimacy of contact (British Columbia and Saskatchewan, Canada, 1966–1971). This analysis clearly demonstrates gradients toward higher rates of tuberculin skin test reactivity among younger contacts on the basis of smear positivity and household exposure; these distinctions diminished in the older age cohorts as a result of lifelong exposures. (Compiled from ref. 22.)

gations; and, given its unreliability in persons with active disease, it is logical to infer fallibility in detecting simple infection).

A recent, highly publicized report of an outbreak in Tennessee and Kentucky typifies some of the ambiguity in these terms (19). The report alludes to "a virulent" strain of *M. tuberculosis,* "the Oshkosh strain." The contact investigations in this setting were quite impressive: overall, 311 (72%) of 429 contacts who were studied had positive TST results. Clearly, this value is much higher than the national averages, both in terms of raw numbers and percentages. Among those deemed infected, a total of 19 cases, excluding the source and index cases, was found.

The authors referred to the remarkable "virulence" of this organism based on mouse studies performed for this report by Orme and colleagues at Colorado State University. When mice were exposed to aerosols of this case strain, "Oshkosh," and a traditional virulent strain, H37Rv, the numbers of bacilli recovered from the lungs were considerably higher with the Oshkosh: at 10 days, 10,000 versus 1,000, and at 20 days, 1 to 10 million versus 100,000 CFUs. The potential flaw that I can find in this design is that inoculum sizes at day 0 were calculated, not measured. If, for some reason, the Oshkosh strain formed fine-particle aerosols more readily, the initial bacillary infestation may have been much greater with that strain than with the H37Rv.

While this may be a true marker of "virulence" in the mouse model, the data from the contact investigations above do not really confirm increased virulence, by my definition. That 19 of roughly 300 (6+%) contacts, presumed to be newly infected, had active disease is not at all a significant departure from other contact investigations. Indeed, Stead (20), in an analysis of tuberculosis among HCWs reported disease rates ranging from 12% to 29% among newly infected HCWs.

There are considerable data derived from animal-model studies which document true variations in the virulence of tubercle bacilli. The most well known of these is a laboratory-bred mutant designated H37R-avirulant (H37Ra), an offshoot of a classic *M. tuberculosis* pathogen, H37R-virulent (H37Rv). H37Ra is far less capable of producing progressive infections in animal models and is not associated with human disease. Also, scientists have demonstrated that strains of *M. tuberculosis* recovered from patients in southern India have generally diminished virulence in the guinea pig model (21). In addition, and not widely recognized in references to the VAH pilot ward project noted above, the organisms from the most infectious patient seen during the studies (a man with laryngeal tuberculosis) showed a disproportionate propensity to produce miliary disease among the guinea pigs. Perhaps this reflected massive inhalational exposure (although the animals showed only the typical single pulmonary tubercle on autopsy); however, exaggerated virulence cannot be excluded. Similarly, one element of tuberculosis contact investigation is not widely appreciated: in a Canadian survey, a modestly higher percentage of contacts infected by smear-positive cases went on to develop active tuberculosis than contacts infected by smear-negative cases (22). In this analysis, the risk of disease was broken down by three variables: index-case smear status, ages of contacts, and closeness of contacts. The data, as adapted in that report, are displayed in Table 3.3. Certainly, the meaning of these modest differences is not clear. A likely interpretation is that contacts to smear-positive cases were infected more intensely (more bacilli inhaled) and over a longer period. However, it is plausible that the bacilli from the sputum smear-positive cases, either because of their own innate properties or because of changes induced by their rapid proliferation in a progressively permissive host, might be somewhat more virulent.

Differences in infectivity are more difficult to demonstrate than altered virulence; yet, it certainly is possible that subtle differences in the physical-chemical nature of the cell walls of tubercle bacilli could alter their ability to be aerosolized, to survive in the environment of droplet nuclei, or to resist local primary defenses within the lung. Parker et al. (23) have demonstrated that, among strains of *M. avium* complex (MAC) recovered from the environment, the strains that were more similar to MAC isolates from human disease went into aerosol significantly more readily than did other strains. In addition, bacilli from the same strain of *M. tuberculosis* may undergo significant changes in their cell walls and colonial morphology following passage through different animals or ex vivo cell cultures (24). Therefore, it is conceivable that strains of *M. tuberculosis* recovered from certain patients may be more virulent or infective because of passage through that patient.

Overall, I conclude that the "infectivity" and "virulence" of strains of *M. tuberculosis* probably are linked but not always identical attributes. Evidence broadly in support of this is the fact that the percentage of contacts who develop overt disease tends to be higher in settings where a higher percentage of exposed persons are infected (e.g., convert their TSTs). While this might suggest that we could use these terms interchangeably, I would prefer to continue to attempt to distinguish between them until we understand the true biology of these processes.

TRANSMISSION FROM NONPULMONARY SOURCES

Although the preponderance of new infections by *M. tuberculosis* occurs by the mechanisms delineated above, we should consider the other circumstances in which transmission has been shown or presumed to occur.

Cutaneous, soft tissue tuberculosis has proven to be a potent source of nosocomial transmission in two recent reports. An extensive outbreak of infection and secondary disease was seen in association with hospital treatment in Arkansas of a patient with a large abscess of the hip and thigh (25). This case study, because it represents so many vital elements in contemporary tuberculosis control, is worth consideration in detail, as follows:

- The index case, in a 67-year-old man, was admitted to a community hospital on January 8, 1985, with pain in the left hip. Important historical points included known prior exposure to tuberculosis, previous gastrectomy, and prolonged corticosteroid therapy in the prior year, 1984. While receiving prednisone, he developed a febrile illness with hilar adenopathy and erythema nodosum; during this period, he received an intramuscular injection with an antibiotic in his left gluteus. Circumstantial evidence makes probable the following scenario: while receiving high-dose prolonged corticosteroid therapy in 1984, the patient probably experienced either primary or reactivation tuberculosis (the febrile illness with hilar adenopathy and erythema nodosum suggest the former). The trauma associated with the intramuscular injection of antibiotic may well have allowed bacteremic tubercle bacilli to seed the left gluteal area by the principle of *locus minoris resistentiae.* This site then became the focus for his 1985 abscess.
- On admission in January 1985, he was found to have a large abscess in the soft tissues of the left thigh. There were no osseous or pulmonary lesions. On January 12, 1985, he underwent surgical debridement and irrigation of the abscess; for 3 days after surgery there was copious drainage from the wound requiring frequent dressing changes. Thereafter, the wound was regularly irrigated with a high-pressure jet system (the Water-Pik oral hygiene appliance); this was performed for 11 days. Smears for acid-fast bacilli of the original debrided material were reported positive 4 days after surgery; antituberculosis therapy was then instituted and given for 10 days before the patient's death.
- During his hospital stay, the patient spent time in the surgical suite and in two ward areas, Station A and the medical intensive care unit (MICU). There was substantial transmission of tuberculosis (tuberculin conversions) in all of these areas: 4 of 5 operating room staff who had participated in the incision and debridement; 28 of 33 exposed employees (85%) from Station A; and 6 of 20 (30%) of exposed MICU staff. The patterns of transmission from Station A were particularly instructive. The room in which the patient had received treatment was found later to be under strongly positive pressure with high rates of airflow into the hallway and other areas of the ward. There was a clear gradient in the intensity of transmission associated with distance from the patient's room (Fig. 3.2). This pattern was similar to that seen in the U.S.S. *Richard E. Byrd*

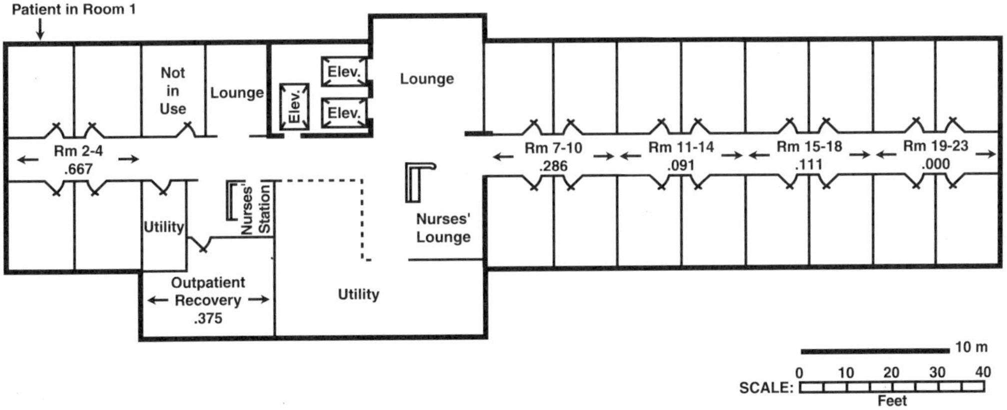

FIG. 3.2. Schematic of hospital floor on which patient with tuberculous hip abscess was treated, and pattern of infection among other patients on ward. The patient was treated for 2 days in Room 1. Room 1 was at positive pressure because of a window-mounted air conditioner. There was an obvious gradient of the likelihood of transmission infection occurring along the distance from Room 1. Some of the infected individuals had spent less than 1 hour in the area. (From ref. 25, with permission.)

epidemic (see above); it strongly suggests a pattern of dilution of infectious particles. This gradient effect was seen as well in other areas for patients and visitors; the fact that visitors who had been in the hospital only for brief periods were infected is compelling testimony to the density of the infectious droplet nuclei. Of note: the temporal sequence of infections among contacts indicated that routine dressing care created highly transmissible particles (e.g., it did not require debridement by the Water-Pik device to generate infectious aerosols).

The authors of the study observed that this epidemic had been potentially preventable, since, by existing American Thoracic Society (ATS) and Centers for Disease Control and Prevention guidelines, the patient would have been a candidate for isoniazid preventive therapy in 1984. They also pointed out that the signal marker of this epidemic had been the large number of tuberculin skin test conversions detected among the hospital staff during a routine surveillance program. By recognizing that this soft tissue infection with tuberculosis had generated such intense transmission to staff, authorities were able to expand the contact investigation and detect many others who were newly infected and at high risk for disease in order to offer them preventive therapy.

Shortly after the Arkansas report, another micro-epidemic occurred in association with a cutaneous tuberculous abscess (26). An elderly woman was treated in a hospital for 31 days for an undiagnosed skin infection; at autopsy, the wound was found to be teeming with tubercle bacilli. Contact investigation of the staff revealed 11 new tuberculin reactors (10 nurses and the surgeon who debrided the wound) among the 43 persons with significant exposure; 9 of the 11 received isoniazid preventive therapy. One nurse who deferred isoniazid because of pregnancy and another nurse whose original TST result had been negative developed tuberculous pleural effusions within 3 months of exposure.

These two reports should alert us to the potential for generating infectious aerosols from skin wounds associated with soft tissue *M. tuberculosis* abscesses. Furthermore, they should alert us to the possibility that communicable droplet nuclei may be generated by manipulation of any material that contains significant numbers of tubercle bacilli. Indeed, another report from Arkansas in 1995 noted that 5 of 5 TST-negative HCWs had become infected while exposed during a 3-hour autopsy of a tuberculous patient (27). In dramatic distinction, none of the 40 TST-negative HCWs caring for the patient in the 3 weeks before his death were infected, despite the presence, on autopsy, of tuberculous pneumonia. The authors speculated that the use of the bone saw, which produced very-high-energy oscillations, resulted in the generation of a highly infectious aerosol with a calculated rate of one quantum per 3.5 cubic feet of air! Two of the TST converters had spent only 10 to 20 minutes in the autopsy suite. And, two of these five HCWs, despite normal chest radiographs, had positive sputum cultures when evaluated 2 months after exposure. See Chapter 14 for additional data regarding transmission in the autopsy suite.

Direct inoculation has been long recognized as one mechanism for tuberculosis contagion. Läennec, who performed hundreds of autopsies on consumptives, was said to have inoculated himself several times during these procedures with resultant local infections. Historically, these cutaneous lesions have become known as prosector's warts. Another opportunity for direct inoculation is the bacteriology laboratory where glass or metalware may puncture the skin of workers. Depending on the inoculum size and host defenses, these local lesions may spontaneously involute, cause chronic local abscesses, spread to local lymph nodes, or even disseminate; a recent report has documented local abscess formation in 10 days following a heavy inoculation in a laboratory accident (28). Another very unusual report described cutaneous tuberculosis attributable to a needlestick injury that had introduced into a nurse's forearm blood contaminated with bacteremic tubercle bacilli from a patient with acquired immunodeficiency syndrome (AIDS) patient (29).

The fiberoptic bronchoscope has also been reported as the vector of tuberculosis transmission. In a 1983 report, following endoscopy of a patient with pulmonary tuberculosis, decontamination with an iodophor solution was apparently inadequate to sterilize the instrument (30). Bronchoscopic washings from the next patient to undergo endoscopy with this instrument yielded positive cultures from *M. tuberculosis* (despite the fact that her underlying disease was shown to be nonmycobacterial bronchiectasis); subsequently, her TST converted to a strongly positive result. Additional data in support of transmission via fiberoptic bronchoscope were published in 1997, one report from South Carolina involving multidrug-resistant strain W (31) and the other from Baltimore with a susceptible strain identified by DNA fingerprinting (32).

SUMMARY

Evidence, which is persuasive in terms of both volume and consistency, indicates that tuberculosis is almost universally spread by fine-particle aerosol. Bacilli are deposited in the lungs of contacts, resulting in local infection, then dissemination.

However, vitally important information is missing from our understanding of the subtleties of this process, including features of the source cases and bacilli that influence the likelihood of this occurring (33). Attributes of the contacts that have an impact on this process are explored in Chapter 4.

REFERENCES

1. Riley RL, O'Grady F. *Airborne infection: transmission and control.* New York: Macmillan, 1961.
2. Corper HJ. Founders of our knowledge of tuberculosis. *Hygeia* 1929;October-November:1–13.
3. Riley R, Wells W, Mills C, et al. Air hygiene in tuberculosis: quantitative studies of infectivity and control in a pilot ward. *Am Rev Tuberc* 1957;75:420–430.
4. Duguid J. The numbers and sites of origin of the droplets expelled during respiratory activities. *Edinburgh Med J* 1945;52:385.
5. Duguid J. Expulsion of pathogenic organisms from the respiratory tract. *Br Med J* 1946;1:245.
6. Wells W. *Airborne contagion and air hygiene.* Cambridge, MA: Harvard University Press, 1955.
7. Wells W, et al. On the mechanism of droplet-nucleus infection, II: quantitative experimental air-borne tuberculosis in rabbits. *Am J Hygiene* 1948;47:11.
8. Riley R, Mills C, O'Grady F, Sultan LU, Wittstadt F, Shivpuri DN. Infectiousness of air from a tuberculosis ward: ultraviolet irradiation of infected air—comparative infectiousness of different patients. *Am Rev Respir Dis* 1962;85:511–525.
9. Bates J, Potts W, Lewis M. Epidemiology of primary tuberculosis in an industrial school. *N Engl J Med* 1965;272:714–717.
10. Houk V, Kent D, Baker J, et al. The Byrd Study. *Arch Environ Health* 1968;16:4–6.
11. Houk V, Baker J, Swensen K, Kent D. The epidemiology of tuberculosis in a closed environment. *Arch Environ Health* 1968;16:26–35.
12. Fennelly KP, Martyny JW. Isolation of viable airborne *Mycobacterium tuberculosis:* a new method to study transmission. *Am J Respir Crit Care Med* 1998;157: A706.
13. Rose C, Zerbe G, Lantz S, Bailey W. Establishing priority during investigation of tuberculosis contacts. *Am Rev Respir Dis* 1979;119:603–609.
14. Capewell S, Leitch AG. The value of contact procedures for tuberculosis in Edinburgh. *Br J Dis Chest* 1984;78: 317–329.
15. Rouillon A, Perdrizet S, Parrot R. Transmission of tubercle bacilli: the effects of chemotherapy. *Tubercle* 1976;57:275–299.
16. Liippo KK, Kulmala K, Tala EOJ. Focusing tuberculosis contact tracing by smear grading of index cases. *Am Rev Respir Dis* 1993;148:235–236.
17. Sultan L, Lyka W, Mills C, et al. Tuberculosis disseminators: a study of the variability of aerial infectivity of tuberculous patient. *Am Rev Respir Dis* 1960;82:358.
18. Loudon RG, Romans WE. Cough frequency and infectivity in patients with pulmonary tuberculosis. *Am Rev Respir Dis* 1969;99:109–111.
19. Valway SE, Sanchez MPC, Shinnick TF, et al. An outbreak involving extensive transmission of a virulent strain of *Mycobacterium tuberculosis. N Engl J Med* 1998;338:633–639.
20. Stead WW. Management of health care workers after inadvertent exposure to tuberculosis: a guide for the use of preventive therapy. *Ann Intern Med* 1995; 122: 906–912.
21. Prabhakar R, Venkataraman P, Vallishayee RS, et al. Virulence for guinea pigs of tubercle bacilli isolated from the sputum of participants in the BCG Trial, Chingleput District, South India. *Tubercle* 1987;68: 3–17.
22. Grzybowski S, Burnett G, Styblo K. Contacts of cases of active pulmonary tuberculosis. *Bull Int Union Tuberc* 1975;60:90–106.
23. Parker BC, Ford MA, Gruft H, Falkinham JO III. Epidemiology of infection by nontuberculous mycobacteria, IV: preferential aerosolization of *Mycobacterium intracellulare* from natural waters. *Am Rev Respir Dis* 1983;128:652–656.
24. Collins FM, Montalbine V. Distribution of mycobacteria grown *in vivo* in the organs of intravenously infected mice. *Am Rev Respir Dis* 1976;113:281–286.
25. Hutton MD, Stead WW, Cauthen GM, Bloch AB, Ewing WM. Nosocomial transmission of tuberculosis associated with a draining abscess. *J Infect Dis* 1990;161: 286–295.
26. Frampton M. An outbreak of tuberculosis among hospital personnel caring for a patient with a skin ulcer. *Ann Intern Med* 1992;117:312–313.
27. Templeton GL, Illing LA, Young L, Cave D, Stead WW, Bates JH. The risk for transmission of *Mycobacterium tuberculosis* at the bedside and during autopsy. *Ann Intern Med* 1995;122:922–925.
28. Genn D, Siegrist HH. Tuberculosis of the thumb fol-

lowing a needlestick injury. *Clin Infect Dis* 1998;26: 210–211.

29. Kramer F, Sasse SA, Simms JC, Leedom JM. Primary cutaneous tuberculosis after a needlestick injury from a patient with AIDS and undiagnosed tuberculosis. *Ann Intern Med* 1993;119:594–595.
30. Nelson K, Larson P, Schraufnagel D, Jackson J. Transmission of tuberculosis by flexible fiberscopes. *Am Rev Respir Dis* 1983;127:97–100.
31. Agerton T, Valway S, Gore B, et al. Transmission of a highly drug-resistant strain (strain W1) of *Mycobacterium tuberculosis:* community outbreak and nosocomial transmission via a contaminated bronchoscope. *JAMA* 1997;278:1073–1077.
32. Michele TM, Cronin WA, Graham NMH, et al. Transmission of *Mycobacterium tuberculosis* by a fiberoptic bronchoscope: identification by DNA fingerprinting. *JAMA* 1997;278:1093–1095.
33. Sepkowitz KA. How contagious is tuberculosis? *Clin Infect Dis* 1996;23:954–962.
34. Shaw JB, Wynn-Williams N. Infectivity of pulmonary tuberculosis in relation to sputum status. *Am Rev Tuberc* 1954;69:724–732.
35. Grzybowski S, Allen EA. The challenge of tuberculosis in decline: a study based on the epidemiology of tuberculosis in Ontario, Canada. *Am Rev Respir Dis* 1964;90:707–720.
36. Van Geuns HA, Meijer J, Styblo K. Results of contact examinations in Rotterdam, 1967–1969: Report No. 3 of TSRU. *Bull Int Un Ag Tuberc* 1975;50:107–121.

4

Immunity and Pathogenesis

TERMINOLOGY

In Chapter 3, the processes by which potentially infectious particles are generated by patients with tuberculosis were reviewed. In the vast preponderance of cases, transmission occurs when patients with pulmonary tuberculosis develop cavitary lesions which results in massive numbers of bacilli being discharged in their respiratory tract secretions. The particles most likely to spread infection are liberated during high-velocity exhalational maneuvers (e.g., coughing, sneezing, singing), which generate fine aerosols; the smaller of these particles undergo rapid dehydration, forming tiny droplet nuclei (1 to 5 μm in diameter) which have so little inertial mass that they may travel with the inhaled air to the periphery of the lungs of exposed persons. In the human lung, there are approximately 25 generations of progressively smaller airways from the carina, which divides the trachea into right and left mainstem bronchi, to the distal alveoli. At each ramification, the incoming airstream undergoes subtle changes in direction; larger particles with greater mass tend to impact the mucous membrane of the airways at these points. Although there may be large numbers of tubercle bacilli in the particles lodging at these sites, animal-model studies cited in Chapter 3 have indicated that invasion and infection rarely occur there. The means by which tubercle bacilli invade the human body, create pulmonary infections, disseminate to cause extrapulmonary disease, and promote spread of infection to other new victims are discussed below. An annotated glossary of modern terminology is displayed in Appendix 4.1.

Twentieth-century scientists studying the host's immunological defenses against tuberculosis have come to recognize certain broad biological patterns to which descriptive titles or names have been given. However, because of lack of clear understanding about the events involved, use of these terms has been quite variable and confusing. Particularly vexing has been the following terminology: **cell-mediated immunity (CMI)** and **delayed-type hypersensitivity (DTH).** In simplest terms, CMI has been generally used to indicate that the host (an experimental animal) was able to withstand initial infection and dissemination of tubercle bacilli, ostensibly through the capacity of its macrophages to inhibit bacillary replication and survival; this was associated with involution of the lesions and diminished bacterial numbers at the primary and remote sites. By contrast, DTH fundamentally was signified by the development of a type IV immune response (induration at the site of intradermal injection 48 hours or more following injection) to tuberculo-protein among subjects infected with *Mycobacterium tuberculosis.* However, there was a broader implication that an intense type of necrotizing inflammation at infected sites was reflective of DTH. The distinction between these terms was fostered in part by the observations that, by use of certain types of antigenic material, one could promote partial immunity against a challenge with tubercle bacilli ("CMI") without causing tuberculin reactivity ("DTH"); that DTH could be produced without a corresponding increase in immunity; and that animals could be desensitized without impairing resistance. [For a succinct discussion of these issues, see Mackaness's 1968 editorial (1) in which he argues for essential relationship between DTH and acquired cellular resistance.]

In the Lurie-Dannenberg rabbit-model system, "CMI" and "DTH" came to be associated with distinctions between strains of rabbits that were "susceptible" or "resistant" to experimental tuberculosis infections (2). Following aerosol challenge, the animals that were deemed genetically resistant to tuberculosis were found at 3 weeks to have 20 to 30 times fewer tubercle bacilli in their lungs, to have fewer mycobacteria within macrophages, to have more lymphocytes in their granulomatous lesions, and to have fewer gross tubercles in their lungs than their "susceptible" brethren. However, Lurie and Dannenberg noted that following 21 days, the numbers of bacilli in the lungs of both strains of rabbits stabilized, both in absolute numbers and in relation to one another. Even the "susceptible animals" had found a means to control the mycobacterial proliferation. The authors inferred from these observations that the "resistant" animals had limited growth of the bacilli by a more effective method, intracellular stasis or killing, while the "susceptible" rabbits had done so by relying on intense destruction of tissue, including the permissive macrophages that were reservoirs for proliferating bacilli. To these phenomena the author assigned the terms CMI and DTH, respectively. However, in Dannenberg's most recent publication—writing in collaboration with Rook (3)—he suggested replacing these terms as follows: CMI to be replaced by **acquired cellular resistance,** referring to the capacity of macrophages to inhibit or kill the mycobacteria, and DTH to be replaced by **tissue-damaging immune responses.** In this system of nomenclature, "delayed-type hypersensitivity" would be used solely to describe the processes involved with the tuberculin skin test response. However, out of both inertia and personal preference, I will continue to employ the older terms of reference.

RELATIONSHIPS BETWEEN THE IMMUNE RESPONSE AND PATHOGENESIS

Tubercle bacilli in vivo have not been noted to elaborate products that are inherently toxic or injurious. (Although "cord factor," recovered when massive numbers of *M. tuberculosis* are cultivated in liquid medium, can produce tissue injury when injected into animals, most authorities do not believe it contributes directly to the pathogenesis of tuberculosis in humans.) Unlike the deleterious endotoxins, exotoxins, or enzymes found in the cellular constituents of many other pathogenic bacteria, *the injurious effects of tuberculosis are largely mediated by the defensive responses that the host's immune system mounts against the bacilli in its tissues.* To examine this process with clarity, this section commences with a simple recounting of the events involved with the primary alveolar infection, the contest between the immune system and the bacilli over local spread and invasion, and the ongoing dynamic battle for dominance in the chronically infected state which is the fate of one-third of the world's population (see Chapter 2). Subsequently, the mechanisms involved in these various stages of pathoimmunity are discussed in greater detail, focusing on cellular and molecular biological mechanisms.

Four-Phase Model: An Overview

The multiphase schema employed in this chapter substantially reflects the work of Arthur M. Dannenberg, Jr., who, four decades ago, commenced his study of tuberculosis with Max B. Lurie (himself a tuberculosis patient who received treatment at the National Jewish Hospital) and has continued his productive scholarship to the present. This process is schematized in Table 4.1.

Phase I: Infection or Not?

Inferential data suggest that not all tubercle bacilli that reach the distal airspaces result in significant "infection." Dannenberg (2), citing the work of Lurie, concluded that under certain circumstances, resident alveolar macrophages could engulf and destroy tubercle bacilli through preimmune or innate properties without permitting the microbial proliferation and inflammation that we deem infection. Critical variables in this initial encounter ostensibly stem from both pathogen and host factors: the "hardiness" of the bacillus (how well it has survived its aerosolization and journey in the droplet nucleus); the inherent virulence of the bacillus; and the in-

TABLE 4.1. *Four-phase model: critical aspects of transmission, immunity, pathogenesis, and retransmission (the cycle)*

	Event
Phase 1	
Transmission	• Diseased person generates aerosol that contains tubercle bacilli. • Smaller particles of aerosol dehydrate to form droplet nuclei. • Droplet nucleus containing bacillus(i) is inhaled by potential host. • Droplet nucleus transits bronchial tree and is deposited in alveolus. • Bacilli are engulfed by nonimmune, resident alveolar macrophages.
Phase II	
initiation of infection, proliferation and dissemination	• Bacilli survive within alveolar macrophages and proliferate intracellularly. • Proliferating bacilli kill alveolar macrophages and are released; chemokines are released and attract additional cells. • New alveolar macrophages and blood monocytes ingest bacilli. • γ/δ lymphocytes, natural killer cells, and T lymphocytes begin to appear in lesions. • Bacilli continue to proliferate, killing host cells and spreading locally. • Bacilli are transported to hilar lymph nodes and spread systemically.
Phase III	
evolution of host immune response	• Host response: macrophages present tuberculosis antigens to T lymphocytes; T cells release cytokines. • Cytokines recruit and activate macrophages; results include protective cellular and tissue-damaging immune responses. • These responses limit proliferation and/or kill, bacilli, resulting in involution of the primary lung lesion and the remote, extrapulmonary foci, or • Host fails to mount effective response and experiences progressive primary disease at initial lung infection and/or extrapulmonary sites.
Phase IV	
liquefaction and accelerated bacillary proliferation	• Pulmonary focus reactivates and undergoes liquefaction with cavity formation. • Extracellular bacilli multiply exponentially during this accelerated bacillary proliferation.
Retransmission	• Patient expectorates bacilli in secretions; another person inhales them; cycle is completed.

hibitory activity of the alveolar macrophage, which probably is the sum of intrinsic, genetically determined properties and prior, nonspecific stimulation by particulate matter or other microbes that have reached the alveoli.

Once the tubercle bacillus initiates the "primary infection," there is set in motion an epic struggle between parasite and host. Before the advent of modern chemotherapy, this affair usually lasted for the lifetime of the host and often resulted in great morbidity and premature mortality.

Phase II: Early Proliferation and Spread

Animal data from Wells (see Chapter 2) and considerations of the physical dimensions of droplet nuclei have indicated that only one to three bacilli typically reach the alveolus in a droplet nucleus. Herein begins one of the seeming paradoxes of tuberculosis: the essential early habitat of *M. tuberculosis* is the macrophage, the same cell that is the primary effector of the host's defensive response. In order to survive, the tubercle bacillus *must promote* its uptake by the macrophages. Once inside the phagosomal vacuole of the alveolar macrophage, the hardy, virulent bacillus commences replication, a process that ultimately destroys the host cell.

The mycobacterium-macrophage struggle results in the elaboration of substances generically referred to as cytokines and chemokines. These substances attract other immune-effector cells including additional alveolar macrophages, dendritic cells, peripheral blood monocytes (PBMs), lymphocytes, and neutrophils to the site. As the fatally damaged macrophages disgorge their burden of bacilli, these recently mobilized and still "incompetent" phagocytic cells engulf the mycobacteria, creating additional breeding capacity for the bacilli.

Tubercle bacilli multiply slowly. Even in the optimal in vitro growth conditions, replication takes roughly 15 to 18 hours. However, the geometric progression of the unchecked bacillary proliferation would soon result in a huge burden of mycobacteria. If we assume replication every 16 hours, one mycobacterium could generate approximately 540,000,000 progeny in 20 days!

During this time frame, the mycobacteria would have been transported via centripetal lymphatics from the site of the primary infection to the hilar lymph nodes. It is likely that the complicated immunological cascade that results in acquired cellular resistance and damaging immune responses is orchestrated largely in the peribronchial and regional lymph nodes rather than at the primary site of infection in the lung parenchyma.

Hematogenous spread of the bacilli would have occurred as well. The mechanism(s) of hematogenous dissemination have not been precisely delineated. Possibilities include (a) free bacilli traveling via mediastinal lymphatics to

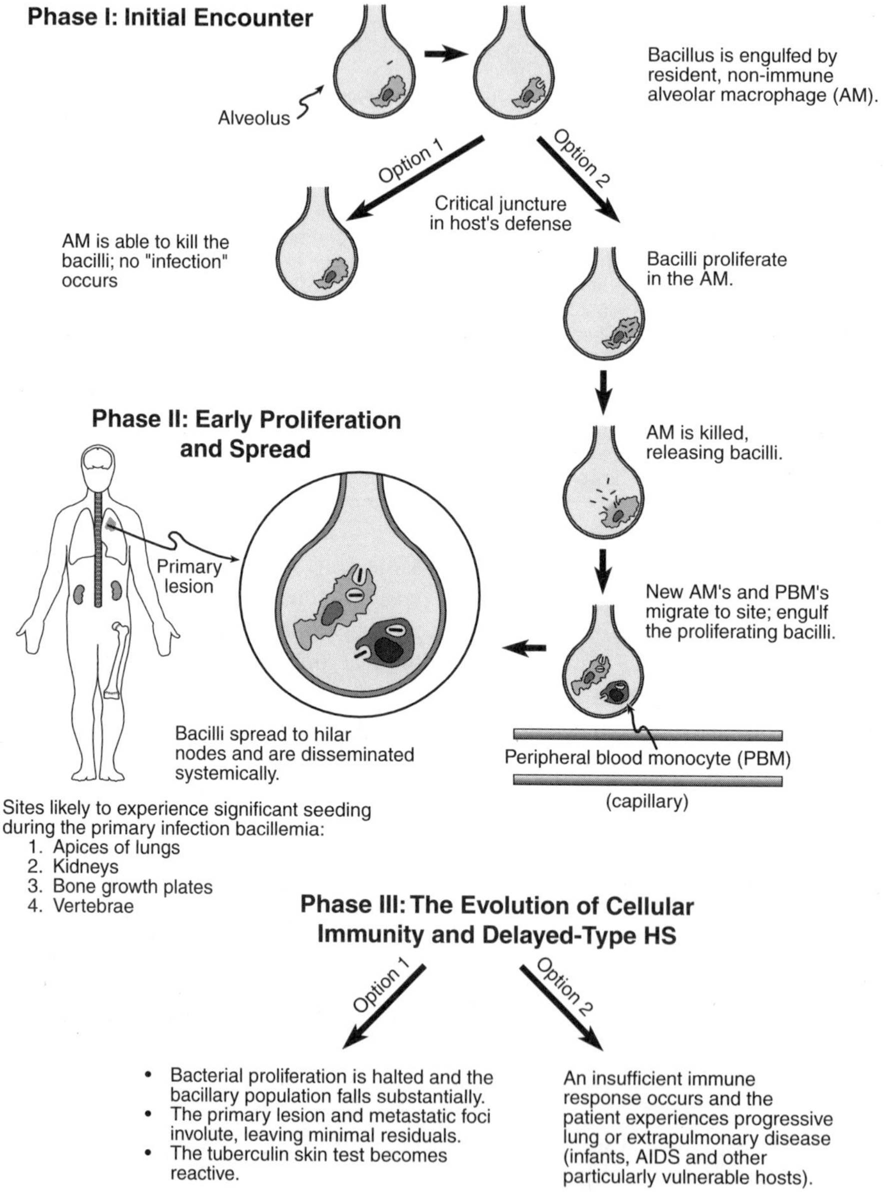

FIG. 4.1. Current conceptualizations of the development of acquired cellular resistance and the tissue-damaging immune response.

the thoracic duct that flows into the left subclavian vein, (b) invasion directly as free bacilli enter into capillaries or other small vessels at the site of primary infection, and (c) hematogenous transportation within monocyte-macrophages or polymorphonuclear phagocytes that have traversed the inflammatory site, engulfed mycobacteria, and returned to the bloodstream. By one or more of these mechanisms, the exponentially proliferating bacilli are widely disseminated in most newly infected hosts.

Phase III: Evolution of Cell-Mediated Immunity and Delayed-Type Hypersensitivity

During the initial days and weeks of this primary tuberculous infection, a complex response is mounted by the host. Although polymorphonuclear leukocytes are attracted (presumably in a nonspecific manner) to this initial site of inflammation, they appear to have an inconsequential role in the host's defenses. Rather, an intracellular pathogen such as *M. tuberculosis* elicits an immunological response that mainly involves two cell lines, the macrophages and lymphocyte series. Humoral or antibody responses, which are central in the defense against usual bacterial pathogens, appear to play a negligible role in protection against tuberculosis, although the complement system apparently contributes to the essential early step of phagocytosis (see below).

Current conceptualizations of the development of CMI and the DTH response are represented in Fig. 4.1 and entail the following. Antigen-presenting cells (APCs), possibly dendritic cells or PBMs that have engulfed tubercle bacilli, exteriorize antigens of the mycobacteria in the form of peptides. These antigen-presenting elements are closely associated geographi-

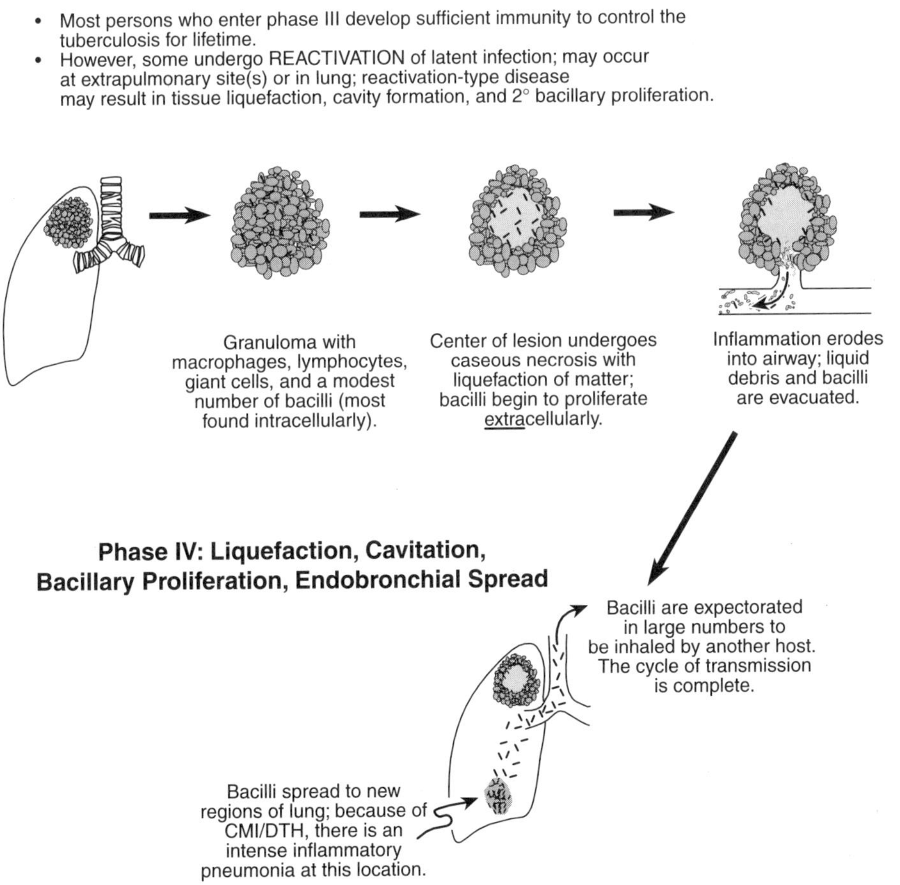
• Most persons who enter phase III develop sufficient immunity to control the tuberculosis for lifetime.
• However, some undergo REACTIVATION of latent infection; may occur at extrapulmonary site(s) or in lung; reactivation-type disease may result in tissue liquefaction, cavity formation, and 2° bacillary proliferation.
Granuloma with macrophages, lymphocytes, giant cells, and a modest number of bacilli (most found intracellularly).
Center of lesion undergoes caseous necrosis with liquefaction of matter; bacilli begin to proliferate extracellularly.
Inflammation erodes into airway; liquid debris and bacilli are evacuated.
Phase IV: Liquefaction, Cavitation, Bacillary Proliferation, Endobronchial Spread
Bacilli are expectorated in large numbers to be inhaled by another host. The cycle of transmission is complete.
Bacilli spread to new regions of lung; because of CMI/DTH, there is an intense inflammatory pneumonia at this location.

FIG. 4.1. *Continued*

cally on the wall of the APC with major histocompatibility (MHC) molecules (Fig. 4.2). The type of MHC molecule, class I or II, determines the type of T cell that recognizes and reacts to the mycobacterial antigen. APCs also elaborate substances—chemokines—that attract additional host cells to their location. The macrophages then "present" these antigens to T lymphocytes, which are induced to manufacture and release a variety of products—cytokines—that attract, stimulate, activate, or otherwise choreograph the behavior of the various effector cells;

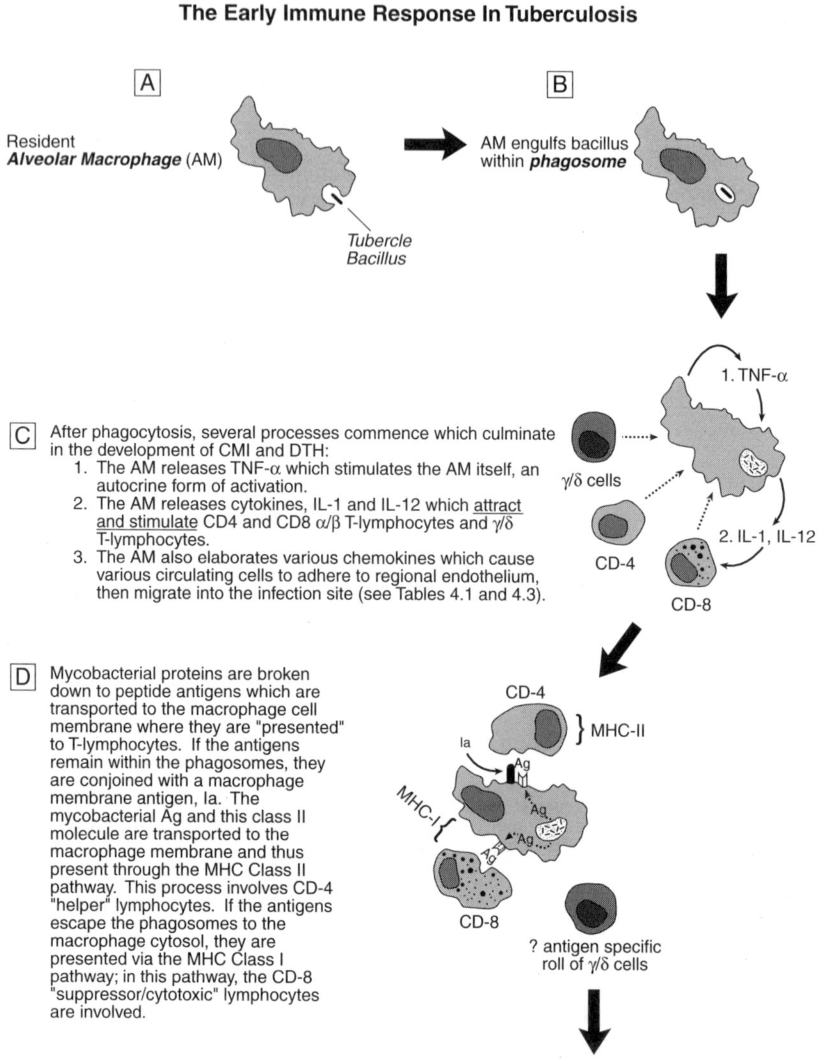
The Early Immune Response In Tuberculosis
A
Resident
Alveolar Macrophage (AM)
Tubercle Bacillus
B
AM engulfs bacillus within *phagosome*
1. TNF-α
γ/δ cells
CD-4
CD-8
2. IL-1, IL-12
C
After phagocytosis, several processes commence which culminate in the development of CMI and DTH:
1. The AM releases TNF-α which stimulates the AM itself, an autocrine form of activation.
2. The AM releases cytokines, IL-1 and IL-12 which attract and stimulate CD4 and CD8 α/β T-lymphocytes and γ/δ T-lymphocytes.
3. The AM also elaborates various chemokines which cause various circulating cells to adhere to regional endothelium, then migrate into the infection site (see Tables 4.1 and 4.3).
D
Mycobacterial proteins are broken down to peptide antigens which are transported to the macrophage cell membrane where they are "presented" to T-lymphocytes. If the antigens remain within the phagosomes, they are conjoined with a macrophage membrane antigen, Ia. The mycobacterial Ag and this class II molecule are transported to the macrophage membrane and thus present through the MHC Class II pathway. This process involves CD-4 "helper" lymphocytes. If the antigens escape the phagosomes to the macrophage cytosol, they are presented via the MHC Class I pathway; in this pathway, the CD-8 "suppressor/cytotoxic" lymphocytes are involved.
CD-4
MHC-II
Ia
Ag
MHC-I
CD-8
? antigen specific roll of γ/δ cells

FIG. 4.2. As a consequence of the early immune response in tuberculosis, the following ensue:

- Activated macrophages become more competent at inhibiting the replication of intracellular mycobacteria [cell-mediated immunity (CMI)].
- Incompetent macrophages that allow rapid bacillary proliferation are destroyed, releasing the mycobacteria to be engulfed by more capable phagocytes [delayed-type hypersensitivity (DTH)].
- These two processes result in a halt in the exponential proliferation of bacilli, bringing to an end the primary infection.

The simplified representation focuses on major, generally agreed upon, elements of the process. Please see text and other tables for more comprehensive discussion of other agents involved.

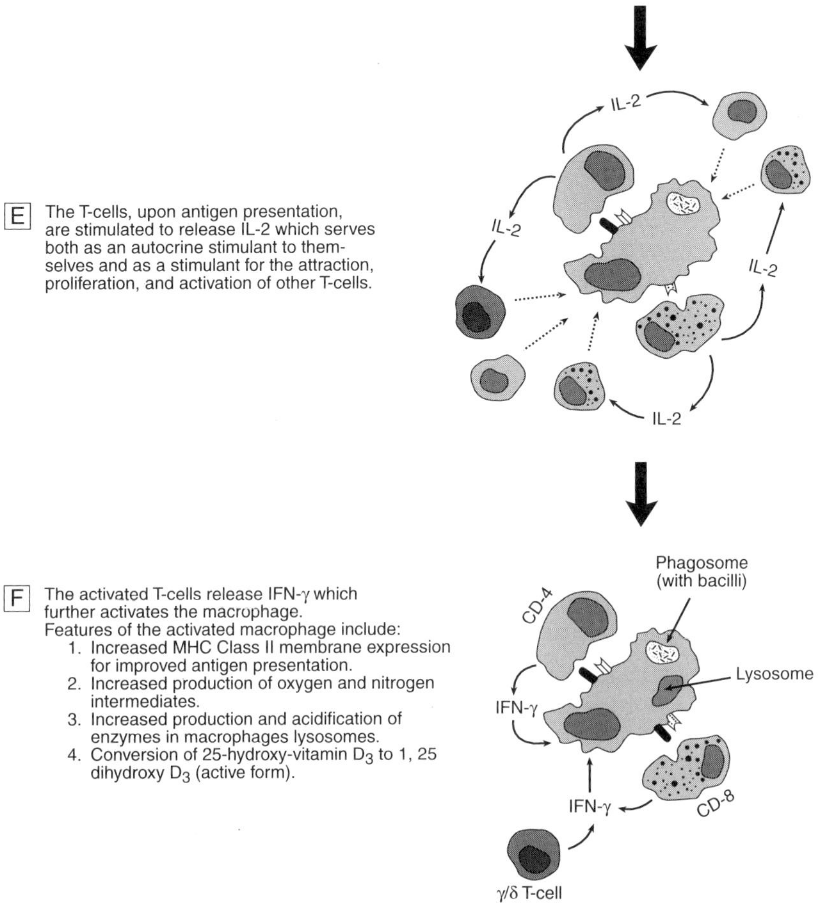

E The T-cells, upon antigen presentation, are stimulated to release IL-2 which serves both as an autocrine stimulant to themselves and as a stimulant for the attraction, proliferation, and activation of other T-cells.
IL-2
IL-2
IL-2
IL-2
F The activated T-cells release IFN-γ which further activates the macrophage.
Features of the activated macrophage include:
1. Increased MHC Class II membrane expression for improved antigen presentation.
2. Increased production of oxygen and nitrogen intermediates.
3. Increased production and acidification of enzymes in macrophages lysosomes.
4. Conversion of 25-hydroxy-vitamin D3 to 1, 25 dihydroxy D3 (active form).
Phagosome (with bacilli)
CD-4
Lysosome
IFN-γ
IFN-γ
CD-8
γ/δ T-cell

FIG. 4.2. *Continued*

the effector cells are responsible for limiting the proliferation and spread of the tubercle bacilli. The chemokines and cytokines thought to play major roles in tuberculous immunopathogenesis are briefly characterized in Table 4.2.

Under the influence of the factors just mentioned, the macrophages that have been attracted to the site(s) of tubercle bacilli proliferation become "activated." Activation is a broad term used to describe a variety of morphological, biochemical, and functional changes including the ability to inhibit bacillary proliferation ("tuberculostatic" activity) or to kill the intracellular microbes ("tuberculocidal" activity). This process eventually gives rise to the phenomenon of DTH—an indurated response at 48 to 72 hours—to tuberculoproteins that have been injected into the skin. This is the basis of the tuberculin skin test, which usually becomes reactive within 3 to 8 weeks after the primary infection.

Lurie and Dannenberg, without the advantage of modern molecular biology techniques, recognized in animal model studies (2) that, over time, the macrophages that appeared in lesions were functionally different. Their observations and theories helped to understand the genesis of the granuloma, the histological marker of tuberculosis. They postulated that the cells that had been summoned to the infection site formed concentric rings, the earlier cells clustered at the center and the latecomers arranged around the periphery. The center of this ring was thought to consist of the debris left by the initial macrophages, which had engulfed the bacilli and been killed by

TABLE 4.2. *Major cytokines and their apparent roles in immunity and pathogenesis of tuberculosis*

Agent	Sources	Roles/comments
Interleukin-1 (IL-1)	• Monocytes • Macrophages • Neutrophils • T and B lymphocytes • NK cells • Various somatic cells	• Promotes T and B lymphocyte proliferation (synergism with other cytokines) • Increases IL-2 receptor expression • Activates NK cells • Acts as an endogenous pyrogen • Multiple effects on CNS and endocrine system • Miscellaneous other
Interleukin-2 (IL-2)	• CD4 (Th1) lymphocytes	• Stimulates proliferation and differentiation of T lymphocytes (autocrine stimulation) • Increases cytolytic activity of NK cells • Stimulates proliferation and immunoglobulin production by B lymphocytes
Interleukin-4 (IL-4)	• T lymphocytes • Macrophages • Mast cells and basophils • B lymphocytes • Bone marrow and stromal cells	• Induces CD4 T cells to differentiate into Th2 cells and suppresses Th1 differentiation • Stimulates proliferation and differentiation of B lymphocytes • Promotes IgE production from B lymphocytes • Diverse other effects on macrophages and granulocytes
Interleukin-8 (IL-8)	• Monocytes • Macrophages • T lymphocytes • Neutrophils • Fibroblasts • Keratinocytes • Endothelial and epithelial cells • Others	• Chemotactic factor for neutrophils, T-lymphocyte subsets, and basophils • Increases adherence of monocytes to endothelial cells • Activates neutrophils to release lysosomal enzymes, undergo a respiratory burst, and degranulate
Interleukin-10 (IL-10)	• T lymphocytes • Macrophages • B lymphocytes • Keratinocytes	• Suppresses functional activity of macrophages • Inhibits production of proinflammatory cytokines by macrophages and monocytes • Increases B-lymphocyte proliferation and immunoglobulin secretion
Interleukin-12 (IL-12)	• Macrophages • B lymphocytes	• Enhances cytolytic activity of cytotoxic T lymphocytes, NK cells, macrophage and lymphokine-activated killer (LAK) cells • Increases proliferation of activated NK cells and T lymphocytes • Induces production of IFN-γ by T lymphocytes • Stimulates differentiation of uncommitted CD4 T lymphocytes into Th1 cells
Interferon-gamma (IFN-γ)	• CD4 (Th 1) lymphocytes • CD8 lymphocytes • γ/δ lymphocytes • NK cells	• A central role in acquired resistance • Activates macrophages and enhances killing of intracellular pathogens • Increases MHC class II surface antigens • Requires TNF-α and 1,25 dihydroxy-vitamin D_3 for maximal effect
Tumor necrosis factor-α (TNF-α)	• Macrophages • Monocytes • T lymphocytes • B lymphocytes • NK cells • Neutrophils • Various somatic cells	• Activation and differentiation of monocytes/macrophages (synergistic with IFN-γ); central role in granuloma formation • Monocyte chemotoxin • Promotes monocyte adhesion to endothelium • Stimulates production of IFN-γ by activated lymphocytes • Activates PMNs • Promotes procoagulant activity by blocking protein C • Diverse effects on many somatic cell lines
Granulocyte-macrophage colony-stimulating factor	• T lymphocytes • Monocytes	• Stimulates physiological activity of monocytes, macrophages, neutrophils, and eosinophils • Promotes growth and differentiation of hematopoietic progenitor cells

TABLE 4.2. *Continued*

Agent	Sources	Roles/comments
(GM-CSF)	• Endothelial cells • Fibroblasts	• Attracts macrophages to granulomas and enhances their ability to slow mycobacterial growth
1,25 Dihydroxy-vitamin D_3 [1,25(OH)2D3]	• Macrophages	• Stimulated by IFN-γ, macrophages convert 25-OH D3 to this active metabolite • Autocrine effect enhances capacity to inhibit intracellular growth of mycobacteria
Monocyte chemotactic and activating factor (MCAF)	• Monocytes • Macrophages • B lymphocytes • Other somatic cells	• Monocyte chemotaxin • Regulates cytokine production in monocytes • Stimulates histamine release from basophils
Macrophage inflammatory protein-1α (MIP-1α)	• T lymphocytes • B lymphocytes • Monocytes • Mast cells and fibroblasts	• Monocyte chemotaxin • T-lymphocyte chemotaxin • Functions as endogenous pyrogen
Macrophage inflammatory protein-1β (MIP-1β)	• T lympocytes • B lymphocytes • Monocyte • Mast cells and fibroblasts	• Monocyte chemotaxin • T-lymphocyte chemotaxin • Promotes T-lymphocyte adhesion to endothelial cells

NK, natural killer; CNS, central nervous system; IgE, immunoglobulin E; IFN-γ, interferon-γ; TNF-α; tumor necrosis factor-α; PMNs, polymorphonuclear neutrophils.

From ref. 76, with permission.

the proliferating microbes. As the immune response evolved, each generation of macrophages that was attracted sequentially to the lesion became more "competent."

Current evidence suggests that some T lymphocytes act to augment the capacity of the macrophages to curtail bacillary proliferation within the cells, while other T cells target the destruction of the incompetent macrophages that are serving as breeding sites. Phenomenologically, these activities have come under the rubric of type 1 T-helper (Th1) versus type 2 T-helper (Th2) activity. The relative contribution of CD4 and CD8 lymphocytes to these functions is discussed below. Under the influences of these activities, the number of bacilli reaches a plateau in animal models. Presumably in humans as well, the bacillary load stabilizes and, in normal hosts, eventually ebbs.

Lurie and Dannenberg posited that the fate of the infection is related to the ability of these "perifocal" (surrounding the granuloma) macrophages to control the proliferation and dissemination of the tubercle bacilli. In most "normal" hosts, the primary lesion in the lung, as well as the distal sites to which the microbes are spread, undergoes involution under the influence of the acquired cellular resistance or CMI. However, some hosts are notably less able to mount an immune response capable of controlling the tuberculosis. These persons experience progressive, uninterrupted invasion by the bacilli, becoming clinically ill with overt tuberculosis within weeks to months following the primary infection. Prominent in this category are infants with immature immune systems, very elderly indivduals whose immune competency has flagged with the advancing decades, and the immunocompromised—most notably, at present, persons with human immunodeficiency virus (HIV) infection or acquired immunodeficiency syndrome (AIDS).

For individuals who withstand the primary infection, there remains an enduring risk of "reactivation" disease attributable to the continuing presence of viable bacilli within old lesions at the various tissue sites. The most common and most significant site for reactivation tuberculosis is the apex of the lungs. The evolution of lesions in this pulmonary location typically represents the fourth stage of the immunopathogenic sequence as delineated by Lurie and Dannenberg.

Phase IV: Intense Inflammation, Liquefaction, Cavity Formation, and Mycobacterial Proliferation

The balance between host defense and microbial domination is a precarious one. Clinicians have long recognized that the evolution of cavitary lesions in the lung signaled supremacy of the tubercle bacillus. Even before chest radiography, which allowed antemortem assessment of the pulmonary lesions, physicians and lay persons had recognized the ominous portent of expectorating red blood, an event which classically is related to cavitation in tuberculosis (see Chapter 1). How these lesions evolve and their implications for the patient and further transmission of tuberculosis are discussed below.

As noted above, interactions between macrophages and T lymphocytes generate two closely related phenomena, both of which serve initially to curtail mycobacterial proliferation. These biological events typically are markers of immunologically competent hosts, and yet, paradoxically, they have been subverted by the microbe to serve its ultimate purposes: bacillary multiplication in such a manner as to promote transmission to new hosts in order to ensure survival of the species (*M. tuberculosis,* not *Homo sapiens*).

As noted above, central elements of the immune response include the capacity to directly limit the proliferation or survival of tubercle bacilli within the activated macrophage (CMI) and the capacity to destroy incompetent macrophages that are acting as permissive habitats for the mycobacteria in order to allow the next generation of more capable macrophages to have access to the bacilli (DTH). Both of these processes entail intense release of cytokines and heavy cellular traffic. Many of these cells, macrophages, and polymorphonuclear leukocytes are destroyed in the battle, releasing large amounts of potent, proteolytic enzymes. In addition to proteolysis, these enzymes, as well as one of the cytokines—tumor necrosis factor-α (TNF-α)—also promote thrombosis of local blood vessels. These factors appear to combine to result in the process of "liquefaction" which, as the word suggests, means the transformation of tissue into a soupy detritus which is eminently supportive and nutritious for the tubercle bacilli. It should be emphasized that the process of liquefaction is *not* the same as caseation. In this schema, caseum is seen as a favorable situation for the host; this environment is thought to be an acidic milieu that inhibits mycobacterial proliferation.

Dannenberg maintained that the appearance of "liquefaction" in the animal models signals a critical transition in the relationship between the host and the parasite. Previously, the bacilli had been limited to the intracellular milieu as an environment to support their multiplication, and in this setting, they were accessible to and limited by cellular defenses. However, in the liquefied debris, the tubercle bacilli for the first time could multiply robustly in an extracellular milieu. As the bacilli replicate, the inflammation intensifies until gross destruction of local tissues ensues, and in this locale, macrophages cannot survive or function. The cascade advances until bronchial structures are invaded; the liquefied matter is evacuated into the airways, leaving behind cavities. This material is expectorated by the host, becoming droplet nuclei to invade the next generation of victims and to ensure propagation of the tubercle bacillus. Incidental to the requirements of the microbe, but often lethal for the host, the liquefied matter may also be transmitted endobronchially to other regions of the lungs. In this manner, there may be progressive damage to the lungs which, untreated, results in respiratory insufficiency, the most common mode of demise for tuberculosis patients.

Detailed Consideration of the Components of Immunopathogenesis

Various components of the sequence noted above have been studied in detail. The current scientific perspectives on these phenomena are briefly delineated below. While it is clear that we have come far in our understanding since Koch's discovery of the tubercle bacillus and his unfortunate efforts at immunotherapy with tuberculin (see Chapter One), there remain large gaps in our understanding of this process.

Uptake of Bacilli by Macrophages

After initial inhalation, it is *essential* that the bacilli be engulfed by macrophages; these phagocytic cells provide a nurturing habitat for the bacilli, which have quite specific growth requirements. Current evidence indicates that bacilli may promote their adhesion to and uptake by macrophages through the following specific mechanisms. First, induced activation of complement component C3 leads to uptake via the macrophage's complement receptor (CR) pathway, which confers a survival advantage (see below) (4). Second, recent observations suggest a novel pathway involving a complement cleavage product, C2a, which binds selectively to *M. tuberculosis* and other pathogenic mycobacteria (but *not* nonpathogenic mycobacteria or nonmycobacterial intracellular pathogens like *Leishmania mexicana* or *Listeria monocytogenes*) to form a C3-cleaving convertase (5). This C2a-mycobacterial moiety cleaves complement C3, resulting in opsonization of the mycobacteria. Inferential evidence suggests that this mechanism of macrophage uptake may also be of ongoing pathogenetic significance: patients with active pulmonary tuberculosis demonstrate complement activation and C2a production (6–8) and circulating immune complexes which result in continuous increased levels of C2a (9). Third, large amounts of molecules are secreted that bind fibronectin to the bacilli, thus promoting uptake via macrophage fibronectin receptors (10).

Evasion of Inhibitory Mechanisms within Macrophages

Electron microscopic studies indicate that the mycobacteria enter the macrophages by conventional phagocytosis: pseudopodia surround the bacillus, the cytoplasm of the monocyte is displaced beneath the site of contact, and the microbe appears to sink into the phagocyte.

Like other intracellular bacterial pathogens, the tubercle bacillus has "learned" to elude or defeat the macrophage's armamentarium of antimicrobial mechanisms. The specific mechanisms by which activated macrophages inhibit or kill intracellular tubercle bacilli have not been clearly identified; therefore, microbial evasion remains poorly characterized. Regardless, *M. tuberculosis* has been shown to possess the following potentially useful attributes: (a) by using the CR pathway for attachment and endocytosis, reactive oxygen intermediate generation is avoided (4); (b) the mycobacteria, when lodged in phagosomes, have a demonstrated capacity to inhibit fusion of this compartment with lysosomes that contain potent enzymes, and this effect is apparently mediated through sulfolipids (11) and ammonia (12); (c) the bacilli, through these pathways, also act to inhibit macrophage priming (13) and the production of reactive oxygen intermediates (14); (d) lipoarabinomannan (LAM) from both *M. tuberculosis* and *Mycobacterium leprae* inhibits priming by interferon-γ (INF-γ) of macrophages (15) [notably, LAM from virulent, but not avirulent, bacilli had this effect (16)]; and (e) virulent strains of *M. tuberculosis* have been reported to disrupt the phagosomal membranes and enter the macrophage cytosol; in this location, they are not subject to lysosomal degradation and their peptide antigens could be presented through the MHC class I pathway to CD8 lymphocytes, potentially triggering a downregulation of the immune response (17) (although an interesting hypothetical model, little evidence has subsequently appeared in support of this theory).

Russell et al. (18) have recently shown that vacuoles containing mycobacteria exclude proton–adenosine triphospatase (proton-ATPase) from their phagosomes, preventing acidification and hydrolysis (18). However, they did not concur with the prior assertion that tubercle bacillus–containing vacuoles were incapable of fusion with the lysosomes (19). Rather, they characterized the vacuoles as being highly dynamic but "extremely selective of the intracellular compartments with which they mix." The capacity of vacuoles containing mycobacteria, in this case *Mycobacterium bovis* Bacille Calmette Guérin (BCG), to resist fusion with lysosomes was shown to be related to properties of living, but not dead, bacilli by another group (20). Rather than inhibition of fusion, this group suggests that the mycobacteria-laden vacuoles are "transported along a route that is distinct from the endocytic pathway."

Although these studies have confirmed that *M. tuberculosis* has acquired the capacity to elude conventional macrophage inhibitory/microbicidal mechanisms, this capacity for intracellular survival is *not* universal among strains of *M. tuberculosis*. Studies in animal models have indicated that catalase-peroxidase enzyme production by the bacilli appears to provide protection against intracellular inhibition or killing (21,22). A recent report (23) has indicated that, in the murine model, this is substantially but not wholly related to the *katG* genetic locus. Although one report (24) suggested that overexpression of an alternative antioxidant mechanism, alkylhydroperoxidase or hydroperoxide reductase *(ahpC),* was a virulence factor for *katG*-deficient bacilli, another study (25) failed to confirm this effect.

These reports focused on the capacity of tubercle bacilli to resist reaction oxygen intermediates; however, another report (26) suggested that in a drug-susceptible strain of *M. tuberculosis,* which was prominently represented in New York City in a recent survey, exceptional virulence was conferred because of its capacity to resist reactive nitrogen intermediates.

On balance, the available information suggests that virulent tubercle bacilli do have the capacity to alter or subvert the normal inhibitory or microbicidal mechanisms of effector phagocytic cells. However, these cells do mount a noxious response that must be neutralized by the bacilli to facilitate pathogenesis.

Immunity (Cell-Mediated Immunity and Delayed-Type Hypersensitivity) and Pathogenesis

The alveolar macrophages and PBM-derived macrophages that engulf the tubercle bacilli during the initial phases of infection are not activated and are generally very permissive for mycobacterial replication. Nevertheless, they play a central role in the initiation of the host's immune response. Subsequently, monocyte-derived macrophages and dendritic cells are prime effector cells. The mechanisms involved in these processes are examined in detail below.

Mycobacterial Antigens and Host Responses

After phagocytizing the bacilli, the macrophages transport various mycobacterial antigens to their exterior cell walls for presentation to T lymphocytes. Kaufmann and Young (27) theorized that, because the early alveolar macrophages, monocyte-derived macrophages, and dendritic cells were not capable of killing the bacilli, the most logical candidates for antigen presentation would be proteins that are secreted by viable but stressed bacilli, not structural proteins that would require microbial disruption for availability (27). Kaufmann and Young (27) and others (28–30) have demonstrated that T lymphocytes from newly infected human contacts, as well as *M. tuberculosis*–infected mice, respond consistently to secreted heat-shock proteins. And, Horwitz et al. (31) have recently demonstrated significant protection in a guinea pig model against aerosol challenge using a vaccine prepared from a 30-kd secretory protein of *M. tuberculosis.*

Orme et al. (35) reported that protective immunity against tuberculosis in a murine model entailed memory T cells that responded to both secreted and cell-wall proteins, suggesting sequential acquisition of the immune repertoire. However, during a rechallenge infection, memory T cells responded only to macrophages displaying low-molecular-weight antigens secreted by viable multiplying bacilli. This indicates different patterns of antigen recognition in the acute host response, in remote protection from exogenous reinfection and, theoretically, in endogenous reactivation (see "Immune Memory and Tuberculosis Reactivation").

Major Histocompatibility Complex (Human Leukocyte Antigen) System and Antigen Presentation

The MHC is a large genetic element with multiple loci on the host's chromosomes. In the mouse, the MHC is referred to as the H-Z complex, while in the human it is commonly denoted as the human leukocyte antigen (HLA) complex. The MHC loci encode for two broad classes of membrane molecules, classes I and II.

Class I molecules are glycoproteins that are found on the membranes of virtually all nucleated cells, associated there with β-2 microglobulin proteins. In the human genome, there are three class I loci (termed A, B, and C); in the mouse, there are two class I loci (K and D). At each of these loci, there are various alleles, which are derived in combinations from the parents.

Unlike class I molecules, class II glycoproteins are not expressed on all nucleated cells;

rather, they appear restricted to specialized APCs. There are three class II loci in humans (DR, DP, and DQ) and two loci in mice (IA and IE). The MHC glycoprotein is composed of two chains, α and β, which are encoded by separate genes. These diverse elements result in a very large number of variations of the MHC complex system that might influence genetically determined resistance or susceptibility to a given infection such as tuberculosis (see "Cellular Immunity and the Human Leukocyte Antigen: Animal Model and Human Observations").

In the MHC class II pathway, the antigens from the tubercle bacilli are presented by the macrophage in conjunction with one of its own endogenous cellular products, the glycoprotein termed Ia (33). Stimulation of macrophages by IFN-γ results in increased expression of the class II cell surface molecules, enhancing their ability to present antigen. Among the variety of T lymphocytes, the CD4 or T-helper cells (see below) are uniquely capable of responding to this method of antigen presentation.

Macrophages also have the capacity to present mycobacterial antigens via a second major pathway, MHC class I, which is the cell's mode of communication with another type of T lymphocyte, the CD8 cytotoxic/suppressor cell (see below) (34). Conventional thought at present holds that the MHC class I pathway presents only antigens that have been deliberately exported from or have escaped from the phagosome into the cytosol of the phagocyte. If, as noted above (17), virulent tubercle bacilli could damage the phagosomal vacuole and escape into the cytosol, the alternate pathway of antigen presentation *could* have profound implications for natural history and pathogenesis of the disease. However, sufficient evidence to support or refute this notion is unavailable.

Lymphocyte Types and Subsets in Immunopathogenesis

Among the lymphocytes that participate in the process of immunopathogenesis, there are, as noted above, distinct roles for the different types or subsets of T cells. There are three stable types of T cells, which are distinguished by their antigen receptors (α/β or γ/δ) and their accessory MHC molecules. The structure and function of the lymphocytes in relationship to tuberculoimmunity are presented in Appendix 4.1.

A 1993 review (35) suggested that in both humans and mice a variety of T cells and cytokines were involved with acute and long-term immunity. As indicated in the review, multiple studies among humans with pulmonary tuberculosis demonstrated a pattern of lymphocytic alveolitis with a variable prominence of CD4 or CD8 lymphocytes with a Th1 phenotype (36–42). The putative functions of these various elements are discussed below.

CD4 Lymphocytes

The MHC class II-restricted CD4 lymphocytes displaying α/β antigen receptors play the central role in tuberculoimmunity, a fact underscored by the extreme vulnerability of CD4-depleted, HIV-infected persons to tuberculosis. Within the CD4 class, Th1 cells appear to function to upregulate immune activity through the production of facilitatory cytokines including interleukin-2 (IL-2), interleukin-12 (IL-12), and IFN-γ. By contrast, Th2 cells seem to have a counterregulatory effect, elaborating interleukin-4 (IL-4), which appears to reduce the capacity of macrophages to elaborate interleukin-1 (IL-1). Recognizing that immune T lymphocytes could produce distinct patterns of cytokine production, Mosmann et al. (43) afforded the initial insights into the Th1/Th2 model. This apparent dichotomy may play a vital role in such events as the natural history of untreated tuberculosis and the efficacy of vaccines, including BCG (44,45). Indeed, by examining the model of the disease leprosy, Modlin (46) argued that factors that influence the balance between Th1 versus Th2 activity may be central to understanding, managing, and preventing an array of illness including tuberculosis. Leprosy has long been recognized to exist along a continuum of clinical and immunological phenomena. Among different patients and within an individual patient whose condition varies over time, there ranges a limited or resistant form of the disease ("tuberculoid") and an overwhelming, susceptible form ("lepromatous"); there are bidirectional "transitional" forms as well. As Modlin noted, the "resistant" manifestation of leprosy—tuberculoid diseases—is clearly associated with a preponderance of Th1 CD4 lymphocyte in the skin and the elaboration of IL-2 and IFN-γ. Modlin (46) and others (47) have related the balance of Th1 versus Th2 activity to the production of IL-12 by macrophages, which appears to preferentially expand the population of lymphocytes with Th1 activity. Kaufmann (48) recently endorsed this model, indicating that the "initial" IL-12 response may largely dictate the subsequent host-parasite relationship.

CD8 Lymphocytes

MHC class I-restricted CD8 lymphocytes, which also display α/β antigen receptors, have been believed generally to play a more circumscribed role in human tuberculoimmunity than do CD4 cells (27). Although CD8 lymphocytes produce IFN-γ, their major contribution has been deemed to be their capacity to induce lysis of immature, incompetent phagocytes that harbor pathogens. However, CD4 lymphocytes have also been shown to have cytotoxic activity, raising questions about the relative responsibilities for these cell lines to disrupt infected macrophages. Inferential evidence in support of a significant role for CD8 lymphocytes has been derived from a mouse "knockout" model (49,50). Mice deficient for β-2 microglobulin, which is functionally linked to the MHC class I CD8 antigen-presenting locus, are quite vulnerable to mycobacterial infections.

Precise and quantitative roles for CD8 lymphocytes in human tuberculoimmunity are lacking or conflicting. Two recent reports (51,52) analyzed the lymphocyte profiles of patients with active tuberculosis, concluding that CD8 cells were prominently represented. Among a group of patients from Los Angeles, levels of IFN-γ could not be correlated with circulating CD4 lymphocytes; thus, by inference, the authors (51) thought CD8 cells, which were present in abundance, were driving this essential cytokine (51). A Canadian group (52) measured cells in bronchoalveolar lavage (BAL) fluid from patients with pulmonary tuberculosis. In the BAL fluid, they found high numbers of CD8 lymphocytes, which correlated with the presence of IL-12 and IFN-γ messenger RNA, inferring a substantial role for these lymphocytes.

On balance, lymphocytes having CD8 markers appear to play an important role in human immunity against tuberculosis. Depending on the timing, extent of disease, and individual genetic factors, these cells may serve to induce lysis or apoptosis of infected cells or to generate cytokine-driven enhanced intracellular inhibition of mycobacteria, or both.

Gamma/Delta Lymphocytes

The role of γ/δ lymphocytes in tuberculoimmunity is not well defined. However, these cells appear to have a high degree of inherent recognition of mycobacterial antigens in normal individuals and exhibit so-called oligoclonal activation (53). Because they can produce IFN-γ, TNF-α, granulocyte-macrophage colony-stimulating factor (GM-CSF) and interleukin-3 (IL-3), it has been speculated that they may play a part in the early response (54). Also, antigen-specific activation of γ/δ T cells has been shown in mycobacterial infections, indicating a possible role in ongoing immune protection (55). Although one study reported increased percentages of $+/\delta$ T cells in the peripheral blood of patients with pulmonary tuberculosis (56), another reported that the proportion and absolute number of CD3 $+/\delta$ T cells were not different between tuberculosis patients and control subjects (57). Subsequently, another group (58) found that only some patients with active tuberculosis demonstrated increased proportions of γ/δ T cells. Among a large number of patients with pulmonary tuberculosis from the United States, China, and Turkey, studies of blood and BAL fluid revealed substantial reductions in a subset of γ/δ $V\gamma9^{+}/V\delta2^{+}$ cells (59). Normally, at a level of 70% to 95% of circulating γ/δ T cells, the mean level fell to 42% in the blood of patients with active tuberculosis and a similarly low proportion of BAL γ/δ lymphocytes. The group also noted that the γ/δ T cells in these patients were unresponsive to in vitro stimulation by mycobacterial antigens. The extent to which these changes are *causes of* or *due to* the active tuberculosis is unclear at this time. At present, a clear picture of the role of γ/δ T cells in human immunity against tuberculosis is not available. Inferring from the available data, an early cellular response role might be suspected—probably cytotoxic—but most evidence in humans indicates a modest role in established disease. A complicated analysis of γ/δ T cells among hospital workers exposed to cases of tuberculosis in Japan found increased numbers of $CD4^+$ $V\gamma2^+$cells (60); the authors inferred that these cells might contribute to effective, ongoing surveillance.

Natural Killer Cells

Lymphocytes that have spontaneous cytotoxic function against various cell lines have been termed natural killer (NK) cells. This function is not dependent on or restricted by MHC molecules. NK cells are distinct from T or B lymphocytes and myeloid cells; possibly, they represent a discrete leukocyte line.

A recent review (61) noted that NK lymphocytes function to promote clearance of viral infected cells, to participate in tumor surveillance and allograft rejection, and to play a role in autoimmune diseases. The review indicated that cytolytic or apoptotic functions are variably shared with T lymphocytes. Yoneda et al. (62) noted that NK cells were lymphokine activated in patients with active tuberculosis. Bermudez and Young (63) demonstrated that human monocyte-derived macrophages infected with *Mycobacterium avium* complex (MAC) were induced to intracellular killing of the mycobacteria when co-incubated with NK cells. Similarly, Yoneda and Ellner (64) recently showed that PBM-derived macrophages infected with *M. tuberculosis* were induced to intracellular killing of mycobacteria when incubated with NK cells, IL-2- activated NK cells, or T cells. Notable aspects of the study included the observation that NK cells or lymphokine-activated NK cells (so-called LAK cells) were more effective at inducing killing of tubercle bacilli than T cells, that this activity was not MHC restricted, and that direct cell-cell contact was not required for the effect—supernatants were adequate. The leading candidate for this soluble factor that promotes intracellular killing is TNF-α. The authors speculated that the NK cell activity had been promoted (in a circular manner) by IL-12 released by the infected monocytes.

Given nature's economy of function(s), it seems probable that NK cells do participate in both early and ongoing protective immunity against tuberculosis. Whether, as suggested by Yoneda and Ellner (64), NK cell function is of particular importance in purified protein derivative (PPD)–negative persons, presumably early in the primary infection phase, is speculative.

Chemokines

As described in two recent reviews (65,66), chemokines are a family of structurally related, small proteins that seem to elicit in-migration of a variety of circulating and tissue leukocytes. In addition to drawing leukocytes into a circumscribed area, these substances may promote leukocyte activation, other antimicrobial functions, and enriched vascularization—all central components of host defense.

This "chemokine system" may be thought of in terms of the following component functions: (a) drawing leukocytes toward the area of interest (chemoattractant or chemotaxis functions); (b) causing changes in the local vascular endothelium that lead to adherence of circulating leukocytes in the vascular channel; and (c) promoting diapodesis of these leukocytes through loosened endothelial junctions.

A partial listing of factors believed to participate in the defense against tuberculosis appears in Appendix 4.1. Given the volume of research and rapidity of change within this field, it is probable that extensive additions or revisions will soon be necessary.

Cytokines

Like the chemokines, as noted above, cytokines are comprised of several groups of low-molecular-weight proteins. These molecules locally mediate inflammation, cell growth, immunity, and tissue repair. Among the cytokine families are interleukins, interferons, tumor necrosis factors, and growth factors (see Table 4.2 for an exposition of cytokines currently held to be active in tuberculous immuno-pathogenesis).

In addition to the overview in Table 4.2, below is a more detailed discussion of three cytokines that appear to have a particularly prominent role in this process. Of additional interest, recent studies have indicated that either normal variations ("polymorphisms") or dysfunctional mutations in these three systems—IFN-γ, TNF-α, or IL-12—cause increased susceptibility to tuberculosis and/or other mycobacterial infections (see "Genetically Determined Immune Deficiencies Associated with Extreme Susceptibility to Mycobacterial Disease: Clinical Observations").

Interferon-γ and 1,25 dihydroxy-vitamin D_3

Clearly, IFN-γ is a major component of the optimal immunity associated with the Th1 pathway. Produced and released primarily by $CD4^+$ T lymphocytes, it may also be generated by NK cells, $CD8^+$ cells and, to a lesser extent, B lymphocytes. Triggers for IFN-γ elaboration include other cytokines such as IL-2 and IL-12. Primary target cells and the effects produced by IFN-γ include the following:

- Macrophages: activation, MHC receptor expression, IL-1, and TNF-α production.
- $CD4^+$ Lymphs: differentiation toward Th1 pathway functions.
- $CD8^+$ Lymphs: enhanced cytotoxic function.
- NK cells: activation, enhanced cytotoxic function, and production of more IFN-γ.

IFN-γ alone has been demonstrated to induce tuberculostasis in the murine macrophage system; however, it does not have comparable effects in human monocytes (67,68) or alveolar macrophages (69). Rook et al. (70) have shown an independent tuberculostatic effect from physiological concentrations of 1,25 dihydroxy- vitamin D_3 [1,25$(OH)_2D_3$] and an additive effect in concert with IFN-γ in young monocytes. Crowle et al. (71) showed a significant impact on tuberculostasis in mature macrophages with concentrations of 1,25 $(OH)_2D_3$ that exceed physiological serum levels but are potentially achievable within granulomas where activated macrophages are converting 25$(OH)D_3$ to the active metabolite. [While this may be far-fetched, these findings raise the possibility that the focus on "heliotherapy" (sunshine) in the latter 19th and early 20th centuries may have been efficacious through the enhancing effects of vitamin D on cellular immune function. Similarly, the wide-spread use in sanatoria of great quantities of milk and cod-liver oil, substances very rich in vitamin D, also may have amplified this effect.]

Two recent clinical studies examined the role of IFN-γ in pulmonary tuberculosis. Taha et al. (52) in Montreal performed bronchoscopy and obtained BAL fluid in 10 patients with active tuberculosis and compared them with 25 subjects deemed to have inactive prior tuberculosis. The authors found among active disease patients increased numbers of circulating $CD8^+$ T cells and significantly higher percentages of BAL cells expressing messenger RNA for IFN-γ and IL-12. The $CD8^+$ preponderance has not been previously noted, but the elevated levels of mRNA for IFN-γ and IL-12 were reported previously (39). The presence of these two cytokines together probably is not coincidental, since IL-12 induces IFN-γ production by T cells and NK cells. Sodhi et al. (51) in Los Angeles studied 106 patients with various forms of pulmonary and extrapulmonary tuberculosis. Unlike the Montreal study, they examined IFN-γ levels in the PBMs. Basically, they observed that, while patients with localized or limited tuberculosis had very high levels of PBM IFN-γ, those with progressively more extensive or disseminated diseases had diminishing levels of this cytokine. Regarding the source of the IFN-γ, they did not find any correlation with $CD4^+$ cell counts, which implied that $CD8^+$ cells had produced it.

Overall, the central role of IFN-γ is readily apparent. However, it is not wholly apparent whether the observation that diminished levels of IFN-γ in patients with more severe tuberculosis is causally related. Certainly, in the patients described later (see "Genetically Determined Immune Deficiencies Associated with Extreme Susceptibility to Mycobacterial Disease: Clinical Observations"), IFN-γ deficiencies played a pivotal role in pathogenesis; however, in the patients described above by Sodhi et al., it is possible that the patients failed to contain their disease for reasons other than limited IFN-γ

production. Also, the lower levels of the cytokine measured in these patients may simply have reflected the suppressor activity noted with far-advanced disease.

Tumor Necrosis Factor-α

TNF-α is primarily produced by monocytes and macrophages. Its elaboration is typically triggered by infectious agents or soluble substances such as IL-1, GM-CSF, platelet activating factor, or interferons. It acts on many cell systems, but in the cellular immune system its primary targets are the T cells. Monocyte-derived macrophages infected with tubercle bacilli elaborate TNF-α, which results in both autocrine stimulation and the attraction of T lymphocytes. Lipoarabinomannan, a constituent of the cell wall of *M. tuberculosis,* is a lipopolysaccharide (LPS) that has properties similar to the LPS of gram-negative bacteria in terms of inducing TNF-α release (16,72,73). However, LAM from virulent strains of *M. tuberculosis* appears to elicit significantly less TNF-α release from monocytes than LAM from avirulent strains (16). This may in fact be a mycobacterial virulence tactic. LAM is not the only constituent of tubercle bacilli to elicit TNF-α production; a 58-kd novel protein caused TNF-α production from human monocytes (74).

The importance of TNF in effective immune responses has been shown via several experimental pathways. In a murine model, anti-TNF antibodies blocked the development of granulomas and bactericidal activity following BCG infection (75). Also, in the murine model, Bloom's group in New York City (76) has recently shown that reducing TNF-α activity by monoclonal antibody to TNF-α or a genetic deficiency of TNF-α receptors was associated with increased vulnerability to infection with *M. tuberculosis,* impaired production of reactive nitrogen intermediates, and abnormal granuloma formulation marked by the absence of "epithelioid cells." Similarly, using a TNF receptor–expressing adenovirus to antagonize TNF activity, another group (77) demonstrated substantial worsening of both acute and chronic tuberculosis in a murine model.

Rom and colleagues (40) in New York have focused interest on the role of TNF-α (and IL-1β) in the pathogenesis of tuberculosis. In 1996, they reported a comparison of the results of BAL studies in 26 patients with tuberculosis and 6 normal volunteers. They found that BAL fluid from focally involved lobes demonstrated increased levels of TNF-α, IL-1β, and IL-6, compared with noninvolved lobes, lobes involved with miliary tuberculosis, or normal controls. Their data are probably divergent from those of the Los Angeles group noted above who found increased mRNA for IFN-γ and IL-12 but *not* for TNF (51); the uncertainty arises in part from methodological differences. Rom's group commented that these elevated cytokine levels presumably represented a granulomatous immune response. Particularly interesting aspects of their observations included extremely high levels of TNF-α from the lobes of three patients in which extensive cavity formation was occurring; this is consistent with the notion that TNF-α, through its potent thrombogenic properties, may precipitate extensive tissue necrosis. Also, the absence of elevated cytokines in the lobes involved with miliary tuberculosis suggests a severely depressed immune response in these cases.

TNF, also referred to as "cachectin" for its capacity to induce profound wasting (78), belongs to a family of ligands with profound biological roles (79). TNF and its related ligands, which activate various receptors, can initiate cellular proliferation or apoptotic death. TNF, as well as lymphotoxin-α, uniquely binds to two receptors (of 55 and 75 kd, respectively). Activation of the 55-kd receptor causes apoptosis and tumor necrosis, and the 75-kd receptor invokes T-cell proliferation. Both can induce fever. Because of the major biological effects of this system, there is ongoing study of methods to modify or block these pathways. Bazzoni and Beutler (79) reviewed this topic in 1996. Other aspects of TNF that merit consideration in relation to tuberculosis include genetic polymorphisms. Vulnerability to a variety of disorders has been related to genetic polymorphisms of TNF including cerebral malaria (80), dermatitis herpetiformis (81), and chronic bronchitis (82). The allele shown to be associated with chronic bronchitis, TNF-α, is associated also with HLA-DR3 (83,84); this may be somehow related to the putative vulnerability to tuberculosis described with HLA-DR2 (see "Cellular Immunity and the Major Histocompatibility Complex: Animal Models and Human Observations").

Interleukin-12

IL-12 is primarily produced by monocytes and macrophages. Its elaboration is promoted by encounters of these cells with intracellular bacteria or parasites. Effects of IL-12 include promoting type 0 T-helper (Th0) cells to proliferate and produce IL-2 and inducing Th1 cells to elaborate IFN-γ and TNF-α. In addition, IL-12 inhibits Th2 cells and thereby suppresses production of IL-4, IL-5, and IL-10. It apparently plays a major role in the development of effective antimycobacterial immunity by (a) promoting the differentiation and proliferation of CD4 Th1 cells from uncommitted T cells and (b) stimulation of IFN-γ production from those Th1 CD4 cells, as well as NK cells. Recently, in a mouse model, genetic susceptibility to disseminated *M. avium* complex infection was found to be associated with decreased IL-12 expression (85). Subsequently, a European group reported on four patients with unexplained disseminated mycobacterioses, *M. avium* complex or BCG, which were associated with defective immunity related to IL-12 receptor deficiency (86,87). The infected subjects were able to form granulomas, but their activated T cells and NK cells had reduced levels of IFN-γ. This information points toward an essential role for IL-12 function in tuberculoimmunity.

Activated Macrophages and Mechanisms of Mycobacterial Inhibition

Presumably, the final or most significant step in the complex choreography described above is the capacity of the principal effector cells of the cellular immune system, PBM-derived macrophages, to engulf/inhibit/kill the invading mycobacteria.

Despite long-standing and intense investigations, the precise mechanisms by which human macrophages perform this task remain incompletely understood. Current debate focuses largely on the potential roles of reactive oxygen intermediates (ROIs) versus reactive nitrogen intermediates (RNIs). There is clear evidence in the mouse model that RNIs play a major, if not exclusive, role in this regard (88–91). However, the contribution of RNIs to human defenses against tuberculosis (and other infections) has been more difficult to demonstrate (92). Although cells isolated from the blood of humans with tuberculosis have consistently failed to express inducible nitric oxide synthetase (iNOS), the keystone to the high-output pathway of RNI generation in the mouse, a recent study of alveolar macrophages obtained by BAL from patients with pulmonary tuberculosis indicated this pathway to be present (93). Using a new antibody marker, 65% of alveolar macrophages from 11 of 11 patients studied were found to express iNOS. In addition, by diaphorase cytochemistry, this group demonstrated presumptive evidence of nitric oxide enzymatic activity. The authors speculated that part of microbial virulence or host susceptibility may be related to the capacity to downregulate or induce this pathway. Additional evidence in support of a role of RNIs in immunity against tuberculosis is the observation from Taiwan of increased levels of nitric oxide in the exhaled gases of patients with active tuberculosis (94). The researchers also noted that the alveolar macrophages of tuberculosis patients had increased expression of inducible NO synthase, which was related to the concentration of exhaled NO. However, another group (95) reported that the ability of human alveolar macrophages to inhibit replication of *M. bovis* or *M. tuberculosis* H37Ra was not found to be related to NO (95). At present, it seems reasonable to infer that the RNIs play some role in the human defenses against tuberculosis, but it is difficult to weigh their contributions compared with ROIs.

Evidence in support of the role of ROIs in human defenses against tuberculosis may be adduced from studies of isoniazid (INH)–susceptible or –resistant strains. As noted in Chapter 11, INH is a pro-drug; its active metabolite is apparently released by the activity of the tubercle bacillus catalase-peroxidase enzymes (96). These enzymes are also critical in protecting the bacilli from direct injury by ROIs. This creates a potential biological dilemma for the bacillus:

what happens if it acquires INH-resistance by deletion of this vital enzyme?

M. tuberculosis acquires resistance to INH via two common mechanisms: (a) mutations/deletions in the *katG* locus, which result in loss of catalase-peroxidase activity and high-level INH resistance, and (b) mutation/deletions in the *inhA* locus, which do not eliminate catalase-peroxidase activity, and result in low-level resistance to INH (see Table 11.2). Of relevance, strains of *M. tuberculosis* with INH resistance associated with loss of catalase-peroxidase activity, presumably mediated by *katG* mutations, have diminished virulence in animal models (97). In support of this concept was the recent demonstration that expression of *katG* by *M. tuberculosis* was associated with the capacity of the bacilli to replicate and persist in two animal models, mice and guinea pigs (23). Further support for the important role of catalase-peroxidase in virulence in humans may be inferred from the lethal epidemic of multidrug-resistant tuberculosis in New York City associated with strain W (98); strain W, despite INH resistance associated with a rare *katG* mutation, retained its catalase-peroxidase activity (see Chapter 11).

From these observations, I infer that in humans ROIs probably play a significant role in the intracellular inhibition/killing of mycobacteria. Additional data in support of some role for ROIs in defense against tuberculosis include a murine knockout model of X-linked chronic granulomatous disease in which neutrophils are incapable of generating ROIs (99); such mice had increased susceptibility to intravenous inoculation with *M. tuberculosis.* Similarly, among eight male long-term survivors of chronic granulomatous disease (CGD) in Hong Kong, six developed recurrent, intractable tuberculosis (100). Of note, deficient oxidative-burst is found not only in neutrophils of patients with CGD, but also in other phagocytic cells.

Endogenous Immunosuppressive Mechanisms and Immunopathogenesis

To prevent excessive tissue damage, all inflammatory pathways have inherent suppressor arms. Exploring this topic has at least two apparent objectives: (a) to determine whether tubercle bacilli, in some instances, cause excessive suppressor activity that works favorably for pathogenesis and (b) to explore means to control tissue injury by downregulating inflammation. The former topic is explored here, and the latter, in Chapter 13.

A European study (101) has demonstrated that human alveolar macrophages produce a substance that inhibits the effects of IL-1, the cytokine produced by these same alveolar macrophages to attract T lymphocytes and facilitate antigen presentation. This substance, interleukin-1 receptor antagonist (IL-1ra), acts by binding to the IL-1 receptor. The investigators found that IL-1ra is normally produced after the macrophage has elaborated IL-1, presumably as an integral, self-limiting measure. However, under stimulation from IL-4 (a substance produced by Th2 CD4 cells) there was early and enhanced production of IL-1ra and reduced production of IL-1, potentially a mechanism to preserve the lung from excessive inflammation. A recent report from the Netherlands (102) showed that among patients with active tuberculosis there were increased serum levels of IL-1ra, but not of another potential inhibitor, soluble IL-1 receptor.

Another mechanism for downregulating immune inflammatory processes entails suppression of the T-cell proliferative response to tuberculoprotein and elaboration of IL-2 through the effects of newly released monocytes and a specific population of lymphocytes (103–108). This response involves, in part, production of increased IL-2 receptors (IL-2r) by these newly released monocytes. The IL-2r molecules, both on the monocyte cell wall membrane and free in the serum, may blunt the effects of IL-2 elaborated by activated T cells. This pattern has been described in anergic patients with active tuberculosis.

Ellner and colleagues in Cleveland, through a series of elegant studies, have identified transforming growth factor-β1 (TGF-β1), a product of activated mononuclear phagocytes, as a potential candidate for the downregulation of the protective immune response. In their initial study (107) of this cytokine in 1994, they noted that PMNs infected with *M. tuberculosis* released both IFN-γ and TGF-β1. They observed that

TGF-β1 antagonized the inhibitory effects of both IFN-γ and TNF-α on intracellular bacillary proliferation and that neutralizing antibodies to TGF-β1 improved monocyte bacteriostasis. Production of TGF-β1 by monocytes from tuberculin-negative individuals when stimulated by PPD was also demonstrated (109). Subsequently, production of TGF-β1 by PBMs and the presence of the cytokine in granulomatous lesions in the lungs of patients with active tuberculosis were documented (110). Of particular interest, it was next shown that an important constituent of the tubercle bacillus cell wall, the lipoarabinomannan moiety, played a central role in the elaboration of TGF-β1 by monocytes/macrophages (111). Intriguing was the observation that LAM from the prototypic laboratory virulent strain, H37Rv, elicited increased TGF-β and limited TNF-α, IL-1, and IL-6 production by the monocytes/macrophages. By contrast, the LAM from the avirulent strain, H37Ra, elicited robust production of both the TGF-β and the proimmunity cytokines. LAM from H37Rv is distinctive for extensive mannosyl capping of the terminal arabinose chains. In 1996, Hirsch et al. (112) reported on a series of tuberculosis patients from Pakistan, observing that, early in the course of treatment, their PBMs manifested depressed responses to antigenic stimulation and diminished production of IFN-γ. This correlated with higher levels of TGF-β. This phenomenon began to subside after treatment for more than one month. The next phase in the group's investigation of the role of TGF-β in facilitating pathogenesis entailed analysis of two naturally occurring inhibitors of TGF-β, decorin and latency-associated peptide (LAP) (113). Both of these molecules restored T-cell response to antigens and mitogens, as well as enhancing production of IFN-γ by PBMs from patients with active tuberculosis. The authors proposed these agents as candidates for immunomodulating therapy.

Other evidence of complementary suppressor activity includes the role of IL-10 in promoting downregulation of proimmune responses (113, 114), circulating serum inhibitors of TNF-α (102); demonstration of impaired T-cell response to various specific peptides from *M. tuberculosis,* which was found to be related to the type and extent of disease (115); and the finding of progressively lower levels of production of IFN-γ by monocytes/macrophages from patients with more severe or disseminated disease (51).

Overall, the evidence clearly documents the presence of counterregulatory mechanisms to limit the inflammatory immune responses to *M. tuberculosis* infection. It might be anticipated that as part of its virulence/survival strategy, the tubercle bacillus would have evolved mechanisms to use these downregulating activities to its advantage. Study of these relationships will certainly afford insight into the pathogenesis of tuberculosis; whether this information can be employed to help with the development of improved vaccines or the immunomodulatory management of patients remains uncertain (116).

Humoral Immunity (Including Complement) in Tuberculosis

As indicated, the great preponderance of evidence and virtually all contemporary authorities indicate that cell-mediated immunity is central to human defenses against tuberculosis. Humoral immunity—and the corollary of "serum therapy"—has essentially been discounted. However, Glatman-Friedman and Casadevall (117) have recently reassessed the 20th century literature on this topic and concluded that there may be relevance and efficacy to these approaches. Among the more plausible linkages are the potential roles of antibodies and complement to promote uptake by macrophages and to influence phagosome-lysosome relations. Also worth reconsideration is the "cause-*or*-effect" relationship between clinical deterioration and the apparent shift to a Th2 pathway with rising antibody titers.

Neutrophils and Platelets

Similar to humoral immunity, the role or contributions of neutrophils to antituberculosis defense have largely been ignored in recent science. However, in an experimental model of tuberculous pleurisy in rabbits, the initial cells elicited into the pleural space are polymorphonuclear leukocytes (118). Other data are consistent also with some circumscribed role(s) for PMNs in the protective response.

Studies in beige mice, which have a variety of immunological defects including poor oxidative burst in PMNs, have indicated that transfusion of neutrophils from their normal immunological kindred, C57BL/6, conferred enhanced capacity to control *M. avium* infection (119). Also, in vitro exposure to granulocyte colony-stimulating factor (G-CSF) or GM-CSF of human neutrophils from both HIV-negative and AIDS patients prompted intracellular inhibition of *M. avium* complex (120).

Riedel and Kaufmann (121) demonstrated that human PMNs, when stimulated by uptake of *M. tuberculosis* or exposure to LAM, release two potent chemokines: IL-8, which attracts a broad array of effector cells, and GRO-α, a specific chemoattractant for PMNs. Similarly, Kasahara et al. (122) demonstrated that PMNs from tuberculin-positive humans, when stimulated with *M. tuberculosis* or PPD, elaborated IL-8 and an additional chemokine, macrophage inflammatory protein-1α. Of particular interest in the latter report, the incubation of PMNs with *M. tuberculosis* or PPD *and* TNF-α induced rapid death of the PMNs.

My interpretation of these data is that PMNs act like early sentries that react to the invading mycobacteria by initiating an inflammatory process with emphasis on chemokines, which summon other more relevant cells to the battle. Their role in the latter phases of the struggle remains uncertain.

The role of thrombocytes or platelets in the defense against or pathogenesis of tuberculosis has long been ignored. A report from France (123) in 1959 described a series of studies in which various animals were injected with tubercle bacilli or *M. bovis* BCG. The authors observed that injected mycobacteria were found agglutinated with platelets in the capillaries of the skin and viscera of the animals. In the 1959 report, it was noted that human platelets ex vivo also clumped with mycobacteria, that this process was facilitated by plasma but not serum, and that immunization with BCG amplified this process.

Recently, Yeaman (124) reviewed the roles of platelets in various infectious conditions noting that platelets exhibited structural and functional characteristics of host defense cells, not simply agents of hemostasis. However, no recent information sheds light on the role(s) of platelets in the immunopathogenesis of tuberculosis.

GENETIC CONTROL OF SUSCEPTIBILITY OR RESISTANCE TO TUBERCULOSIS

Mouse and rabbit models of tuberculosis document substantial differences in susceptibility/resistance to the infection among various animal strains, phenomena which are clearly under the hosts' genetic controls (2). Among humans, tightly defined genetic pedigrees and controlled exposures are not possible. Therefore, any estimation of the genetic bases for human resistance/susceptibility must be based on an amalgam of epidemiological and biological observations. And, given the multitude of nonbiological factors that play upon the probabilities of primary infection, reinfection, and progression to active disease, the "truly genetic" susceptibility/resistance must be at least partially obscured under real-life conditions.

Epidemiological Observations

Like many other infectious diseases, tuberculosis, when introduced into a population not previously exposed, typically produces an intense epidemic with high morbidity and mortality (108,125). The potential implications of tuberculosis epidemics for population genetics can be seen from the following observations.

During acute outbreaks, postadolescent individuals have been seen to be particularly prone to disease, women slightly more than men. In the prechemotherapy era, patients with moderate- to far-advanced pulmonary disease had 5-year survival rates of less than 50%. Thus, persons who were "genetically susceptible" were more likely to die of the disease and, because of their age, be precluded from reproducing. In this darwinian scenario, there would be a selective advantage for the resistant phenotype, dramatically referred to as "survival of the fittest." Over time, then, populations would shift toward a collectively less vulnerable gene pool, and one would predict the subsidence of the epidemic. In the case of tuberculosis, this sequence plays out over a considerably longer period than acute, lethal epidemics like the bubonic plague, cholera, or influenza. Indeed, in large populations like Europe or North America, the epidemic cycles during the prechemotherapy era entailed several centuries (108).

This natural selection process presumably works *within* racially uniform groups to promote the resistant phenotypes (*intragroup* selection). But it might also be expected to operate to promote differences in susceptibility/resistance between races or ethnic groups, if these populations have disparate exposures to the infectious agent (*inter-group* variation). Hence, differences in susceptibility to tuberculosis could be anticipated in this model among 20th century European/North American whites (among whom epidemic tuberculosis—"consumption"—had been operating for over 300 years) and African blacks (into whom tuberculosis was substantially introduced only in the 19th century) (126,127). Clinicians in the United States had suspected that African Americans were more vulnerable to tuberculosis, but it was very difficult to separate biological factors from socioeconomic, environmental, and nutritional components.

Stead et al. (128), in analyzing patterns of tuberculin skin test reactivity in nursing homes and prisons, made a fascinating observation: given comparable levels of exposure to infectious cases, blacks were twice as likely to become infected (as reflected by skin test conversion). Once "infected," both populations developed active tuberculosis at the same rates. The authors' inference from these data, with which I concur, was that there is a significant intergroup, genetically controlled difference in susceptibility/resistance to tuberculosis. Direct data that might support this hypothesis are seen in a report from The Gambia in West Africa (129), in which certain allelic variations in the *NRAMP1* gene were associated with susceptibility to tuberculosis. Of note, one of these *NRAMP1* polymorphisms is far more common in Africans than Europeans (see below).

The most persuasive line of evidence in support of a genetic role in susceptibility is the study of twins and other family members. Kallman and Reisner (130) reported in 1943 the results of a large and remarkably sophisticated analysis of this topic from New York City. Studying 308 twin pairs (78 monozygotic and 230 dizygotic), along with 930 full siblings, 74 half-siblings, 688 parents, and 266 marriage partners of the twins, the authors observed that "the chance of developing tuberculosis increases in strict proportion to the degree of blood relationship to a tuberculous index case." It was 3.5 times more likely for both monozygotic twins than for both dizygotic twins to have tuberculosis. The authors concluded that "the morbidity distribution in the sibling groups indicate that resistance to tuberculosis is modified by a heredoconstitutional mechanism which seems to be multifactorial in its genetic nature."

By contrast, a study of the influence of twinship on the risk of tuberculosis in the United Kingdom, part of the Prophit Survey, concluded *initially* that the association among monozygotic twins was not genetically mediated, but due to greater contact, more sputum smear-positive disease, and a higher percentage of females who were deemed more vulnerable among the monozygotic twins (131). However, Comstock (132) reanalyzed these data employing multiple-regression analysis and concluded that concordance for tuberculosis was significantly higher for monozygotic than for dizygotic twins—a twofold excess risk.

Macrophages and Preimmune Resistance: Animal Models and Human Observations

Assuming that the apparent variable in susceptibility/resistance among blacks in the United States is the propensity to become infected when exposed, the mouse model, of *M. bovis* (BCG) infection is worth consideration as a *possible* analogue. In the murine model, the vulnerability to *infection* per se has *not* been examined. Rather, the defining trait has been a quantitative difference in organ loads of bacilli following standard intravenous challenge (this is the same phenomenon noted by Lurie and Dannenberg in the rabbit model). Following intravenous injection of BCG, various strains of mice demonstrate widely differing levels of resistance to invasion by and proliferation of bacilli (133).

These differences apparently manifest themselves in *two phases*. The first phase is discussed in this section; the latter phase is discussed below (see "Cellular Immunity and the Major Histocompatibility Complex: Animal Models and Human Observations").

The *initial phase*, 0 to 3 weeks after infection, is shown by either rapid proliferation or substantial curtailment of the numbers of bacilli in the reticuloendothelial system (134); this phenomenon has been subsequently shown to reside in the mononuclear phagocyte/macrophage cell line and to be under genetic control of a locus on murine chromosome 1 (135). The two alleles of this locus were named Bcg_r (resistant) and Bcg_s (susceptible). Later studies in the mouse model found that the genetic locus Bcg_r was associated with resistance to two other unrelated intracellular pathogens, *Salmonella typhimurium* and *Leishmania donovani* (133). Ongoing studies (136) identified a candidate gene for this phenotype, the *n*atural *r*esistance-*a*ssociated *m*acrophage *p*rotein *(Nramp)*. The authors presented evidence that *Nramp* was a cell-membrane–associated transporter protein and speculated that it might function in relationship to intracellular movement of reactive nitrogen intermediates (136).

These observations on early, preimmune resistance in mice are consistent with the observations of Stead et al. (128) on the epidemiology of tuberculosis among black and white humans in the United States. As noted above, observing rates of conversion of the tuberculin skin test among residents of nursing homes and inmates of prisons as the indictor of "new infection," Stead et al. concluded that blacks were roughly twice as likely to become infected following a known exposure. If, indeed, there were a genetic resistance factor analogous to the Bcg_r which was unequally distributed among whites and blacks (and other persons of color), this might *partially* explain the disparate rates of tuberculosis among these groups. (And, if this resistance factor conferred protection against other intracellular pathogens, it might also be an element in the apparently greater resistance of whites against diseases such as leprosy and coccidiomycosis.) Assuming an innately more competent alveolar macrophage, inhaled tubercle bacillus that reached the alveolus of a white individual might be engulfed and inhibited before a sufficiently extensive infection could be established to provoke the remainder of the cellular immune response that results in DTH (e.g., a positive tuberculin skin test result would not ensue) (127). Circumstantial evidence in support of this hypothetical model includes the observations by Crowle and Elkins (137) that macrophages derived from peripheral blood mononuclear cells from a small number of whites were *less* permissive for intracellular replication by *M. tuberculosis* than were macrophages from a few blacks.

Given the above observations and issues, the report of increased susceptibility to tuberculosis among blacks from The Gambia with certain allelic variations of the *NRAMP1* gene (the human equivalent to the murine *Nramp* gene) is of great interest (129). Whether the *NRAMP1* gene mediates this effect through RNI pathways or other mechanisms relating to phagolysosomal function is unclear (138). Susceptibility to leprosy also has been linked to *NRAMP1* polymorphism among a population of Vietnamese (139); however, failure to find such linkage among other races suggests that human resistance to mycobacterial infections is polygenic.

Cellular Immunity and the Major Histocompatibility Complex: Animal Models and Human Observations

As noted above (see "Lymphocyte Types, Subsets, and Function in Immunopathogenesis"), the MHC genetic loci may have potentially powerful influences on the nature and capability of a host's immune response to a given pathogen.

In "Macrophages and Preimmune Reistance: Animal Models and Human Observations," genetic control of the mouse's preimmune, macrophage-dependent defense against BCG invasion was shown to reside on chromosome 1. The resistant allele, Bcg_r, was associated with control of the number of bacilli in the animal's reticuloendothelial system during weeks 0 to 3 after infection. By contrast, during the *late phase,* 3 to 6 weeks after infection, resistance is manifested by varying levels of protection against subsequent rechallenge with BCG and *L. monocytogenes,* the vigor with which granulomas are formed, and the extent and duration of DTH reactions to PPD (140). Paradoxically, it was found that the Bcg_s strain of mice had relatively greater capacity for these *late-phase* elements of cellular immunity, including DTH, granuloma formation, and protection against reinfection with homologous or heterologous pathogens (141). The authors contended that this component of host defense is not under control of the macrophage-dependent *Bcg* locus, but rather, appears to be determined by genetically derived MHC variables (141).

Multiple studies have analyzed groups of tuberculosis patients and variably suitable control populations for the presence of MHC human leukocyte antigen (HLA) determined markers of susceptibility or resistance to the disease. Widely diverse outcomes have been reported, and it is very difficult to draw strong conclusions from these data. As noted in Appendix 4.1, the genetic control of the MHC Class II system resides in three genes, HLA-DR, HLA-DQ, and HLA-DP.

One interesting, recurrent theme is the apparent association of HLA-DR2 with vulnerability to tuberculosis. Among families in India with extensive patterns of tuberculosis, DR2 was found in excess among family members with active disease (142). Subsequently, among patients with sputum smear-positive tuberculosis in Indonesia, HLA-DR2 and HLA DQwl were found in excessive frequencies (143); of added interest, high titers of antibodies to two epitopes of the 38-kd protein were found in association with DR2. Another study from India (144) also indicated that DR2 was not only associated with apparent risk for active tuberculosis, but also with a particular risk for far-advanced, smear-positive disease. An additional study from India (145) indicated similar findings: HLA-DR2 was present more frequently in tuberculosis patients than in a control population. Among tuberculosis patients, HLA-DR2 was associated with higher rates of treatment failure (relative risk, 3.7). These latter reports raise the possibility that DR2 is associated with an immune response dominated by the Th2 cell, which—in leprosy—is associated with relatively ineffectual cellular immunity, bacillary proliferation, extensive tissue damage, and a prominent humoral immune response. A survey of children from the former Soviet Republic of Tuva also noted increased frequencies of HLA-DR2 and HLA-DRw53 in association with tuberculosis (146).

A recent study from Cambodia (147) found another apparent association between a different allele, HLA-DQB1*0503, and vulnerability to tuberculosis. Notably, this analysis did *not* find an association between two TNF-α alleles and the risk of tuberculosis.

One of the studies from India (144) and others (148–150) have reportedly found associations between the MHC class I determining loci HLA-A or HLA-B. However, other studies have failed to confirm such an association (151,152).

Overall, it seems probable that MHC cell membrane elements are associated at some level with the risk of developing active tuberculosis once infected, and also with the form and severity of disease that ensues. However, given the number of other biological variables (e.g., nutrition, associated diseases) and clinical variables (e.g., time from onset of illness to diagnosis and treatment, adequacy of chemotherapy and other supportive care), it is unlikely that these elements will play dominant roles in the epidemiology and manifestations of tuberculosis in the present era. Nonetheless, further investigations into this arena may shed considerable light on the important variables in the defense against this disease, possibly with implications for vaccine development.

Genetically Determined Immune Deficiencies Associated with Extreme Susceptibility to Mycobacterial Infections: Clinical Observations

Among practitioners of tuberculosis the strong impressions of familial (genetic) susceptibility to the disease have existed over the ages, including such dramatic examples as the deaths from consumption of an entire generation of the famous Brontë children. However, with the exception of the studies of twins and the MHC/HLA analyses cited earlier, few studies have analyzed direct or surrogate markers of genetically controlled immune capacity in families, the presumption being that clustered morbidity reflected extensive exposures or particularly virulent strains of tuberculosis.

However, when disseminated disease or familial clusters of disease occur as a result of nontuberculous mycobacteria (NTM) (organisms of substantially less pathogenic capacity than *M. tuberculosis*), attention has been given to the immune systems of these patients. Two recent reports of familial clusters of disseminated disease attributable to NTM offer insights into the roles of various cell lines and cytokines in our defenses against mycobacteria. Holland et al. (153) from the National Institutes of Health reported seven patients with refractory, disseminated infection with NTM; four cases were unrelated and were associated with idiopathic CD4 lymphopenia and three cases were from a single family. Studies of the family members demonstrated reduced production of both IL-2 and INF-γ by cultured PBMs when stimulated in vitro by phytohemagglutinin. Also, all of these cases responded well to therapy with IFN-γ. Similarly, Levin et al. (154) reported on two familial clusters of childhood disseminated NTM disease in three patients from Malta and two of Greek Cypriot origin. Among the patients and parents in the latter report a variety of abnormalities was found in mononuclear phagocyte and cytokine studies, including the following: (a) Like the NIH patients, peripheral blood mononuclear cells produced lower amounts of IFN-γ when stimulated (in this case, by both recall and mycobacterial antigens); and (b) whole-blood aliquots, when stimulated by IFN-γ, produced abnormally low amounts of TNF-α. In this report, total T-cell numbers and subsets were noted, as well as B cells, NK cells, and monocytes. T-cell proliferation to phytohemagglutinin (PHA) assays among patients was initially normal in four of six patients; in one of the two patients with a low response during illness, T-cell proliferation normalized after treatment, which included anti-microbials and IFN-γ.

The authors of the latter report initially suggested that they might have identified a genetic anomaly similar to the Bcg_s murine locus described above. Subsequently, though, they reported that it was a mutation of the IFN-γ receptor gene that promoted the susceptibility (155). They demonstrated that this receptor defect resulted in failure of macrophages to upregulate production of TNF-α after exposure to IFN-γ. This group (156) also reported another case wherein a Tunisian infant with the IFN-γ–receptor deficiency died of disseminated BCG infection. Another report (157) documented a French child with IFN-γ–receptor deficiency who died of a disseminated nontuberculous mycobacterial infection attributable to *Mycobacterium smegmatis*.

Reviewing these cases in the aggregate, one is led to believe that these accidents of nature highlight the critical role of certain elements of the hosts' defenses against mycobacteria. The relationship of these cases to tuberculosis in normal hosts is unclear. Regarding the prominence of BCG or NTM infections rather than tuberculosis in these series, it is likely that such persons simply are much more likely to come into contact with these potentially pathogenic mycobacteria than with the *M. tuberculosis*.

LOCALIZATION OF IMMUNITY WITH THE LUNGS

One of the truly remarkable aspects of tuberculosis is a phenomenon that clinicians see routinely but rarely comment on. In the prechemotherapy era or, more recently, in cases with drug-resistant disease refractory to treatment, some patients have demonstrated prolonged localization of disease to one lobe (or segment) of the lung, despite spewing hundreds of thousands of bacilli about their bronchial tree during daily fits of coughing. Sputum from patients with smear-positive disease contains, routinely, 1 to 10 million mycobacteria per milliliter (see Chapter 2 for details). Cough helps propel secretions out of the airways, but a paroxysm of coughing only partially expels this matter. Also, every fit of coughing is inevitably followed by a deep, rapid inspiration. This process inevitably must lead to the dispersed delivery of droplets and phlegm laden with mycobacteria through other regions of the lungs, including the terminal airspaces. Yet, no evident disease appears in these regions, while inches away, identical bacilli are prospering in cavities and progressively injuring the abutting lung tissue.

This may seem mundane, but I believe there is rich scientific capital in this observation. A group from Bellevue Hospital in New York City (42) recently explored this issue, reporting on local immune responses within the lungs of tuberculosis patients. The researchers noted diverse cell populations in the various regions or within the same anatomical region at different stages of disease. To follow patients (or suitable animal models) in order to determine why the disease remains localized in some cases and in other cases it spread should provide an extraordinary laboratory of immunopathogenesis. What is the role of bleeding in propagation of the infection? Is it merely that the hemorrhagic fluid is more easily nebulized within the lungs, or does the iron from the hemoglobin enrich mycobacterial growth and interfere with monocyte/macrophage function? What local shifts in cellular or cytokine constituents presage the evolution of a new disease focus?

Perhaps there are simple mechanical explanations for the seeming paradox (e.g., the number of bacilli or size of particles delivered), but I suspect that truly significant insights into the disease reside in this clinical conundrum.

IMMUNE MEMORY AND TUBERCULOSIS REACTIVATION

Most of Chapter 4 has addressed the immediate immune response to a new infection or the struggle between a host and active disease. However, a more important question concerns the puzzle of remote reactivation of a latent tuberculous infection. The clear majority of cases of tuberculosis in adults are due to reactivation of an infection with *M. tuberculosis* that was acquired and *successfully dealt with* years or decades earlier. In some instances, the cause is apparent: vitiation of cellular defenses by an immunosuppressive disease or treatment (e.g., AIDS, organ transplantation). In other cases, however, the cause is not readily apparent. In Chapter 5, epidemiological observations on risk factors for reactivation are discussed. However, it is important, as well, to consider direct observations on long-term cellular immunity in animal models.

Orme and other researchers at Colorado State University (CSU) have conducted a series of studies on the mechanisms of antituberculosis immunity memory in mice and the effects of aging on this process. In 1987, Orme (158) reported that older mice succumbed to a relatively small inoculum of *M. tuberculosis,* which was tolerated by younger mice; he inferred, at that time, that the "defect" in the older mice was an inability to produce $CD4^+$ lymphocytes capable of elaborating IFN-γ. However, this theory was subsequently amended by the observation that the older mice did produce capable $CD4^+$ lymphocytes, but that these lymphocytes were lacking cell-surface markers that facilitated vascular adhesion and immigration into sites of active infection (159). Another study by Orme (160) represented his effort to create a murine model for reactivation or recrudescent tuberculosis. Administration of a low-dose aerogenic inoculan created a subclinical chronic condition in the young mice; however, with the passage of time, the colony counts in the mouse lungs gradually rose and the mean survival times for the infected mice were significantly shorter than for noninfected controls. While indicating waned immunity with time, this model probably was not a good analogue to the human situation, in which a long-term culture-positive state is not sustained.

Orme et al. (28) and Anderson and Heron (32) studied mice to determine which lymphocyte cell line(s) conveyed immune memory for tuberculosis and to which mycobacterial antigens these cells responded. The CSU group (28) determined that protective immunity emerged early in the course of infection, while the mycobacteria were still multiplying logarithmically, and inferred that the T cells that conveyed such protection were responding to secreted antigens. By contrast, Anderson and Heron (32) demonstrated that memory T cells reacted with both secreted and somatic or cell-wall antigens; however, memory T cells differed from those involved with the primary infection by delays in proliferation and lymphokine production on stimulation by tubercle bacilli. Also, their data indicated that on rechallenge with tuberculosis infection these memory T cells did not expand symmetrically, but to a limited repertoire of low-molecular-weight, secreted antigens.

Collectively, these data clearly demonstrate age-related changes in susceptibility to tuberculosis in animals. This is wholly consistent with the epidemiology of tuberculosis in humans (see Chapter 5 for detailed discussion). It is very likely that these observations relate to inherent aspects of aging in the immune system—immunosenescence, if you will—but the possible influence of dietary (or other interventions) on retarding this process should not be ignored (161).

SUMMARY

Immunity to tuberculosis should probably be seen as comprising two broad elements that are under separate genetic controls. Early defense against infection is the task of alveolar macrophages. Their innate capacity to cope with newly inspired/ingested tubercle bacilli probably determines whether infection occurs and, if so, how rapidly and widely the bacilli are allowed to proliferate and disseminate. At the present time, this process probably should be considered analogous to the murine-resistant phenotypes, bcg_r or bcg_s (see "Macrophages and Preimmune Resistance: animal Models and Human Observations").

By contrast, once the infection has been implanted within the body, more complicated immune mechanisms come into play involving elaborate interplay between T lymphocytes, NK cells, and monocyte-derived macrophages. This process presumably is influenced by other genetically controlled variables, including the HLA antigen–presenting system and many other components enumerated above. Bellamy et al. (129), in their review of genetic susceptibility to tuberculosis, offer a list of candidate genes, all of which have known polymorphisms: HLA; *NRAMP1;* TNF; IFN-γ receptor; IL-1α, IL-1β, and IL-1 receptor antagonist; iNOS; and IL-6.

The pathogenesis of tuberculosis seems almost inextricably linked to immunity. Tissue damage, even with optimal immunity, derives inevitably to some degree from the host's encounter with the pathogen. However, the pursuit of interventions that might lessen tissue injury without critically compromising adequate immunity is an obvious goal for research.

The ultimate goal of our ongoing research must be to understand more clearly the process so that an effective vaccine(s) may be developed. For, without a vaccine, prospects for global control of tuberculosis are dismal (see Chapter 13).

APPENDIX 4.1. GLOSSARY OF TUBERCULOSIS IMMUNITY: TERMS AND FUNCTIONS

I. Antigen-presenting cells (APCs)	By processing and presenting mycobacterial antigens (Ags) to T lymphocytes in the context of major histocompatability complex (MHC) membrane molecules, APCs promote lymphocyte activation; other essential functions of APCs include adhesion receptor molecules (so APCs and lymphocytes can "embrace") and co-stimulatory signals (to promote activation of effector cells).
A. Alveolar macrophages	As preimmune, nonspecific scavengers of alveoli and distal airways, alveolar macrophages are first cells to encounter tubercle bacilli. Rudimentary APC function; probably serve to initiate local inflammation. Initiation of immune cascade probably done via dendritic cells (below).
B. Peripheral blood monocyte-derived macrophages (PBMs)	PBMs are attracted into site of primary infection; probably a major element in formation of granulomas. Major function is probably immune effector cell to inhibit (or kill) mycobacteria.
C. Dendritic cells	Phagocytic cells found normally in alveolar septa, lung interstitium, and airway epithelium. Perhaps the major APCs. May be responsible for transport of engulfed bacilli to hilar nodes where "immunity" evolves. Can express MHC class I or II molecules.

continues

APPENDIX 4.1. *Continued*

D. Major histocompatibility complex (MHC) system	To be immunogenic, APCs must present the peptide antigens in the physical context of cell membrane molecules. These serve as physicochemical keys to specify the type of T lymphocytes with which the APCs can interact.
1. MHC class I	Specific interaction with CD8 T lymphocytes (see below). Presents Ags that are located in cytosol of APC. MHC class I molecules are found on membranes of all nucleated cells; these molecules are linked to β-2 microglobulin.
2. MHC class II	Specific interaction with CD4 T lymphocytes (see below). Presents Ags that are retained within phagocytic vacuoles of APCs. MHC class II molecules are restricted to only APCs. Genes that determine MHC class II molecules are HLA-DR, HLA-DQ, and HLA-DP (see text for genetic control of immunity).
3. T-cell receptors (TcRs)	TcRs are MHC-determined elements on membranes of APC, which determine the type of T lymphocyte(s) with which the APC can interact; see MHC classes I and II. Corresponds with α/β chains of CD4 and CD8 lymphocytes.
4. Adhesion molecules (AMs)	Found on the surface of T lymphocytes, these molecules allow the T cell to embrace the APC while it interrogates the MHC locus for Ags. The lymphocyte AMs attach to specific ligand sites of APCs.
5. Co-stimulatory molecules	There are complementary accessory molecules at MHC sites on APCs and T lymphocytes, which mediate effector cell responses. The CD28 T-cell locus is critical for interleukin 2 (IL-2) production and lymphocyte activation.
II. Lymphocytes A. B lymphocytes	Derived from embryonic bursal or bone-marrow–derived cell line, the B lymphocytes are involved with production of antibodies or humoral immunity. Very limited role in tuberculoimmunity. Antibody production is increased in treatment failure cases; see Th2 below.
B. T lymphocytes	Thymus-derived T cells play dominant role in effective immunity against tuberculosis. Subtypes of T cells play specific roles in process; cell membrane molecules define these subtypes and influence their functions.
1. T-helper (Th) (CD4) cells	The CD4 molecule is a membrane glycoprotein that interacts with the T-cell receptor (above) to facilitate Ag presentation by the MHC class II system. The "helper" designation alludes to apparent role of CD4 cells in promoting more effective inhibition of mycobacteria within macrophages. Given consistent patterns of antigenic stimulation, CD4 lines may evolve with differing patterns of cytokine production; see Th pathways below. CD4 cells can have cytotoxicity activity.
2. T-cytotoxic (Tc) (CD8) cells	The CD8 molecule was the cell surface glycoprotein used to mark the T-cell subset. CD8 cells interact specifically with MHC class I APCs. CD8-positive T cells have very potent cytotoxic functions. One model of tuberculommunity posits that this cytotoxicity is primarily directed against naïve macrophages, which harbor and nurture proliferating tubercle bacilli. CD8 lines may also evolve with differing patterns of cytokine production; see Th and Tc pathways below.
3. Th and Tc pathways	Depending upon the type of Ag with which it is stimulated, a line of CD4 or CD8 lymphocytes may manifest different patterns of cytokine production. For CD4 helper cells, these lines are designated "Th," and for CD8 cytotoxic cells, "Tc."
a. Th1 and Tc1	Lymphocytes produce IL-2, interleukin 12 (IL-12), and interferon-γ (IFN-γ). These cytokines promote macrophage activation, CMI, and DTH activity.
b. Th2 and Tc2	Lymphocytes produce interleukins 4, 6, and 10 (IL-4, IL-6, and IL-10), which promote expansion and differentiation of B-lymphocyte population (see below).
c. Th0 and Tc0	Apparently undifferentiated or mixed population of lymphocytes, which produce mixture of cytokines above.
4. Gamma/delta lymphocytes	Unlike CD4 or CD8 cells, γ/δ lymphocytes do not have α/β chains for interacting with APCs; role in protection against tuberculosis is undermined. No clear evidence of antimycobacterial activity. May downregulate immune-mediated inflammation.
C. Natural killer (NK) cells	A discrete cell line, probably of lymphocytic origin. NK cells have spontaneous cytotoxicity versus an array of altered or foreign cells. May function to promote or enhance cytotoxic activity against APCs that are infected with tubercle bacilli.

continues

APPENDIX 4.1. *Continued*

II. Cytokines	Low-molecular-weight protein mediators that influence cell growth, inflammation, immunity, and repair. Unlike hormones, which typically have systemic effects, cytokines typically act in narrowly localized arenas. Under this rubric are various groups of agents (see below).
A. Interleukins	A subset of cytokines that modulate interactions between leukocytes.
1. IL-1	Released by alveolar macrophages and other APCs. IL-1 has an autocrine stimulating effect upon the parent cells, as well as attracting and stimulating CD4 lymphocytes.
2. IL-2	Released by CD4 lymphocytes after Ag presentation. IL-2 causes autocrine stimulation, as well as attraction and activation of additional lymphocytes.
3. IL-4	Produced by macrophages, downregulates T-cell functions, and promotes eosinophil and B-cell functions.
4. IL-6	Produced by macrophages as a co-stimulatory factor; activates CD4 cells.
5. IL-10	Produced by macrophages, works with IL-4 and transforming growth factor-β (TGF-β) to downregulate CD4 functions and stimulate B-cell function.
6. IL-12	Produced by macrophages, IL-12 plays a major role in immunity by fostering Th1-pathway lymphocyte differentiation.
B. Interferon-γ (IFN-γ)	Produced by CD4, CD8, NK cells and γ/δ lymphocytes, IFN-γ plays a major role in upregulating production of tumor necrosis factor-α (TNF-α) and Ag processing and regulation by macrophages. Vital component of immunity.
C. Tumor necrosis factor-α (TNF-α)	TNF-α is produced by infected macrophages. Autocrine stimulates these cells; also attracts and activates T lymphocytes. A critical component of immunity.
D. Transforming growth factor-β (TGF-β)	TGF-β is produced by macrophages to downregulate or suppress CD4 lymphocyte function; presumably a modulator of inflammation, excessive TGF-β production may impair host defense. Interferes with IL-2, IL-12, and IFN-γ.
E. Granulocyte-macrophage colony-stimulating factor (GM-CSF)	GM-CSF is produced by T cells, attracting monocytes and stimulating their proliferation and activity. May be central to maturation of dendritic cells to function as APCs.
IV. Chemokines	Small proteins that function to attract leukocytes to localized tissue sites. A critical element of host defenses versus infections. Grouped into 40 families according to chemical structures.
A. Leukocyte adhesion molecules	Elements on leukocytes that promote adhesion to vascular endothelium as they circulate through tissue.
B. Vascular endothelial ligands	Elements on vascular endothelium that retain circulating leukocytes. Coupled with leukocyte adhesion molecules, function like a "Velcro" system.
C. Type CC or CXC chemokines	Members of two of the four chemokine families, these substances attract the effector cells that participate in the host defense against tuberculosis.
1. Monocyte chemotactic protein (MCP-1)	Attracts dendritic cells, activated T cells, NK cells, and peripheral blood monocytes.
2. Macrophage inflammatory protein (MIP-1)	Attracts dendritic cells, activated T cells, NK cells, and peripheral blood monocytes.
3. RANTES	Acronym for *R*egulated on *A*ctivation *N*ormal *T*-cell *E*xpressed and *S*ecreted; known to attract peripheral blood monocytes, NK cells, eosinophils, and basophils.
4. Interferon-inducible protein-10	Attracts T cells and NK cells. Promotes adhesion, chemotaxis, and cytotoxicity.
5. Interferon-inducible monokine	Attracts peripheral blood monocytes, activated T cells, and NK cells. Mainly promotes chemotaxis.
6. Interleukin-8 (IL-8)	Attracts T cells and NK cells; also promotes superoxide release and killing functions.

REFERENCES

1. Mackaness G. The immunology of antituberculous immunity [editorial]. *Am Rev Respir Dis* 1968;97:337–344.
2. Dannenberg AM. Delayed-type hypersensitivity and cell-mediated immunity in the pathogenesis of tuberculosis. *Immunol Today* 1991;12:228–233.
3. Dannenberg AM Jr, Rook GAW. Pathogenesis of pulmonary tuberculosis: an interplay of tissue-damaging and macrophage-activating immune responses—dual mechanisms that control bacillary multiplication. In: BR Bloom, ed. *Tuberculosis: pathogenesis, protection, and control.* Washington DC: ASM Press, 1994.
4. Schlesinger LS, Bellinger-Kawahara CG, Payne NR, Horwitz MA. Phagocytosis of *Mycobacterium tubercu-*

losis is mediated by human monocyte complement receptors and complement component C3. *J Immunol* 1990;144:2271–2280.
5. Schorey JS, Carroll MC, Brown EJ. A macrophage invasion mechanism of pathogenic mycobacteria. *Science* 1997;277:1091–1093.
6. Schlesinger LS. Macrophage phagocytosis of virulent but not attenuated strains of *Mycobacterium tuberculosis* is mediated by mannose receptors in addition to complement receptors. *J Immunol* 1993;150:2920–2930.
7. Stokes RW, Haidl ID, Jefferies WA, Speert DP. Mycobacteria-macrophage interactions: macrophage phenotype determines the nonopsonic binding of *Mycobacterium tuberculosis* to murine macrophages. *J Immunol* 1993;151:7067–7076.
8. Brostoff J, Lenzini L, Rottoli P, Rottoli L. Immune complexes in the spectrum of tuberculosis. *Tubercle* 1981;62:169–173.
9. Sai Baba KSS, Moudgil KD, Jain RC, Srivastava LM. Complement activation in pulmonary tuberculosis. *Tubercle* 1990;71:103–107.
10. Abou-Zeid C, Ratliff TL, Wikes HG, Harboe M, Bennedsen J, Rook GAW. Characterization of fibronectin-binding antigens released by *Mycobacterium tuberculosis* and *Mycobacterium bovis* BCG. *Infect Immun* 1988;56:3046–3051.
11. Goren MB, D'Arcy Hart P, Young MR, Armstrong JA. Prevention of phagosome-lysosome fusion by sulfatides from *Mycobacterium tuberculosis. Proc Natl Acad Sci U S A* 1976;73:2510–2514.
12. Gordon AH, D'Arcy Hart P, Young MR. Ammonia inhibits phagosome-lysosome fusion in macrophages. *Nature* 1980;286:79–80.
13. Pabst MJ, Gross JM, Brozna JP, Goren MB. Inhibition of macrophage priming by sulfatide from Mycobacterium tuberculosis. *J Immunol* 1988; 140: 634–640.
14. Zhang L, Goren MB, Holtzer TJ, Anderson BR. Effect of *Mycobacterium tuberculosis*-derived sulfolipid 1 on human phagocytic cells. *Infect Immun* 1988;56:2876–2883.
15. Sibley LD, Hunter SW, Brennan PJ, Krahenbuhl JL. Mycobacterial lipoarabinomannan inhibits gamma interferon-mediated activation of macrophages. *Infect Immun* 1988;56:1232–1236.
16. Chatterjee D, Robert AD, Lowell K, Brennan PJ, Orme IM. Structural basis of capacity of lipoarabinomannan to induce secretion of tumor necrosis factor. *Infect Immun* 1992;60:1249–1253.
17. Myrvik Q, Leake E, Wright M. Disruption of phagosomal membranes of normal alveolar macrophages by the H37Rv strain of *Mycobacterium tuberculosis:* a correlate of virulence. *Am Rev Respir Dis* 1984;129: 322–328.
18. Russell DG, Dant J, Sturgill-Koszycki S. *Mycobacterium avium-* and *Mycobacterium tuberculosis*-containing vacuoles are dynamic, fusion-competent vesicles that are accessible to glycosphingolipids from the host cell plasmalemma. *J Immunol* 1996;156:4764–4773.
19. Clemens DL, Horwitz MA. Characterization of the *Mycobacterium tuberculosis* phagosome and evidence that phagosomal maturation is inhibited. *J Exp Med* 1995;181:257–270.
20. Hasan Z, Schlax C, Kuhn L, et al. Isolation and characterization of the mycobacterial phagosome: segregation from the endosomal/lysosomal pathway. *Mol Microbiol* 1997;24:545–553.
21. Collins FM, Miller TE. Growth of a drug-resistant strain of *M. bovis* (BCG) in normal and immunized mice. *J Infect Dis* 1969;120:517–533.
22. Ordway DJ, Sonnenberg MG, Donahue SA, Belisle JT, Orme IM. Drug-resistant strains of *Mycobacterium tuberculosis* exhibit a range of virulence for mice. *Infect Immun* 1995;63:741–743.
23. Li Z, Kelley C, Collins F, Rouse D, Morris S. Expression of *katG* in *Mycobacterium tuberculosis* is associated with its growth and persistence in mice and guinea pigs. *J Infect Dis* 1998;177:1030–1035.
24. Sherman DR, Mdluli K, Hickey MJ, et al. Compensatory *ahpC* gene expression in isoniazid-resistant *Mycobacterium tuberculosis. Science* 1996;272:1641–1643.
25. Heym B, Stavropoulos E, Honoré N, et al. Effects of overexpression of the alkyl hydroperoxide reductase *ahpC* on the virulence and isoniazid resistance of *Mycobacterium tuberculosis. Infect Immun* 1997;65: 1395–1401.
26. Friedman CR, Quinn GC, Kreiswirth BN, et al. Widespread dissemination of a drug-susceptible strain of *Mycobacterium tuberculosis. J Infect Dis* 1997;176: 478–484.
27. Kaufmann SHE, Young DB. Vaccination against tuberculosis and leprosy. *Immunobiology* 1992;184: 208–229.
28. Orme IM, Miller ES, Roberts AD, et al. T-lymphocytes mediating protection and cellular cytolysis during the course of *Mycobacterium tuberculosis* infection. *J Immunol* 1992;148:189–196.
29. Andersen P, Askgaard D, Ljungqvist L, Weis Bentzon M, Heron I. T-cell proliferative response to antigens secreted by *Mycobacterium tuberculosis. Infect Immun* 1991;59:1558–1563.
30. Daugelats S, Gulle H, Schoel B, Kaufmann SHE. Secreted antigens of *Mycobacterium tuberculosis:* characterization with T-lymphocytes from patients and contacts after two-dimensional separation. *J Infect Dis* 1992;166:186–190.
31. Horwitz M, Lee B, Dillon B, Harth G. Protective immunity against tuberculosis induced by vaccination with major extracellular proteins of *Mycobacterium tuberculosis. Proc Natl Acad Sci U S A* 1995;92: 1530–1534.
32. Anderson P, Heron I. Specificity of a protective memory immune response against *Mycobacterium tuberculosis. Infect Immun* 1993;61:844–851.
33. Harding CV. Cellular and molecular aspects of antigen processing and the function of class II MHC molecules. *Am J Respir Cell Mol Biol* 1993;8:461–467.
34. Townsend A, Ohlen C, Bastin J, Ljunggren H, Foster L, Karre K. Association of class I major histocompatibility heavy and light chains induced by viral peptides. *Nature* 1989;340:443–448.
35. Orme IM, Andersen P, Boom WH. T cell response to *Mycobacterium tuberculosis. J Infect Dis* 1993;167: 1481–1497.
36. Dhand R, De A, Ganguly NK, et al. Factors influencing the cellular response in bronchoalveolar lavage and peripheral blood of patients with pulmonary tuberculosis. *Tubercle* 1988;69:161–173.

37. Ozaki T, Nakashira S, Toni K, Ogushi F, Yasouka S, Ogura T. Differential cell analysis in bronchoalveolar lavage fluid from pulmonary lesions of patients with tuberculosis. *Chest* 1992;102:54—59.
38. Ainslie GM, Solomon JA, Bateman ED. Lymphocyte and lymphocyte subset numbers in blood and bronchoalveolar and pleural fluid in various forms of human pulmonary tuberculosis at presentation and during recovery. *Thorax* 1992;47:513–518.
39. Robinson DS, Ying S, Taylor IK, et al. Evidence for a Th1-like bronchoalveolar T-cell subset and predominance of interferon-gamma gene activation in pulmonary tuberculosis. *Am J Respir Crit Care Med* 1994;149:989–993.
40. Law KF, Jagirdar J, Weiden MD, Bodkin M, Rom WN. Tuberculosis in HIV-positive patients: cellular response and immune activation in the lung. *Am J Respir Crit Care Med* 1996;153:1377–1384.
41. Lai CKW, Ho S, Chan CHS, et al. Cytokine gene expression profile of circulating $CD4^+$ T cells in active pulmonary tuberculosis. *Chest* 1997;111:606–611.
42. Condos R, Rom WN, Liu YM, Schluger NW. Local immune responses correlate with presentation and outcome in tuberculosis. *Am J Respir Crit Care Med* 1998;157:729–735.
43. Mosmann T, Cherwinski H, Bond M, Giedlin M, Coffman R. Two types of murine helper T-cell clones, I: definition according to profiles of lymphokine activities and secreted proteins. *J Immunol* 1986;136:2348–2357.
44. Orme I. Processing and presentation of mycobacterial antigens: implications for the development of a new improved vaccine for tuberculosis control. *Tubercle* 1991;72:250–252.
45. Rook GAW. Mobilising the appropriate T-cell subset: the immune response as taxonomist? *Tubercle* 1991; 72:253–254.
46. Modlin RL. Th-1 Th-2 paradigm: insights from leprosy. *J Invest Dermatol* 1994;102:828–832.
47. Cooper AM, Roberts AD, Rhoades ER, Callahan JE, Getzy DM, Orme IM. The role of interleukin-12 in acquired immunity to *Mycobacterium tuberculosis* infection. *Immunol* 1995;84:423–432.
48. Kaufmann S. Conference report. 9th International Congress of Immunology: San Francisco. *Lancet* 1995;346:434–435.
49. Flynn JL, Goldstein MM, Triebold KJ, Koller B, Bloom BR. Major histocompatibility complex class I-restricted T cells are required for resistance to *Mycobacterium tuberculosis* infection. *Proc Natl Acad Sci U S A* 1992;89:12013–12017.
50. Flynn JL, Goldstein MM, Triebold KJ, Bloom BR. Major histocompatibility complex class I-restricted T cells are necessary for protection against *M. tuberculosis* in mice. *Infect Agents Dis* 1993;2:259–262.
51. Sodhi A, Gong J-H, Silva C, Qian D, Barnes PF. Clinical correlates of interferon γ production in patients with tuberculosis. *Clin Infect Dis* 1997;25:617–620.
52. Taha RA, Kotsimbos TC, Song Y-L, Menzies D, Hamid Q. IFN-γ and IL-12 are increased in active compared with inactive tuberculosis. *Am J Respir Crit Care Med* 1997;155:1135–1139.
53. Born W, Harshan K, Modlin R, O'Brien R. The role of gamma/delta T lymphocytes in infection. *Curr Opin Immunol* 1991;3:455–459.
54. Barnes PF, Grisso CL, Abrams JS, Band H, Rea TH, Modlin RL. γ/δ T lymphocytes in human tuberculosis. *J Infect Dis* 1992;165:506–512.
55. Munk ME, Gatrill AJ, Kaufmann SHE. Target cell lysis and IL-2 secretion by γ/δ T lymphocytes after activation with bacteria. *J Immunol* 1990;145: 2434–2439.
56. Ito M, Kojiro N, Ikeda T, Ito T, Funada J, Kokubu T. Increased proportions of peripheral blood γ/δ T cells in patients with pulmonary tuberculosis. *Chest* 1992;102: 195–197.
57. Tazi A, Bouchonnet F, Valeyre D, Cadranel J, Battesti J, Hance A. Characterization of γ/δ T lymphocytes in the peripheral blood of patient with active tuberculosis. *Am Rev Respir Dis* 1992;146:1216–1221.
58. Balbi B, Valle M, Oddera S, et al. T-lymphocytes with γ/δ^+ Vδ 2^+ antigen receptors are present in increased proportions in a fraction of patients with tuberculosis or with sarcoidosis. *Am Rev Respir Dis* 1993;148: 1685–1690.
59. Li B, Rossman MD, Imir T, et al. Disease-specific changes in γ/δ T cell repertoire and function in patients with pulmonary tuberculosis. *J Immunol* 1996;157: 4222–4229.
60. Ueta C, Tsuyuguchi I, Kawasumi H, Takashima T, Toba H, Kishimoto S. Increase of γ/δ T cells in hospital workers who are in close contact with tuberculosis patients. *Infect Immun* 1994;62:5434–5441.
61. Liu C-C, Young LHY, Young JD-E. Lymphocyte-mediated cytolysis and disease. *N Engl J Med* 1996;335: 1651–1659.
62. Yoneda T, Kasai M, Ishibashi J, Tokunaga T, Mikami R. NK cell activity in pulmonary tuberculosis. *Br J Dis Chest* 1983;77:185–188.
63. Bermudez LEM, Young LS. Natural killer cell-dependent mycobacteriostatic and mycobactericidal activity in human macrophages. *J Immunol* 1991;146:265–270.
64. Yoneda T, Ellner JJ. $CD4^+$ T cell and natural killer cell-dependent killing of *Mycobacterium tuberculosis* by human monocytes. *Am J Respir Crit Care Med* 1998;158:395–403.
65. Adams DH, Lloyd AR. Chemokines: leucocyte recruitment and activation cytokines. *Lancet* 1997;349: 490–495.
66. Luster AD. Chemokines-chemotactic cytokines that mediate inflammation. *N Engl J Med* 1998;338:436–445.
67. Douvas GS, Looker DL, Vatter AE, Crowle AJ. Gamma interferon activates human macrophages to become tumoricidal and leishmanicidal but enhances replication of macrophage-associated mycobacteria. *Infect Immun* 1985;50:1–8.
68. Rook GAW, Steele J, Ainsworth M, Champion BR. Activation of macrophages to inhibit proliferation of *M. tuberculosis:* comparison of the effects of recombinant gamma-interferon on human monocytes and murine peritoneal macrophages. *Immunology* 1986;59: 333–338.
69. Steele J, Flint KC, Pozniak AL, Hudspith B, Johnson NM, Rook GAW. Inhibition of virulent *Mycobacterium tuberculosis* by murine peritoneal macrophages and human alveolar lavage cells: the effects of lymphokines and recombinant gamma interferon. *Tubercle* 1986;67:289–294.

70. Rook GAW, Steele J, Fraher L, et al. Vitamin D3, gamma interferon and control of proliferation of *Mycobacterium tuberculosis* by human monocytes. *Immunology* 1986;57:159–163.
71. Crowle AJ, Ross EJ, May MH. Inhibition by 1,25 (OH)2-vitamin D3 of the multiplication of virulent tubercle bacilli in cultured human macrophages. *Infec Immun* 1987;55:2945–2950.
72. Ogawa T, Ushida H, Kusumoto Y, Mori Y, Yamanura Y, Hamada S. Increase in tumor necrosis factor α and interleukin-6–secreting cells in peripheral blood mononuclear cells from subjects infected with *Mycobacterium tuberculosis. Infect Immun* 1991;59: 3021–3025.
73. Zhang Y, Doerfler M, Lee TC, Guillemin B, Rom WN. Mechanisms of stimulation of interleukin-1β and tumor necrosis factor-α by *Mycobacterium tuberculosis* components. *J Clin Invest* 1993;91:2076–2083.
74. Wallis RS, Paranjape R, Phillips M. Identification by two-dimensional gel electrophoresis of a 58-kilodalton tumor necrosis factor-inducing protein of *Mycobacterium tuberculosis. Infect Immun* 1993;61:627–632.
75. Kindler V, Sappino I, Grau G, Piguet P, Vassolli P. The inducing role of tumor necrosis factor in the development of bactericidal granulomas during BCG infection. *Cell* 1989;56:731–740.
76. Flynn JL, Goldstein MM, Chan J, et al. Tumor necrosis factor-α is required in the protective immune response against *Mycobacterium tuberculosis* in mice. *Immunity* 1995;2:561–572.
77. Adams L, Mason C, Kolls J, Scollard D, Krahenbuhl J, Nelson S. Exacerbation of acute and chronic murine tuberculosis by administration of a tumor necrosis factor receptor-expressing adenovirus. *J Infect Dis* 1995; 171:400–405.
78. Beutler B, Greenwald D, Hulmes JD, et al. Identity of tumour necrosis factor and the macrophage-secreted factor cachectin. *Nature* 1985;316:552–554.
79. Bazzoni F, Beutler B. The tumor necrosis factor ligand and receptor families. *N Engl J Med* 1996;334: 1717–1725.
80. McGuire W, Hill AVS, Allsopp CEM, Greenwood BM, Kwjatkowski D. Variation in the TNF-α promoter region associated with susceptibility to cerebral malaria. *Nature* 1994;371:508–511.
81. Messer G, Kick G, Ranki A, Koskimies S, Reunala T, Meurer M. Polymorphism of the tumor necrosis factor genes in patients with dermatitis herpetiformis. *Dermatology* 1994;189:135–137.
82. Huang S-L, Su C-H, Chang S-C. Tumor necrosis factor-α gene polymorphism in chronic bronchitis. *Am J Respir Crit Care Med* 1997;156:1436–1439.
83. Cox A, Gonzalez M, Wilson AG, et al. Comparative analysis of the genetic associations of HLA-DR3 and tumor necrosis factor alpha with human IDDM. *Diabetologia* 1994;37:500–503.
84. Wilson AG, Gordon C, di Giovine FS, et al. A genetic association between systemic lupus erythematosus and tumor necrosis factor alpha. *Eur J Immunol* 1994; 24:191–195.
85. Kobayashi K, Yamazaki J, Kasama T, et al. Interleukin (IL)-12 deficiency in susceptible mice infected with *Mycobacterium avium* and amelioration of established infection by IL-12 replacement therapy. *J Infect Dis* 1996;174:564–573.
86. Altare F, Durandy A, Lammas D, et al. Impairment of mycobacterial immunity in human interleukin-12 receptor deficiency. *Science* 1998;280:1432–1435.
87. de Jong R, Altare F, Haagen I-A, et al. Severe mycobacterial and *Salmonella* infections in interleukin-12 receptor-deficient patients. *Science* 1998;280:1435–1438.
88. Chan J, Tanaka K, Carroll D, Flynn J, Bloom BR. Effects of nitric oxide synthase inhibitors on murine infection with *Mycobacterium tuberculosis. Infect Immun* 1995;63:736–740.
89. Flesch IEA, Kaufmann SHE. Mechanisms involved in mycobacterial growth inhibition by gamma interferon-activated bone marrow macrophages: role of reactive nitrogen intermediates. *Infect Immun* 1991;59:3213–3218.
90. Flynn JL, Chan J, Triebold KJ, Dalton DK, Stewart TA, Bloom BR. An essential role for interferon γ in resistance to *Mycobacterium tuberculosis* infection. *J Exp Med* 1993;178:2249–2254.
91. Arias M, Rojas M, Zabaleta J, et al. Inhibition of virulent *Mycobacterium tuberculosis* by Bcg^r and Bcg^s macrophages correlates with nitric oxide production. *J Infect Dis* 1997;176:1552–1558.
92. Denis M. Human monocytes/macrophages: NO or no NO? *J Leukoc Biol* 1994;55:682–684.
93. Nicholson S, Almeida-Bonecini M, Lapa e Silva J. Inducible nitric oxide synthase in pulmonary alveolar macrophages from patients with tuberculosis. *J Exp Med* 1996;183:2293–2302.
94. Wang C-H, Liu C-Y, Lin H-C, Yu C-T, Chung KF, Kuo H-P. Increased exhaled nitric oxide in active pulmonary tuberculosis due to inducible NO synthase upregulation in alveolar macrophages. *Eur Respir J* 1998;11:809–815.
95. Aston C, Rom WN, Talbot AT, Reibman J. Early inhibition of mycobacterial growth by human alveolar macrophages is not due to nitric oxide. *Am J Respir Crit Care Med* 1998;157:1943–1950.
96. Wengenack NL, Uhl JR, St Amand AL, et al. Recombinant *Mycobacterium tuberculosis* KatG(S315T) is a competent catalase-peroxidase with reduced activity toward isoniazid. *J Infect Dis* 1997;176:722–727.
97. Cohn ML, Kovitz C, Oda U, Middlebrook G. Studies on isoniazid and tubercle bacilli, II: the growth requirements, catalase activities, and pathogenic properties of isoniazid-resistant mutants. *Am Rev Tuberc* 1954;54:641–664.
98. Frieden TR, Sherman LF, Maw KL, et al. A multi-institutional outbreak of highly drug-resistant tuberculosis: epidemiology and clinical outcomes. *JAMA* 1996; 276:1229–1235.
99. Adams LB, Diauer MC, Morganstern D, Krahenbuhl. Phagocytic burst oxidase plays a role in the host response to Mycobacterium tuberculosis. *Am Soc Microbiol* 1997:548.
100. Lau YL, Chan GCF, Ha SY, Hui YF, Yuen KY. The role of phagocytic respiratory burst in host defense against *Mycobacterium tuberculosis. Clin Infect Dis* 1998;26:226–227.
101. Galve de Rochemonteix B, Nicod L, Chicheportice R, Lacraz S, Baumberger C, Dayer J-M. Regulation of interleukin-1ra, interleukin-1g, and interleukin-1β production by human alveolar macrophages with phorbal myrislate acetate, lipopolysaccharide, and interleukin-4. *Am J Respir Cell Mol Biol* 1993;8:160–168.
102. Juffermans NP, Verbon A, van Deventer SJH, van

Deutekom H, Speelman P, van der Poll T. Tumor necrosis factor and interleukin-1 inhibitors as markers of disease activity of tuberculosis. *Am J Respir Crit Care Med* 1998;157:1328–1331.
103. Ellner JJ. Suppressor adherent cells in human tuberculosis. *J Immunol* 1978;121:2573–2578.
104. Toossi A, Kleinhenz ME, Ellner JJ. Defective interleukin-2 production and responsiveness in human pulmonary tuberculosis. *J Exp Med* 1986;163:1162–1172.
105. Toossi A, Edmonds KE, Tomford WJ, Ellner JJ. Suppression of PPD-induced interleukin-2 production by interaction of Leu-11 (CD 16) positive lymphocytes and adherent mononuclear cells in tuberculosis. *J Infect Dis* 1989;159:352–356.
106. Toossi Z, Lapurga JP, Ondash RJ, Sedor JR, Ellner JJ. Expression of functional IL-2 receptors by peripheral blood monocytes from patients with active pulmonary tuberculosis. *J Clin Invest* 1990;85:1777–1784.
107. Hirsch CS, Yoneda T, Averill L, Ellner JJ, Toossi Z. Enhancement of intracellular growth of *Mycobacterium tuberculosis* in human monocytes in transforming growth factor-β1. *J Infect Dis* 1994;170:1229–1237.
108. Grigg ERN. The arcana of tuberculosis with a brief epidemiologic history of the disease in the U.S.A. *Am Rev Tuberc Pulm Dis* 1958;78:151–172; 426–453; 583–603.
109. Toossi Z, Young T-G, Averill LE, Hamilton BD, Shiratsuchi H, Ellner JJ. Induction of transforming growth factor β1 by purified protein derivative of *Mycobacterium tuberculosis. Infect Immun* 1995;63:224–228.
110. Toossi Z, Gogate P, Shiratsuchi H, Young T, Ellner JJ. Enhanced production of TGF-β by blood monocytes from patients with active tuberculosis and presence of TGF-β in tuberculous granulomatous lung lesions. *J Immunol* 1995;154:465–473.
111. Dahl KE, Shiratsuchi H, Hamilton BD, Ellner JJ, Toossi Z. Selective induction of transforming growth factor β in human monocytes by lipoarabinomannan of *Mycobacterium tuberculosis. Infect Immun* 1996;64:399–405.
112. Hirsch CS, Hussain R, Toossi Z, Dawood G, Shahid F, Ellner JJ. Cross-modulation by transforming growth factor β in human tuberculosis: suppression of antigen-driven blastogenesis and inteferon γ production. *Proc Natl Acad Sci U S A* 1996;93:3193–3198.
113. Hirsch CS, Ellner JJ, Blinkhorn R, Toossi Z. In vitro restoration of T cell responses in tuberculosis and augmentation of monocyte effector function against *Mycobacterium tuberculosis* by natural inhibitors of transforming growth factor β. *Proc Natl Acad Sci U S A* 1997;94:3926–3931.
114. Gong J-H, Zhang M, Modlin RL, et al. Interleukin-10 downregulates *Mycobacterium tuberculosis*-induced Th1 responses and CTLA-4 expression. *Infect Immun* 1996;64:913–918.
115. Wilkinson RJ, Vordermeier HM, Wilkinson KA, et al. Peptide-specific T cell response to *Mycobacterium tuberculosis:* clinical spectrum, compartmentalization, and effect of chemotherapy. *J Infect Dis* 1998;178:760–768.
116. Ellner JJ. Review: The immune response in human tuberculosis: implications for tuberculosis control. *J Infect Dis* 1997;176:1351–1359.
117. Glatman-Freedman A, Casadevall A. Serum therapy for tuberculosis revisited: reappraisal of the role of antibody-mediated immunity against *Mycobacterium tuberculosis. Clin Microbiol Rev* 1998;11:514–532.
118. Antony VB, Sahn SA, Antony AC, Repine JE. Bacillus Calmette Guérin stimulated neutrophils release chemotaxins for monocytes in rabbit pleural spaces and in vitro. *J Clin Invest* 1985;76:1514–1521.
119. Appelberg R, Castro AG, Gomes S, Pedrosa J, Silva MT. Susceptibility of beige mice to *Mycobacterium avium:* role of neutrophils. *Infect Immun* 1995;63:3381–3387.
120. Newman GW, Guarnaccia JR, Remold HG, Kazanjian PH Jr. Cytokines enhance neutrophils from human immunodeficiency virus-negative donors and AIDS patients to inhibit the growth of *Mycobacterium avium* in vitro. *J Infect Dis* 1997;175:891–900.
121. Riedel DD, Kaufmann SHE. Chemokine secretion by human polymorphonuclear granulocytes after stimulation with *Mycobacterium tuberculosis* and lipoarabinomannan. *Infect Immun* 1997;65:4620–4623.
122. Kasahara K, Sato I, Ogura K, Takeuchi H, Kobayashi K, Adachi M. Expression of chemokines and induction of rapid cell death in human blood neutrophils by *Mycobacterium tuberculosis. J Infect Dis* 1998;178:127–137.
123. Copley AL, Maupin B, Baléa T. The agglutinant and adhesive behaviour of isolated human and rabbit platelets in contact with various strains of mycobacteria. *Acta Tuberc Scand* 1959;37:151–161.
124. Yeaman MR. The role of platelets in antimicrobial host defense. *Clin Infect Dis* 1997;25:951–970.
125. Blower SM, McLean AR, Porco TC, et al. The intrinsic transmission dynamics of tuberculosis epidemics. *Nat Med* 1995;1:815–821.
126. Budd W. The nature and the mode of propagation of phthisis. *Lancet* 1867;2:451–452.
127. Stead W. Genetics and resistance to tuberculosis: could resistance be enhanced by genetic engineering? *Ann Intern Med* 1992;116:937–941.
128. Stead W, Senner J, Reddick W, Lofgren J. Racial differences in susceptibility to infection by *Mycobacterium tuberculosis. N Engl J Med* 1990;322:422–427.
129. Bellamy R, Ruwende C, Corrah T, McAdam KPWJ, Whittle HC, Hill AVS. Variations in the *NRAMP1* gene and susceptibility to tuberculosis in West Africans. *N Engl J Med* 1998;338:640–644.
130. Kallmann FJ, Reisner D. Twin studies on the significance of genetic factors in tuberculosis. *Am Rev Tuberc* 1943;47:549–574.
131. Simonds B. *Tuberculosis in twins.* London: Pitman Medical Publishing, 1963.
132. Comstock G. Tuberculosis in twins: a re-analysis of the Prophit Survey. *Am Rev Respir Dis* 1978;117:621–624.
133. Skamene E, Pistrangeli C. Genetics of the immune response to infectious pathogens. *Curr Opin Immunol* 1991;3:511–517.
134. Gros P, Skamene E, Forget A. Genetic control of natural resistance to *Mycobacterium bovis* (BCG) in mice. *J Immunol* 1981;127:2417–2421.
135. Gros P, Skamene E, Forget A. Cellular mechanisms of genetically controlled host resistance to *Mycobacterium bovis* (BCG). *J Immunol* 1983;131:1966–1972.
136. Vidal S, Malo D, Vogan K, Skamene E, Gros P. Natural resistance to infection with intracellular parasites: isolation of a candidate for *Bcg. Cell* 1993;73:469–485.
137. Crowle A, Elkins N. Relative permissiveness of macrophages from black and white people for virulent tubercle bacilli. *Infect Immun* 1990;58:632–638.

138. Supek F, Supekova L, Nelson H, Nelson N. A yeast manganese transporter related to the macrophage protein involved in conferring resistance to mycobacteria. *Proc Natl Acad Sci U S A* 1996;93:5105–5110.
139. Abel L, Sánchez FO, Oberti J, et al. Susceptibility to leprosy is linked to the human *NRAMP1* gene. *J Infect Dis* 1998;177:133–145.
140. Pelletier M, Forget A, Bourassa D, Gros P, Skamene E. Immunopathology of BCG infection in genetically resistant and susceptible mouse strains. *J Immunol* 1982;129:2179–2185.
141. Brett S, Orrell J, Swanson-Beck J, Ivanyi J. Influence of H-2 genes on growth of *Mycobacterium tuberculosis* in the lungs of chronically infected mice. *Immunol* 1992;76:129–132.
142. Singh S, Mehra N, Dingley H, Pande J, Vaidya M. Human leukocyte antigen (HLA)-linked control of susceptibility to pulmonary tuberculosis and association with HLA-DR types. *J Infect Dis* 1983;148:676–681.
143. Bothamley G, Beck J, Schreuder G, et al. Association of tuberculosis and *M. tuberculosis*-specific antibody levels with HLA. *J Infect Dis* 1989;159:549–555.
144. Brahmajothi V, Pitchappan RM, Kakkanaiah VN, et al. Association of pulmonary tuberculosis and HLA in South India. *Tubercle* 1991;72:123–132.
145. Rajalingam R, Mehra NK, Jain RC, Myneedu VP, Pande JN. Polymerase chain reaction-based sequence-specific oligonucleotide hybridization analysis of HLA class II antigens in pulmonary tuberculosis: relevance to chemotherapy and disease severity. *J Infect Dis* 1996;173:669–676.
146. Pospelov LE, Matrakshin AG, Chernousova LN, et al. Association of various genetic markers with tuberculosis and other lung diseases in Tuvinian children. *Tuberc Lung Dis* 1996;77:77–80.
147. Goldfeld AE, Delgado JC, Thim S, et al. Association of an HLA-DQ allele with clinical tuberculosis. *JAMA* 1998;279:226–228.
148. Al-Arif L, Goldstein R, Affronti L, Janicki B. HLA-Bw 15 and tuberculosis in North American black population. *Am Rev Respir Dis* 1979;120:1275–1278.
149. Selby R, Barnard J, Buehler S, Crumley J, Larsen B, Marshall W. Tuberculosis associated with HLA-B8, Bfs in a Newfoundland community study. *Tissue Antigens* 1978;11:403–408.
150. Zervas J, Constantopoulos C, Toubis M, Anagnostopoulos D, Cotsovoulon V. HLA-A and B antigens and pulmonary tuberculosis in Greeks. *Br J Dis Chest* 1987;81:147–149.
151. Papiha S, Singh B, Lanchbury J, et al. Association of HLA and other genetic markers in South Indian patients with pulmonary tuberculosis. *Tubercle* 1987;68:159–167.
152. Hawkins B, Higgins D, Chan S, Lowrie D, Mitchison D, Girling D. HLA typing in the Hong Kong Chest Service/British Medical Research Council study of factors associated with the breakdown to active tuberculosis of inactive pulmonary lesions. *Am Rev Respir Dis* 1988;138:1616–1621.
153. Holland SN, Eisenstein EM, Kuhns DB, et al. Treatment of refractory disseminated nontuberculous mycobacterial infection with interferon gamma. *N Engl J Med* 1994;330:1348–1355.
154. Levin M, Newport M, D'Souza S, et al. Familial disseminated atypical mycobacterial infection in childhood: a human mycobacterial susceptibility gene? *Lancet* 1995;345:79–83.
155. Newport MJ, Huxley CM, Huston S, et al. A mutation in the interferon-γ-receptor gene and susceptibility to mycobacterial infection. *N Engl J Med* 1996;335:1941–1949.
156. Jouanguy E, Altare F, Lamhamedi S, et al. Interferon-γ-receptor deficiency in an infant with fatal Bacille Calmette-Guérin infection. *N Engl J Med* 1996;335:1956–1961.
157. Pierre-Audigier C, Jouanguy E, Lamhamedi S, et al. Fatal disseminated *Mycobacterium smegmatis* infection in a child with inherited interferon γ receptor deficiency. *Clin Infect Dis* 1997;24:982–984.
158. Orme IM. Aging and immunity to tuberculosis: increased susceptibility of old mice reflects a decreased capacity to generate mediator T lymphocytes. *J Immunol* 1987;138:4414–4418.
159. Orme IM, Griffin JP, Roberts AD, Ernst DN. Evidence for a defective accumulation of protective T cells in old mice infected with *Mycobacterium tuberculosis. Cell Immunol* 1993;147:222–229.
160. Orme IM. A mouse model of the recrudescence of latent tuberculosis in the elderly. *Am Rev Respir Dis* 1988;137:716–718.
161. Meydani SN, Meydani M, Blumberg JB, et al. Vitamin E supplementation and in vivo immune response in healthy elderly subjects: a randomized controlled trial. *JAMA* 1997;277:1380–1385.

5

Tuberculosis Epidemiology

Tuberculosis infection and disease patterns among different populations are extremely heterogeneous. Understanding the epidemiology of this disease is, therefore, vitally important as an aid to diagnosis, prevention, and public health program development.

My aims in developing this chapter are as follows: (a) to assist public health planners to appreciate the magnitude and form of the tuberculosis problem in order to allocate resources for treatment and prevention; (b) to aid clinicians with diagnosis of active disease—more than with many disorders, the diagnosis of tuberculosis is greatly enhanced by recognition of epidemiological risk factors; and (c) to help identify individuals or groups with latent tuberculosis infection as candidates for preventive chemotherapy.

THE TRADITIONAL ELEMENTS OF EPIDEMIOLOGY

- Who: identifiable populations at risk.
- What: the scope and impact of the infections.
- When: temporal trends in infection patterns.
- Where: geographical locations.
- How: reservoirs and mechanisms of transmission.
- Why: risk factors—why do some become infected and/or diseased and others not?

CONTEMPORARY TERMINOLOGY OF TUBERCULOSIS

As an introduction, the classic terminology of this disease should be reviewed.

Tuberculosis, Infected

This is the state of harboring viable tubercle bacilli within one's body without manifesting signs or symptoms of overt disease. The great majority of normal hosts who are exposed to and infected with *M. tuberculosis* enjoy this status throughout their entire lives.

Tuberculosis, Diseased

This is the state of suffering from active, progressive invasion of an organ or organs by *M. tuberculosis*. This typically is manifested by constitutional symptoms or signs or symptoms that relate to a specific organ system. In most cases, a tuberculin skin test is reactive, but this test is neither specific nor sensitive for disease status. Ideally, bacteriological confirmation (cultivation of *M. tuberculosis* from the sputum, tissues, or fluids of the patient) is desired, but—depending on the form of the disease and local diagnostic resources—substantial numbers of cases are identified by inferential means.

Current American Thoracic Society/Centers for Disease Control (CDC) Classification System

Largely for public health communication and reporting, U.S. authorities have developed a system to classify persons with known or suspected disease and individuals being evaluated in contact investigations surrounding new cases (1). Information gathered in this system forms the backbone of case reporting, although the CDC has recently expanded data gathering to enhance

TABLE 5.1. *Current ATS/CDC classification of persons exposed to and/or infected with M. tuberculosis (1)*

Class	Definition	Comment
0	No known exposure to TB and a negative tuberculin test	Typically, in a contact investigation some persons are deemed not have been exposed or infected.
1	Tuberculosis exposure, no evidence of infection	Person known to have been exposed but tuberculin test is negative. If infant, may also include negative chest x-ray. May require follow-up at 3 months to confirm.
2	Tuberculous infection, no disease	Persons with significant tuberculin reaction but no clinical, radiographic, or bacteriologic evidence of disease.
	[Chemotherapy status]	[To clarify ongoing risk, notation about preventive chemotherapy is to be made.]
3	Tuberculosis, clinically active [Location] [Bacteriologic status] [Chemotherapy status]	Includes all patients with clinically active tuberculosis whose diagnostic studies are adequate to confirm the diagnosis; if inconclusive, should list as class 5.
	± [Chest x-ray findings] ± [Tuberculin reaction]	[Essential data include site(s) involved, culture results, and treatment status for patients with negative cultures but an inferential diagnosis; chest x-ray and tuberculin status must be included.]
4	Tuberculosis, not clinically active	A history of previous episode(s) of tuberculosis or abnormal but stable chest x-ray, positive TST, negative bacteriology (if done), and no clinical or radiographic signs of disease.
	[Chemotherapy status]	[Must note if person has received treatment for disease, preventive chemotherapy, or none.] Until active disease is excluded, should list as class 5.
5	Tuberculosis suspect (diagnosis pending)	Persons in whom active tuberculosis is suspected on basis of clinical, radiographic, and/or epidemiologic factors. Use this status for up to 3 months while complete evaluation is pending.
	[Chemotherapy status]	[Note whether treatment is underway.]

our understanding of the epidemiology of tuberculosis. The various classifications are delineated in Table 5.1.

Smear-Positive (Bacillary) Case

This refers to a patient with tuberculosis of the respiratory tract whose airway secretions, when examined by special stains and microscopy, demonstrate tubercle bacilli. This is a highly significant finding, for the probability of transmitting tuberculosis infection to others is strongly related to the presence of bacilli in the respiratory secretions (see Chapter 3). Some authorities refer to these as "bacillary" cases.

Smear-Negative Pulmonary Case

This refers to a patient with pulmonary disease whose sputum microscopy examination fails to demonstrate bacilli. The diagnosis of disease is established by symptomatology, positive cultures, progressive changes on chest radiograph deemed to reflect disease activity, and/or other supporting data such as tuberculin skin test reactivity, epidemiological features, and—for infants and children—a history of exposure. In some nations with extremely marginal resources, such patients may be designated for less extensive regimens, that is, fewer and/or less potent medications and/or shortened duration.

Extrapulmonary Disease

This is the case of a patient whose clinical illness presents with active inflammatory tuberculosis in organs outside the lungs. Strictly speaking, even endobronchial or pleural disease may be regarded as "extrapulmonary." (In the United States, pleural disease is categorized as "extrapulmonary"; in Canada and the United Kingdom, it is classified as "pulmonary"). Depending on age, race, and immunological competency, 5% to 70% of patients who develop active tuberculosis will manifest it primarily in organs other than the lungs. Most patients have either pulmonary or extrapulmonary tuberculosis; a minority manifest simultaneous disease in both systems. Although extrapulmonary and smear-negative pulmonary cases are both clearly components of the overall morbidity of tuberculosis, they are less significant epidemiologically than sputum smear-positive cases, which act as the primary vectors of transmission to others.

Incidence Rate

The incidence rate is the number of new infections or new cases of active disease (events) occurring in an identified population over a time period. New infections are measured by the rate of newly positive tuberculin skin-test reactions, whereas new cases are defined by the criteria above. Generally, tuberculosis morbidity is referred to in events per 100,000 population per year.

Prevalence of Disease

Prevalence is the percentage or number of those manifesting infection or disease in a population at a given time, e.g., a point survey. Prevalence thus reflects the cumulative morbidity from tuberculosis. If all new cases were promptly "cured" by treatment, the incidence and prevalence of disease would be closely approximate. But if patients are lost from therapy or partially treated, cases of chronic tuberculosis will accumulate, causing gross disparities in the incidence and prevalence values.

Annual Rate of Infection

The annual rate of infection (ARI) is the yearly incidence of new tuberculous infections among "eligible" (tuberculin-negative, not previously infected) members of a population, manifested primarily by tuberculin skin test conversion rates. The ARI has been employed as an indirect or inferential marker of the prevalence of sputum smear-positive (communicable) cases within a population (2). By following a group of individuals known to be nonreactive to tuberculin and observing the frequency with which their skin tests become reactive through time, authorities have attempted to estimate the total tuberculosis morbidity within that community by comparison with established data bases. This technique has been employed primarily in developing nations that lack the resources for consistent diagnosis and case tabulations. Although the logic of ARI appears sound, its actual capacity to quantify transmission rates is problematic because of the inevitable variability in tuberculin skin-test surveys.

GLOBAL AND CONTINENTAL EPIDEMIOLOGY

Introduction

The profile of tuberculosis in the world today has been developed by a mix of direct observations and inferential means such as the annual risk of infection (ARI), as detailed above. Because tuberculosis is most extensive in impoverished nations, which typically have inadequate health information systems, much of the information is indirect.

Styblo developed the ARI model by employing data from both developed and developing nations to calculate a relationship between the incidence of sputum smear-positive cases within a population and the risk to other members of that population of acquiring infection with the tubercle bacillus. The model estimates that 1% of the eligible population will be newly infected annually for every 49 cases of sputum smear-positive tuberculosis (3).

Overview

The World Health Organization (WHO) published in 1995 an overview of the global pattern of tuberculosis (4); estimated case rates and numbers by region are displayed in Table 5.2. Overall, WHO estimated that one in three persons alive today is infected with the tubercle bacillus, that there were nearly 8 million new cases of active tuberculosis and approximately 2.6 million deaths from tuberculosis in 1990, making it the leading etiological agent among lethal infectious diseases of adults in the world.

By contrast with the overall annual incidence of 143 cases per 100,000 in these regions, the overall incidence for the United States in 1997 was 7.4 (5). Actual case "notifications" to the WHO for 1984–1986 and 1989–1991 for the var-

TABLE 5.2. *Estimated global tuberculosis incidence and mortality in 1990*

	Tuberculosis Incidence		Tuberculosis mortality	
	Cases	Rate[a]	Deaths	Rate[a]
Southeast Asia	3,106,000	237	1,087,000	84
Western Pacific[b]	1,839,000	136	644,000	48
Africa	992,000	191	393,000	76
Eastern Mediterranean	641,000	165	249,000	64
Americas[c]	569,000	127	114,000	25
Eastern Europe	194,000	47	29,000	7
Industrialized countries[d]	196,000	23	14,000	2
All regions	7,537,000	143	2,530,000	48

These data represent WHO estimates for cases and rates in various regions for 1990.
[a] Incidence and mortality per 100,000 population.
[b] All countries of region except Australia, Japan, and New Zealand.
[c] All countries of region except Canada and the United States.
[d] Western Europe plus Australia, Canada, Japan, New Zealand, and the United States.

ious regions as defined by WHO and estimated by the methods noted above are found in Table 5.3. Because of deficiencies in reporting in the areas where tuberculosis is most prolific, these numbers are far lower. But increasing cases and rates were demonstrable for much of the world.

Looking at longitudinal trends for tuberculosis, Murray, Styblo, and Rouillon noted a clear divergence between the industrialized nations, where incident case numbers and rates steadily and substantially declined, and the developing world, where the number of reported cases remained stable or rose (3). In the developing nations, if incidence rates declined, they did so only as a result of the dilutional effects of explosive population growth.

Tuberculosis: The Impact of HIV Infection

It is vital to realize that these 1990 WHO data did not yet substantially reflect the influence of HIV infection, with only 316,000 of the 7,537,000 cases calculated to be attributable to HIV. Current trends of the coexisting epidemics, HIV and tuberculosis, in sub-Saharan Africa are alarming and suggest that the data for 1990 substantially underrepresent the future morbidity and mortality from these infections (6). As the WHO analysis re-

TABLE 5.3. *Tuberculosis case notifications and average notification rates by World Health Organization region*

	1984 through 1986, average			1989 through 1991, average			Percent change 1984 through 1986 and 1989 through 1991	
WHO region	Cases	Total, %[a]	Rate[b]	Cases	Total, %[a]	Rate[b]	Cases	Rate[b]
African	264,037	9	66.8	365,465	10	79.6	38.4	19.0
American	227,277	8	34.2	207,790	5	32.7	−8.6	−4.5
Eastern Mediterranean	212,872	7	64.9	281,182	8	74.7	32.1	15.1
European	307,617	10	37.4	242,643	6	29.6	−21.1	−20.8
Southeast Asian	1,338,896	45	115.5	1,874,950	49	146.2	39.9	26.6
Western Pacific	600,185	20	42.6	826,507	22	54.5	37.7	27.9
Global	2,950,884	100	61.8	3,798,537	100	74.6	28.7	20.8

Actual case notifications received by WHO substantially underreport the incidence of tuberculosis, particularly in the developing nations where the disease is most common but public health systems are grossly inadequate. In the period from 1984 through 1991, cases subsided modestly in the American and European regions but rose elsewhere. Indeed outside the American and European regions, cases actually increased by nearly 39%, not 28.7%, in this period.
[a] Percentages may not total 100 because of rounding.
[b] Rate per 100,000 population.

vealed, the overall African population is significantly younger than its Western European counterpart. Because of the high ARI in Africa, large portions of the population aged 15 to 49 are infected with the tubercle bacillus. This sexually active age group is also proving very vulnerable to HIV-1 infection. Another dangerous element of this pattern is the fact that both HIV and tuberculosis are more common in crowded urban areas where tuberculosis transmission is more likely to occur.

As alarming as the African data are, the long-range impact of the coepidemic will likely be greater in the Western Pacific countries and Southeast Asia, where HIV infection is just beginning to make substantial incursions. Confluence of the following elements make the situation there potentially incendiary with regard to tuberculosis: (a) these areas represent the highest prevalence of latent tuberculosis reported by WHO—43.8% and 34.3%, respectively; (b) a larger percentage of the populations there are congregated in crowded urban environments than in Africa, (c) flourishing tourism and commercial sex raise the potential for dramatic increases in the prevalence of HIV infection, and (d) these regions suffer from extremely high rates of drug-resistant strains of *M. tuberculosis,* which will predictably interfere with treatment and prevention of tuberculosis (see Chapter 11). The epidemiological relationships between HIV and tuberculosis are explored further in Chapter 8.

UNITED STATES EPIDEMIOLOGICAL PATTERNS

Remarkably little has been written about tuberculosis in colonial America. However, Holmberg, in reviewing a variety of original source material, concluded that consumption was highly prevalent in America before 1820 (7). Thus, we may infer that, in addition to a taste for independence, the early immigrants to America brought with them the seeds of tuberculosis. Presumably, 18th and 19th Century America experienced a prolonged pandemic cycle of tuberculosis analogous to that described in Europe.

Trends of the 20th Century

Tuberculosis case and mortality rates have declined steadily throughout the 20th Century in the United States. In 1900, the incidence rate was approximately 250, and the death rate in excess of 100, per 100,000 annually. These numbers subsided in the first half of the century (Fig. 5.1),

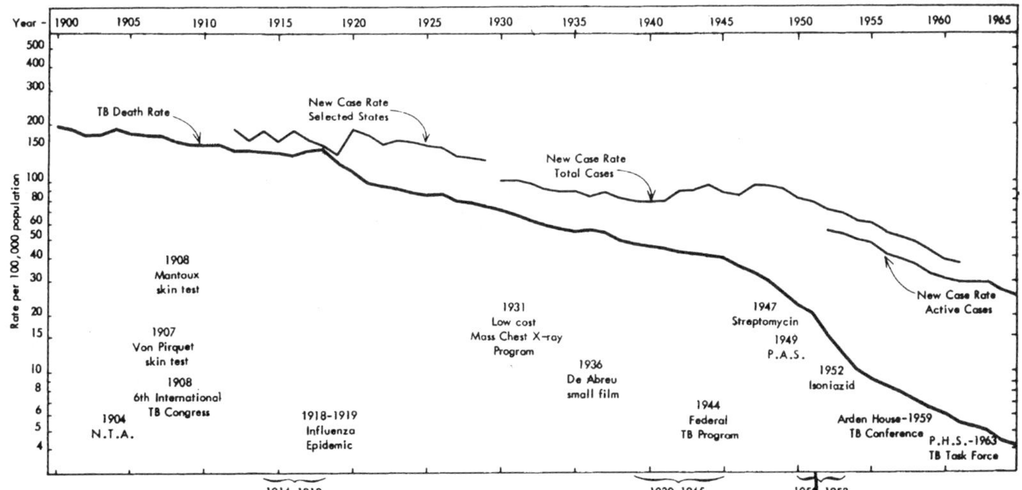

FIG. 5.1. At the turn of the century, only deaths, not cases, of tuberculosis were recorded. At that time, the disease was one of the leading causes of death in the United States. From 1920 to 1950, there was a steady decline in mortality. The sources of this improvement are not clear, but presumed elements would include the impact of the sanatorium movement, improved social, economic, housing, and dietary conditions and, possibly herd immunity. With the advent of curative therapy in the early 1950s, both mortality and morbidity began a steeper decline.

TABLE 5.4. *Trends for the United States of the steep drop in death rates and accelerated decline in incidence rates with the advent of curative chemotherapy, circa 1950*

	1953	1963	1973	1983	1993
Number of cases	84,304	54,042	30,998	23,846	25,287
Case rate[a]	53	28.7	14.8	10.2	9.8
Number of deaths	19,707	9,311	3,875	1,779	1,670
Death rate[a]	12.4	4.9	1.8	0.8	<0.54

Data compiled by the Centers for Disease Control.
[a] Rates are per 100,000 population.

the decline presumably driven by these factors: (a) a predictable reduction associated with the evolution of genetically mediated resistance to the disease—in a continuously exposed population, a darwinian selective process would be natural (see Chapter 4); (b) improved socioeconomic conditions resulting in better housing and nutrition; (c) reduced transmission in the communities secondary to isolation of progressive numbers of active cases in sanatoria (see Chapter 1); and (d) the predictable decline in an epidemic when, because of the factors above, each new case failed to generate a case (or cases) to replace itself.

The advent of curative chemotherapy, circa 1950, induced a steep drop in death rates and an accelerated decline in incidence rates. These trends for the United States are highlighted by the data compiled by the Centers for Disease Control in Table 5.4. As would be expected, chemotherapy had a greater impact on mortality rates (23-fold reduction) than on case rates (5.4-fold reduction) from 1953 to 1993.

Recent Resurgence

However, this steady decline in tuberculosis case rates, which averaged roughly 5.5% yearly, began leveling off in 1984. From that time to 1993, there was an upturn in the incidence of cases, resulting in a surplus of roughly 70,000 cases above those anticipated between 1985 and 1993 (Fig. 5.2). The causes of this upturn have not been fully quantified. However, analysis of the data indicates that the following elements contributed:

Immigration

An analysis of case rates among foreign-born persons in the United States from 1986 to 1993 indicates that the absolute number of cases rose from 4,925 cases in 1986 to 7,346 in 1993 (8). During this period, foreign-born cases comprised a steadily increasing portion of the total morbidity, 21.6% rising to 29.6% in 1993. Federal authorities estimated that the burgeoning cases among the foreign-born were responsible for 60% of the total increase in the period 1986–1992 (9).

HIV Infection

The rising tuberculosis case rates were coincident temporally, geographically, and demographically with the appearance of HIV/AIDS in the United States, rising throughout the decade 1982–1992, affecting primarily large urban populations, involving disproportionate numbers of persons aged 25 to 44, and afflicting substantially African-American and Hispanic minorities. Because there are incomplete data on HIV serology reporting, it is not possible to establish comprehensive linkage between these coepidemics. However, the available information indicated that HIV/AIDS was responsible for approximately 30% of the excess morbidity (10).

Deteriorating Public Health Services

Although it is difficult to quantify the effect of this factor, many observers of urban health in America have concluded that budgetary disruptions within its large cities, which resulted in

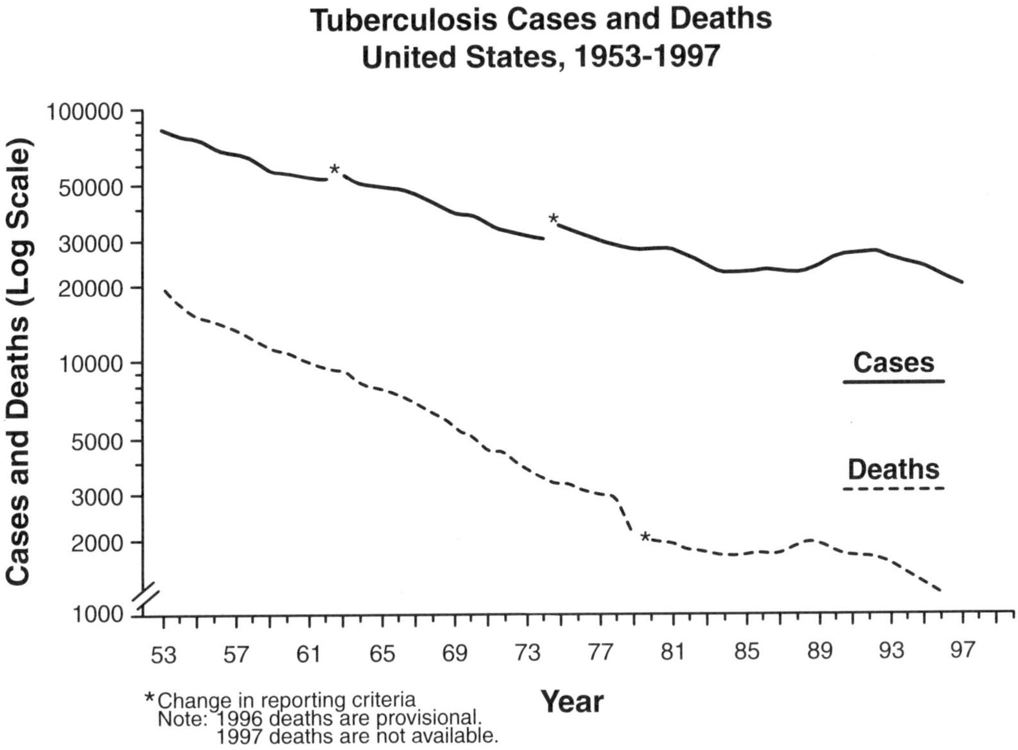

FIG. 5.2.

curtailment of preventive health, medical, and social services, contributed to the worsening tuberculosis morbidity (11). Coupled with homelessness and substance abuse, the truncation of tuberculosis treatment and control programs resulted in fertile breeding grounds for tuberculosis.

New York City: A Case Study

To illustrate these elements in resurgence, one may examine tuberculosis in New York City over the past 25 years as a case study. In many respects, New York City represents a vivid example of contemporary forces that are influencing American public health and tuberculosis. As a major port of entry for immigration, a community always rich with minority groups and the United States' densest urban aggregation, New York has experienced documented high rates of tuberculosis throughout the entire 20th Century. However, inspired by the vision of Herman Biggs, New York—both city and state—led the way in the early decades of the century with beneficial public health regulations and the development of sentinel tuberculosis treatment and prevention programs. Resources in the battle against tuberculosis included neighborhood tuberculosis clinics, specialty hospital facilities, a network of sanatoria for long-term care, a comprehensive information system, efficient laboratory support, and a dedicated cadre of specialty workers—physicians, nurses, technicians, and administrators. However, with the advent of curative therapy and the presumed demise of tuberculosis as a public health menace, authorities rapidly eliminated these programs and reallocated the assets to other, "more pressing" problems.

This situation is reflected in a report by Brudney and Dobkin of tuberculosis care at Harlem Hospital in 1988 that ranks, in my estimation, as one of the more significant studies in contemporary medicine (11). The document focuses on the abysmal failure of the municipal tuberculosis program to conduct adequate therapy for 224 patients, the great majority of whom suffered from combinations of alcoholism, drug abuse, homelessness, unemployment, and HIV/AIDS. Critically, the authors reviewed the decisions and policies that were at the roots of this failed program. Highlights of their findings were as follows:

1. In 1968, New York City (NYC) spent $40,000,000 on tuberculosis; there were 21 tuberculosis specialty clinics run by the city Health Department, seven "combined" clinics run jointly by the Health and the Hospital Departments, and over 1,000 beds in NYC hospitals plus a number of beds in upstate hospitals designated for tuberculosis care.
2. A community task force in 1968 urged reduction in the hospital care of tuberculosis patients, an appropriate plan given the demonstrated efficacy of outpatient treatment. They urged that 100 of the tuberculosis beds be closed annually and that resources be shifted to outpatient care, recommending $18,000,000 per year for that purpose by 1973.
3. The task force advocated that the outpatient program feature flexible clinic hours, trained workers from the community, home care, domiciliary facilities for special patients, and integration of tuberculosis programs with alcohol and substance abuse clinics.
4. However, 10 years later, in 1978, tuberculosis patients were increasingly under the care of private practitioners, who generally did not have the temperament or the resources to deal with noncompliance or to perform contact investigations and carry out preventive therapy.
5. The combined city and state 1978 expenditures for tuberculosis control were only $2,000,000; the outpatient treatment system was grossly inadequate in terms of both capacity and assets.

Given this scenario, it is not surprising that New York City tuberculosis case rates had begun to rise in 1979, mainly as a result of these socioeconomic factors. This was well before the impact of HIV/AIDS. To worsen matters, in 1979, New York State terminated its tuberculosis control contract with the City, money that had supported 50% of the metropolitan program (12); as seen in Fig. 5.3, cases and rates began rising in the late 1970s. Case rates for central Harlem in the 1980s were comparable to those of impoverished, Third-World countries.

The saga noted above documents the deterioration that befell New York's program; similar stories could be told for many of the United States' larger cities. None were protected from the economic turbulence that buffeted America's urban centers. But, unlike prior episodes of municipal distress, neither state administrations nor the federal government were able or willing to come to their aid in this era.

On this weakened urban fabric then fell the two major cofactors in the resurgence of tuberculosis in the United States: HIV/AIDS and immigration. Again, examining the New York City experience may inform us of the nature of these problems.

The contribution that HIV infection made to increases in tuberculosis case rates in New York City or other regions cannot be strictly quantified because HIV serology testing was not performed systematically. However, the individuals most dramatically affected by the resurgent tuberculosis were demographically very closely linked to the HIV/AIDS epidemic. Brudney and Dobkin showed that 71% of the 224 adult tuberculosis patients from Harlem Hospital had HIV risk factors; of the 140 who submitted to testing, 112 (80%) were positive. By 1993, among men with tuberculosis in NYC, 36% were known to be HIV-positive; among those whose serologic status was known, 70% were seropositive (13). Among females, these figures were 28% and 61%, respectively (13).

The impact of immigrant tuberculosis morbidity is easier to delineate than that of HIV. In 1993, 27% of all newly reported cases in New York City occurred in persons from outside the continental United States; this pattern had been consistent for the previous seven years, averaging approximately 25% of the annual morbidity (13). The Caribbean area accounted for 44% of this group in 1993.

TB Cases in New York City, 1921 - 1994

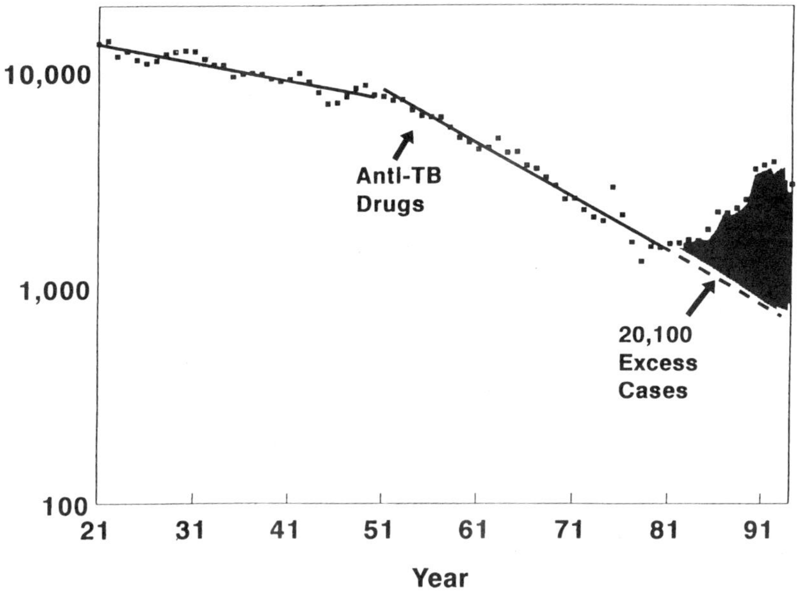

FIG. 5.3. Mirroring the national trends, case rates began a steeper decline with the advent of curative chemotherapy circa 1950. However, in the early 1980s, well before the national upturn in cases, New York City case numbers rose. Indeed, of the approximate 75,000 national surplus cases seen between 1984 and 1994, New York City produced roughly one-third of these cases.

In summary, the case study of New York City—a microcosm of American life—indicates that the triad of urban deterioration, AIDS, and immigration had a dramatic effect on tuberculosis: in 1991, New York, with roughly 3.5% of the United States population, experienced 14% (3,673 cases) of the total United States tuberculosis morbidity. In the decade of the 1980s, New York City alone suffered an excess of over 12,000 cases above predicted. The incidence rate of 50.2 for New York City was roughly fivefold higher than the national level of 10.2 cases per 100,000. Because the upsurge was largely among men in the sexually active ages of 25 to 44 years, there was spillover of the epidemic to involve women of slightly younger ages. Also involved were the children of these individuals' families: in 1991, there were 159 cases in those under 15 years of age, a 115% increase over the number from 1989.

In response to this extraordinary upturn in tuberculosis morbidity and mortality, new personnel and programs were brought into the battle in New York City (14). These heroic (and expensive) measures bore fruit: overall case rates have fallen substantially, with the greatest reductions occurring among blacks, Hispanics, homeless, and HIV-infected persons. Approximately 450 cases of multidrug-resistant (MDR) tuberculosis occurred in 1992, falling to roughly 50 in 1997. These results clearly indicate curtailment of recent transmission of infection. A major contributor to this improvement was the widened use of directly observed therapy (DOT). In 1985, fewer than 5% of eligible patients were on DOT; this figure rose to over 60% by 1996 (see Chapter 10 for extended discussion of impact of DOT programs).

The dramatic improvement in New York City's TB statistics is very gratifying. Elements involved with this turnaround clearly include expanded DOT, reductions in nosocomial transmission as a result of improved policies and facilities, and a natural but tragic attrition of MDR TB carriers because of high mortality rates among persons with AIDS. But this remedial campaign was extremely expensive. Authorities calculate that New York City spent roughly $1,000,000,000 in the early 1990s to regain control of tuberculosis (15).

A critical take-away message from this saga is that the improvement occurred despite the continued HIV/AIDS epidemic among TB-vulnerable subjects and ongoing immigration from areas endemic for tuberculosis. *The only real difference in the eras 1982–1992 ("rampant") and 1993–1997 ("subsiding") were competent detection/treatment programs and improved infection control practices and facilities.*

As this sad period recedes, we may anticipate that authorities will begin to whittle away at commitments. Rather than sustain high-quality programs until we might truly contemplate elimination, cuts will probably be made that will again unleash this destructive disease.

> "What experience and history teach is this—that people and governments never have learned anything from history, or acted on principles deduced from it" (Georg Wilhelm Friedrich Hegel, *Philosophy of History*, 1832).

CURRENT EPIDEMIOLOGY IN THE UNITED STATES

Overall, there have been recent divergent trends in the United States: (a) rising case rates in high-prevalence areas and (b) remarkable reductions elsewhere with increasing numbers of counties that report no cases in a given year. Woven into this polarity are a number of general observations:

- Minorities suffer disproportionately from tuberculosis
- Socioeconomic factors play a dominant role in the disproportionate morbidity among these groups
- Recent immigrants constitute a very high-risk population
- Tuberculosis among Hispanics and blacks predominantly involves younger persons; among whites, it is largely a disease of the elderly
- Readily identifiable groups are at high risk for tuberculosis

The following section examines patterns by state, city, age, sex, race, country of origin, and special risk factors.

States

Case numbers and rates in 1997 for the states and District of Columbia are displayed in Table 5.5 (5); they are compared with data from 1992. In terms of raw numbers, California (4,059), New York (2,265), Texas (1,992), Florida (1,400), Illinois (974), New Jersey (718), and Georgia (696) alone yielded a total of 12,104 cases or 61% of the total national morbidity in 1997. Of note, these states had produced 17,320 cases 5 years earlier; the difference represents a 36% reduction in these seven states over the 5-year interval. Leading the way among these states were New York (−50%) and California (−25%); these data were part of an overall national reduction of −26%. In this period, 11 states had increased case numbers, one was unchanged, and 39 states enjoyed reduced numbers. From 1996 to 1997 there was a −7% reduction in cases.

Cities

In 1994, a typical year in which to calculate these relationships, United States cities with populations in excess of 500,000 (97 communities) reported 18,040 cases (16). Thus, among these areas—which had a total population of 161,058,347—the annual case rates averaged 11.2 per 100,000. By contrast, among the other 99,282,653 residents who live in smaller communities or rural areas, there were 6,321 cases, for a case rate of 6.3. Urban dominance may be seen as well in the 1997 data. Sixty-four cities yielded 40% of the total national morbidity, and in the seven leading states noted above, a disproportionate share of cases were derived from their major cities (5).

Age

The distribution of 1997 tuberculosis cases by age is as follows: under 5, 3.8%; 5 to 14, 2.6%;

TABLE 5.5. *Number of reported tuberculosis cases, percentage change in number of cases, and case rates by state and year, United States, 1992 and 1997*

	No. cases		Change (%) from 1992	Case rate	
State	1992	1997	to 1997	1992	1997
Alabama	418	405	−3%	10.1	9.4
Alaska	57	78	37%	9.7	12.8
Arizona	259	296	14%	6.8	6.5
Arkansas	257	200	−22%	10.7	7.9
California	5,382	4,059	−25%	17.4	12.6
Colorado	104	94	−10%	3.0	2.4
Connecticut	156	128	−18%	4.8	3.9
Delaware	55	39	−29%	8.0	5.3
District of Columbia	146	110	−25%	24.8	20.8
Florida	1,707	1,400	−18%	12.7	9.6
Georgia	893	696	−22%	13.2	9.3
Hawaii	273	167	−39%	23.5	14.1
Idaho	26	15	−42%	2.4	1.2
Illinois	1,270	974	−23%	10.9	8.2
Indiana	247	168	−32%	4.4	2.9
Iowa	49	74	51%	1.7	2.6
Kansas	56	78	39%	2.2	3.0
Kentucky	402	199	−50%	10.7	5.1
Louisiana	373	406	9%	8.7	9.3
Maine	24	21	−13%	1.9	1.7
Maryland	442	340	−23%	9.0	6.7
Massachusetts	428	268	−37%	7.1	4.4
Michigan	495	374	−24%	5.2	3.8
Minnesota	165	161	−2%	3.7	3.4
Mississippi	281	245	−13%	10.7	9.0
Missouri	245	248	1%	4.7	4.6
Montana	16	18	13%	1.9	2.0
Nebraska	28	22	−21%	1.7	1.3
Nevada	99	112	13%	7.5	6.7
New Hampshire	18	17	−6%	1.6	1.4
New Jersey	984	718	−27%	12.6	8.9
New Mexico	88	71	−19%	5.6	4.1
New York	4,574	2,265	−50%	25.2	12.5
North Carolina	604	463	−23%	8.8	6.2
North Dakota	11	12	9%	1.7	1.9
Ohio	358	286	−20%	3.2	2.6
Oklahoma	216	212	−2%	6.7	6.4
Oregon	145	161	11%	4.9	5.0
Pennsylvania	758	528	−30%	6.3	4.4
Rhode Island	54	38	−30%	5.4	3.9
South Carolina	387	328	−15%	10.7	8.7
South Dakota	32	19	−41%	4.5	2.6
Tennessee	527	467	−11%	10.5	8.7
Texas	2,510	1,992	−21%	14.2	10.2
Utah	78	36	−54%	4.3	1.7
Vermont	7	6	−14%	1.2	1.0
Virginia	457	350	−23%	7.2	5.2
Washington	306	305	0	6.0	5.4
West Virginia	92	54	−41%	5.1	3.0
Wisconsin	106	130	23%	2.1	2.5
Wyoming	8	2	−75%	1.7	0.4
Total	26,673	19,855	−26%	10.5	7.4

These data demonstrate vividly the substantial decline in case numbers, 26%, and case rates, 30%, during this 5-year period. During this time, utilization of directly-observed therapy rose nationally from less than 5% to over 40%. Case rates are per 100,000 population.

15 to 24, 8.5%; 25 to 44, 34.8%; 45 to 64, 26.7%; and 65 or older, 23.6%. The data are also broken down according to race and ethnicity, revealing an extraordinary disparity between minorities and non-Hispanic whites. The pattern for blacks, Hispanics, and Asian/Pacific Islanders reveals that 49% of cases are amassed between ages of 15 and 44, whereas among non-Hispanic whites only 26% of the cases occur in this age range. There are also gross discrepancies at the extremes of age according to race. Only 96 of the 747 cases among children under 5 occurred among whites, accounting for 12.9% of the morbidity in this group. By contrast, 2,077 of the cases in persons 65 or older, 44.3% of the morbidity, occurred among whites. Overall case rates by age in 1997 were as follows: under 5, 3.9; 5 to 14, 1.3; 15 to 24, 4.6; 25 to 44, 8.3; 45 to 64, 9.6; and 65 or older, 13.8/100,000/year.

Sex

Throughout the 20th century in the United States there has been a consistent pattern of excess tuberculosis morbidity among men. Recent data reaffirm that finding: in 1985, 65%, and, in 1997, 62% of cases were male. The numbers according to race in 1997 are fairly consistent: among whites, 66% were male; blacks, 63%; Hispanics, 64%; Asian/Pacific Islanders, 55%; and among American Indians/Alaskan Natives, 55% were male. Of note, among infants and children up to age 14, case rates are equal by sex or tend toward a slight female preponderance. By age 65 or older, however, there is a roughly 2:1 male-to-female ratio in all racial groups.

Race

Tuberculosis in the United States is not an equal-opportunity disease. Over the 40 years that comprehensive public health statistics on tuberculosis have been kept, there has been a steady, progressive disparity in the proportion of tuberculosis morbidity borne by minorities.

Largely, this reflects diminishing case rates among whites without commensurate reductions in those for persons of color. The incident rates for the American racial/ethnic groups in 1997 are listed in Table 5.6 (5). The decade of the 1980s witnessed for the first time the majority of new cases occurring among America's minorities; by 1997, 75.5% of the cases involved these groups (Fig. 5.4).

TABLE 5.6. *Incidence rates for the American racial/ethnic groups in 1997*

Group	Incidence/per 100,000 population	Relative risk[a]
Non-Hispanic whites	2.5	1.0
Black, non-Hispanic	20.5	8.2
Hispanic	14.4	5.8
Asian/Pacific Islander	40.6	16.2
Native American/ Alaskan Native	13.4	5.4

[a] The ratio of the case rates for other groups compared to non-Hispanic whites.

The factors leading to these high relative risk ratios for minorities in the United States were recently analyzed with adjustments made for socioeconomic status (17). By using demographic data and a sophisticated multivariate analysis, the authors attempted to relate tuberculosis rates to six socioeconomic status (SES) indicators: crowding, income, public assistance, poverty, unemployment, and education. Predictably, they found that case rates overall went up as these SES indicators went down. Crowding was a potent risk factor, particularly among black Americans. In the aggregate, adjusting for these SES risk factors accounted for approximately *one-half* the increased rates seen among the groups noted above. Although these extrinsic factors clearly play an immense role in the disproportionate tuberculosis morbidity in these groups, "poverty's penalty" (18), consideration should be given to differences in genetic susceptibility as well (see Genetic Susceptibility below).

Foreign Birth

In 1986, 4,925 cases of tuberculosis were reported among foreign-born persons in the United States, 21.6% of the national morbidity. By 1997, this number had risen to 7,702 cases and 38.8% of the total morbidity (5). This trend is illustrated in Fig. 5.5. The proportion of for-

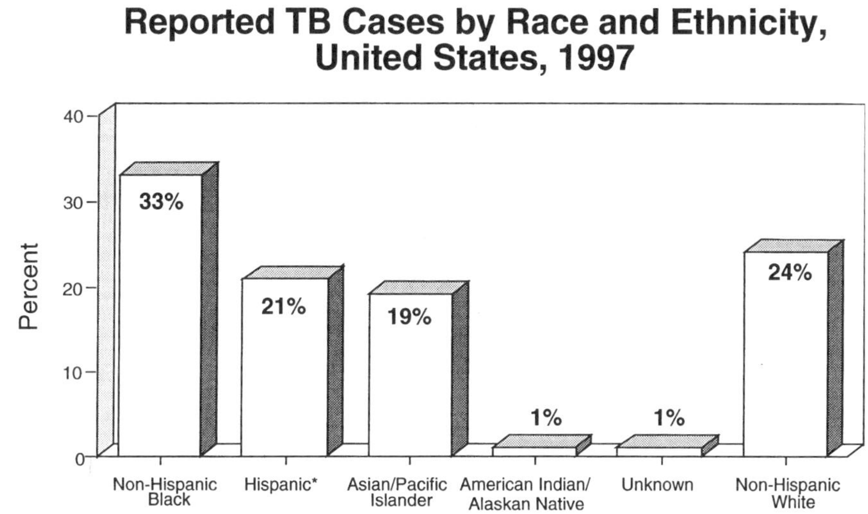

FIG. 5.4. Approximately one-fourth of cases now occur in white Americans, whereas a decade earlier, one-half of the morbidity involved this group. This shift reflects diminishing risks in whites, stable risks in indigenous persons of color, and a rising number of cases among immigrant minorities over this period.

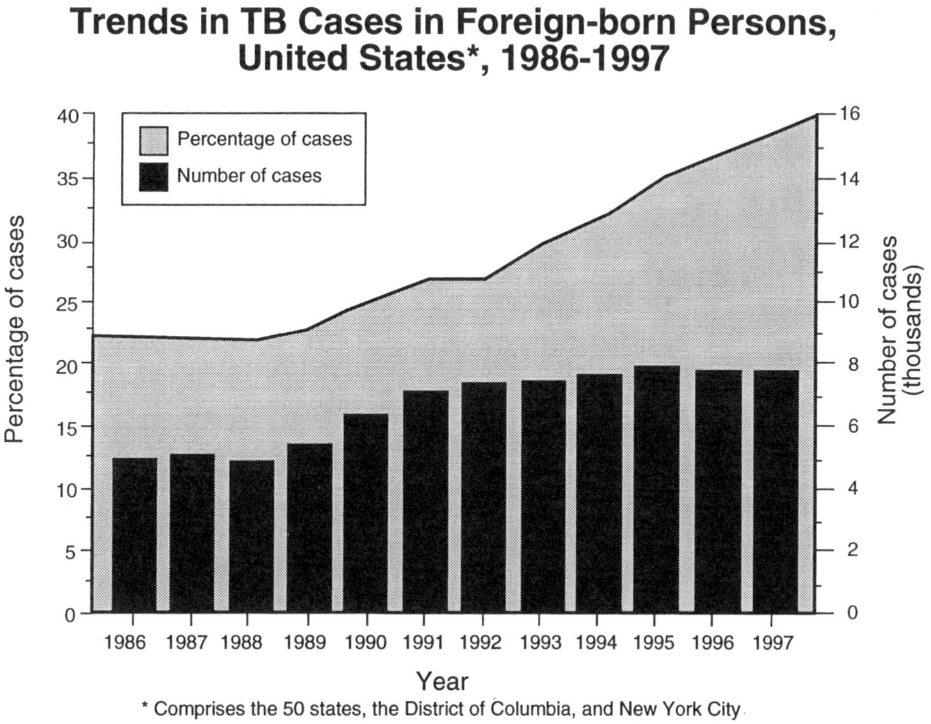

FIG. 5.5. Over this 12-year period, cases among persons born in the United States fell substantially while the number of cases among the foreign-born, residing in the United States, actually rose. This increase occurred despite significant efforts on the part of the Immigration and Naturalization Service to screen more thoroughly. Many factors were involved with this trend; please see text.

eign-born cases varies widely by state. The highest percentages for 1997 were reported from Hawaii (75%), Massachusetts (69%), California (69%), and Washington (63%). By contrast, among states with high case rates among the indigenous populations, a much lower proportion of foreign-born cases was seen, for example, Alabama (5%), Arkansas (8%), Kentucky (7%), Louisiana (6%), Mississippi (4%), and Tennessee (9%).

The countries from which these cases were derived include the following: Mexico (1,685), Philippines (1,054), Vietnam (817), India (465), Republic of China (386), Haiti (284), and Republic of Korea (260) (Fig. 5.6). These seven countries yielded a total of 4,951 cases or 65% of all foreign-born cases. State-by-state distribution by country of origin for 1997 is available (5).

Factors associated with the high rates of disease among foreign-born subjects have been explored in a variety of reports. The methods and problems with overseas screening of immigrants and refugees were noted in a 1996 report from Centers for Disease Control and Prevention (19); notable in this report are the lack of sensitivity and specificity of screening tools as well as the high percentage of cases in certain communities such as Los Angeles, occurring among persons who have not been screened, e.g., undocumented or illegal aliens.

Another report from the CDC examined the utility of the 1991 guidelines in detecting/predicting cases in Hawaii (20). These guidelines use chest x-rays and sputum examinations to categorize subjects as class A infectious tuberculosis (abnormal x-ray, positive smear); class B1 active tuberculosis, not infectious (abnormal x-ray, negative smear); class B2 inactive tuberculosis (x-ray abnormal but not suggestive of active disease, smear negative); class B3 calcified granuloma only; and no TB. They observed that of 124 cases of active disease occurring within one year of arrival among these immigrants and refugees, 14% were among those classified as B2, and 23% among "normals." Similarly, a report from Seattle documented that 5% of 924 immigrants and refugees coming to this community had active disease within a few years of arrival and that a very high percentage, 34%, of

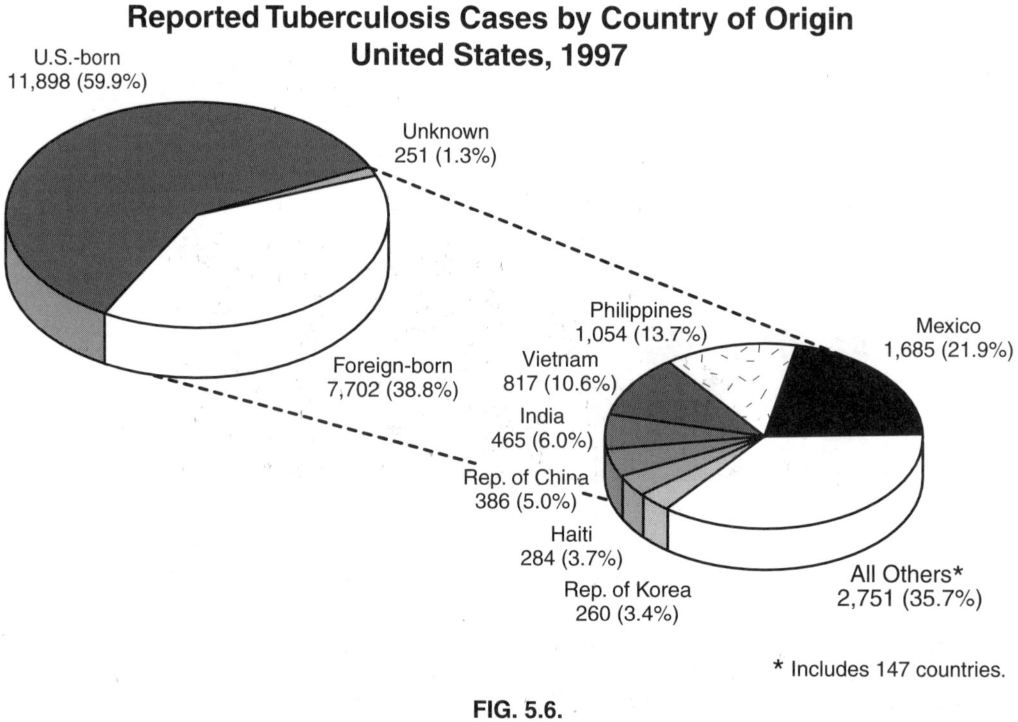

FIG. 5.6.

this population were candidates for preventive chemotherapy (21). And, among 893 immigrants and refugees coming to San Francisco from 1992 through 1993, 7% were found to have active disease, and 40% were candidates for preventive chemotherapy at their time of arrival (22). All of these reports emphasize the critical importance of early evaluation and interventions for these populations. An analysis of tuberculosis among foreign-born persons in Los Angeles, 1992–1994, noted extreme morbidity in immigrants and refugees but reached different conclusions regarding the utility of screening and intervention (23). Although foreign-born comprised 60% of the cases in this period, most of them came from Mexico and Central America, were undocumented, and, therefore, were not accessible for screening.

One particularly alarming report of tuberculosis among foreign-born described Tibetan refugees who immigrated from camps in India and Nepal to Minnesota in 1992–1995 (24). Among 191 subjects screened, a total of 16 cases (8.4%) were noted within 1.5 years of arrival, and 98% overall were tuberculin reactors. Ominously, six of the nine cases involved drug-resistant strains, with three of these six yielding MDR TB strains.

Of note, recent reports from Canada (25), England and Wales (26), the Netherlands (27), Denmark (28), and Australia (29) all indicate substantial numbers of tuberculosis cases among their foreign-born populations.

A 1997 report from the CDC offered very useful insights into patterns of tuberculosis among foreign-born persons in the United States (30). Among the cohort of cases reported from 1986–1994, 32.6% of the cases were among the foreign-born, roughly one-fourth of these from Mexico and almost one-half from Asia. The authors noted that immigrants who arrived after their fifth birthday had tuberculosis rates two- to sixfold higher than comparably aged persons who had arrived before their fifth birthday, suggesting that infection had generally occurred before arrival in the United States. Nearly two-thirds of this group had been eligible for preventive chemotherapy but had not been identified or treated. And because of inadequate screening or local programs, immigrants from several countries had annual case rates greater than 20 per 100,000 up to 20 years after arrival in the United States.

One particularly thorny aspect of tuberculosis among foreign-born persons is the care of "illegal" or "undocumented" aliens. In response to perceived heavy burdens of social and medical services for these individuals, the citizens of California voted for "Proposition 187," which would have substantially curtailed many benefits to them, including treatment for all but emergent forms of disease including tuberculosis. Never enacted, the Proposition remains in adjudication. But, the ethical implications of acceding to these regulations were explored in a 1995 essay (31). However, the issues are not uncomplicated; it is one thing for physicians to provide their services freely, it is another for them to expend potentially large sums of *public* money against legally established regulations (32).

INDIVIDUAL RISK FACTORS

In the introduction to this chapter, the "why" of epidemiology was noted. This issue involves identifying particular features of individuals that make them more likely to develop tuberculosis. Potential factors in this process include (a) extrinsic risk factors in promoting the acquisition of new infections, (b) intrinsic vulnerability to the acquisition of new infection, and (c) intrinsic risk factors for progressive disease or reactivation of the latent tuberculous infection. In this section, these risk factors are described as biological or environmental, although there well may be interrelations between these phenomena.

Extrinsic: Settings That Influence Risk of Acquisition of Infection

There are readily identifiable environments in which the probability of a person being exposed to and infected with tubercle bacilli are substantially greater than in other walks of life. These are worth careful notation because these situations are epidemiologic clues that should direct clinicians to consider the possibility of tuberculous disease or infection. Some of the more

TABLE 5.7. *Risk factors for acquiring infection with M. tuberculosis*

Situation/group	Comments
Correctional facilities	Inmates and staff at risk. Major contributors include high percentages of minority and immigrant inmates, crowding, and HIV infection.
Nursing homes	Residents and staff at risk. Common elements include delayed diagnosis, poor ventilation, and reluctance to use INH preventive therapy.
Homeless shelters/SRO hotels	Crowding, poor ventilation, malnutrition, alcohol, and HIV infection all contribute to risks.
Health care workers	Exposure in hospitals and clinics.
Substance abuse	Seen with IDU and "crack" cocaine use; high-risk minorities.
Immigrant camps	High-risk national origins, crowding, stress, and lack of access to health care.
Migrant worker camps	High-risk national origins; crowding.

prominent risk settings are delineated in Table 5.7.

Correctional Facilities

Tuberculosis outbreaks have been noted in multiple correction facilities in the United States over the past 20 years. Stead described an epidemic arising in an Arkansas prison, potentially involving nearly 90% of the state's entire male tuberculosis morbidity (33); infection rates in the prison were 6.5-fold higher than those in the general population. In 1988–1990, 24% of the tuberculosis cases in Nassau County, NY were associated with the county jail (34). Three outbreaks of MDR TB were recorded in the New York state prisons, involving both HIV-infected and noninfected persons (35). And, autopsies on a series of patients in Texas with AIDS found those with histories of incarceration were significantly more likely to have tuberculosis (36). Similar findings have been described in foreign correctional facilities (37,38).

Prisons and jails in the United States are particularly hazardous environments in this era for the following reasons: (a) the majority of inmates come from minority populations, which are at high risk for tuberculosis, (b) the vast preponderance of inmates are men aged 20 to 44, the highest-risk ages within these minority populations for active disease, (c) substance abuse, an independent risk factor for tuberculosis, is highly prevalent in the prison/jail populations, (d) HIV/AIDS is relatively common among inmates of correctional facilities, and (e) because of the explosive increase in the number of persons sentenced to correctional facilities, prisons and jails are densely crowded, potentiating the risk for transmission of tuberculosis (39); also, the frequent transfers used to control gang activities have interfered with surveillance and transmission control (40). Among inmates of the New York State prison system the incidence of tuberculosis increased from 15.4 in 1976–1978 to 105.5 per 100,000 in 1986, a 685% rise in a decade; 56% of those inmates with tuberculosis in 1985–1986 were HIV infected (41). A 1984–1985 survey of 29 state prison systems showed that the tuberculosis incidence for prisoners was 30.9, a rate 3.9-fold higher than the general populations of these states (42).

Nursing Homes

Nursing homes have also proven themselves to be high risk environments for the transmission of tuberculosis. A substantial proportion of America's population 65 years and older harbor latent tuberculosis infections, reflecting the fact that persons who were alive during the first three decades of this century, when tuberculosis was widely prevalent, faced a very great likelihood of being exposed to and infected with tubercle bacilli in their childhood and youth. Unlike today, tuberculosis then did not observe neat boundaries, afflicting persons of all races and economic classes. Most of these individuals have survived without any manifest illness attributable to tuberculosis. However, as they advance in years, there is predictable senescence of cell-mediated immunity (43–45). Among the manifestations of this process is progressive waning of tuberculin skin test reactivity and increased risk for reactivation. Diminishing rates of tuberculin reactivity were reported in two recent studies: (a) among a group of Canadian men aged 65 to 74, 50% were tuberculin positive, whereas only 26.7% of a contemporary group aged 85 to 94 were positive (46), and (b) a survey in Arkansas revealed similar findings, with 54% of men 60 to 69 having significant reactions while only 35% in the age range 80 to 89 were positive (47). The diminishing rates of skin-test reactivity presumably reflect an impairment of cellular immune capacity, which is responsible for heightened vulnerability to tuberculosis.

Increasing risks for reactivation with age are demonstrated in 1984 data (chosen to reflect the patterns before the impact of HIV/AIDS) for the United States, shown in Fig. 5.7A. The national

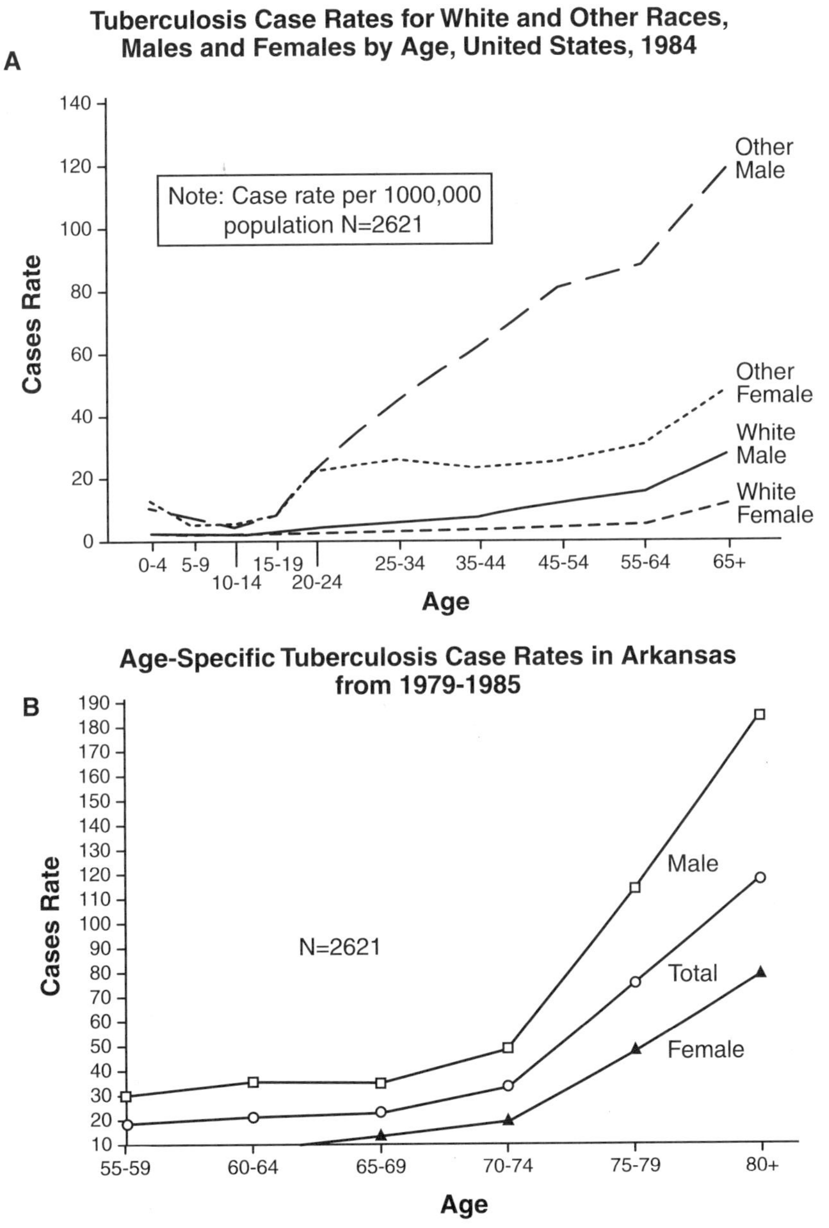

FIG. 5.7. A sharp increase is apparent at about age 70. In states with a large minority or refugee population, the increase in the elderly may be less apparent.

data reveal a "hockey-stick" upturn in case rates beginning in the age range 55 to 64 for white men, white women, and "other" women; by contrast, the pattern for "other" men rises from age 20 to 24, with the suggestion of a second acceleration in case rates for this group at age 55 to 64. These national data may be viewed in contrast to data from Arkansas, where age-related incidence rates from 1979 to 1985 show a clear demarcation of case rates at age 70 (Fig. 5.7B). There are many variables to consider in analyzing these data. I interpret the disparity in case rates between the United States and Arkansas in this manner. There clearly is a biological phenomenon associated with aging that renders persons vulnerable to reactivation tuberculosis. However, at a national level, young minority men are subjected to a variety of environmental and biological influences, including homelessness, substance abuse, and HIV infection, which increase their risks for acquiring active tuberculosis. These factors are arguably less prevalent in Arkansas society, allowing the normal age-related vulnerability to be seen more clearly.

Nursing home placement appears to exacerbate this tendency to increased tuberculosis vulnerability with age (48). Factors that are likely to contribute to this propensity to tuberculosis include intercurrent illnesses, loss of home, and separation from spouse—stresses that may well have substantial impact on homeostasis and immunity, thus promoting endogenous reactivity (see Social/Environmental Variables, below). In addition to these elements, the possibility of adverse effects on tuberculoimmunity of reduced serum levels of vitamin D might be considered. Among a large group of elderly Europeans, vitamin D levels fell to inadequate levels during the winter months, when their activity and exposure to sunlight were curtailed (49); unfortunately, these factors are common among nursing home residents.

In addition to reactivation tuberculosis, nursing homes have been the scene of large scale epidemics (50). An important aspect of the epidemics among these nursing home populations was the extraordinary rapidity with which active disease developed in the newly infected in the Arkansas report: 11.7% of men and 7.6% of women with newly positive tuberculin skin tests following exposure went on to develop active disease within 6 months. Such vulnerability is matched only by infants and persons with AIDS. Of note: INH preventive therapy was well tolerated and effective among newly infected contacts. The high risk of fatal outcomes with tuberculosis in the elderly is documented by data from the Netherlands (51), further justifying the small risk of hepatitis from INH.

Homelessness, Shelters, and Single-Room-Occupancy (SRO) Hotels

These facilities are prominent among contemporary environments that entail particularly high risks for transmission of tuberculosis (52). A 1980 survey of tuberculosis among residents of a SRO hotel found that 98 of 191 (51%) screened were tuberculin skin test positive, 13 (7%) had active, culture-positive disease, and another 21 were candidates for isoniazid preventive therapy (53). A later study from New York City's Men's Shelter (1982–1988) revealed that 38.6% of the men tested were tuberculin reactors and another 6% had active disease (54); a more recent survey of persons seeking social services in New York City found over 40% to be tuberculin reactors, with residence in a congregate setting to be a risk factor (55). An epidemic of tuberculosis occurred in a shelter for homeless men in Seattle from 1985 to 1987. It involved 20 cases, many of which appeared related to recent transmission in the shelter (56). Elements that promoted transmission included a relatively stable client pool, close proximity of bedding, and a closed-recirculating ventilation system—elements common to virtually all such facilities. Similar outbreaks in six other shelters were reported to the CDC between 1984 and 1988 (52). Also, a state-wide RFLP analysis of tuberculosis strains in Alabama identified a large, ongoing epidemic among the homeless in Birmingham (57). In addition to time spent in such institutions, persons living in these circumstances are likely to socialize in bars where wholesale transmission of tuberculosis has been shown to occur (58).

Additional objective data indicating a probable direct role for homelessness and residency in shelters in promoting tuberculosis may be found in molecular epidemiology reports that indicate high rates of strain clustering among homeless men in Los Angeles (59) and New York (60,61). Also, patterns of drug resistance strongly indicated transmission of tuberculosis among the homeless in Boston (62) and Texas (63).

Health Care Workers

Health care workers historically have always been at risk for tuberculosis. Because of their more extended exposures to patients, nurses and physicians have borne the major portion of this morbidity. From 1920 to 1953, as many as 9% of the patients at the Trudeau Sanatorium in New York State were medical students or physicians (64). (Ironically, the disease, by afflicting physicians, has recruited some of the most astute scientists ever to do battle with the microorganism: Gaspard Laurent Bayle and Rene Theophile Hyacinthe Läennec in the 18th century, Edward Livingston Trudeau in the 19th century, and a remarkable group of 20th-century scholars including Drs. J. Burns Amberson, James J. Waring, Allen K. Krause, Esmond Ray Long, Roger Mitchell, Gerald Baum, Glenn Lillington, Georges Canetti, Jacques Chretien, and Jacques Grosset.)

Two surveys of tuberculosis among physicians in the United States inform us of modern trends. Barrett-Connor studied 6,425 physicians on the rosters of seven California medical schools in 1974–1975 (65). Salient findings of the survey included these: (a) students matriculating in 1975 had a 70% lower prevalence of tuberculin reactivity than those doing so in 1950, and following matriculation, the 1975 students experienced 78% less tuberculin reactivity; (b) 69 of 669 (10.3%) physicians who graduated between 1966 and 1975 had been infected after beginning medical school; (c) among those physicians who had not been immunized with BCG and had been infected after entering medical school, 83 of 842 (9.9%) developed active tuberculosis, with 75% of the active cases appearing between ages 20-35, (d) surveillance practices among physicians, e.g., tuberculin skin testing and chest x-rays, were very erratic; two-thirds did not have annual skin tests (3), and 56% of recent tuberculin converters did not take isoniazid preventive therapy. Geiseler and colleagues performed a similar analysis on 4,575 physicians who graduated from the University of Illinois Medical School between 1938 and 1981 (66). Their findings were strikingly similar to those of Barrett-Connor: 66 cases were seen, including 23 occurring between 1970 and 1981. The age at morbidity was virtually equal to that of the California survey, with 73% of the cases (48 of 66) occurring between 25 and 34 years of age. The overall incidence for physicians within 6 years of graduation was 140 per 100,000 person years. Both of these studies reported substantially reduced morbidity among those physicians who had received BCG vaccination, 80% less in California and 40% less in Illinois. However, methodologic variables prevented absolute comparisons of these groups (see Chapters 12 and 13 for a more complete review of prevention strategies).

Obviously, the risks for physicians to become infected vary with the particular disciplines they pursue as well as the community or hospital in which they practice. A recent survey of physicians completing specialty training (fellowship) in pulmonary and infectious disease medicine revealed that 7 of 62 (11%) pulmonary trainees had experienced tuberculin skin test conversion, whereas only 1 of 42 (2.4%) contemporary infectious disease fellows in the same institutions did so, suggesting that time spent doing invasive procedures and intensive care increased the risk (67).

Historically, nurses who spent more time in close contact with patients than did physicians suffered very high rates of tuberculosis (68). Nearly all of the young women who completed nursing training in the United States in the 1920s and 1930s became tuberculin reactive (69). In the modern era, nurses and other health care workers in direct patient contact have been shown to be at considerable risk of tuberculosis infection and disease during recent outbreaks (70).

Health care workers (HCWs) with tuberculosis in six New York City hospitals were shown to be at significantly increased risk of infection with clustered strains (71). These findings, noted in the absence of nosocomial outbreaks in these institutions, suggest unrecognized work-site transmission. This trend was particularly prominent among HIV-infected HCWs: eight of nine such cases were clustered.

Multiple studies have recently documented nosocomial transmission to HCWs in hospitals or clinics (72–77) or autopsy suites (78,79). A CDC review of cases from 29 states for the period 1984–1985 indicated that, although HCWs overall had case rates similar to the general public, inhalation therapists and low-paid HCWs had statistically higher rates (80). Regarding the latter group, an analysis from St. Louis suggested that socioeconomic status markers other than employment may have contributed to rate differentials in tuberculin reactivity (81); by contrast, tuberculin skin test reactivity among HCWs at St. Clare's Hospital in New York City was strongly related to occupations with patient exposure (82). Several reviews of tuberculosis among HCWs have recently been published (83–85). One novel report described a situation wherein HCWs both suffered from and participated in nosocomial transmission of tuberculosis (86).

Thus, we again must be greatly concerned that a generation of physicians, nurses, and other health care workers is at significant risk of being infected with the tubercle bacillus. And, if history is a valid instructor, we may anticipate substantial numbers of active cases among these recently exposed young men and women in the decades to come (87,88). Issues surrounding prevention (chemotherapy or immunization) are discussed in detail in Chapters 12 and 13, and limiting transmission within institutions is addressed in Chapter 14.

Intrinsic: Vulnerability to New Infections

Biological factors that predispose to the development of tuberculosis generally may do so by altering the host's immune competency to prevent local reactivation or spread of a previously established infection with *M. tuberculosis* (see below). However, data have recently been presented suggesting that there also may be significant differences in the propensity of persons to acquire such infections. Stead, in examining the results of contact investigations in nursing homes and prisons, found that under similar circumstances, blacks were significantly more likely to undergo tuberculin skin test conversion (presumably a manifestation of new infection) than were whites (89). The range of relative risks for blacks to acquire new infections in these settings was from 1.5 to 3.0, the usual range being about 1.6 to 1.9. Of great interest, this group found that among blacks who entered the institutions with significant tuberculin skin test reactions or who developed newly positive tuberculin tests while in the institution, the risk of progressing to clinically active tuberculosis was no greater than that for whites under analogous conditions. The authors cited a theoretical scientific basis for these observed differences: (a) murine studies that indicate that genetically determined differences in resistance to mycobacterial infection lie in the ability of resident, preimmune macrophages to control multiplication of the bacilli and (b) *ex vivo* studies of human monocyte-derived macrophages that showed increased susceptibility of macrophages from black persons to intracellular multiplication of *M. tuberculosis* (see Chapter 4 for more complete discussion). Subsequently, Stead reviewed the historical relationships of tuberculosis to black and white populations and made an intelligent case for darwinian selective pressure creating a relatively more tuberculosis-resistant gene pool among Caucasians (90).

Although the material cited above indicates interracial differences in vulnerability to tuberculosis, there is a likelihood of great variation of individuals within races regarding susceptibility to this infection. Comstock's reanalysis of the Prophit Survey, a long-standing survey of tuberculin reactivity in Great Britain, showed that concordance for tuberculosis was significantly higher for monozygotic than dizygotic twin pairs, indicating "that inherited susceptibility is an important risk factor for tuberculosis among humans" (91).

Overall, there is reasonable evidence to believe that genetic resistance/susceptibility to tuberculosis plays variable roles in the epidemiology of the disease. Whether it lies primarily in the preimmune macrophage function or in antigen-specific cellular immunity is not wholly delineated. And, in the era of highly effective chemotherapy and proven public health modalities of prevention and control, the size of this effect on the patterns of disease is likely to be relatively small.

Intrinsic: Risk Factors That Promote Reactivation

The struggle for dominance between the tubercle bacillus and the human host is tightly contested. In a widely cited contemporary model, we are taught the following: among 100 adults with "normal" immunity who are newly infected with *M. tuberculosis,* fewer than 15 will typically develop active disease during their lifetimes. Assuming a typical distribution of ages among those persons infected, five to ten will experience overt disease within the first 2 years following infection. The factors that select for those who experience the early appearance of disease are not well delineated. However, the following elements are assumed to be influential: (a) the more bacilli inhaled, the "inoculum size," the higher the probability of progressive infection, (b) innate, preimmune defenses determine the initial proliferation and spread of inhaled bacilli, and (c) the genetically controlled immune pathways also influence the host's response against *M. tuberculosis.* Less well studied, but possibly contributing in this selection process, is the relative virulence of the infecting strain of bacillus (see Chapter 2 for discussion). Or, prior cross-immunization from subclinical exposure to environmental mycobacteria other than *M. tuberculosis* may provide some protection (92) (see Chapter 4 for detailed review).

For those persons newly infected with *M. tuberculosis* who pass through this high-risk-for-disease 3-year period, the annual risk of endogenous reactivation falls substantially. This section subsequently examines those factors that increase the probability of individuals experiencing tuberculosis during these following years. Arbitrarily, for a basis of comparison, I have chosen data from the Danish Tuberculosis Index that indicate that for tuberculin-reactive Caucasian adults between the ages of 15 and 44 years without special risk factors, the annual reactivation rate was 29/100,000 or 0.029% (93). At the risk of making some artificial distinctions, I have broken risk factors for reactivation into three categories: normal biological variables, illness/medical variables, and social/situational variables. I presume that all of these components ultimately work through one final effector mechanism, i.e., diminished cellular immune capacity. However, for the purposes of clinical understanding and public health programming, I believe there is utility to this categorization (Table 5.8). These factors are discussed in detail below.

Normal Biological Variables

Among these elements are features that appear to reflect phenomena that fall within the "normal range" of human health rather than indicating a diseased or anomalous state.

Genetic Susceptibility

The potential effects of race on vulnerability to acquisition of infection are discussed above (see "Race" and "Extrinsic: Settings That Influence Risk . . ."). The risk of progression from infection to overt disease is another story. Certainly, in murine models, genetic differences in susceptibility/resistance to tuberculosis have been well and quantitatively documented (see Chapter 4). Moreover, there is emerging evidence that humans may also experience genetic variability in their ability to withstand tubercle bacilli. This factor is discussed in relation to HLA typing in Chapter 4. Body habitus may be a surrogate for genetic factors influencing susceptibility to tuberculosis, although it is possible that pulmonary structure exerts nonimmunological effects on vulnerability to tuberculosis (see Physical Habitus, below, for further discussion).

Apical Scarring

One of the most straightforward markers for higher risk of reactivation is the presence or absence of chest radiographic sequelae of the "primary" infection. At the time of the initial exposure to infection with *M. tuberculosis,* there occurs a bacillemia with variable seeding of organs remote from the lung as well as a recircula-

TABLE 5.8. *Risk factors for endogenous reactivation of latent tuberculosis (see text for references)*

Factor	Comments
Normal biological variables	
Genetic susceptibility	Elements may include intra- and interracial immune phenomena. This may also be involved with the asthenic phenotype noted below.
Chest x-ray status	Apical fibronodular scarring is a high-risk marker; Ghon foci and pleural thickening are not significant risk factors.
Asthenic habitus	May be a phenotypic marker of vulnerability ... "tall and slender."
Extremes of age	Preschool children are at very high risk for progressive primary tuberculosis, not truly reactivation disease. Sharp increase in risk around age 65–70 (possible alterations in T-lymphocyte profiles or vitamin D levels).
Pregnancy/parturition	Probable immunosuppression to promote placental tolerance; possible nutritional stresses.
Illness/medical variables	
HIV infection/AIDS	Progressive vulnerability with decline in CD4 counts.
Diabetes mellitus	Insulin-dependent diabetes a significant risk factor.
Renal failure/azotemia	Probable association with impaired function of macrophages.
Silicosis	Probable association with impaired function of macrophages.
Corticosteroid therapy	Impact of glucocorticoids alone difficult to ascertain; risks increase with addition of cytotoxic drugs or immunosuppressive illnesses.
Undernutrition	A variety of disturbances may induce this condition.
Cigarette smoking	Cigarette smoking may be associated with increased risk of both acquiring new infection and then experiencing reactivation from tuberculosis. May affect macrophage function.
Others	Cancer: Both solid tumors and lymphatic or hematologic malignancies; increased risk attendant with chemotherapy.
	Transplantation: Massive, sustained immunosuppression required to prevent organ rejection.
	Illicit drug use.
	Alcoholism.
Social/environmental variables	
Marital status	Single and widowed men with twofold higher risk than married males; divorced men with fourfold risk; similar, but less pronounced findings in women.
Stress	Although tightly woven into many of the factors noted above, stress itself may cause sufficient perturbation of immunity to increase the risk of tuberculosis.
Immigration[a] Incarceration[a] Homelessness[a]	Immense disruption of personal homeostasis.

[a] These individuals, because of social/environmental circumstances, are also at high risk for exogenous reinfection, which would increase their risk of overt disease.

tion of the microbes diffusely through the lungs. The mycobacteria generally are eliminated from the tissues as effective cellular immunity evolves (see Chapter 4). However, in some persons there is enough inflammation (presumably subclinical "disease") that fibronodular scarring remains visible on subsequent chest x-rays. Why some persons emerge from the primary infection with these lesions (called "Simon foci") and others with normal chest radiographs is unclear. Potential factors theoretically include inoculum size, innate or immunological resistance, and microbial virulence. Whatever the cause, persons with these radiographic abnormalities are at greatly increased risk of reactivation tuberculosis (estimated 30-fold) than similar tuberculin reactors with normal chest films (93).

Physical Habitus

An individual's height, weight, and other body characteristics as risk markers for tuberculosis reactivation generally have been overlooked recently despite substantial evidence of their validity. Clinicians throughout the ages observed that a certain type of person seemed vulnerable to consumption: the slender, asthenic, or delicate. This very probably was a component of the conception that "artists" or "geniuses" were particularly vulnerable to tuberculosis, this habitus being associated popularly with such gifts. Two independent surveys among Caucasian populations have demonstrated significant associations among increased height, low weight, and risk for tuberculosis. Inspired in part by an observational study of U.S. Army personnel in World War II that suggested that tall, thin men were more prone to tuberculosis, a study of U.S. Naval enlistees was conducted from 1949 through 1951; it determined that among 100,000 white males, there were significant associations among increased height, leanness, and the propensity to experience reactivation-type tuberculosis (Fig. 5.8) (94). Tall, slender, asthenic individuals were not more likely to be tuberculin reactors at enlistment; rather, those who were tuberculin reactors simply experienced higher rates of clinically active tuberculosis than their tuberculin-positive counterparts.

The tendency for taller men to have more tuberculosis, although suggestive, was not statistically significant. However, as the authors stated:

> the lighter men appear to have generally higher tuberculosis rates than the heavier ones. The difference is significant at the 5 per cent level for those with tuberculin reactions of 10 mm or more. With respect to the index of the relationship between height and weight. . .section C. . . these associations are statistically significant at the 1 per cent level. (94)

Subsequently, Tverdal reported on a long-term study of tuberculosis risk among a large cohort of the population of Norway (95). Because of the national data base, health statistics were available on the entire population from birth. This study yielded results similar to those obtained from the previous U.S. Navy recruits, including the following: (a) persons of lower body weight had higher rates of all forms of tuberculosis, (b) women of greater than average

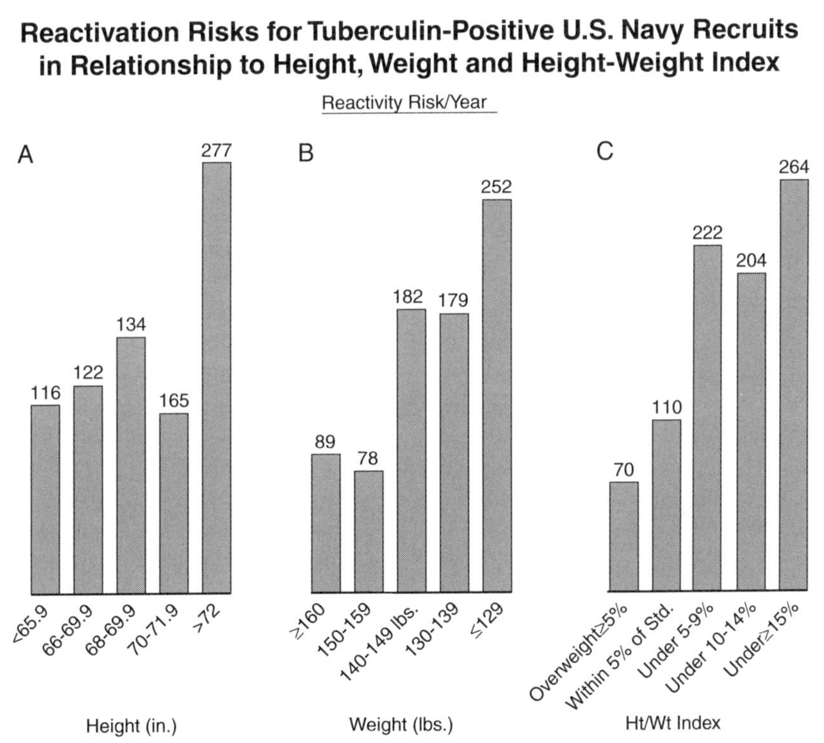

FIG. 5.8. Reactivation risks for tuberculin-positive U.S. Navy recruits in relation to **(A)** height, **(B)** weight, and **(C)** height–weight index. These recruits, 1949–1951, were tuberculin reactors on enlistment. There was no tendency for higher rates of skin-test positivity among the tall and/or slender sailors, but the risk of reactivation clearly tended to increase with this habitus.

height had higher rates of all forms of tuberculosis, and (c) obversely, for patients with bone–joint tuberculosis, persons of less than average height were vulnerable at a statistically significant level.

These findings about phenotype and apparent risk for tuberculosis are fascinating but obviously have limited programmatic implications (one is not likely to offer preventive chemotherapy to someone on the basis of weight). Biologically, though, these observations raise numerous questions. Probably related to this habitus is the observation that, among patients with pulmonary disease caused by *M. avium* complex seen recently at the National Jewish Medical and Research Center, there was a remarkably high prevalence of pectus excavatum deformity of the sternum or otherwise abnormal narrowing of the anterior–posterior dimension of the thorax (96). Notably, the patients with *M. avium* pulmonary disease had more pronounced narrowing than did patients with *M. tuberculosis.* Other findings among the *M. avium* patients included a high frequency of thoracic scoliosis and mitral valve prolapse. Various elements of this body shape and thoracic configuration were used by Hippocrates to define the "phthisical habitus." Although it is merely conjecture at this time, I believe that a pathophysiological basis for the relatively high vulnerability to mycobacterial infections of slender, tall, asthenic individuals will be found.

Extremes of Age

Age is another normal biological variable that influences the risk of reactivation-type tuberculosis. Specific age-related factors that predispose to tuberculosis are not well delineated. Infants and preschool children are clearly at higher risk for tuberculosis, including disseminated, life-threatening diseases, but many of these cases represent progressive primary infection, not reactivation. In later years, the risk for both reactivation and rapid progression to disease are increased. The cause for heightened risk in the elderly is unclear. However, a substantial reduction in the number and percentage of $CD4^+$ helper lymphocytes in the eighth decade has been noted (43,44), and impaired proliferative responses have been noted (45). Also, a survey in Europe recently revealed inadequate serum levels of vitamin D in elderly persons in Europe (49). See "Age," above, for a detailed analysis of age-related epidemiology.

Pregnancy

Pregnancy historically has been deemed a perilous situation for women with consumption. However, modern surveys have failed to show a clear correlation; there is variable evidence to suggest that women may be slightly predisposed to reactivation of their tuberculosis during the postpartum period (97). One recent study from Kenya indicated that pregnancy in HIV-infected women may promote tuberculosis (98); however, a later study from the Dominican Republic failed to confirm this effect (99).

Nonetheless, recently described alterations of immune status, including variations in Th1 versus Th2 lymphocyte activity during pregnancy, suggest that this period might entail increased risk for some persons. Evidence is accumulating that Th2 cytokines, which can be produced in the placenta and are found in dominant concentrations at the placental interface, are protective against loss of the fetus (100,101). (See Chapter 4 for a review of Th1 and Th2 cytokines.) This effect may be mediated by sustained exposure to progesterones, which favor Th2 pathway development and suppress lymphocyte proliferation, NK-cell activation, and TNF production (102). The possible role of pregnancy-induced altered immunity in causing a life-threatening infection with *Bartonella henselae* may be partially analogous to tuberculosis (103,104).

However, even if pregnancy is not shown to be a major risk factor for tuberculosis reactivation, tuberculosis screening programs for pregnant women from high-risk groups including minorities or immigrants may be programmatically efficient (105). This occasion may be the only time these individuals may encounter the health care system, providing a unique opportunity to diagnose and treat early tuberculous disease or to offer preventive chemotherapy (106).

Illness/Medical Variables

A variety of illnesses, sometimes abetted by therapy given for the condition, predispose to reactivation of latent tuberculosis.

Human Immunodeficiency Virus

By far the most powerful element in promoting reactivation of tuberculosis is infection with the human immunodeficiency virus (HIV). For a more complete exposition of the relationship between HIV infection, AIDS, and tuberculosis, see Chapter 8.

Diabetes Mellitus

Diabetes mellitus was recognized by Avicenna (a.d. 950–1027) as a predisposition to phthisis; this association has been confirmed by clinical observers ever since. Banyai authored a classical review of this topic in 1931 (107). Estimates for the relative risk of insulin-dependent diabetes as a predisposition for tuberculosis vary widely. Root in 1934 indicated that juvenile diabetics were tenfold more likely to develop tuberculosis (108). However, data from the Danish Tuberculosis Index indicated only a threefold risk, probably a more realistic measure in the modern era of insulin use and a diminished prevalence of tuberculosis (93). A study from Korea in 1995 noted substantially increased tuberculosis case rates among subjects noted in insurance records to be diabetic (109). In this series, rates among diabetics for all forms of tuberculosis were 1,061 versus 306/100,000/year for nondiabetic controls, a relative risk of 3.5; for sputum smear-positive cases, the rates were 231 versus 33, a relative risk of 7.0.

The mechanism of risk has not been identified with certainty. The literature relating to cellular immune function in diabetes mellitus is swamped with discussions of cellular autoimmunity in relation to the pathogenesis of the endocrine disorder but relatively bereft of studies of immune function versus infections such as tuberculosis.

Bloom reported on 47 men admitted to the San Diego Naval Hospital from 1967 to 1968 with newly diagnosed pulmonary tuberculosis; 34% were found to have abnormal glucose tolerance curves (110). Zack in 1973 showed that 41% of 256 patients admitted to a tuberculosis ward had, on glucose tolerance testing, 2-hour concentrations in the diabetic range (111); only 15 of these 105 patients had clinically recognized diabetes before the diagnosis of tuberculosis. Unfortunately, neither Bloom nor Zack systematically reported whether the glucose intolerance persisted after the tuberculosis had been treated. Based on limited observations, I suspect that many of these persons had abnormal glucose metabolism under the physiological stress of active, inflammatory tuberculosis and were not independently "diabetic."

End-Stage Renal Disease

End-stage renal disease (ESRD) has been identified as a risk factor for tuberculosis. A 1980 report from San Francisco identified 10 of 172 patients undergoing long-term hemodialysis between 1967 and 1977 who developed tuberculosis (112). Notable findings of this series included a remarkable overrepresentation of minorities: only one of the ten tuberculosis victims was white despite the fact that 48% of the dialysis patients were Caucasian. A decade after that report, other investigators found impaired splenic macrophage Fc-γ receptors among all 56 ESRD patients undergoing hemodialysis and speculated that this may be a factor in the vulnerability of uremic patients to infection (113). However, the primary known role for these macrophage receptors is clearance of IgG-coated antigens and immune complexes, so their particular role in tuberculosis is not apparent. Other pathophysiological factors such as malnutrition, other metabolic deficiencies, or high levels of endogenous glucocorticoids must be considered as well.

Silicosis

A relationship between tuberculosis and mining has been noted for centuries. In an excellent review of the topic in 1978, Snider observed that there has been a consistent association between silicosis and tuberculosis that has varied in intensity depending on temporal, demographic, and methodological factors (114). Salient findings of the analysis included: (a) tuberculosis has always been a major cause of morbidity and death among silicotics; (b) the rate of tuberculosis among silicotics is always higher than surrounding populations, (c) the risk of tuberculosis is higher among silicotics than those with other pneumoconioses, and (d) the risk of tuberculosis increases with more advanced forms of silicosis. Interference with alveolar macrophage function by the silica particles is presumably the primary pathophysiological mechanism involved with heightened vulnerability.

Two recent reports from South Africa clearly identified silicosis among black gold miners to be a powerful risk factor for tuberculosis. Cowie, in a surveillance program for miners, noted the annual risk of tuberculosis for miners without silicosis to be 981/100,000 while that for silicotic miners was 2,707/100,000, a relative risk of 2.8 (115). The risk of tuberculosis increased with the severity of the radiographic findings of silicosis. Although these data suggest that the severity of lung damage from silicates is the cause for higher rates of tuberculosis, they may also simply reflect longer periods spent in mines, where the ongoing risk of tuberculosis transmission is very high. Murray and colleagues, in an autopsy series of South African miners dying from unnatural causes between 1974 and 1991, found that the prevalence of tuberculosis during this period increased from 0.9 to 3.9% (116). They also noted that the risk of tuberculosis increased with the severity of silicosis. They ascribed the increasing rate of tuberculosis to prolonged patterns of employment during this era. A recent report on silicosis in the state of Michigan profiled risk factors for the pneumoconiosis and noted that 13% had been told of either "tuberculosis" or a positive tuberculin test (117).

The American Thoracic Society published an official statement on the "Adverse Effects of Crystalline Silica Exposure" in 1997 (118); this document contains recommendations regarding the therapy of silicotuberculosis with which I disagree (please see Chapter 10).

Corticosteroid Therapy

The role of corticosteroid therapy in reactivation of tuberculosis in humans is uncertain. Early animal model studies showed that administration of glucocorticoids to some species of animals substantially potentiated tuberculosis infection, resulting in disseminated disease (119). However, the applicability of such data to humans was unclear then (120) and remains so now because there are substantial differences in steroid pharmacokinetics and susceptibility of lymphocytes to steroids between these model animals and humans. Human data regarding steroids and tuberculosis consist exclusively of anecdotal case reports or methodologically weak surveys. Sahn and Lakshminarayan identified 13 patients with 14 episodes of tuberculosis associated temporally with the administration of corticosteroids among patients at the National Jewish Hospital between 1963 and 1973 (121). Because of the nature of their survey, they were unable to establish incidence data for tuberculosis. Remarkable findings in this study included that the majority of patients had other diseases or conditions that also may have impaired immunity, including three renal transplant recipients, one chronic lymphocytic leukemia case, five with rheumatoid arthritis, one systemic lupus erythematosus case, and—among the above—four patients who were taking additional immunosuppressive drugs. An often-quoted survey of tuberculosis among asthmatic patients receiving oral steroids, also published in 1976, reported no association with reactivation (122); unfortunately, limitations of the numbers of patients and years observed did not allow exclusion of a significant risk of reactivation. Other reports that concern the potential relationship of corticosteroids and tuberculosis reactivation are noted for interest (123–125).

Overall, I believe that corticosteroids given in sufficient doses for long enough periods of time would surely exert an immunosuppressive effect adequate to promote reactivation of an endogenous focus of tuberculosis. However, currently available data do not allow us to determine the hazardous dose–time constant. The 1994 ATS/CDC Guidelines indicate that more than 15 mg per day of prednisone for 2 to 3 weeks is the presumed threshold for increased risk of tuberculosis; although this is reasonable, there is little direct evidence to support it. The anecdotal data available as well as clinical intuition suggest that the underlying disease or condition for which steroids are given and other potentially immunosuppressive medications may also play substantial roles in risk enhancement.

Undernutrition

Gastrectomy alone was at one time considered an independent risk factor for the reactivation of tuberculosis and was included in the American Thoracic Society's Guidelines as an indication in tuberculin reactors for isoniazid preventive therapy. However, closer analysis of the data revealed that tuberculosis was of increased prevalence mainly among those gastrectomy patients who were significantly underweight (126). Hence, current policies identify rapid weight loss or chronic undernutrition as high-risk markers (127). In addition to gastrectomy patients, those who have undergone intestinal bypass surgery for obesity or who suffer from various malabsorption syndromes or short-bowel syndromes associated with intestinal resections would be included under this rubric.

Cigarette Smoking

Two recent case-control studies from Spain reported a highly significant relationship between cigarette smoking and active tuberculosis (128,129). These reports readdressed this practice as a potential risk factor, a phenomenon reported in several prior studies (130–134). The Alcaide report was criticized on the bases of methodology and the lack of a credible hypothesis to explain a causal relationship (135). Regarding the latter issue, various recent observations can be linked to offer a credible relationship between cigarette smoking and vulnerability to tuberculosis reactivation. Bronchoalveolar lavage of the lungs of smokers and nonsmokers shows there to be substantially increased concentrations of extracellular ferritin-bound iron, particularly in the upper lobes of smokers (136). Three reports describe impaired human macrophage function against intracellular organisms, *M. avium* or *Candida albicans* in the presence of increased iron (137–139). Although there clearly are confounding variables in the putative association of cigarette smoking and tuberculosis, including alcoholism, homelessness, and other socioeconomic status factors, this relationship deserves serious consideration.

Other Factors

Miscellaneous conditions or disorders such as various cancers (140), organ transplantation (141–149), and illicit drug use (150–152) have been reported in association with active tuberculosis. In support of a causal link between drug use and tuberculosis, inhaled marijuana and cocaine have both been shown to impair alveolar macrophage function (153). Arguably, alcoholism and drug abuse pose substantial exposure risks for the acquisition of infection as well as the propensity to experience progression to active disease or reactivation (153).

Social/Environmental Variables

Certain features of social conditions seem to be consistently associated with the risk of tuberculosis. Some of them are clearly situational, probably associated with high levels of stress or disturbed homeostasis. Others involve these situational stressors in combination with substantial risks of exogenous infection as a result of being placed in environments where there are unusually high rates of communicable tuberculosis.

In the former category, data from the Danish Tuberculosis Index revealed that single and widowed men were twice as likely to develop tuberculosis as married men; divorced men were four times more likely to suffer active tuberculosis (154). In the United States, Holmes and colleagues in Seattle compiled considerable circumstantial evidence linking the risk of tuberculosis to "stressors" or "life events" (155–157). This work was well reviewed in a recent essay by Lerner (158).

In the category of simultaneous stressors and increased environmental risks are such circumstances as homelessness, incarceration, immigration, and life in time of war (159). Although there is no doubt that these conditions may also involve increased risk of contracting new infection, it seems equally or more compelling to reason that these experiences, which surely are among the most intense perturbations of personal homeostasis an individual can know, are by themselves potentiators of tuberculosis reactivation. As we advance our understanding of the relationships between psychological stress and immunity, endocrine function, and behavior (160), these connections between social disruption and tuberculosis will become more comprehensible. If the absence of social ties can predispose to the common cold, why not tuberculosis (161)?

SUMMARY

For the United States, the tide of tuberculosis that immersed the nation throughout the 18th and 19th centuries has slowly ebbed throughout the 20th century. As it receded, this remarkable infection has left behind smaller tide pools of disease primarily involving minorities, immigrants, the socioeconomically disadvantaged, and the elderly. A recent resurgence reminded us of our ongoing vulnerability to an illness that has always taken advantage of individual and societal frailties. A contemporary CDC report that analyzed the factors statistically associated with diminished case rates in 1993 and 1994 compared with 1991 and 1992 identified these contributing factors: (a) diminished rates in persons with AIDS, probably as a result of curtailed transmission in hospitals and shelters, (b) improvements in treatment completion and sputum conversion rates, probably related to vastly increased programs of directly observed therapy, and (c) enhanced programs of contact tracing and INH preventive therapy (162).

However, for both the United States and the world, we must appreciate that the corpus of tuberculosis is immense in scale and relentless in momentum. Blower and colleagues in an extremely sophisticated model have shown that epidemic tuberculosis evolves over decades and centuries (163). Unless we are delivered chemotherapy or vaccines of presently unimaginable potency, we may anticipate that the 21st century will remain a global battleground against consumption.

REFERENCES

1. American Thoracic Society/Centers for Disease Control. Diagnostic standards and classification of tuberculosis. *Am Rev Respir Dis* 1990;142:725–735.
2. Styblo K, Meijer J, Sutherland I. The transmission of tubercle bacilli. Its trend in a human population. *Bull Int Union Tuber* 1969;42:5–104.
3. Murray CJL, Styblo K, Rouillon A. Tuberculosis in developing countries: burden, intervention and cost. *Bull IUAT* 1990;65:1–20.
4. Raviglione MC, Snider DE, Kochi A. Global epidemiology of tuberculosis. Morbidity and mortality of a worldwide epidemic. *JAMA* 1995;273:220–226.
5. Centers for Disease Control and Prevention–Division of Tuberculosis Elimination. Tuberculosis morbidity–United States, 1997. *MMWR* 1998;47:253–257.
6. Berkley S. HIV in Africa: what is the future? *Ann Intern Med* 1991;116:339–340.
7. Holmberg SD. The rise of tuberculosis in America before 1820. *Am Rev Respir Dis* 1990;142:1228–1232.
8. McKenna MT, McCray E, Onorato I. The epidemiology of tuberculosis among foreign-born persons in the United States, 1986–93. *N Engl J Med* 1995;332:1071–1076.
9. Cantwell MF, Snider DE Jr, Cauthen GM, Onorato IM. Epidemiology of tuberculosis in the United States, 1985 through 1992. *JAMA* 1994;272:535–539.
10. Burwen DR, Bloch AB, Griffin LD, Ciesielski CA, Stern HA, Onorato IM. National trends in the concurrence of tuberculosis and acquired immunodeficiency syndrome. *Arch Intern Med* 1995;155:1281–1286.
11. Brudney K, Dobkin J. Resurgent tuberculosis in New York City. Human immunodeficiency virus, homelessness, and the decline of tuberculosis control programs. *Am Rev Respir Dis* 1991;144:745–749.
12. Reichman L. The U-shaped curve of concern. *Am Rev Respir Dis* 1991;144:741–742.
13. New York City Department of Health–Bureau of Tuberculosis Control. *Tuberculosis in New York City, 1993. Information summary.* New York: New York City, 1994.
14. Frieden TR, Fujiwara PI, Washko RM, Hamburg MA. Tuberculosis in New York City—turning the tide. *N Engl J Med* 1995;333:229–233.
15. Garrett L. *The coming plague. Newly emerging diseases in a world out of balance.* New York: Penguin Books, 1994.
16. Centers for Disease Control and Prevention. *Tuberculosis case rates by state: United States, 1994.* Atlanta: CDC, 1994.
17. Cantwell MF, McKenna MT, McCray E, Onorato IM. Tuberculosis and race/ethnicity in the United States. Impact of socioeconomic status. *Am J Respir Crit Care Med* 1997;157:1016–1020.
18. Weiss KB, Addington WW. Tuberculosis. Poverty's penalty (editorial). *Am J Respir Crit Care Med* 1998;157:1011.

19. Binkin NJ, Zuber PLF, Wells CD, Tipple MA, Castro KG. Overseas screening for tuberculosis in immigrants and refugees to the United States: current status. *Clin Infect Dis* 1996;23:1226–1232.
20. Zuber PLF, Binkin NJ, Ignacio AC, et al. Tuberculosis screening for immigrants and refugees. Diagnostic outcomes in the state of Hawaii. *Am J Respir Crit Care Med* 1996;154:151–155.
21. Wells CD, Zuber PLF, Nolan CM, Binkin NJ, Goldberg SV. Tuberculosis prevention among foreign-born persons in Seattle—King County, Washington. *Am J Respir Crit Care Med* 1997;156:573–577.
22. DeRiemer K, Chin DP, Schecter GF, Reingold AL. Tuberculosis among immigrants and refugees. *Arch Intern Med* 1998;158:753–760.
23. Zuber PLF, Knowles LS, Binkin NJ, Tipple MA, Davidson PT. Tuberculosis among foreign-born persons in Los Angeles County, 1992–1994. *Tuberc Lung Dis* 1996;77:524–530.
24. Truong DH, Hedemark LL, Mickman JK, Mosher LB, Dietrich SE, Lowry PW. Tuberculosis among Tibetan immigrants from India and Nepal in Minnesota, 1992–1995. *JAMA* 1997;277:735–738.
25. Wang J-S, Allen EA, Enarson DA, Grzybowski S. Tuberculosis in recent Asian immigrants to British Columbia, Canada: 1982–1985. *Tubercle* 1991;72: 277–283.
26. Doherty MJ, Spence DPS, Davies PDO. The increase in tuberculosis notifications in England and Wales since 1987. *Tuberc Lung Dis* 1995;76:196–200.
27. van Deutekom H, Gerritsen JJJ, van Soolingen D, van Ameijden EJC, van Embden JDA, Coutinho RA. A molecular epidemiological approach to studying the transmission of tuberculosis in Amsterdam. *Clin Infect Dis* 1997;25:1071–1077.
28. Wilcke JTR, Poulsen S, Askgaard DS, Enevoldsen HK, Rønne T, Kok-Jensen A. Tuberculosis in a cohort of Vietnamese refugees after arrival in Denmark 1979–1982. *Int J Tuberc Lung Dis* 1998;2:219–224.
29. Heath TC, Roberts C, Winks M, Capon AG. The epidemiology of tuberculosis in New South Wales 1975–1995: the effects of immigration in a low prevalence population. *Int J Tuberc Lung Dis* 1998;2: 647–654.
30. Zuber PLF, McKenna MT, Binkin NJ, Onorato IM, Castro KG. Long-term risk of tuberculosis among foreign-born persons in the United States. *JAMA* 1997; 278:304–307.
31. Ziv TA, Lo B. Denial of care to illegal immigrants. Proposition 187 in California. *N Engl J Med* 1995;332:1095–1098.
32. Iseman MD, Starke J. Immigrants and tuberculosis control. *N Engl J Med* 1995;332:1094–1095.
33. Stead WW. Undetected tuberculosis in prison. Source of infection for community at large. *JAMA* 1978; 240:2544–2547.
34. Pelletier AR, DiFerdinando GT Jr, Greenberg AJ, et al. Tuberculosis in a correctional facility. *Arch Intern Med* 1993;153:2692–2695.
35. Valway SE, Greifinger RB, Papania M, et al. Multidrug-resistant tuberculosis in the New York State prison system, 1990–1991. *J Infect Dis* 1994;170: 151–156.
36. Lyon R, Haque AK, Asmuth DM, Woods GL. Changing patterns of infections in patients with AIDS: a study of 279 autopsies of prison inmates and nonincarcerated patients at a university hospital in eastern Texas, 1984–1993. *Clin Infect Dis* 1996;23:241–247.
37. Martin V, Gonzalez P, Cayl JA, et al. Case-finding of pulmonary tuberculosis on admission to a penitentiary centre. *Tuberc Lung Dis* 1994;74:49–53.
38. Drobniewski F. Tuberculosis in prisons—forgotten plague. *Lancet* 1995;346:948–949.
39. MacIntyre CR, Kendig N, Kummer L, Birago S, Graham NMH. Impact of tuberculosis control measures and crowding on the incidence of tuberculous infection in Maryland prisons. *Clin Infect Dis* 1997;24:1060–1067.
40. Glaser J, Greifinger R. Correctional health care: a public health opportunity. *Ann Intern Med* 1993;118: 139–145.
41. Braun MM, Truman BI, Maguire B, et al. Increasing incidence of tuberculosis in a prison inmate population. Association with HIV infection. *JAMA* 1989; 261:393–397.
42. Snider D, Hutton M. Tuberculosis in correctional institutions. *JAMA* 1989;261:436–437.
43. Mackall CL, Fleisher TA, Brown MR, et al. Age, thymopoiesis, and $CD4^+$ T-lymphocyte regeneration after intensive chemotherapy. *N Engl J Med* 1995;332: 143–149.
44. Weinberg K, Parkman R. Age, the thymus, and T-lymphocytes (editorial). *N Engl J Med* 1995;332:182–183.
45. Saltzman RL, Peterson PK. Immunodeficiency of the elderly. *Rev Infect Dis* 1987;9:1127–1139.
46. Dorken E, Grzybowski S, Allen E. Significance of the tuberculin test in the elderly. *Chest* 1987;92:237–240.
47. Stead W, To T. The significance of the tuberculin skin test in elderly persons. *Ann Intern Med* 1987;107: 837–842.
48. Stead WW. Tuberculosis among elderly persons: an outbreak in a nursing home. *Ann Intern Med* 1981;94:606–610.
49. van der Wielen R, Löwik M, van den Berg H, et al. Serum vitamin D concentrations among elderly people in Europe. *Lancet* 1995;346:207–210.
50. Stead W, Lofgren J, Warren E, Thomas C. Tuberculosis: an endemic and nosocomial infection among the elderly in nursing homes. *N Engl J Med* 1985;312: 1483–1487.
51. Borgdorff MW, Veen J, Kalisvaart NA, Nagelkerke N. Mortality among tuberculosis patients in the Netherlands in the period 1993–1995. *Eur Respir J* 1998; 11:816–820.
52. Schieffelbein C, Snider D. Tuberculosis control among homeless populations. *Arch Intern Med* 1988;148: 1843–1846.
53. Sherman M, Brickner P, Schwartz M, et al. Tuberculosis in single-room-occupancy hotel residents: a persisting focus of disease. *NY Med Q* 1980;Fall:39–41.
54. McAdam JM, Brickner PW, Scharer LL, Crocco JA, Duff AE. The spectrum of tuberculosis in a New York City men's shelter clinic 1982–1988. *Chest* 1990;97: 798–805.
55. Schluger NW, Huberman R, Wolinsky N, Dooley R, Rom WN, Holzman RS. Tuberculosis infection and disease among persons seeking social services in New York City. *Int J Tuberc Lung Dis* 1997;1:31–37.
56. Nolan CM, Elarth AM, Barr H, Saeed AM, Risser DR. An outbreak of tuberculosis in a shelter for homeless

men. A description of its evolution and control. *Am Rev Respir Dis* 1991;143:257–261.
57. Kimerling ME, Benjamin WH, Lok KH, Curtis G, Dunlap NE. Restriction fragment length polymorphism screening of *Mycobacterium tuberculosis* isolates: population surveillance for targeting disease transmission in a community. *Int J Tuberc Lung Dis* 1998;2:655–662.
58. Kline SE, Hedemark L, Davies SF. Outbreak of tuberculosis among regular patrons of a neighborhood bar. *N Engl J Med* 1995;333:222–227.
59. Barnes PF, El-Hajj H, Preston-Martin S, et al. Transmission of tuberculosis among the urban homeless. *JAMA* 1996;275:305–307.
60. Frieden TR, Woodley CL, Crawford JT, Lew D, Dooley SM. The molecular epidemiology of tuberculosis in New York City: the importance of nosocomial transmission and laboratory error. *Tuberc Lung Dis* 1996;77:407–413.
61. Friedman CR, Quinn GC, Kreiswirth BN, et al. Widespread dissemination of a drug-susceptible strain of *Mycobacterium tuberculosis. J Infect Dis* 1997;176: 478–484.
62. Nardell E, McInnis B, Thomas B, Weishaas S. Exogenous reinfection with tuberculosis in a shelter for the homeless. *N Engl J Med* 1986;315:1570–1575.
63. Morris JT, McAllister CK. Homeless individuals and drug-resistant tuberculosis in South Texas. *Chest* 1992;102:802–804.
64. Myers JA. *Tuberculosis. A half century of study and conquest.* St Louis: Warren H Green, 1970.
65. Barrett-Connor E. The epidemiology of tuberculosis in physicians. *JAMA* 1979;241:33–38.
66. Geiseler J, Nelson K, Crispen R, Moses V. Tuberculosis in physicians: a continuing problem. *Am Rev Respir Dis* 1986;133:773–778.
67. Malasky C, Jordan T, Potulski F, Reichman L. Occupational tuberculous infections among pulmonary physicians in training. *Am Rev Respir Dis* 1990;142: 505–507.
68. Mikol E, Horton R, Lincoln N, Stokes A. Incidence of pulmonary tuberculosis among employees of tuberculosis hospitals. *Am Rev Tuberc* 1952;66:16–27.
69. Israel H, Hetherington H, Ord J. A study of tuberculosis among students of nursing. *JAMA* 1941;117: 839–844.
70. Sepkowitz K. Tuberculosis and the health-care worker: a historical perspective. *Ann Intern Med* 1994;120: 71–79.
71. Sepkowitz KA, Friedman CR, Hafner A, et al. Tuberculosis among urban health care workers: a study using restriction fragment length polymorphism typing. *Clin Infect Dis* 1995;21:1098–1102.
72. Dooley SW, Villarino ME, Lawrence M, et al. Nosocomial transmission of tuberculosis in a hospital unit for HIV-infected patients. *JAMA* 1992;267:2632–2635.
73. Pearson ML, Jereb JA, Frieden TR, et al. Nosocomial transmission of multidrug-resistant *Mycobacterium tuberculosis.* A risk to patients and health care workers. *Ann Intern Med* 1992;117:191–196.
74. Beck-Sagu C, Dooley SW, Hutton MD, et al. Hospital outbreak of multidrug-resistant *Mycobacterium tuberculosis* infections. Factors in transmission to staff and HIV-infected patients. *JAMA* 1992;268:1280–1286.
75. Griffith DE, Hardeman JL, Zhang Y, Wallace RJ, Mazurek GH. Tuberculosis outbreak among healthcare workers in a community hospital. *Am J Respir Crit Care Med* 1995;152:808–811.
76. Jereb JA, Klevens M, Privett TD, et al. Tuberculosis in health care workers at a hospital with an outbreak of multidrug-resistant *Mycobacterium tuberculosis. Arch Intern Med* 1995;155:854–859.
77. Wenger PN, Otten J, Breeden A, Orfas D, Beck-Sague CM, Jarvis WR. Control of nosocomial transmission of multidrug-resistant *Mycobacterium tuberculosis* among healthcare workers and HIV-infected patients. *Lancet* 1995;345:235–239.
78. Templeton GL, Illing LA, Young L, Cave D, Stead WW, Bates JH. The risk for transmission of *Mycobacterium tuberculosis* at the bedside and during autopsy. *Ann Intern Med* 1995;122:922–925.
79. Ussery XT, Bierman JA, Valway SE, Seitz TA, DiFerdinando GT Jr, Ostroff SM. Transmission of multidrug-resistant *Mycobacterium tuberculosis* among persons exposed in a medical examiner's office, New York. *Infect Control Hosp Epidemiol* 1995;16:160–165.
80. McKenna MT, Hutton M, Cauthen G, Onorato IM. The association between occupation and tuberculosis. A population-based survey. *Am J Respir Crit Care Med* 1996;154:587–593.
81. Bailey TC, Fraser VJ, Spitznagel EL, Dunagan WC. Risk factors for a positive tuberculin skin test among employees of an urban, midwestern teaching hospital. *Ann Intern Med* 1995;122:580–585.
82. Louther J, Rivera P, Feldman J, Villa N, DeHovitz J, Sepkowitz KA. Risk of tuberculin conversion according to occupation among health care workers at a New York City hospital. *Am J Respir Crit Care Med* 1997; 156:201–205.
83. Nolan CM. Tuberculosis in health care professionals: Assessing and accepting the risk. *Ann Intern Med* 1994;120:964–965.
84. Menzies D, Fanning A, Yuan L, Fitzgerald M. Tuberculosis among health care workers. *N Engl J Med* 1995;332:92–98.
85. Sepkowitz KA. AIDS, tuberculosis, and the health care worker. *Clin Infect Dis* 1995;20:232–242.
86. Zaza S, Blumberg HM, Beck-Sagu C, et al. Nosocomial transmission of *Mycobacterium tuberculosis:* role of health care workers in outbreak propagation. *J Infect Dis* 1995;172:1542–1549.
87. Sepkowitz KA. Occupationally acquired infections in health care workers. Part I. *Ann Intern Med* 1996; 125:826–834.
88. Sepkowitz KA. Occupationally acquired infections in health care workers. Part II. *Ann Intern Med* 1996; 125:917–928.
89. Stead W, Senner J, Reddick W, Lofgren J. Racial differences in susceptibility to infection by *Mycobacterium tuberculosis. N Engl J Med* 1990;322:422–427.
90. Stead W. Genetics and resistance to tuberculosis. *Ann Intern Med* 1992;116:937–941.
91. Comstock G. Tuberculosis in twins: a re-analysis of the Prophit Survey. *Am Rev Respir Dis* 1978;117:621–624.
92. Smith DW. Protective effect of BCG in experimental tuberculosis. In: Fox W, Grosset J, Styblo K, eds. *Ad-*

vances in tuberculosis research. Basel: Karger, 1985: 1–97.
93. Horwitz O. The risk of tuberculosis in different groups of the general population. *Scand J Respir Dis* 1970;72[Suppl]:55–60.
94. Palmer C, Jablon S, Edwards P. Tuberculosis morbidity of young men in relation to tuberculin sensitivity and body build. *Am Rev Tuberc* 1957;76:517–534.
95. Tverdal A. Height, weight, and incidence of tuberculosis. *Bull IUAT* 1988;63:16–17.
96. Iseman MD, Buschman DL, Ackerson LM. Pectus excavatum and scoliosis: thoracic anomalies associated with pulmonary disease due to *M. avium* complex. *Am Rev Respir Dis* 1991;144:914–916.
97. Hamadeh M, Glassroth J. Tuberculosis and pregnancy. *Chest* 1992;101:1114–1120.
98. Gilks CF, Brindle RJ, Otieno LS, et al. Extrapulmonary and disseminated tuberculosis in HIV-1 seropositive patients presenting to the acute medical service in Nairobi. *AIDS* 1990;4:981–985.
99. Espinal M, Reingold A, Lavandeva M. Effect of pregnancy on the risk of developing active tuberculosis. *J Infect Dis* 1996;173:488–491.
100. Wegmann TG, Lin H, Guilbert L, Mosmann TR. Bidirectional cytokine interactions in the maternal foetal relationship: is successful pregnancy a Th2 phenomenon? *Immunol Today* 1993;14:353–356.
101. Hill JA, Polgar K, Anderson DJ. T-helper 1-type immunity to trophoblast in women with recurrent spontaneous abortion. *JAMA* 1995;273:1933–1936.
102. Raghupathy R. Th1 type immunity is incompatible with successful pregnancy. *Immunol Today* 1997;18:478–482.
103. McCormack G, Fenelon LE, Sheehan K, McCormick PA. Postpartum coma (case report). *Lancet* 1998; 351:1700.
104. Reid TMS. Striking a balance in maternal immune response to infection. *Lancet* 1998;351:1670–1671.
105. Centers for Disease Control and Prevention. Tuberculosis among pregnant women—New York City, 1985–1992. *MMWR* 1993;42:605–612.
106. Carter E, Mates S. Tuberculosis during pregnancy: the Rhode Island experience, 1987 to 1991. *Chest* 1987; 106:1466–1470.
107. Banyai AL. Diabetes and pulmonary tuberculosis. *Am Rev Tuberc* 1931;24:650–667.
108. Root HF. The association of diabetes and tuberculosis. *N Engl J Med* 1934;210:1–13,78–92,127–147,192–206.
109. Kim SJ, Hong YP, Lew WJ, Yang SC, Lee EG. Incidence of pulmonary tuberculosis among diabetics. *Tuberc Lung Dis* 1995;76:529–533.
110. Bloom JD. Glucose intolerance in pulmonary tuberculosis. *Am Rev Respir Dis* 1969;100:38–41.
111. Zack M, Fulkerson C, Stein E. Glucose intolerance in pulmonary tuberculosis. *Am Rev Respir Dis* 1973;108: 1164–1169.
112. Andrew OT, Schoenfeld PY, Hopewell PC, Humphreys MH. Tuberculosis in patients with end-stage renal disease. *Am J Med* 1980;68:59–65.
113. Ruiz P, Gomez F, Schreiber A. Impaired function of macrophage Fc-gamma receptors in end-stage renal disease. *N Engl J Med* 1990;322:717–722.
114. Snider D. The relationship between tuberculosis and silicosis. *Am Rev Respir Dis* 1978;118:455–460.
115. Cowie RL. The epidemiology of tuberculosis in gold miners with silicosis. *Am J Respir Crit Care Med* 1994;150:1460–1462.
116. Murray J, Kielkowski D, Reid P. Occupational disease trends in black South African gold miners. An autopsy-based study. *Am J Respir Crit Care Med* 1996;153: 706–710.
117. Rosenman KD, Reilly MJ, Kalinowski DJ, Watt FC. Silicosis in the 1990s. *Chest* 1997;111:779–786.
118. American Thoracic Society. Adverse effects of crystalline silica exposure. *Am J Respir Crit Care Med* 1997;155:761–765.
119. Dye WE, Hobby GL, Middlebrook G, Princi F, Youmans GP. The effect of cortisone and/or corticotropin on experimental tuberculous infections in animals. *Am Rev Tuberc* 1952;66:257–259.
120. American Trudeau Society. The effect of cortisone and/or corticotropin on tuberculous infection in man. *Am Rev Tuberc* 1952;66:254–256.
121. Sahn S, Lakshminarayan S. Tuberculosis after corticosteroid therapy. *Br J Dis Chest* 1976;70:195–205.
122. Schatz M, Patterson R, Kloner R, Falk J. The prevalence of tuberculosis and positive tuberculin skin tests in a steroid-treated asthmatic population. *Ann Intern Med* 1976;84:261–265.
123. Mayfield RB. Tuberculosis occurring in association with corticosteroid treatment. *Tubercle* 1962;43:55–60.
124. Bottiger LE, Nordenstam HH, Wester PO. Disseminated tuberculosis as a cause of fever of obscure origin. *Lancet* 1962;1:19–20.
125. Smyllie HC, Connolly CK. Incidence of serious complications of corticosteroid therapy in respiratory disease. *Thorax* 1968;23:571–581.
126. Snider DE Jr. Tuberculosis and gastrectomy. *Chest* 1985;87:414–415.
127. American Thoracic Society. Treatment of tuberculosis and tuberculosis infection in adults and children. *Am J Respir Crit Care Med* 1994;149:1359–1374.
128. Alcaide J, Altet MN, Plans P, et al. Cigarette smoking as a risk factor for tuberculosis in young adults: a case-control study. *Tuberc Lung Dis* 1996;77:112–116.
129. Altet MN, Alcaide J, Plans P, et al. Passive smoking and risk of pulmonary tuberculosis in children immediately following infection. A case-control study. *Tuberc Lung Dis* 1996;77:537–544.
130. Lowe CR. An association between smokng and respiratory tuberculosis. *Br Med J* 1956;ii:1081–1086.
131. Edwards JH. Contribution of cigarette smoking to respiratory disease. *Br J Prev Soc Med* 1957;11:10–21.
132. Adelstein A, Rimington J. Smoking and pulmonary tuberculosis: an analysis based on a study of volunteers for mass miniature radiography. *Tubercle* 1967; 48:219–226.
133. Yu G, Hsieh C, Peng J. Risk factors associated with the prevalence of tuberculosis among sanitary workers in Shanghai. *Tubercle* 1988;69:105–112.
134. Doll R, Peto R, Wheatley K, Gray R, Sutherland I. Mortality in relation to smoking: 40 years' observations on male British doctors. *Br Med J* 1994;309: 901–911.
135. Levy MH, Connolly MA, O'Brien RJ. Cigarette smoking as a risk factor for tuberculosis in young adults: a case-control study (comments). *Tuberc Lung Dis* 1996;77:570.

136. Nelson ME, O'Brien-Ladner AR, Wesselius LJ. Regional variation in iron and iron-binding proteins in the lungs of smokers. *Am J Respir Crit Care Med* 1996;153:1353–1358.
137. Douvas GS, May MH, Crowle AJ. Transferrin, iron, and serum lipids enhance or inhibit *Mycobacterium avium* replication in human macrophages. *J Infect Dis* 1993;167:857–864.
138. Douvas GS, May MH, Pearson JR, Lam E, Miller L, Tsuchida N. Hypertriglyceridemic serum, very low density lipoprotein, and iron enhance *Mycobacterium avium* replication in human macrophages. *J Infect Dis* 1994;170:1248–1255.
139. Mencacci A, Cenci E, Boelaert JR, et al. Iron overload alters innate and T helper cell responses to *Candida albicans* in mice. *J Infect Dis* 1997;175:1467–1476.
140. Kaplan M, Armstrong D, Rosen P. Tuberculosis complicating neoplastic disease. A review of 201 cases. *Cancer* 1974;33:850–858.
141. Lichtenstein IH, MacGregor RR. Mycobacterial infections in renal transplant recipients: report of five cases and review of the literature. *Rev Infect Dis* 1983; 5:216–226.
142. Jereb JA, Burwen DR, Dooley SW, et al. Nosocomial outbreak of tuberculosis in a renal transplant unit: application of a new technique for restriction fragment length polymorphism analysis of *Mycobacterium tuberculosis* isolates. *J Infect Dis* 1993;168:1219–1224.
143. Hall CM, Willcox PA, Swanepoel CR, Kahn D, Van Zyl Smit R. Mycobacterial infection in renal transplant recipients. *Chest* 1994;106:435–439.
144. Miller RA, Lanza LA, Kline JN, Geist LJ. *Mycobacterium tuberculosis* in lung transplant recipients. *Am J Respir Crit Care Med* 1995;152:374–376.
145. Ridgeway AL, Warner GS, Phillips P, et al. Transmission of *Mycobacterium tuberculosis* to recipients of single lung transplants from the same donor. *Am J Respir Crit Care Med* 1996;153:1166–1168.
146. Schulman LL, Scully B, McGregor CC, Austin JHM. Pulmonary tuberculosis after lung transplantation. *Chest* 1997;111:1459–1462.
147. Muñoz P, Palomo J, Muñoz R, Rodríguez-Creixéms M, Pelaez T, Bouza E. Tuberculosis in heart transplant recipients. *Clin Infect Dis* 1995;21:398–402.
148. Körner MM, Hirata N, Tenderich G, et al. Tuberculosis in heart transplant recipients. *Chest* 1997;111: 365–369.
149. Fishman JA, Rubin RH. Infection in organ-transplant recipients. *N Engl J Med* 1998;338:1741–1751.
150. Reichman L, Felton C, Edsall J. Drug dependence—a possible new risk factor for tuberculosis disease. *Arch Intern Med* 1979;139:337–339.
151. O'Donnell AE, Selig J, Aravamuthan M, Richardson MSA. Pulmonary complications associated with illicit drug abuse—an update. *Chest* 1995;108:460–463.
152. Daley CL, Hahn JA, Moss AR, Hopewell PC, Schecter GF. Incidence of tuberculosis in injection drug users in San Francisco. Impact of anergy. *Am J Respir Crit Care Med* 1998;157:19–22.
153. Baldwin GC, Tashkin DP, Buckley DM, Park AN, Dubinett SM, Roth MD. Marijuana and cocaine impair alveolar macrophage function and cytokine production. *Am J Respir Crit Care Med* 1997;156:1606–1613.
154. Horwitz O. Tuberculosis risk and marital status. *Am Rev Respir Dis* 1971;104:22–31.
155. Clarke ER Jr., Zahn DW, Holmes TH. The relationship of stress, adrenocortical function, and tuberculosis. *Am Rev Tuberc* 1954;69:351–369.
156. Hawkins NG, Holmes TH. Environmental considerations in tuberculosis: ecologic factors in tuberculosis morbidity. *Trans Natl Tuberc Assoc* 1954;50: 233–238.
157. Hawkins NG, Davies R, Holmes TH. Evidence of psychosocial factors in the development of pulmonary tuberculosis. *Am Rev Tuberc Lung Dis* 1957;75:768–780.
158. Lerner BH. Can stress cause disease? Revisiting the tuberculosis research of Thomas Holmes, 1949–1961. *Ann Intern Med* 1996;124:673–680.
159. Barr RG, Menzies R. The effect of war on tuberculosis. *Tuberc Lung Dis* 1994;75:251–259.
160. Ader R, Cohen N, Felten D. Psychoneuoimmunology: interactions between the nervous system and the immune system. *Lancet* 1995;345:99–103.
161. Cohen S, Doyle WJ, Skoner DP, Rabin BS, Gwaltney JM. Social ties and susceptibility to the common cold. *JAMA* 1997;277:1940–1944.
162. McKenna MT, McCray E, Jones JL, Onorato IM, Castro KG. The fall after the rise: tuberculosis in the United States, 1991 through 1994. *Am J Public Health* 1998;88:1059–1063.
163. Blower SM, McLean AR, Porco TC, et al. The intrinsic transmission dynamics of tuberculosis epidemics. *Natl Med* 1995;1:815–821.

6

Clinical Presentations

Pulmonary Tuberculosis in Adults

In countries or communities with high prevalences of tuberculosis, a person's initial encounter with *M. tuberculosis* usually occurs during childhood or adolescence. Thus, most of the clinical literature regarding initial infection or "primary" tuberculosis relates to these age groups. However, even in these high-prevalence areas, most overt tuberculosis morbidity or disease occurs in young adults and is caused by reactivation or "postprimary" forms of tuberculosis. Therefore, this chapter deals briefly with "primary" forms of tuberculosis; this general topic is dealt with more fully under pediatric tuberculosis (Chapter 9) and pathogenesis and immunity (Chapter 4). Tuberculosis that occurs in persons with HIV infection or AIDS has such distinctive epidemiological, clinical, laboratory, treatment, and prevention aspects that it will be dealt with in a separate chapter (Chapter 8).

PRIMARY INFECTION IN ADULTS

Strictly speaking, primary infection means the first biologically significant encounter with the tubercle bacillus. Conversion of the tuberculin skin test from "negative," "unreactive," or "insignificant," to "positive," "reactive," or "significant" is the most common marker of this event because most episodes have minimal symptomatic or radiographic manifestations. Traditionally, "primary" tuberculosis has been regarded as all clinical manifestations occurring up to 5 years following the initial infection (1). I believe, however, that this schema misrepresents the biological events involved and should be abandoned. The true primary forms of tuberculosis are those disorders that entail continuous, uninterrupted mycobacterial proliferation without a period of involution or quiescence. As noted, such primary disease is most likely to occur in infants and children before 5 years of age. Recently, progressive primary tuberculosis has been noted also to occur commonly in adults with advanced HIV infection or AIDS.

Relatively little is known about the biology and clinical manifestations of primary infection with *M. tuberculosis* in immunologically normal adults. Stead and colleagues presented a review of 37 cases that they deemed "primary tuberculosis in adults," defining the condition by one or more of these criteria: (a) known recent tuberculin conversion in 22 cases, (b) a mid- or lower-zone parenchymal infiltrate associated with hilar adenopathy in eight cases, (c) tuberculous pleurisy in young adults with clear underlying lung involvement on radiography in three cases, and (d) parenchymal lesions limited to the lower lobes or anterior segments that cleared with antituberculosis therapy in four cases (2). The study was flawed by the circular logic that defined the last three groups: the authors deemed them primary by their nature, without consistent evidence of new or "primary" infection. However, overall, the study probably affords sound observations on the phenomenon.

Salient clinical findings in the Stead report included the following: (a) degree of clinical illness, none 11, mild 15, moderate 10, and severe 1; (b) chest x-ray findings, hilar adenopathy 16/37 (43%), pleural effusions 14/37 (38%). Of note is that among those with hilar adenopathy, seven of ten blacks (70%) had enlarged nodes while only 9 of 27 whites (33%) had this finding. Regarding pleural effusions, six of ten blacks (60%) had significant collections, whereas only 8 of 27 whites (30%) had detectable effusions. In this highly selected group (many of the patients had been referred to a sanatorium in Milwaukee), 16 persons had gone on to develop pulmonary parenchymal disease within a few months or years. The study does not provide "denominator" data to inform us how frequently these clinical outcomes result from primary infection in adults. Surely, the great majority of newly infected adults follow a much more benign course, never becoming ill enough to come to medical attention. However, for the less fortunate, this study also delineates the potential manifestations.

Table 6.1 is a representation of the natural history of primary tuberculosis in adults. The factors that determine the course of the initial infection in "normal" hosts are not clearly delineated. Certainly, there are well-defined risk factors such as HIV infection, diabetes mellitus, extremes of age, and others (see Chapter 5) that increase the probability of morbidity; but, for other persons, it is unclear whether inoculum size, strain virulence, subtle genetic vulnerability, or other elements mark those who are more likely to experience an unfavorable course. Certainly, the most readily detectable marker of those at higher risk of future pulmonary tuberculosis is the appearance of upper lung zone fibronodular infiltration on the chest x-ray. Known eponymically as "Simon foci," these abnormalities are in fact the breeding ground for much of the reactivation-type pulmonary disease that these persons experience throughout the remainder of their lives. The presence of these findings in a person with a positive tuberculin reaction increases that individual's subsequent risk of pulmonary tuberculosis 30-fold in comparison to a similar individual with tuberculin reactivity but a normal chest x-ray (3).

REACTIVATION-TYPE PULMONARY TUBERCULOSIS

The lungs are not only the portal of entry for the tubercle bacillus, but they are the organ most likely to be involved clinically by the microbe. However, in most cases, the lung disease is not the immediate consequence of the primary infection but rather is a delayed or "postprimary" sequela of the bacillemia that typically occurs as part of the primary infection (see Chapter 4). During this bacillemia, many organs presumably are seeded; however, the lungs—particularly the

TABLE 6.1. *The natural history of primary tuberculosis in adults*

Event	Time	Comments
Alveolar deposition of tubercle bacilli	0	Engulfed by alveolar macrophage; proliferate intracellularly
Bacilli proliferate and disseminate; normal immune response results in involution of infection	3–8 weeks	Protective and tissue-damaging immunity evolve (Chapter 4); tuberculin skin test becomes reactive; some experience chest x-ray abnormalities, fever, and/or hypersensitivity phenomena (*erythema nodosum* or *induratum*, phylectenular conjunctivitis, Poncet's arthritis)
A modest number of patients develop pleurisy; smaller numbers develop miliary disease	8–26 weeks	Pleural tuberculosis usually undergoes spontaneous involution but signals persons at high risk for reactivation
High-risk period for pulmonary and extrapulmonary disease	26–156 weeks	5–15% of newly infected adults develop overt disease within 3 years

After 3 years, persons with new tuberculosis infections join those with remote infection in terms of risk for active tuberculosis disease. Risk factors for endogenous reactivation then include residual chest x-ray abnormalities and other features (see Chapter 5).

upper lobes—are especially vulnerable to significant lodgement of the bacilli.

Why the Predilection for Upper Zones?

Speculation regarding upper zone predisposition includes the following:

- Tubercle bacilli are obligate aerobes. The upper zones of the lung have a substantially higher mean oxygen tension than the lower zones because of the relative paucity of "venous" blood circulated in the pulmonary artery system to the apical regions. As calculated by West and Dollery, at sea level the arterial oxygen tension (partial pressure, alveolar, or P_{aO2}) at the level of the first rib would be 132 mm Hg, falling to 89 mm Hg at the level of the xiphi-sternum (4). However, as Goodwin and Des Prez note, this factor alone is insufficient to explain the apical predilection of tuberculosis because high-altitude dwellers, throughout whose lungs the oxygen tensions are uniformly reduced below 89 mm Hg, have been shown to be very vulnerable to tuberculosis (5). Thus, although this explanation is commonly offered to explain apical tuberculosis, it probably is not of biological significance.
- Dock proposed in 1946 that tuberculosis localized in the apex of the lungs because of diminished lymph generation and impaired tissue clearance (6). The reduced lymph fluid generation results from the same physiological phenomenon as the oxygen tension differential: diminished pulmonary artery/capillary flow in the upper zones. Because lymph is produced by extravasation of serum where hydrostatic pressure exceeds the oncotic pressure, there can be only minimal lymphatic flow in the apices (7). Goodwin and Des Prez make a persuasive analogy in the pathogenesis of silicosis: despite the fact that most inhaled silica particles are deposited in the lower zones (where ventilation is greatest), most silicotic lesions occur in the upper zones, probably because of impaired lymphogenous clearance (5).
- Recently, another potential explanation for the apical predilection of tuberculosis has been offered: human macrophages appear less capable of inhibiting intracellular mycobacterial proliferation in oxygen-rich environments than in physiologically hypoxic environments (8). The advocates of this theory were puzzled by the consistent inability of human monocyte-derived macrophages, even under pharmacological stimulation, to substantially inhibit the replication of tubercle bacilli (9,10). They hypothesized that macrophage function might be favorably altered in an environment that more closely simulated the tissue milieu common to most organs, that is, lower oxygen tension. They thus compared macrophage physiology and capacity to inhibit mycobacterial replication in 20% and 5% oxygen environments. The macrophages cultivated at the lower oxygen tension spread more widely and, on stimulation, elaborated more reactive oxygen intermediates; these cells also permitted significantly less mycobacterial growth. To control for the possiblity that the relative hypoxia was inhibiting the mycobacterial growth, they compared growth of tubercle bacilli in vitro in 20% and 5% oxygen environments and found no differences. The authors therefore concluded that the oxygen-rich environment of the lung apices (and other tissues with rich arterial plexuses) may well have an adverse effect on local macrophage performance, resulting in increased risk for mycobacterial invasion of that organ.
- Another potential factor in the predilection for apical disease is tissue-specific adaptation by the microbes. As noted in Chapter 2, animal model studies indicate that *M. tuberculosis* recovered from the lungs of animals has a greater tendency to localize in the lungs (as opposed to liver or spleen) of animals subsequently infected by the intravenous route than tubercle bacilli that had simply been cultivated in vitro (11). Presumably, the mycobacteria undergo some adaptations to the pulmonary environment that make them more viable in the lungs. Because tuberculosis is almost always transmitted from cavitary lung disease, there may be some subtle preadaptations that result in more intensive lung infestation during the primary phase in the newly infected host.

- A complex model to explain apical localization was recently offered by a group from the University of Wisconsin (12). This model is based on the assumptions of an initial low primary infection inoculum, bacillemic seeding of all lung zones at this time, and apical localization with endogenous reactivation because of preferential bacillemia seeding of the upper zones. By contrast, apical predilection in exogenous reinfection is deemed to result from preferential airway delivery. The critical premise underlying this model is that, in areas with very high prevalences of tuberculosis, a substantial majority of cases—even in adults—result from exogenous reinfection. But, despite this route of pathogenesis, the great preponderance of these patients manifest apical disease. The logic of this model seems rather strained.

Evidence for Endogenous Reactivation

Most pulmonary tuberculosis is the result of endogenous reactivation of latent foci; this is supported by both epidemiological and microbiological findings. Essential points of this logic are as follows: (a) most patients who develop tuberculosis have been infected for long periods before the disease becomes manifest; (b) patients with prior tuberculosis infection (known tuberculin reactors) are relatively resistant to reinfection/disease after heavy exposure when compared to tuberculin-negative subjects (13); and (c) apical fibronodular lesions (Simon foci) are much more likely to contain viable tubercle bacilli than are solitary lower-zone primary-focus lesions or hilar lymph nodes (Ghon lesion or Ranke complex) (14). Stead estimated from a literature review that postprimary, quiescent apical lesions yielded viable tubercle bacilli in about 20% of such cases studied at autopsy (13).

These findings, coupled with epidemiological patterns, indicate that most cases of adolescent/adult pulmonary tuberculosis result when one or more of these upper-zone chronic fibronodular lesions undergoes transition from quiescent to progressive activity. There are numerous elements involved with the risk of reactivation, all of which presumably act through the final pathway of immunological impairment (see Chapter 5 for risk factors).

SIGNS AND SYMPTOMS

Patients with active pulmonary tuberculosis experience a wide gamut of manifestations. Some are extremely ill, progressing rapidly to a life-threatening condition; this fulminant sequence was referred to in the past as "galloping consumption." Other patients have minimal complaints, living for extended periods with very modest and static findings; such persons were deemed "good chronics" in the preche-motherapy era.

Symptoms may be either respiratory or constitutional. Common complaints are noted in Table 6.2. The clear preponderance of patients with active pulmonary tuberculosis are symptomatic at the time of diagnosis, yet for many the chronicity of their complaints lulls both the patient and the clinician into underestimating their importance. There are clear exceptions, but tuberculosis tends to be a more rapidly progressive illness among genetically vulnerable groups. As noted by Stead in his review of racial susceptibility to tuberculosis, when *M. tuberculosis* was initially introduced into Africans, the disease was explosive with a "typhoidal" course commonly resulting in death in a matter of weeks (15).

Physical examination is often quite unremarkable. Characteristically, there are minimal adventitious sounds in the lungs until the disease is

TABLE 6.2. *Typical symptoms in pulmonary tuberculosis*

Respiratory	Constitutional
Cough (initially dry; later productive)	Malaise
Chest pain (with both primary and reactivation)	Lassitude/weakness
Hemoptysis (sparse early; heavy with cavitation)	Feverishness
Shortness of breath (with advancing disease)	Sweats
Hoarseness (severe with laryngeal involvement)	Anorexia

Some patients have profound, rapidly progressive signs and symptoms, whereas others have a paucity of complaints despite extensive disease. Despite complaints of feverishness ± sweats, a modest proportion of patients do not have objective fever under clinical observation (see text).

quite advanced. Localized rales or posttussive rales may suggest tuberculosis infiltration but are not consistent findings. Pleural friction rubs are rare in postprimary tuberculosis, even with pleuritic chest pain. Dullness to percussion and limited thoracic excursions usually are associated with old pleural thickening, presumably from primary tuberculous pleurisy or other disorders. Regional lymphadenopathy is quite uncommon, either intrathoracically (seen on chest x-ray) or in the supraclavicular or cervical chains. Hepatomegaly and/or splenomegaly are rarely found in postprimary tuberculosis. Digital clubbing is very infrequent among patients presenting with recent-onset tuberculosis; however, among those who have suffered from active disease for years, a rising percentage will manifest clubbing. Cutaneous abnormalities such as erythema nodosum, erythema induratum, or erythema annulare centrifugum are quite rare among patients in the United States with postprimary pulmonary tuberculosis.

Fever is not found universally among patients with active, untreated tuberculosis. The percentage of patients hospitalized for treatment of tuberculosis who were febrile ranged from 55% (44 of 80), to 66% (106 of 161), to 79% (59 of 75) in recent reports (16–18). In the first series noted above, 3 of the 80 patients had miliary disease; the others in that report and all of those in the other studies had pulmonary disease. Factors associated with fever in the second report above included male sex and alcoholism. However, these findings were not duplicated in the third study; rather, this article associated fever significantly with younger age. The predisposition of younger patients to have fever more frequently than those 65 years or older was confirmed in a recent report from Canada (19). In two of the above studies, there was a tendency toward higher and more prolonged fever with radiographically advanced, strongly sputum smear-positive cases (17,18). In one report, there was an association between febrility and hyponatremia and hypoalbuminemia, both markers of chronicity and severity of the tuberculosis (18). The definitions of fever in the above series (16–18) included temperatures of 100.0°F, 37.6°C (99.7°F), and 37.8°C (100.0°F), respectively. A substantial number of patients who were "afebrile" in these studies may well have complained of feeling "feverish" but were not febrile by these strict criteria. However, it is important for clinicians to keep in mind that 45%, 21%, and 34% of hospitalized patients with proven tuberculosis did not demonstrate pyrexia in those series (16–18): *lack of fever does not exclude or even render substantially improbable the diagnosis of tuberculosis.* For more data on the course of fever under treatment, see Chapter 10.

DIAGNOSTIC/LABORATORY STUDIES

Clinicians may obtain a variety of studies to aid with the diagnosis and management of patients with tuberculosis. These studies include those that are variably specific to tuberculosis (smears, cultures, skin tests) and those that are nonspecific but inferentially helpful in determining the probability of a given patient's suffering from active tuberculous disease (ESR, sodium level, albumin concentration, etc.). These studies are listed in Tables 6.3 and 6.4.

Tuberculin Skin Testing

In 1890, Koch announced a substance that he believed would cure tuberculosis. Unfortunately, this material—which became known as tuberculin—proved generally harmful as a therapeutic agent (see Chapter 1). However, Clemens von Pirquet recognized that this substance had utility as a diagnostic agent, and throughout the 20th century, tuberculoproteins have been employed to elicit a delayed-type hypersensitivity reaction among those infected with *M. tuberculosis.* Although extremely useful from an epidemiological perspective, the tuberculin test has been found to lack both sensitivity and specificity in other applications. Regarding sensitivity, four modern studies have demonstrated substantial rates of false negativity to a contemporary tuberculin preparation, purified-protein derivative stabilized with Tween (PPD-T): 17% in New York in 1971 (20), 21% in New York in 1976 (21), 25% in Texas in 1980 (22), and 19% in Canada in 1994 (19). A recent national survey found that 32% of persons with active tubercu-

TABLE 6.3. *Tests with partial specificity for tuberculosis*

Test	Positive result and meaning	Negative result and meaning
Tuberculin skin test	Positive in 68–83% of cases of pulmonary TB; false positives occur with nontuberculous mycobacterial (NTM) infections and prior BCG vaccination. In some cases, people have a true positive TST but do not have active TB.	False negatives occur in 17–32% of cases of active TB. Two-step testing is of no utility in this setting. Tests may become positive after treatment is initiated and the severity of illness lessens.
Sputum smear	Usually positive in cavitary cases. However, positive is not specific for *M. tuberculosis* (NTM and *Nocardia* are also acid-fast). Overall, positive in roughly 50–70% of cases of proven pulmonary TB.	Negative smears in cases with gross cavitation suggest other diagnoses. Cases of smear-negative culture-positive pulmonary TB are less contagious than those that are positive/positive; see Chapter 3.
Sputum culture	The gold standard for diagnosis; positive culture for *M.* tuberculosis is always regarded as indicative of disease and an indication for treatment (contrast with NTM, which may be saprophytic).	Roughly 10–15% of pulmonary cases that are ultimately deemed "active" by x-ray progression, symptoms, and/or response to therapy will not yield positive sputum cultures.
Chest x-ray	Abnormal in virtually all cases. However, findings may be subtle or atypical. Computed tomography more sensitive than plain radiographs	Very rare cases of sputum-positive disease with "normal" chest x-ray; usually caused by endobronchial disease or peribronchial node with fistula.

These comments apply to adult patients without HIV infection or AIDS. The sensitivity of all of these diagnostic techniques diminishes in the presence of AIDS (see Chapter 8).

losis failed to yield a positive reaction (≥10 mm induration) to PPD-T (23). Similarly, two recent reports from Saudi Arabia (24) and Ethiopia (25) using different preparations included lack of tuberculin reactivity in 17% and 20%, respectively. By contrast, a recent study from the United States found significant tuberculin reactivity in 51 consecutive HIV-negative adults with "culture-confirmed active tuberculosis" (26). Although these results at first appear discrepant with the above reports, the patients in the latter series were not tested at the time they presented with an acute, undiagnosed illness but several months or more after treatment had been initiated.

The failure of persons, known to have active disease with *M. tuberculosis,* to respond to intradermal infection of tuberculin has been termed "anergy." However, one should not confuse this use of the label with understanding of the mechanism(s) involved. Although there are some general patterns that seem associated with anergy—advanced age, extreme wasting, overwhelming or disseminated tuberculosis—there are enough exceptions to leave the mechanistic explanations in doubt. Pesanti recently reviewed "negative" tuberculin skin tests including the issues of anergy testing and HIV infection (27); this analysis clearly documents the lack of utility of using more potent ("second strength") tuberculin tests.

Regarding specificity, some persons who are not infected with *M. tuberculosis* but are infected by mycobacteria other than tuberculosis (MOTT) will demonstrate a strong reaction to PPD-T or other tuberculins. The probabiltiy of obtaining false-positive reactions to PPD-T will vary in a Beyesian manner, given the prevalences of true *M. tuberculosis* infections and MOTT infections in a given population. In a multicenter survey from the United States published in 1991, PPD-T reactions had a specificity of 90% (23). Notably, patients infected with *M. scrofulaceum* and *M. kansasii* were most likely, among persons with nontuberculous mycobacterial infection, to have substantial reactions to PPD-T. Similarly, among 44 persons, who 12 years previously had had cutaneous disease caused by *M. marinum,* 23 had strongly positive reactions (14 mm or more induration) to PPD-S, the standard tuberculosis antigen used before PPD-T (28). Preliminary results comparing a "sensitin" prepared from *M. avium* simultaneously with "tuberculin" prepared from *M. tuberculosis* (PPD RT-23) indicate that dual skin testing may be quite useful in distinguishing infections with MAC (29). Use of this or similar

TABLE 6.4. *Nonspecific abnormalities associated with pulmonary tuberculosis*

Test	Comment
Anemia	Many patients with severe or long-standing tuberculosis develop mild "anemia of chronic disease."
Erythrocyte sedimentation rate (ESR)	Commonly see elevations into range of 40–80 mm/hr. Usually declines with treatment.
Albumin	Low concentrations associated with chronic, wasting illness and more severe course, prolonged fever, and debility.
Serum sodium	Hyponatremia usually secondary to syndrome of inappropriate antidiuretic hormone secretion because of pulmonary involvement.
Abnormal liver function tests (LFTs)	Abnormal LFTs may result from hepatic tuberculosis, nonspecific inflammatory effect, or chronic passive congestion caused by cor pulmonale in far-advanced disease. [Occasionally related to existent alcohol abuse or viral hepatitis.]
Leukocytosis	Most common pattern is modest increase in WBC count without left shift; monocytosis in distinct minority. Eosinophilia very rare.
Hypercalcemia	Modest elevations of serum calcium are seen in significant proportion of patients receiving supplemental calcium and/or vitamin D; rare without such repletion.

antigens might restore some specificity to skin testing.

Thus, one must employ the results of tuberculin skin testing in clinical medicine with a keen appreciation of their limitations. The most vital issue, I believe, is to appreciate that an insignificant reaction does not allow a clinician to exclude active tuberculosis in a patient, even in the absence of factors known to produce anergy, such as HIV infection, debility, or extremes of age. Nor does a significant reaction prove that the illness that has brought a patient to medical attention is tuberculosis: the tuberculin reactivity could reflect a latent infection with *M. tuberculosis* that is totally unrelated to the present illness, or it could be caused by active or prior infection with nontuberculous mycobacteria or by prior BCG vaccination. Certainly, a positive or negative result can be seen to alter the probabilities of tuberculous disease; however, tuberculin skin testing is at best a diagnostic aid, not a diagnosis.

Sputum and Other Respiratory Secretions

Sputum specimens are of central importance in the diagnosis of pulmonary tuberculosis. Great effort should be made to obtain good quality specimens of lower respiratory tract secretions for analysis. Early morning sputum is considered ideal because patients tend not to cough as frequently or forcefully while asleep, allowing mycobacteria-laden secretions to accumulate.

For patients who are unable to spontaneously produce sputum, induction of cough by inhalation of a heated saline nebulization may be of utility. Bronchial irritation typically causes the patient to cough deeply, and the fluid deposited by the aerosol may help provide a liquid base for the expulsion of secretions. It should be noted that sputum induction for patients with possible tuberculosis offers substantial potential hazard for transmission and should be conducted only in areas with well-controlled ventilation and/or ultraviolet germicidal irradiation.

If patients are unable to provide such specimens because of a lack of secretions or inability to cooperate with induction, gastric aspiration has proven of modest utility (30). Gastric aspiration is based on the overnight accumulation of respiratory secretions in the stomach as bronchial ciliary clearance propels respiratory mucus into the pharynx where it is reflexively swallowed. The technique is most effective early in the morning before peristalsis is initiated by food or the anticipation of same. Formerly, it was believed that because of commensal mycobacteria in the stomach, smears of gastric aspirates were nonspecific and of no value; however, recent studies have shown that readily positive smears in patients who were suspected of having tuberculosis were of significant diagnostic utility (31–33).

The next level of intervention in the pursuit of diagnostic material is bronchoscopy. In general, I believe it is appropriate to pursue the other modalities before resorting to this procedure because of both the risks and discomfort for the patient and the unavoidable hazards of transmission to health-care workers during this cough-intensive, intimate-exposure procedure. If, however, bronchogenic neoplasms are prominent in the differential diagnosis, early bronchoscopy is indicated. A reasonable algorithm for the utilization of these would be as follows:

1. Obtain spontaneous sputum.
2. If patient is unable to produce sputum, induce by irritant aerosol, or, if patient is unable to cooperate with induction procedure, go directly to gastric aspiration.
3. If induction fails or the specimen is of poor quality and is negative on microscopy, obtain early morning gastric aspirate (gastric aspiration is more practical and effective for hospitalized patients because the procedure can be done immediately on awakening).

If the above specimens are of poor quality or sparse or are negative on microscopic examination, bronchoscopy should be considered. However, if the specimens have been inoculated into a rapid cultivation system, it may be appropriate to wait for a week to see if mycobacterial growth is occurring; if so, bronchoscopy may be averted. If not, flexible fiberoptic bronchoscopy may enhance the diagnostic yield. In one series from Michigan, 41 patients with ultimately demonstrated pulmonary tuberculosis were studied; 37 of them had three negative sputum smears, and four were unable to produce sputum (34). In 14 of 41, bronchoscopic aspirates were the sole source of microscopy-positive material; bronchial washings and postbronchoscopy each yielded exclusively positive microscopy in two cases; brushings contributed no uniquely positive material. Regarding culture results, bronchoscopic aspirates were uniquely positive in 19 of 41, while washings and postbronchoscopy sputa were the sole source of positive cultures in five cases each. Obviously, this series was selected on the basis of positive bronchoscopy findings and does not include those persons with active pulmonary tuberculosis in whom endoscopy also failed to yield a diagnosis. Similar results were noted in a large survey of patients from the Walter Reed Army Medical Center who underwent bronchoscopy for undiagnosed pulmonary disease. Among 25 patients ultimately shown to have tuberculosis, bronchoscopic aspirates/washings were culture positive in 24 of 25 and were the sole source of positive bacteriology in 10 of 25 cases (35). Culture of bronchial aspirates increased isolation of *M. tuberculosis* by 30% in another series of 70 patients undergoing endoscopy (36). Bronchoscopy resulted in accelerated diagnosis of 18 of 67 patients reported in a series from Japan (37). Bronchoalveolar lavage (BAL; washing out a localized region of the lung with 120–240 ml of saline) was reported to enhance the yield of bronchoscopy in a series of patients from Cincinnati (38); however, because of methodological issues, it was difficult to ascertain how much BAL contributed to the sensitivity of endoscopy. A recent report from Canada that compared the yields of sputum induction and subsequent bronchoscopy found that induction was generally more sensitive (87% vs. 71%) and had a comparable negative predictive value (96% vs. 91%) (39).

Overall, there are limited but significant roles for bronchoscopy in the diagnosis of pulmonary tuberculosis. I would summarize these indications in the following manner: (a) routine diagnosis in patients from whom it is not possible to obtain adequate sputum, induced sputum, or gastric aspirates or in whom these specimens are negative but the suspicion for tuberculosis remains high; (b) patients in whom there is a substantial risk of drug-resistant tuberculosis and in whom initial routine studies are negative; in such cases, a presumptive diagnosis is insufficient to initiate optimal therapy—in vitro susceptibility testing is vital to guide choice of drugs, and this requires a positive culture; and (c) patients in whom there is suspicion of endobronchial tuberculosis; many of these patients have very unusual chest x-rays, negative sputum smears, and complicated clinical courses (see below).

Molecular Biology Techniques and Diagnosis

For detection of mycobacteria in sputum or other respiratory secretions, microscopy is relatively insensitive, and culture is frustratingly slow, even when it employs modern systems. Hence, there is great enthusiasm for the development of methods such as nucleic acid amplification techniques to provide one-day tests to give the diagnosis of tuberculosis. Theoretically, such a method could be more sensitive even than culture techniques, could distinguish mycobacterial species, and might even identify drug-resistant strains in less than 48 hours. Numerous commercial and research facilities are currently attempting to bring such technology to the clinic or bedside. However, the routine applicability and cost-effectiveness of these systems has yet to be proven. For a more comprehensive review of these systems, please see Chapter 2.

Conventional Chest Radiography

Shortly after Roentgen's discovery of x-rays in the 1890s, radiologic studies of the lungs were employed in tuberculosis. Characteristic abnormalities are extremely valuable in estimating the probability of a given patient suffering tuberculosis. However, in the vast majority of situations, the radiographic findings are only an inferential aid in diagnosis. As noted above, following the primary infection with *M. tuberculosis,* most persons emerge with a normal chest x-ray. A minority of persons are left with apical or biapical fibronodular shadowing (referred to as "Simon foci"); these findings mark individual tuberculin reactors as being at high risk for reactivation or postprimary-type tuberculosis. Others are left with minor findings such as an isolated small fibrocalcific lesion or Ghon focus. This type of lesion, coupled with an ipsilateral, calcified hilar lymph node, constitutes a Ranke complex (Fig. 6.1). Other abnormalities include thickening of the apical pleura or blunting of the costophrenic sulcus; these findings—

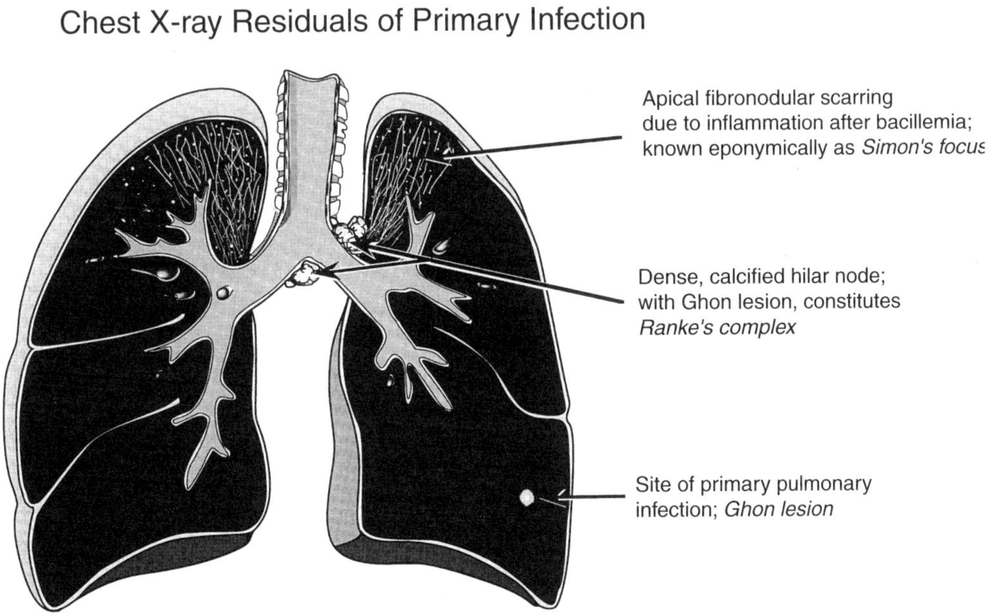

FIG. 6.1. The pulmonary site of the primary infection may heal without any visual sequelae, or it may result in a spherical shadow or "nodule" that, over time, usually one year or longer, may calcify. This lesion is known eponymically as a "Ghon focus." Occasionally, the hilar/mediastinal lymph nodes to which the primary focus drains will undergo a similar process. The finding of the calcified primary focus in the parenchyma coupled with a calcified ipsilateral hilar node is referred to as "Ranke's complex." Epidemiologically, neither of these processes marks an individual as being at greater risk of subsequent active tuberculosis than does a positive tuberculin skin test. By contrast, the presence of uni- or bilateral apical fibronodular shadows, historically known as "Simon's foci," do indicate a substantially greater risk of subsequent pulmonary tuberculosis (see Chapter 12). These lesions are believed to reflect subclinical (undetected) active inflammation in this region that involuted with the acquisition of more competent immunity.

usually indicative of remote tuberculous infection—do not mark individuals as being at higher risk for reactivation disease.

Because most pulmonary tuberculosis is of the postprimary type, it usually involves the upper lung zones. Below are listed typical radiographic features of pulmonary disease:

- *Location:* apical and/or posterior segment of RUL, apicoposterior segment of LUL, or superior segment of either lower lobe
- *Infiltrate:* fibronodular, irregular shadowing with variable coalescence and cavitation
- *Cavities:* thick, moderately irregular walls; air–fluid levels very uncommon
- *Volume:* progressive, often rapid loss of volume within the segment(s) or lobe(s) involved.

Schematically, these features would appear as in Fig. 6.1. Early in the course of the disease, there tends to be unilateral involvement, the most common site involved being the apical/posterior segments of the right upper lobe (RUL). However, with the passage of time, bilateral involvement becomes increasingly probable, and the risk of endobronchial spillage of cavity contents to the lower zones rises (see Chapter 4 on pathogenesis).

Although a consistent preponderance of patients with pulmonary tuberculosis present with variable combinations of the above "typical" features, it is important to emphasize that a significant number of persons present with unusual or "atypical" radiographic findings. Among these unusual findings are lower zone infiltration, prominent pleural effusions, mass lesions, solitary pulmonary nodules, miliary shadowing, hilar/paratracheal/mediastinal lymphadenopathy, pneumothorax, and normal chest x-rays. The proportion of patients with "atypical" findings seems rather consistent at about one-third in the reports summarized in Table 6.5.

Is the chest x-ray of a sufficiently characteristic nature that it allows presumptive diagnosis and therapy? Certainly in many instances, clinicians do initiate treatment based on a complex of symptoms, epidemiologic profiles, and radiographic findings, even in the presence of negative smears. A San Francisco group reported their experience with a series of 139 such patients (40). Eventually, 68 (48%) of them were deemed to have active tuberculosis by various criteria: 16 by positive cultures, 43 by improvement of chest x-rays on therapy, and seven by clinical improvement. However, the practicality of this approach varies, obviously, with the skill of radiographic interpretation and the prevalence of tuberculosis in the population seen. However, as the authors indicate, this approach—in the right setting—is an appropriate practice.

If, as above, the chest x-ray's improvement during chemotherapy can be used as a criterion for diagnosis, what can be concluded when an x-ray deteriorates while a patient is on treatment? While gross worsening is a cause for concern, clinicians should appreciate that, up to several months into what is eventually "successful" treatment, chest x-rays may show progression. This may take the form of enlarging infiltrates, evolving cavitation, new lung zones involved, and the appearance of pleural effusions (41,42).

TABLE 6.5. *Radiographic features in adult pulmonary tuberculosis*

Series (ref.)	Patients (*n*)	"Atypical"	Lower zone	Miliary	Nodular	Effusion or adenopathy
Khan (66)	88	34%	7%	5%	9%	14%
Miller (67)	88	34%	4%	7%	7%	11%
Farman (68)	51	33%	6%	–	16%	18%
Korzeniewska-Kosela (19)	211	31%	6%	3%	8%	(?)
Jones (43)	103	38%	6%	4%	2%	23%

These five series of patients from the United States with pulmonary tuberculosis show strikingly similar findings in terms of the distribution of findings. Only the last group (Jones et al.) had an admixture of HIV-infected persons; this was responsible for the modestly increased frequency of "atypical" and effusion/adenopathy in this report.

Can the pattern of chest x-ray abnormality distinguish between recent and temporally remote infection? Certainly, clinicians have long agreed (including some passages in this chapter) that there are findings typical of primary or reactivation-type disease. Bolstered by RFLP strain fingerprinting, Jones and colleagues tested this hypothesis (43). Assuming that RFLP clustering suggested recent transmission, they characterized x-ray findings of 103 adults in Los Angeles. Aside from mediastinal lymphadenopathy and pleural effusions in HIV-infected persons, no distinctions could be made. These findings are mindful of the group from Wisconsin's hypothesis for upper lung zone predilection, as noted above.

Computed Tomography

Computed tomography (CT) of the lung yields far more detailed images than conventional techniques. This includes the presence or absence of cavities, the nature and extent of airspace filling processes, bronchiectasis, atelectasis, or pleural disorders. In most advanced cases of tuberculosis, such studies are not necessary for diagnosis or management. However, in diagnostically elusive cases or in complicated treatment situations, CT scans may prove very useful.

A Korean group authored a series of articles describing CT scan findings of various aspects of tuberculosis (44–47). These reports describe various typical findings both in terms of characteristic abnormalities and anatomical distribution; however, in the majority of situations, the findings do not allow diagnosis or exclusion of tuberculosis with sufficient predictive power to supplant a conventional evaluation. Cases in which CTs may be considerably more sensitive than conventional radiography include early miliary disease (48,49).

A more recent report from Canada employed CT scans along with detailed spirometric and arterial blood gas determinations to assess the physiological sequelae of tuberculosis (50). Among the salient findings in this report are the following: (a) typical reactivation-type tuberculosis progresses from focal nodular shadows to confluent pneumonia; where this process undergoes necrosis, cavities form, and endobronchial spread occurs; (b) plain radiography consistently underrepresents the severity and extent of disease; (c) although much of the parenchymal shadowing cleared during the course of chemotherapy, the badly involved areas remained physiologically inert in terms of both ventilation and perfusion; and (d) despite curative therapy, cavities persisted in eight, and bronchiectasis evolved in 9 of 11 patients. In terms of global physiological consequences of pulmonary tuberculosis, it was impressive that there were very modest reductions in airflow, diffusing capacity, oxygen transport, and carbon dioxide elimination in the majority of those patients (who were chosen for the absence of underlying lung disorders). The fact that disturbances of ventilation and perfusion tended to be matched helps explain why even with advanced tuberculosis many patients are not hypoxemic at rest.

LOWER LUNG ZONE PULMONARY TUBERCULOSIS

Lower lung zone tuberculosis (LLZ TB) represents a particularly troublesome subset of patients for two reasons: it is frequently misdiagnosed, and it is commonly associated with peribronchial lymphadenitis and endobronchitis, which complicate the outcome. The series included in Table 6.5 noted LLZ TB in 7%, 4%, 6%, 6%, and 6% of pulmonary tuberculosis patients; other reports found it to be present in 6.9% (51) and 5.1% (52) of cases. Both of these latter reports, which focused on LLZ TB, emphasized the following features of this problem: (a) the infiltrates were much more likely to appear as homogeneous, pneumonic consolidation than upper zone disease; (b) diabetes mellitus appeared to be modestly associated as a predisposition; (c) cough was the most prominent presenting complaint; (d) there was a relative paucity of tubercle bacilli in the respiratory secretions; and (d) bronchoscopy with biopsy and lavage was commonly required to establish the diagnosis (53). It is my clinical impression, not supported by careful comparative studies, that

LLZ TB is relatively more common among Asian patients than others.

ENDOBRONCHIAL TUBERCULOSIS

Endobronchial tuberculosis was commonly observed in the two series of LLZ TB noted above (51,52). Both reports suggested that peribronchial lymphadenitis with invasion of the bronchus by fistula formation was central in the pathogenesis of a large percentage of the LLZ TB cases. In the series from Taiwan, endobronchial involvement was seen in 32 of 42 patients undergoing endoscopy; prominent findings included ulcerative granulomata, fibrotic stenosis of the airway, and submucosal infiltration (52). Subsequently, this group reported their extended experience with LLZ TB, noting the major importance of bronchoscopy in the diagnosis and management of these cases (53). In this 1991 article, the authors noted that patients with atelectasis, consolidation, and radiographically prominent lymphadenopathy were at high risk for endobronchial disease and that this group was at considerable risk for a complicated course. Other recent reports have confirmed the high risk of complications (54–57), the capacity for the bronchial narrowing to masquerade as asthma [the original source of the adage, "all that wheezes is not asthma" (McConkey)] (58), the propensity for endobronchial involvement in elderly patients with tuberculosis (59), and a significant predilection for right-sided involvement, particularly the upper lobe in a series of patients from Korea (60). A "barking cough" (61%), localized wheeze (19%), and normal chest x-ray (8.3%) were common findings among 121 Korean patients with endobronchial tuberculosis (60). An uncommon subset of endobronchial tuberculosis is tracheal involvement (61,62).

For patients in whom chest radiographs, physical signs, or symptoms suggest the possiblity of endobronchial tuberculosis, fiberoptic bronchoscopy is indicated. Because of the potential utility of corticosteroid therapy in acutely reducing lymph node and mucosal swelling, this procedure should be done promptly. No systematic approach to management of these cases has been studied. However, bronchoscopic curettage of the proximal pseudomembrane coupled with systemic steroid therapy was reported to enhance drainage among selected patients in the Korean series (60). Among a smaller number of patients from Hong Kong, steroids did not appear to influence the outcome (54). However, based on the reasonable analogy to primary tuberculosis in children with lymphadenopathy-induced atelectasis (Chapter 9), a course of corticosteroids (prednisone, 1 mg/kg daily for 4 to 6 weeks) appears justified in younger patients ($\leq$35 years of age) with endobronchial tuberculosis. The purpose of this treatment is twofold: (a) acutely reduce the bronchial narrowing to promote drainage and reduce the extent of post-stenotic lung damage, and (b) reduce the long-term evolution of high-grade bronchial stenosis. Despite such therapy, these patients remain at high risk for complications, most notably chronic infection with mycobacteria or other pathogens behind an obstructed bronchus (53). In a series of elderly patients from Belgium, endobronchial tuberculosis was relatively common, and its presence signaled high risk for complicated courses, often requiring surgical intervention (59).

HEMOPTYSIS: ORIGINS AND MANAGEMENT

Massive hemoptysis is uncommon in the era of chemotherapy but is a potentially disastrous complication of pulmonary tuberculosis. As tissue destruction occurs (see Chapter 4 on pathogenesis), minor blood vessels are damaged, and small amounts of blood may be expectorated along with the phlegm; approximately one-third of pulmonary tuberculosis patients expectorate some blood during their illness. However, as cavities form, bigger arteries become involved with the possible hazard of large-volume, life-threatening hemorrhage. In the prechemotherapy era, 4% in one series of patients were noted to succumb to bleeding from grossly dilated pulmonary arteries—Rasmussen's aneurysms—in cavity walls (63). In another series of tuberculosis patients dying of pulmonary hemorrhage, 29 of 49 were found to have a Rasmussen aneurysm

(64). However, it is important to note that hemorrhage in tuberculosis may originate from the bronchial artery circuit as well. Stimulated by chronic inflammation, the local bronchial artery(ies) may undergo substantial hypertrophy dilation, becoming capable of profuse hemorrhage. In some cases, fistulas develop between the bronchial and pulmonary vascular circuits and can result in compound bleeding sources. Large-scale hemorrhage occurs relatively more commonly in patients with active or recurrent tuberculosis of long standing; in fact, in a recent hemoptysis series, 6 of 12 patients were "retreatment" cases (65).

Efforts to quantify the amount of hemorrhage for purposes of management and prognosis have been somewhat arbitrary and uncontrolled. Terms such as "major" (200 ml of blood in 24 hours) or "massive" (1,000 ml in 24 hours) have been applied without clear documentation of their implications (64). It is logical that the more hemorrhage in a period of time, the greater the risk to the patient. However, it is impossible to isolate this variable because other factors have strong influences on therapeutic, diagnostic, and prognostic considerations.

Hemoptysis poses two major immediate risks to a patient: exsanguination or respiratory failure. Because of the availability of transfusions or blood-volume support, the former is relatively uncommon in developed countries. Indeed, abrupt respiratory failure from filling of airways and airspaces with blood is the typical mode of death for such patients. Hence, the management of tuberculous patients who are expectorating blood may be approached in this manner:

- Acute therapy
  - Reassurance/calming: these patients are generally frightened, near panic, and need continuous, attentive hospital care
  - Oxygen supplementation: high-flow nasal oxygen is indicated to maximize arterial oxygen transport
  - Cough suppression: although never proven in a controlled study, logic suggests that violent coughing may precipitate or prolong the hemorrhage; the patient should be coached to try to clear his throat gently, not cough explosively. Also, low-dose intravenous morphine may be titrated to suppress cough without altering the sensorium.
  - Intravenous access for potential volume support or transfusions (no food or drink to minimize complications at endoscopy or general anesthesia).
- Diagnostic (identifying site of bleeding)
  - History: some patients can clearly identify and localize the inception of the bleeding; descriptions may include rushing sensations, localized sharp chest pain, gurgling, or warm feelings within specific areas of the chest.
  - Chest x-ray: in some cases, the disease is so clearly localized on prehemorrhage films that it is justifiable to assume that the bleeding is issuing from a specific locale. In other cases, posthemorrhage chest films may indicate the probable site of bleeding by the appearance of a large, confluent infiltrate or "blood pneumonia." However, one must be aware that these infiltrates may appear remote from the bleeding site as a result of endobronchial spread of the blood. If the probable site of bleeding can be established by these methods, we generally attempt to have the patient lie on the side of the hemorrhage. In this way, the blood will tend to collect in the diseased lung and not spill so readily into the other, presumably functional, lung. In some cases, this is not tolerated because of adverse effects on ventilation–perfusion relationships and arterial blood gases.
  - Bronchoscopy: for patients in whom the site of bleeding is undetermined, endoscopy may be indicated. In general, I think this is appropriate only if one is planning invasive interventions such as arterial embolization or resectional surgery. The inherent problem with bronchoscopy is that it is most useful if performed while the patient is actively hemorrhaging. In this manner, one can occasionally see fresh blood issuing from a particular orifice. However, this may be problematic for the following reasons: (a) bloody matter may be deposited throughout the lung and give the false appearance of issuing from a bronchus as a result of air movement; (b) such patients may be unstable with regard to ventilatory reserve; and

(c) bronchoscopy may provoke violent, paroxysmal coughing. Therefore, I recommend that patients who are hemorrhaging heavily and/or having poor respiratory reserve undergo bronchoscopy only in an operating room, under airway management by an anesthesiologist, and with the availability of competent thoracic surgical support. For patients who are bleeding heavily, a rigid bronchoscope is the preferred instrument because of its greater capacity to rapidly evacuate blood from the airways. For patients with lesser hemorrhage and better respiratory reserve, conventional fiberoscopy in less restrictive settings may be adequate.

- Ongoing management
  - Quantify blood loss by measuring volume of hemoptysis and following hemoglobin/hematocrit levels; replete by transfusion if blood volume falls to physiologically significant levels.
  - Blood gas assessment by initial arterial blood gas and continued monitoring of oximetry.
  - Assess for either arterial embolization procedure or resectional surgery if hemorrhage persists. No controlled randomized studies have been performed comparing the utility of these two interventions. Recent studies have suggested that embolization with Gel-foam via pulmonary artery and/or bronchial artery catheters may be sufficient to terminate even massive hemorrhage (64). However, this technology requires highly experienced angiographers and may not be available in many communities and regions. Resectional surgery also is fraught with problems and hazards. Extirpating badly damaged, massively scarred and distorted lung tissue in chronic tuberculosis is extremely difficult, even under "optimal" conditions (see Chapter 10). Attempting to do so in a patient who is destabilized by acute bleeding and whose tuberculosis may not be under good chemotherapeutic control is extremely dangerous. Therefore, unless radiographically directed therapeutic embolization is available, it is my opinion that patients with substantial, continuing hemorrhage should be managed with conservative observation. If the volume and progression of blood loss are ominous, these patients should be transferred to specialty centers where sophisticated radiographic and surgical services are available.

SUMMARY

The lungs remain the main site of clinical tuberculosis as well as the portal of entry for primary infections. The upper zones, particularly the apical posterior segments of the upper lobes and the superior segments of the lower lobes, are the most common loci of disease. The mechanisms underlying this predilection are uncertain. The signs and symptoms vary widely, ranging from chronic cough without constitutional symptoms to "galloping consumption." Bacteriological studies are central to diagnosis and must be pursued aggressively; radiography including CT scans may be helpful in difficult cases. Other "nonspecific" tests may be helpful in assessing the probability of disease; the tuberculin skin test suffers from lack of both sensitivity and specificity. Clinical awareness is critical for prompt diagnosis and timely therapy.

REFERENCES

1. Lucas SB. Mycobacteria and the tissues of man in the biology of mycobacteria. In: Rutledge C, Stanford J, Grange JM, eds. *Clinical aspects of mycobacterial disease.* New York: Academic Press, 1989:120–122.
2. Stead WW, Kerby GR, Schlueter DP, Jordahl CW. The clinical spectrum of primary tuberculosis in adults. *Ann Intern Med* 1968;68:731–745.
3. Horwitz O. The risk of tuberculosis in different groups of the general population. *Scand J Respir Dis* 1970; 72[Suppl]:55–60.
4. West J, Dollery C. Distribution of blood flow and ventilation–perfusion ratios in the lung, measured with radioactive CO_2. *J Appl Physiol* 1960;15:405–410.
5. Goodwin R, DesPrez R. Apical localization of pulmonary tuberculosis. Chronic pulmonary histoplasmosis and progressive massive fibrosis of the lung. *Chest* 1983;83:801–805.
6. Dock W. Apical localization of phthisis. *Am Rev Tuberc* 1946;53:297–305.
7. Lauweryns JM, Baert JH. Alveolar clearance and the role of the pulmonary lymphatics. *Am Rev Respir Dis* 1977;115:625–683.
8. Meylan P, Richman DD, Kornbluth RS. Reduced intracellular growth of mycobacteria in human macrophages at physiologic oxygen pressure. *Am Rev Respir Dis* 1992;145:947–953.
9. Rook G, Steele J, Ainsworth M, Champion B. Activation of macrophages to inhibit proliferation of M. tuberculosis: comparison of the effects of recombinant gamma-interferon on human monocytes and murine

peritoneal macrophages. *Immunology* 1986;59:333–338.
10. Douvas G, Looker D, Vatter A, Crowle A. Gamma interferon activates human macrophages to become tumoricidal and leishmanicidal but enhances replication of macrophage associated mycobacteria. *Infect Immun* 1989;57:840–844.
11. Collins FM, Montalbine V. Distribution of mycobacteria grown in vivo in the organs of intravenously infected mice. *Am Rev Respir Dis* 1976;113:281–286.
12. Balasubramanian V, Wiegeshaus EH, Taylor BT, Smith DW. Pathogenesis of tuberculosis: pathway to apical localization. *Tuberc Lung Dis* 1994;75:168–178.
13. Stead WW. Pathogenesis of a first episode of chronic pulmonary tuberculosis in man: recrudescence of residuals of the primary infection or exogenous reinfection? *Am Rev Respir Dis* 1967;95:729–744.
14. Feldman W, Baggenstoss A. The residual infectivity of the primary complex of tuberculosis. *Am J Pathol* 1938;14:473.
15. Stead W. Genetics and resistance to tuberculosis. *Ann Intern Med* 1992;116:937–941.
16. Berger H, Rosenbaum I. Prolonged fever in patients treated for tuberculosis. *Am Rev Respir Dis* 1968;97:140–143.
17. Barnes P, Chan L, Wong S. The course of fever during treatment of pulmonary tuberculosis. *Tubercle* 1987;68:255–260.
18. Kiblawi S, Jay SJ, Stonehill RB, Norton J. Fever response of patients on therapy for pulmonary tuberculosis. *Am Rev Respir Dis* 1981;123:20–24.
19. Korzeniewska-Kosela M, Krysl J, Muller N, Black W, Allen E, FitzGerald JM. Tuberculosis in young adults and the elderly. A prospective comparison study. *Chest* 1994;106:28–32.
20. Holden M, Dubin MR, Diamond PH. Frequency of negative intermediate-strength tuberculin sensitivity in patients with active tuberculosis. *N Engl J Med* 1971;285:1506–1509.
21. Rooney J, Crocco J, Kramer S, Lyons H. Further observations on tuberculin reactions in tuberculosis. *Am J Med* 1976;60:517–522.
22. Nash D, Douglas J. Anergy in active pulmonary tuberculosis. *Chest* 1980;77:32–37.
23. Huebner RE, Schein MF, Cauthen GM, et al. Evaluation of the clinical usefulness of mycobacterial skin test antigens in adults with pulmonary mycobacterioses. *Am Rev Respir Dis* 1992;145:1160–1166.
24. Teklu B, Al-Wabel A. Tuberculin reaction in pulmonary tuberculosis in the Asir Region of Saudi Arabia. *Tuberc Lung Dis* 1993;74:20–22.
25. Teklu B. Symptoms of pulmonary tuberculosis in consecutive smear-positive cases treated in Ethiopia. *Tuberc Lung Dis* 1993;74:126–128.
26. Duchin JS, Jereb JA, Nolan CM, Smith P, Onorato IM. Comparison of sensitivities to two commercially available tuberculin skin test reagents in persons with recent tuberculosis. *Clin Infect Dis* 1997;25:661–663.
27. Pesanti EL. The negative tuberculin test. Tuberculin, HIV, and anergy panels. *Am J Respir Crit Care Med* 1994;149:1699–1709.
28. Judson FN, Feldman RA. Mycobacterial skin tests in humans 12 years after infection with *M. marinum*. *Am Rev Respir Dis* 1974;109:544–547.
29. von Reyn CF, Williams DE, Horsburgh CR Jr, et al. Dual skin testing with *Mycobacterium avium* sensitin and purified protein derivative to discriminate pulmonary disease due to *M. avium* complex from pulmonary disease due to *Mycobacterium tuberculosis*. *J Infect Dis* 1998;177:730–736.
30. Hsing CT, Ma YT. A comparative study of the efficacy of the laryngeal swab, bronchial lavage, gastric lavage, and direct sputum examination methods in detecting tubercle bacilli in a series of 1,320 patients. *Am Rev Respir Dis* 1962;86:16–20.
31. Strumpf IJ, Tsang AY, Schork MA, Weg JG. The reliability of gastric smears by auramine-rhodamine staining technique for the diagnosis of tuberculosis. *Am Rev Respir Dis* 1976;114:971–976.
32. Klotz SA, Penn RL. Acid-fast staining of urine and gastric contents is an excellent indicator of mycobacterial disease. *Am Rev Respir Dis* 1987;136:1197–1198.
33. Berean K, Roberts F. The reliability of acid fast stained smears of gastric aspirate specimens. *Tubercle* 1988;69:205–208.
34. Danek S, Bower J. Diagnosis of pulmonary tuberculosis by flexible fiberoptic bronchoscopy. *Am Rev Respir Dis* 1979;119:677–679.
35. Russell M, Torrington K, Tenholder M. A ten-year experience with fiberoptic bronchoscopy for mycobacterial isolation. *Am Rev Respir Dis* 1986;133:1069–1071.
36. Tevola K. Bronchial aspiration in the diagnosis of pulmonary tuberculosis. *Scand J Respir Dis* 1974;89 [Suppl]:151–154.
37. Fujii H, Ishihara J, Fukama A, et al. Early diagnosis of tuberculosis by fiberoptic bronchoscopy. *Tuberc Lung Dis* 1992;73:167–169.
38. Baughman R, Dohn M, London R, Frame P. Bronchoscopy with bronchoalveolar lavage in tuberculosis and fungal infections. *Chest* 1991;99:92–97.
39. Anderson C, Inhaber N, Menzies D. Comparison of sputum induction with fiber-optic bronchoscopy in the diagnosis of tuberculosis. *Am J Respir Crit Care Med* 1995;152:1570–1574.
40. Gordin FM, Slutkin G, Schecter G, Goodman PC, Hopewell PC. Presumptive diagnosis and treatment of pulmonary tuberculosis based on radiographic findings. *Am Rev Respir Dis* 1989;139:1090–1093.
41. Bobrowitz ID. Reversible roentgenographic progression in the initial treatment of pulmonary tuberculosis. *Am Rev Respir Dis* 1980;121:735–742.
42. Neff TA, Buchanan BD. Tension pleural effusion. A delayed complication of pneumothorax therapy in tuberculosis. *Am Rev Respir Dis* 1975;111:543–548.
43. Jones BE, Ryu R, Yang Z, et al. Chest radiographic findings in patients with tuberculosis with recent or remote infection. *Am J Respir Crit Care Med* 1997;156:1270–1273.
44. Lee KS, Song KS, Lim TH. Adult-onset pulmonary tuberculosis: findings on chest radiographs and CT scans. *Am J Roentgenol* 1993;160:753–758.
45. Im J-G, Itoh H, Shim Y-S. Pulmonary tuberculosis: CT findings—early active disease and sequential change with antituberculous therapy. *Radiology* 1993;186:653–660.
46. Lee KS, Im J-G. CT in adults with tuberculosis of the chest: characteristic findings and role in management. *Am J Roentgenol* 1995;164:1361–1367.
47. Lee KS, Hwang JW, Chung MP, Kim H, Kwon OJ. Utility of CT in the evaluation of pulmonary tuberculosis in patients without AIDS. *Chest* 1996;110:977–984.

48. McGuinness G, Naidich DP, Jagirdar L. High resolution CT findings in miliary lung disease. *J Comput Assist Tomogr* 1992;16:384–390.
49. Oh Y-H, Kim YH, Lee NJ. High-resolution CT appearance of miliary tuberculosis. *J Comput Assist Tomogr* 1994;18:862–866.
50. Long R, Maycher B, Dhar A, Manfreda J, Hershfield E, Anthonisen N. Pulmonary tuberculosis treated with directly observed therapy. Serial changes in lung structure and function. *Chest* 1998;113:933–943.
51. Berger H, Granada M. Lower lung field tuberculosis. *Chest* 1974;65:522–526.
52. Chang S-C, Lee P-Y, Perng R-P. Lower lung field tuberculosis. *Chest* 1987;91:230–232.
53. Chang S-C, Lee P-Y, Perng R-P. The value of roentgenographic and fiberbronchoscopic findings in predicting outcome of adults with lower lung field tuberculosis. *Arch Intern Med* 1991;151:1581–1583.
54. Ip MSM, So SY, Lam WK, Mok CK. Endobronchial tuberculosis revisited. *Chest* 1986;89:727–730.
55. Smith L, Schillaci R, Sarlin R. Endobronchial tuberculosis. Serial fiberoptic bronchoscopy and natural history. *Chest* 1987;91:644–647.
56. Albert RK, Petty TL. Endobronchial tuberculosis progressing to bronchial stenosis: fiberoptic bronchoscopic manifestations. *Chest* 1987;70:537–539.
57. Tse CY, Natkunam R. Serious sequelae of delayed diagnosis of endobronchial tuberculosis. *Tubercle* 1988; 69:213–216.
58. Williams D, York E, Norbert E, Sproule B. Endobronchial tuberculosis presenting as asthma. *Chest* 1988;93:836–838.
59. van den Brande P, Van de Mierop F, Verbeken E, Demedts M. Clinical spectrum of endobronchial tuberculosis in elderly patients. *Arch Intern Med* 1990; 150:2105–2108.
60. Lee JH, Park SS, Lee DH, Shin DH, Yang SC, Yoo BM. Endobronchial tuberculosis. Clinical and bronchoscopic features in 121 cases. *Chest* 1992;102:990–994.
61. Wathen CG, Kerr KM, Cowan DL, Douglas AC. Tuberculosis of the trachea. *Tubercle* 1987;68:225–228.
62. Watson JM, Ayres JG. Tuberculous stenosis of the trachea. *Tubercle* 1988;69:223–226.
63. Auerbach O. Pathology and pathogenesis of pulmonary artery aneurysm in tuberculous cavities. *Am Rev Tuberc* 1939;39:99–115.
64. Plessinger V, Jolly P. Rasmussen's aneurysms and fatal hemorrhage in pulmonary tuberculosis. *Am Rev Tuberc* 1949;60:589–603.
65. Muthuswamy PP, Akbik F, Franklin C, Spigos D, Barker WL. Management of major or massive hemoptysis in active pulmonary tuberculosis by bronchial arterial embolization. *Chest* 1987;92:77–82.
66. Khan MA, Kovnat DM, Bachus B, Whitcomb M, Brody JS, Snider GL. Clinical and roentgenographic spectrum of pulmonary tuberculosis in the adult. *Am J Med* 1977;62:31–38.
67. Miller WT, MacGregor RR. Tuberculosis: frequency of unusual radiographic findings. *Am J Roentgenol* 1978; 130:867–875.
68. Farman D, Speir WA Jr. Initial roentgenographic manifestations of bacteriologically proven *M. tuberculosis.* Typical or atypical? *Chest* 1986;89:75–77.

7

Extrapulmonary Tuberculosis in Adults

Tuberculosis has been classically regarded as a pulmonary disorder. In fact, the Greek designation, *phthisis,* or the Western term, consumption, referred essentially to the destructive disease of the lungs. Läennec was the first to clearly and explicitly recognize the common etiology of the diverse forms of tuberculosis, including a multiplicity of sites outside the thorax (see Chapter 1). For various reasons, extrapulmonary tuberculosis (XPTB) has come to constitute a progressively more significant share of the total morbidity from tuberculosis during the 20th century. Furthermore, given the striking propensity for tuberculous involvement of organs other than the lungs among those with HIV infection or AIDS, XPTB presumably will represent an even greater portion of this picture in the future. Because the clinical manifestations of tuberculosis in HIV-infected/AIDS patients are often significantly different from those among other persons, this topic, including extrapulmonary manifestations, is dealt with in Chapter 8. Extrapulmonary disease is also a major portion of tuberculosis among infants and children; this topic is covered in Chapter 9.

The diagnostic consideration of XPTB comes into play in two fairly unique settings: individuals with fever of unknown origin and patients with biopsy demonstration of granulomatous inflammation in an organ or other infected site. The differential diagnosis in either of these settings is extensive and has been well discussed in recent reviews (1–3).

PATHOGENESIS OF EXTRAPULMONARY TUBERCULOSIS

During an individual's initial encounter with the tubercle bacillus, the primary infection, there typically occurs a bacillemia during which mycobacteria are deposited in widely scattered sites throughout the body (see Chapter 4 for details of transmission and pathogenesis). However, with the evolution of an effective host response—protective cellular immunity—these local sites typically undergo involution. Although protective, the host response is often insufficient to sterilize these foci. Therefore, small numbers of viable bacilli remain in these tissues, controlled by a consortium of macrophages and T lymphocytes. The sites most commonly involved in XPTB typically have a rich arterial blood supply that, it has been believed, favors infection by both facilitating bacillary delivery and maintaining a high local oxygen tension, which enhances mycobacterial growth. Recent evidence, however, suggests a different role of the oxygen-rich environment: macrophages are significantly impaired in their ability to inhibit intracellular proliferation of tubercle bacilli in the presence of high oxygen tension (4).

Most forms of XPTB among infants, children, and adolescents represent recent infection with rapid progression to overt disease. Among older persons, except those with AIDS, most cases of XPTB represent late reactivation, remote in time from the primary infection.

EPIDEMIOLOGY AND PERTINENT VARIABLES

Extrapulmonary disease has gradually but steadily risen as a percentage of the total tuberculosis morbidity in the United States from 1963 to the present. This rising proportion reflects the fact that during the 1960s and 1970s the absolute number of pulmonary cases had fallen while the

TABLE 7.1. *Extrapulmonary TB cases in the United States (1975, 1980, 1985, and 1990)*

	Cases (*n*)	XPTB (*n*)	XPTB (%)	Pleural (%)	Lymph (%)	B/J (%)	GU (%)	Miliary (%)
1975	33,989	4,589	13.5%	23%	22%	9.5%	15.5%	9%
1980	27,749	3,947	14.2%	23%	26%	8.4%	15.5%	9%
1985	22,201	3,757	16.9%	23%	30%	10.3%	11.7%	8%
1990	25,701	4,600	17.9%	24%	30%	10.2%	8.7%	7.8%

Data from Centers for Disease Control. *Tuberculosis statistics in the United States (1990).* Atlanta: US Department of Health and Human Services, 1992. Over the 15-year period, the proportion of morbidity at extrapulmonary sites slowly rose. Mostly notably, the greatest increase was in lymphatic disease, which is the most frequent sign in HIV-infected persons and in women from Asia or India. The greatest reduction occurred in genitourinary disease, a condition most common in elderly whites. B/J, bone–joint; GU, genitourinary; XP, extrapulmonary.

number of XPTB cases reported remained remarkably constant. The causes for this changing pattern are not clearly defined. However, a 1990 analysis from the Centers for Disease Control (CDC) suggested that broad changes in the demographic profile of tuberculosis during this period played the dominant role in the altered epidemiology (5). Data from 1975, 1980, 1985, and 1990 in Table 7.1 demonstrate a modest rise in the percentage of XPTB cases over this 15-year period, presumably reflecting shifts in race and age. As tuberculosis has receded among Caucasian Americans, a greater portion of the morbidity has occurred among racial and ethnic minorities, including recent immigrants, who are, on average, younger than recent Caucasian tuberculosis patients. Similar findings were noted in a recent review from Alberta, Canada (6); from 1990 to 1994, 351 cases of tuberculosis were seen in this region. Remarkably, 46% of patients had XPTB. Lymph node disease was most common, particularly among young Asians. HIV infection/AIDS undoubtedly contributed to the rising numbers of XPTB cases seen in 1985 to 1990, although fewer than 2% of the cases in the Canadian series were HIV infected.

Age

Age tends to influence the overall risk for XPTB in a manner analogous to its impact on pulmonary tuberculosis: high vulnerability from infancy to roughly age 5, a period of significantly less risk from age 5 through puberty, a rapid upturn in risk through the teenage and early child-bearing years, a plateau extending approximately from age 35 to 65, then a progressively heightened risk in the seventh decade and beyond. Data from a 1979 CDC review of XPTB (Fig. 7.1) indicate that there were occasional deviations from that pattern among the diverse forms of XPTB in the United States from 1969 to 1973. Notable in this survey were the propensity of the age group 0 to 4 years for meningeal disease and of those 65 years and older for disseminated disease (7).

Another CDC review of XPTB in the United States reported data for the year 1986 (5). These findings deviated modestly from the earlier study, probably reflecting both demographic shifts and the influence of HIV infection. Patients in the age group 0 to 14 years had the highest proportion of XPTB among their total tuberculosis morbidity: 25.2% of all cases involved sites outside the lungs versus 17.5% for the entire population. This pattern always has been typical for this age range because, for unknown reasons, classic pulmonary disease is relatively uncommon in this group. The relative proclivity for XPTB of both the 25–34 and 35–44 years age groups (21.3% and 19.7% versus the national proportion of 17.5%) suggests the influence of HIV infection. The impact of age on the specific forms of XPTB is discussed below.

Sex

Gender patterns for XPTB differ substantially from that of pulmonary disease. In the 1969–1973 survey noted above, women comprised 45% of the total XPTB cases versus only 33.4%

of the pulmonary cases. In terms of incidence, the male and female annual rates of pulmonary disease were 20.6 and 9.8, a ratio of 2.1:1, whereas for XPTB the rates were 2.4 and 1.9, a ratio of only 1.3:1. In 1986, XPTB comprised 21.8% of all tuberculosis in women but only 15.2% in men; this was a statistically significant difference. The influence of sex on the individual forms of XPTB is reviewed below. Overall, there is a striking and consistent relative propensity for women with tuberculosis to manifest their infections at an extrapulmonary site. The causes of this phenomenon are unknown.

Race and Ethnicity

These factors also have substantial influence on the epidemiology of XPTB. In the 1969–1973 CDC survey noted above (7), both pulmonary and extrapulmonary tuberculosis were substantially more prevalent among blacks and others than whites. While the majority of cases of both forms of tuberculosis still occurred among whites, the incidence was much higher among minorities. Comparing the incidence rates for the various forms of tuberculosis among blacks and whites in this era, the relative risk for XPTB among blacks was considerably greater than for pulmonary tuberculosis. The proportion of XPTB among Amerinds (25.2%) and blacks (18.9%) was higher than other groups, including whites (16.1%). The explanation for this disparity is not clear. To some extent, it presumably reflects the fact that tuberculosis among minorities occurs at a significantly younger age than among whites in America and that children and adolescents are more likely to have XPTB. However, as the CDC survey for 1986 indicates, even after adjustments for age, XPTB is still more likely in black, Asian, and Native American patients (5). The influence of race/ethnicity on particular forms of XPTB is reviewed subsequently.

Country of Origin

Nativity also influenced the probability of XPTB. In the 1986 CDC survey, foreign-born persons experienced 19.7% of their tuberculosis disease at extrapulmonary sites versus 16.9% of U.S.-born cases, a statistically significant difference (5). Perhaps the most striking aspect of

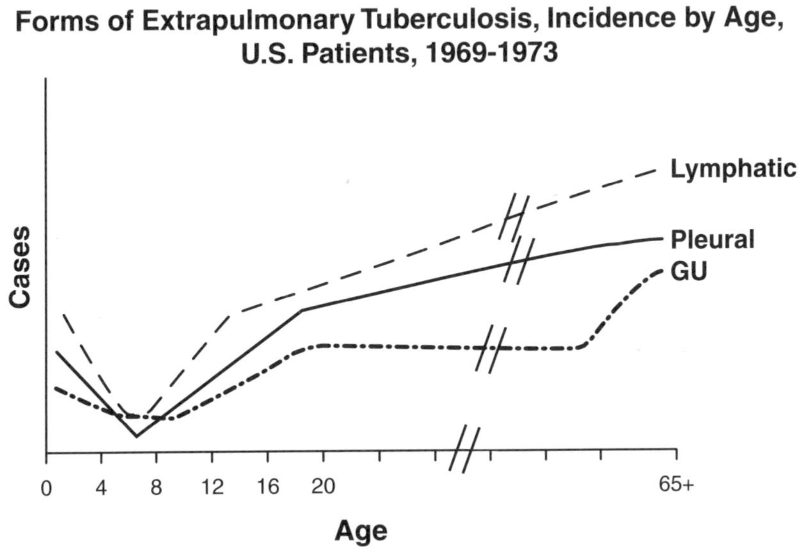

FIG. 7.1. During this 5-year period, the CDC carefully tracked XPTB in the United States. As with pulmonary disease, infants and children aged 0–4 were quite vulnerable. Children of primary school age, 5 to 10 years, were relatively protected. With puberty and adolescence, case rates rose substantially. Most forms of XPTB rose considerably at ages 65 and above; GU disease was particularly prominent in the older age groups. From Farer et al. (7).

XPTB in the foreign-born and minorities is the disproportional number of cases of cervical lymphadenitis among women from Asia and the Indian subcontinent. This pattern was clearly apparent in the Canadian series cited above (6).

GENERAL MANIFESTATIONS OF XPTB

Proteus was a sea god of Greek mythology who was said to be capable of assuming many forms; hence, things that have a varied nature or great diversity are said to be protean. This term is used frequently in reference to XPTB with good reason: the tubercle bacillus causes disease in a wide array of human organs or tissues, and, within these organs or tissues, the resulting disorders have many forms.

In reviewing the signs and symptoms that are associated with XPTB, it is important to stress that a majority of such patients have only subtle or minimal constitutional manifestations. Among a series of patients from Los Angeles reported in 1977, only 34% reported feverishness, 15% weight loss, and 8% chills or sweats (8). In another series of patients from Connecticut with XPTB reported in 1985, 34% reported malaise, 31% fever, 31% weight loss, and 26% fatigue (9).

The tuberculin skin test is a potentially useful diagnostic aid in XPTB. However, a modest but clinically meaningful number of persons with active disease will not have a significant reaction to the 5-tuberculin-unit (intermediate strength) skin test with PPD-T. In the California series above, 21% of the patients' tuberculin reactions were less than 10 mm (8); among the Connecticut patients, 9% of the patients tested had negative results (9). For patients with XPTB who have coexisting immunosuppressive conditions (HIV infection, renal failure, organ transplantation, etc.), the probability of a false-negative tuberculin test will be substantially increased (see Chapter 8).

Simultaneous pulmonary tuberculosis is a highly valuable diagnostic clue for XPTB. However, this coincidence is relatively uncommon. Aside from patients with miliary disease (in whom lung disease is an inherent part of the disorder), active pulmonary disease is found in a distinct minority of cases. Among the California patients, 12 of 62 (19%) were found to have positive sputum cultures (8); in the Connecticut series, 7 of 38 (18%) had positive sputum cultures (9). In the 1969–1973 CDC survey, 1,423 of 7,891 (18%) of cases with extrapulmonary disease had active pulmonary disease (7). In the 1997 CDC report, 1,410 of 4,964 (28%) XPTB patients had coexisting pulmonary disease (Fig. 7.2). The criteria for activity were not stipulated in these CDC reports, and it is difficult to ascertain why the proportion of cases with simultaneously active pulmonary disease has recently risen, although HIV infection and the demographic shifts noted above may contribute.

SPECIFIC ORGAN INVOLVEMENT IN XPTB

In the 1969–1973 CDC survey of XPTB, detailed information was provided on the relative frequency of organ involvement (7). The data were broken down to provide information on the relationship of race/ethnicity, sex, and age to the specific forms of XPTB. Table 7.2 compares the frequencies of the more common forms according to race. Notable among these data are the apparent vulnerability of blacks to disseminated disease and of others, mostly Asians, to lymph node tuberculosis.

The relationship of sex to the various forms of XPTB in the 1969–1973 survey demonstrated a modest male preponderance for all forms except abdominal, in which the frequencies were equal, and lymphatic tuberculosis, for which there was a 5:3 female preponderance.

There were distinct differences in the age distribution for various forms of XPTB in this 1969–1973 CDC analysis. As seen in Fig. 7.1, most of the isolated meningeal disease occurred in ages 0–4; the greatest share of the disseminated disease occurred in those 65 and older; and genitourinary was most prevalent in those 35 and older. Striking is the extraordinarily low incidence of all forms of XPTB in the 5- to 14-year-old age group. Long recognized as the favored age of childhood, there is no clear understanding for this transient period of apparently heightened resistance to tuberculosis. Similarly low rates of pulmonary disease are seen in this age range, as well.

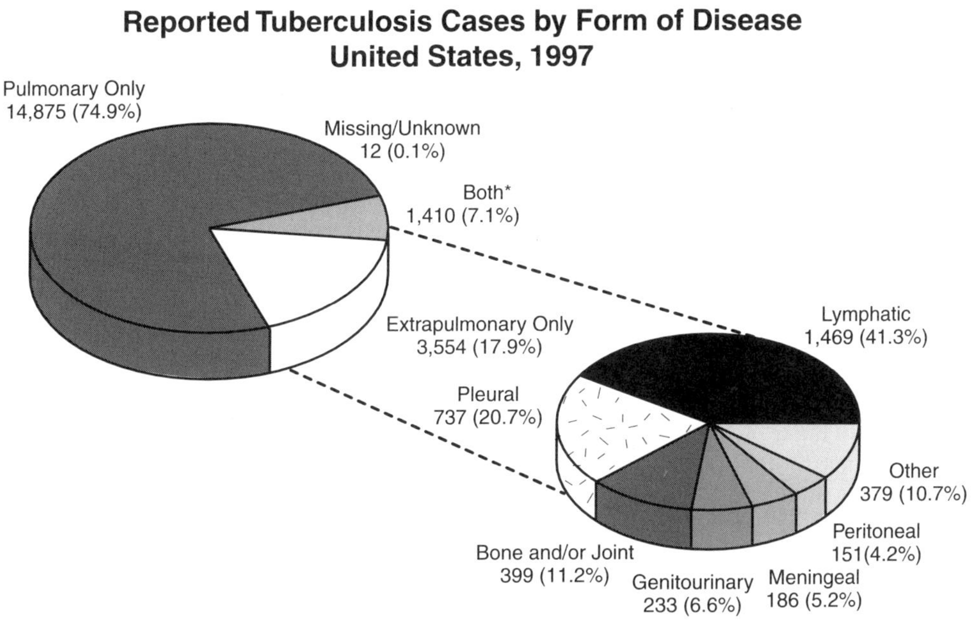

FIG. 7.2. The CDC reported that 4,964 cases of XPTB occurred in the United States in 1997. 3,554 patients whose sole disease site was outside the lungs constituted 17.9% of the total tuberculosis case load. Another 1,410 patients had simultaneous disease in the lungs and at extrapulmonary sites, 7.1% of the total morbidity (369 of these patients had miliary disease).

Comparing the CDC data from 1969-1973 with those from 1986 (5) demonstrates modest but interesting shifts in profile of XPTB in the United States. The relative proportions of the various forms of XPTB are contrasted in Table 7.3. Although the factors involved with the shifting patterns cannot be easily ascertained, several hypotheses could be considered. Changing ages of the XPTB population could alter the disease site profile; as noted in Fig. 7.1, organ involvement is clearly related to age. However, there was only a minor downward shift in the median ages of the XPTB cases from 1969–1973 (ap-

TABLE 7.2. *Various forms of extrapulmonary TB and race, United States, 1969–1973*

	Overall (%)	White (%)	Black (%)	Other (%)
Pleural	26.5	23.7	30.0	18.3
Lymphatic	21.3	20.0	18.5	38.9
Genitourinary	17.9	22.0	10.3	17.9
Disseminated	10.6	9.8	15.5	6.9
Bone–joint	8.8	9.1	9.2	4.6
CNS	4.7	4.9	5.2	3.1
Abdominal	3.8	2.4	5.6	4.7

Of all of the XPTB seen among these racial/ethnic groups, differential percentages of disease were seen at these various sites. In this era, pleural involvement was more common than lymphatic (contrast with Table 7.1). Of particular interest, black Americans consistently manifested a higher proportion of their extrapulmonary tuberculosis as disseminated disease than did whites, Hispanics, or others. CNS, central nervous system.

TABLE 7.3. *Comparison of the proportion of common forms of XPTB, 1969–1973 versus 1990 and 1997*

	1969–1973	1990	1997
Pleural	26.5%	24%	20.7%
Lymphatic	21.3%	30%	41.3%
Genitourinary	17.9%	8.75%	6.6%
Miliary	10.6%	7.8%	7.4%
Bone—joint	8.8%	10.2%	11.2%
CNS	4.7%	6.1%	5.2%
Abdominal	3.8%	3.4%	4.2%

Over this 28-year period of time, lymphatic disease has risen substantially, presumably in large measure because of the influence of HIV. Reductions have been most pronounced in genitourinary and pleural disease. CNS, central nervous system.

proximately 43 years) to that of the XPTB cases in 1986 (approximately 42 years). Gender differences in the two populations are likely not significant because the overall ratios of male to female patients in these two studies were also remarkably similar: 55 to 45 in the earlier study, 56 to 44 in the latter. In terms of race and ethnicity, comparison of these two studies reveals the following: in the 1969–1973 survey, 45% of the XPTB cases occurred in non-Hispanic whites, whereas in the 1986 report, only 29.8% of the cases were in whites. Thus, I infer that the changing profile of XPTB in the United States is associated with the evolving demographic mixture, augmented by the impact of HIV infection/AIDS. Certainly, the rise in the proportion of lymphatic XPTB is very suggestive of the influence of HIV. But because of the absence of systematic HIV serology data for tuberculosis patients, this putative association remains uncertain.

Rieder, Snider and Cauthen's analysis of XPTB in the United States in 1986 employed an innovative method for calculating the relative propensities for XPTB to occur among the many demographic groupings studied (5). Using a computer program, they were able to estimate adjusted proportions among various age, race/ethnicity, sex, and country-of-origin groups. These data were displayed in graphic form for seven common forms of XPTB with the others lumped into one group. Because it was such a unique means of analyzing the data, I have included the entire description of their methodology:

> In 1986, 22,764 patients with tuberculosis with known major site of disease were reported to the Centers for Disease Control, of which 3,991 (17.5%) had an extrapulmonary site reported as the major site. After exclusion of 262 patients with incomplete information, 22,506 (98.9%) with known age, race/ethnicity, sex, and country of birth were available for analysis. Patients were divided by major site of disease into pulmonary and eight extrapulmonary categories: lymphatic, pleural, genitourinary, bone and joint, miliary, meningeal, and all other forms combined. Patients were also stratified by age, race/ethnicity, sex, and country of origin. For each of these demographic characteristics, the stratum with the most cases of pulmonary tuberculosis was arbitrarily chosen as the reference stratum for comparing disease site distributions in terms of relative odds. For example, among female patients, 6,119 sites were pulmonary, and 174 were bone and joint as the major site of disease; among male patients, 12,445 sites were pulmonary and 211 were bone and joint. Thus, the observed odds of bone and joint to pulmonary cases was 174/6,119 among female and 211/12,445 among male patients. If male patients are used as the reference category, the observed relative odds were thus (174/6,119)/(211/12,445) = 1.68 among female patients relative to male patients and (211/12,445)/(211/12,445) = 1 among male patients relative to male patients by definition. This can be interpreted as showing that female patients with tuberculosis are 1.68 times more likely to have bone and joint tuberculosis than are male patients.
>
> To isolate the effect of the variable of interest, the observed relative odds were adjusted (adjusted relative odds, ARO) to control for the effects of other variables. For example, foreign-born patients with tuberculosis do not have the same age, race/ethnicity, and sex characteristics as do U.S.-born patients; therefore, adjustment for differences in age, race/ethnicity, and sex is necessary to artificially make U.S.-born and foreign-born patients comparable with regard to age, race/ethnicity, and sex in order to isolate the effect of being foreign born. Adjusted relative odds were estimated by the maximal likelihood method in a log-linear categorical model of the proportions with disease at each site (7,8). Significance tests and 95% confidence intervals were also derived from the model. (5)

Because of the unique quantitative perspective that this system allows, these graphic analyses are displayed in Fig. 7.3. It is important to emphasize that the adjusted relative odds do *not* indicate the percentage of the total XPTB mor-

FIG. 7.3. Extrapulmonary TB in the United States: demographic variables according to form of the disease. Workers from the CDC analyzed these demographic variables among patients previously presenting with these forms of XPTB in 1986. The likelihood of individuals to have such disease was expressed as adjusted relative odds (ARO); please see text for derivation of these data. **A,** Lymphatic (1,219 cases); **B,** pleural (905); **C,** genitourinary (469); **D,** bone/joint (385); **E,** miliary (289); **F,** meningeal (183); **G,** peritoneal (132); **H,** all other forms combined (360). From Rieder et al. (5).

Extrapulmonary Tuberculosis In The United States; Demographic Variables According To Form Of Disease

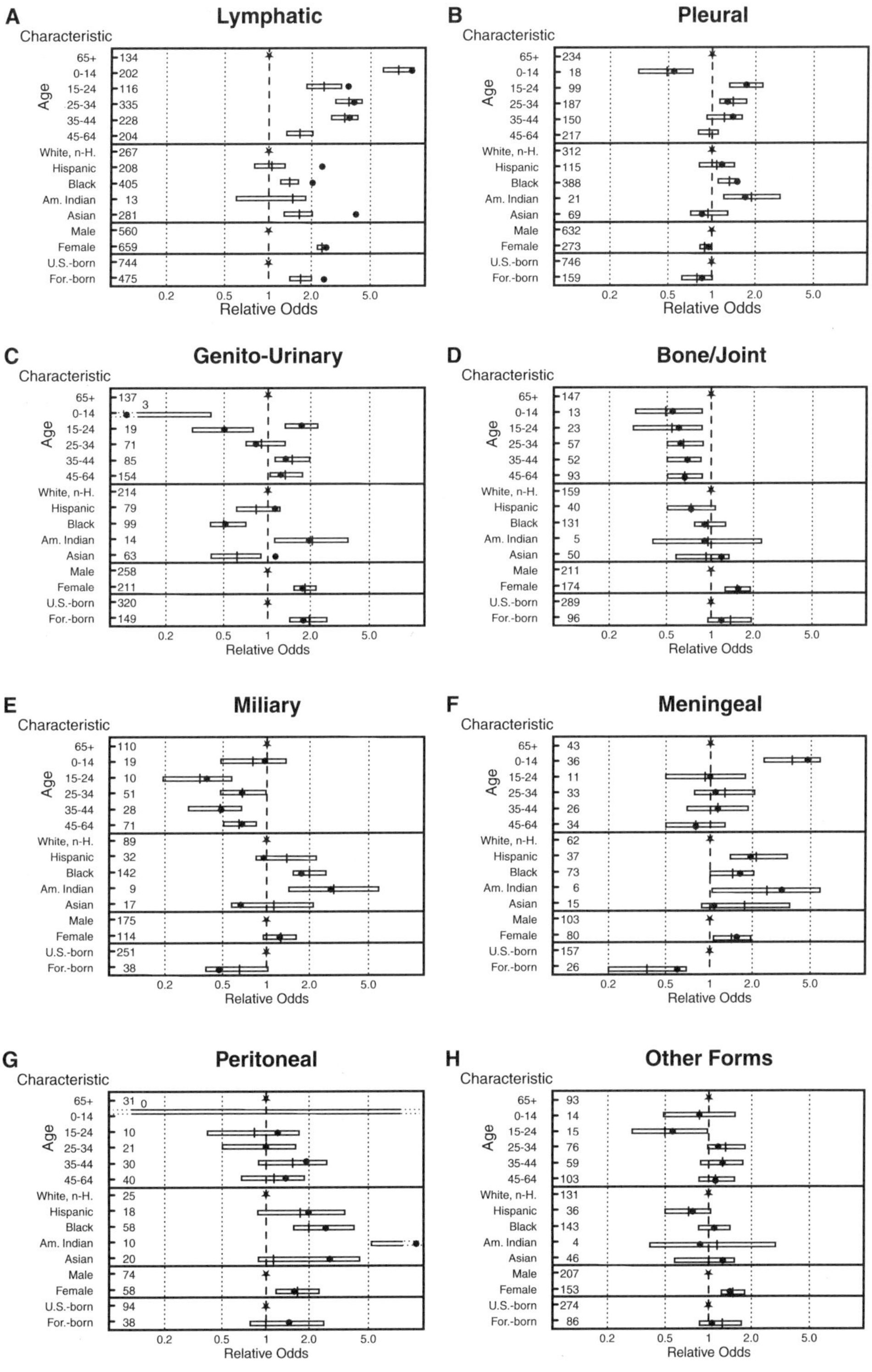

bidity constituted within that demographic grouping but rather the impact that particular variable has on the probability of a certain form of XPTB occurring in persons within that group.

LYMPHATIC TUBERCULOSIS

Known historically as "scrofula" or "the King's evil" (for the alleged power of European regents to cure by touch), tuberculous involvement of the superficial lymphatics, especially those of the neck, has plagued mankind throughout recorded history (10). No doubt many of the cases in the past were caused by *M. bovis* or by other mycobacteria such as *M. avium, M. intracellulare,* or *M. scrofulaceum.* However, this section focuses exclusively on disease caused by *M. tuberculosis.*

Epidemiologically, the adjusted relative odds patterns of lymph node tuberculosis in the United States in 1986 are displayed in Fig. 7.3. The adjusted relative odds (ARO) indicate that lymphatic tuberculosis was strongly associated with female sex (ARO 2.2), foreign birth (ARO 1.7), and Asian/Pacific Island nationality. Although the adjusted relative odds for lymphatic tuberculosis associate this disorder with ages 14 or younger, it is important to reiterate that the greatest number of cases of lymph node disease from *M. tuberculosis* are seen in patients ages 25 to 64. The high ARO for younger persons merely means that, for patients in this age range, lymphatic disease constitutes a large proportion of their tuberculous morbidity.

Clinically, tuberculous lymphadenitis is most often found in the head and neck region. The posterior cervical and supraclavicular chains are the sites most commonly involved; less frequently diseased are the submandibular or preauricular nodes. Tuberculous lymphadenitis involving the axillary or inguinal nodes is rare, probably fewer than 10% of cases. Regarding the localization, Yew and Lee analyzed a series of 111 patients from Taiwan with lymphadenitis of the cervical region and offered an interesting hypothesis (11). Anatomically, they observed 45% on the right, 28% on the left, and 27% with bilateral disease; 78% had multiple nodes, and 22% had solitary nodes. Of these patients, 41% were found to have simultaneously active pulmonary tuberculosis. Based on the relationship between the location of the lymphadenitis and the pulmonary foci, they conjectured that many of their cervical sites were seeded by lymphatic drainage from the right lung and left lower lobe, not the oropharynx. In support of this, they noted that the majority of the tuberculous lymph nodes were found in the supraclavicular fossa, lower anterior cervical chain, or posterior triangle of the neck, chains known to be contiguous with intrathoracic lymphatics. This distribution should be contrasted with the nodes typically involved with nontuberculous lymphadenitis; in these cases, believed to usually represent invasion via the oropharynx by environmental mycobacteria, preauricular and submandibular nodes are more commonly involved (12). Although this pulmonary–cephalad pathway may explain a large portion of tuberculous lymphadenitis, involvement of other nodes by *M. tuberculosis* must entail different mechanisms (12,13). Presently, a highly virulent form of disseminated lymphatic tuberculosis is being seen in patients with AIDS; this entity is reviewed in Chapter 8.

Mediastinal, peribronchial, and paratracheal lymph node tuberculosis is most often seen in the United States as part of primary disease in children or disseminated disease in immunocompromised hosts; they are described in Chapters 9 and 8, respectively. Clinically and radiographically apparent disease caused by mediastinal tuberculous lymphadenitis among HIV-negative Caucasian adults is rare; however, this entity is not uncommon among persons of color (14–18). To the extent that such adenopathy compresses and invades the large airways, it is discussed in Chapter 6 under "Endobronchial Tuberculosis".

The typical scenario for superficial nodal disease is gradual, painless enlargement over several weeks to months. Initially, the overlying skin is not inflamed, but with the passage of time the epidermis may become shiny, pink to red, and faintly tender and warm to touch. Eventually, if left untreated, the skin may be breached and a fistula formed that discharges matter that ranges in nature from serous to purulent, caseous debris. Usually, an isolated lymphatic chain is involved, although in a minority of cases bilateral disease or simultaneous involvement of adjacent, ipsilateral chains occurs (11,19). Physical examination findings vary according to the acuity or chronicity of the process. Early peripheral tuberculous adenopathy is usually firm, discrete, and mobile. As the infection progresses, the chronic inflammation results in matting of the adjacent nodes as well as adherence to subcutaneous tissues, reducing mobility. In the more advanced stages, multiple nodes in a chain may be involved, and, as caseation occurs, the nodes may soften; sinus tracts may form with long-standing disease.

Among patients with active disease that is limited to a single regional chain, constitutional symptoms such as fever, chills, sweats, weight loss, or malaise are rare and should, in fact, suggest the possibility of a more extensive form of tuberculosis or a coexisting disease. Among the exotic disorders that should be included in the differential diagnosis are Kichuchi's disease, or necrotizing, histiocytic lymphadenitis, a disorder found most often in young Asian girls (20); Castleman's disease, a complex disorder associated with mediastinal and peripheral lymphadenopathy, highly variable clinical features, and a propensity for appearing in *New England Journal of Medicine* Clinico-Pathological Conferences (21); Kimura's disease, a chronic inflammatory disorder of unknown etiology, endemic in Asia, most common among young to middle-aged adults, male predominant, marked by adenopathy or tumor-like skin nodules, and associated frequently with elevated IgE and eosinophilia (22); and *Corynebacterium pseudotuberculosis* lymphadenitis, a zoonosis reported among Australian sheepherders (23).

Diagnosis is made absolutely only by culture identification of the microbe. Other valuable components of the diagnostic process include epidemiological features, chest x-rays, and skin testing. Of note, false-negative tuberculin skin tests are quite rare among HIV-negative patients with tuberculous lymphadenitis (see below).

Epidemiology

As noted, there is a high-risk profile that should suggest the probability of tuberculosis. The great majority of children with lymph node tuberculosis have a history of exposure to a person with pulmonary tuberculosis, and many have radiographic residuals of the primary infection (see below). The major confounding disorder today is lymphadenitis from mycobacteria other than tuberculosis, which shares many of the clinical manifestations with disease caused by *M. tuberculosis.* Distinction between these etiologic agents is aided by epidemiological consideration. A survey in Massachusetts reported in 1984 demonstrated an age-related trend among patients with mycobacterial disease of the nodes (24). Among persons older than 12 years, 147 of 154 (95%) cultures yielded *M. tuberculosis;* thus, an individual in this age range with granulomatous lymph node disease, especially with caseation and/or microscopically demonstrated acid-fast bacilli, even without cultural confirmation, should be presumed to have tuberculosis, particularly if epidemiological risk factors and the tuberculin skin test are positive. By contrast, among those 12 years or younger, the obverse was seen: only 5 of 60 (8%) cultures yielded *M. tuberculosis,* the remainder being positive for *M. avium-intracellulare* (75%) or *M. scrofulaceum* (17%). A similar relationship between age and etiologic agent was found in a review of mycobacterial adenitis in Australia: for children 6 years or younger, tuberculosis caused only 4% of the disease, whereas in those patients 15 years and older, tuberculosis was responsible for 89% of the cases (25). However, it is not acceptable to assume, based on this probability, that a child with mycobacterial adenitis is infected with MOTT. Although the likelihood of MOTT disease is greater, the implications of not treating a child with tuberculosis are potentially so profound that extra diagnostic steps should be taken, including repeat biopsy if lymphadenitis persists (12).

Although the patient's age is an imperfect tool to distinguish between tuberculosis and NTM etiology, it may be used well in the following situation. In any immunocompetent adult with biopsy evidence of granulomatous inflammation of a lymph node and stain-demonstrated mycobacteria, there is an immensely greater likelihood that the etiologic agent is *M. tuberculosis.*

The Tuberculin Skin Test

The skin test may be falsely negative in up to 20–25% of normal hosts with pulmonary tuberculosis, but the probability of negative tests in persons with localized tuberculous adenitis is less than 10% (13,26,27). Thus, a positive skin test may be seen to support the diagnosis and a negative test to substantially reduce the likelihood of tuberculosis. Formerly, dual skin testing with antigens from the other mycobacteria and *M. tuberculosis* sensitive (PPD-S or PPD-T) was believed useful in distinguishing the etiological agent in childhood lymphadenitis (28). But, because of their inability to meet FDA standards for skin test products, the NTM antigens are no longer available in the United States for intradermal testing. Recent experience in Australia comparing responses to *M. tuberculosis* antigens with those to *M. avium* complex antigens indicated poor specificity and sensitivity with the technique (25). However, another recent report suggested that dual testing with PPD-T and a different *M. avium* sensitin have substantial power to discriminate (29).

The Chest X-Ray

Both to exclude intrathoracic disease and to support a diagnosis of tuberculosis, a chest radiograph should be obtained for all persons with proven or suspected tuberculous lymphadenitis. In cases where the diagnosis remains in doubt (a compatible biopsy but a negative culture), findings on the chest film suggestive of active or healed tuberculosis would be supportive evidence for tuberculous etiology.

Biopsy and Culture

The preferred method for diagnosis is biopsy of the involved node. An excisional biopsy is greatly preferred over incisional because of the risk of poor healing with fistula formation from the latter technique. In addition to histological study of the solid portion of the node, substantial portions of the caseous debris, pus, or involved tissue should be sent for culture.

The histopathologic findings in tuberculosis of the lymph nodes are quite diverse and due to their similarity to disease due to mycobacteria other than tuberculosis are rarely considered diagnostic. However, a recent report from England indicated that careful scrutiny of the histopathology of cervical lymph nodes could distinguish adenitis caused by *M. tuberculosis* from that due to other mycobacteria (30). Irregularities of the granulomata and variations in the distribution of polymorphonuclear leukocytes were cited as distinguishing features. But, until this system is proven reliable in other centers, it should be employed with caution. Mycobacteria cannot be found in most specimens that are ultimately proven to be tuberculous in etiology.

Optimal yield from culture efforts entails sending as much inflammatory matter or tissue as feasible, avoiding dehydration of the specimen by immersion in small volumes of normal saline or liquid culture medium, and cultivation in liquid medium such as the Bactec system.

Alternative Diagnostic Methods

A diverse array of methods have been studied to aid with the diagnosis of tuberculosis. Techniques specific for local disease include polymerase chain reaction tests of the tissue to identify tubercle bacilli; see Chapter 2 for a detailed review. Preliminary results look promising although this methodology is not ready for general clinical use. Tests not specific for lymph node disease but generic for tuberculosis infection include serological testing or detection of antigen–antibody complexes. Unfortunately, these techniques have not been known to have sufficient sensitivity or specificity to be of real utility; see Chapter 2.

Management

Chemotherapy is the keystone to treatment. In cases of proven or strongly suspected tuberculous lymphadenitis, medication should be initiated promptly. Current recommendations of the American Thoracic Society (31) and the British Thoracic Society (32) call for use of the usual short-course chemotherapy regimens for patients with lymph node tuberculosis. Details of regimens, dosage, duration, toxicity, and monitoring are discussed in Chapter 10.

Notable, though, among patients with tuberculous lymphadenitis is the potential for delayed or suboptimal response to chemotherapy. Although the disease is a paucibacillary form of tuberculosis, a small proportion of the patients may experience continued local inflammatory activity several months into therapy. This may take the form of the appearance of freshly involved nodes, enlargement of the initially inflamed nodes, and/or the development of sinus tracts at or away from the biopsy site. The peculiar tendency of this to occur with lymphatic disease was highlighted in a 1971 report wherein 5 of 15 patients with cervical lymphadenitis failed to respond to therapy (33). Although the medical therapy in these patients (isoniazid, PAS, and short courses of streptomycin) was not very potent by modern standards, the refractoriness of the lymphatic disease was highlighted by clinical improvement in other involved organ systems but the nodal disease was paradoxically worsening in 3 of the 5 cases. Among a series of 108 patients from the United Kingdom, fresh nodes appeared during treatment in 12%, existing nodes enlarged in 13%, fluctuation developed in 11%, and drainage or sinus tracts appeared in 7%; excisional surgery or aspiration was performed in 19% after commencing drug treatment (34). A modern series of 45 cases of presumed tuberculous lymphadenitis from India also indicated a suboptimal response to a regimen of isoniazid, rifampin, and ethambutol (35). Only 68.8% of the patients had resolution after 9 months of therapy; drug treatment had to be extended in 14 cases and 5 of the poor responders eventually underwent surgical drainage and excision. Among 48 patients from Taiwan with tuberculous lymphadenitis, 10% developed new or enlarging nodes while on therapy, and 10% had residual adenopathy after 9 months of chemotherapy (19). Although there were not ideal culture and susceptibility data to exclude drug-resistant tuberculosis or NTM infection and adherence with therapy was not assured, these studies, as well as a report from Arkansas (36), indicate that some portion of patients with tuberculous adenitis will follow a complicated course during treatment. Explanations for this sometimes anomalous response are wanting. Possible elements include infection with NTM (which are naturally more drug resistant), undetected drug-resistant *M. tuberculosis,* poor drug penetration into the lymph nodes, unfavorable local milieu, or exaggerated delayed hypersensitivity reactions as disrupted mycobacterial antigens are released during treatment.

In most cases, response to therapy should be acceptable. However, close clinical monitoring is indicated. Careful attention should be paid to the location, nature, and size of involved nodes at the inception of treatment to document response objectively. Scrupulous efforts should be made to culture the etiological agent and, if it is *M. tuberculosis,* to obtain prompt susceptibility testing. If there is worsening after 8 weeks of treatment, consideration for *en bloc* resection of the involved chain is appropriate. If the nodes are located in a cosmetically sensitive area, the relative acceptability of a surgical scar versus possible sinus tract scarring should be weighed. Although some have suggested systemic steroids to reduce inflammation during the early phase of drug therapy for lymphatic tuberculosis in cosmetically sensitive areas, the safety and utility of this approach are unproven, and this treatment should be viewed cautiously.

Pleural Tuberculosis

Inflammation of the pleural space has classically been associated with the primary pulmonary tuberculosis infection. Unlike other forms of XPTB, wherein an organ is thought to be seeded during the primary-phase bacillemia, traditional wisdom holds that the pleural process results from contiguous spread of the pulmonary inflammation across the visceral pleura as delayed-type hypersensitivity evolves (37,38). Although this mechanism is surely valid in some cases and was formerly associated with the great preponderance of tuberculous pleurisy, the current epidemiology of pleural tuberculosis suggests that other pathogenetic mechanisms are operating in a large proportion of cases. Specifically, among older patients who experience pleural disease in association with reactivation-type pulmonary tuberculosis, one must suspect actual spread of infection into the pleural space rather than simply invoking an evolving immunological reaction to tuberculous antigens as in the primary infection model. A severe form of the direct spread of infection occurs when a subpleural lesion actually ruptures into the pleural space, resulting in a pneumothorax complicated by tuberculous empyema. An unusual variant of this latter pattern is the consequence of remote pneumothorax collapse therapy (see Chapter 1). In addition to these pathways of pleural tuberculosis, tuberculosis-induced pleural effusions may occur in association with osseous tuberculosis of the ribs or vertebrae that abut the pleural surfaces, with miliary/disseminated tuberculosis or with peritoneal tuberculosis that invades the thorax through diaphragmatic fenestrations. For the purposes of this chapter, the following forms of pleural tuberculosis are considered:

- Pleuritis/effusion complicating primary pulmonary tuberculosis
- Pleuritis/effusion complicating reactivation-type pulmonary tuberculosis
- Effusion associated with extrapulmonary tuberculosis
- Chronic empyema associated with pneumothorax

This organization, in addition to considerations of pathogenesis, has important implications for management (see below).

Epidemiologically, pleural tuberculosis has constituted a major portion of the XPTB morbidity in the United States. (Note: in the United Kingdom, pleural disease is traditionally *not* included with XPTB but is counted with pulmonary disease.) As noted above, pleural disease constituted 26.5% of the XPTB in the United States during a 5-year period from 1969 to 1973; by 1997, the pleural component of XPTB had fallen to 20.7%, a 22% reduction (39). In the adjusted relative odds analysis for XPTB in 1986, the most notable findings were the paucity of pleural disease among those 0 to 14 years of age and the relatively great risk for pleural tuberculosis among Amerind/Alaskan native patients.

Clinically, there is a wide array of manifestations of pleural tuberculosis. A recent report contrasted the presentation of patients with primary ("classic") and reactivation-type tuberculous pleuritis (40). Among these groups, there was a significant difference in the duration of symptoms before diagnosis. The primary cases were considerably more acute, the duration of signs and symptoms ranging from means of 4.7 to 17.5 days compared to 10.1 to 62 days for patients with reactivation disease. However, it should be noted that among the reactivation patients, some had experienced a very abrupt illness. This is consistent with the findings of an earlier series wherein two-thirds of the patients, including a number of older individuals who presumably had reactivation-type pleural involvement, experienced an acute illness mindful of bacterial pneumonia (41). The appearance of symptomatic pleurisy with radiographic evidence of effusion weeks to months into a course of chemotherapy, being given for active pulmonary tuberculosis, is an uncommon event, but it is worthy of note because of the clinical confusion it may engender (42).

The most common related symptoms are cough and chest pain. Typically, the cough is nonproductive unless it is associated with underlying parenchymal tuberculosis. The chest pain typically is pleuritic in character—sharp, stabbing, and associated with respiration. However, some patients experience a duller, less well localized variety of pain. Feverishness is very common; 63% of those in the earlier series noted above exhibiting temperatures in the 100–103°F range, and another 18% in the range of 103.1–104.6°F (41). Dyspnea, chills, sweats, weight loss, and malaise occur more commonly with advanced disease and may reflect underlying parenchymal disease.

Physical examination of patients with uncomplicated pleural tuberculosis typically reveals minimal abnormalities. Friction rubs are found in fewer than 20% of patients. Dullness to percussion and diminished breath sounds are found with larger fluid collections; however, whispered pectoriloquy and egophony are rarely present. Rales and rhonchi are uncommon except in instances of active pulmonary lesions. Digital clubbing is seen only with long-standing—years to decades—disease.

Diagnosis of pleural tuberculosis ideally involves culture of the tubercle bacilli from the site. Supportive elements in establishing the diagnosis include the following. *Epidemiologically,* many persons with pleuritis associated with primary infection come from high-risk social, ethnic, socioeconomic, or employment groups. *Radiographically,* tuberculous pleuritis classically is seen as a unilateral effusion of modest scale. Bilateral tuberculous effusions are quite rare and should suggest disseminated or peritoneal tuberculosis. Typically, the effusion occupies less than a quarter of the volume of the hemithorax (500–1,000 ml), although massive fluid collections are occasionally reported, particularly in persons with AIDS (see Chapter 8). Underlying parenchymal lesions have been identified in 20% to 50% of patients by plain chest radiographs; with more sophisticated modern imaging techniques, such as computed tomography, a greater percentage of patients will have demonstrable pulmonary abnormalities. Certainly, the presence of cavitary or fibronodular parenchymal shadows in the lung region abutting an effusion is strong circumstantial evidence in favor of tuberculous etiology (noteworthy in this regard, pleural effusions rarely occur with pulmonary disease caused by *M. avium* complex, *M. kansasii, M. chelonae,* or other pulmonary mycobacterioses). Early in their development, tuberculous effusions tend to be free flowing; however, with the passage of time, adhesions develop that can trap or loculate the fluid.

As with all forms of tuberculosis, *the tuberculin skin test* is falsely negative in a substantial proportion of patients with pleural disease. In the 1973 series cited above (41), 31% of the patients had a negative tuberculin reaction on initial testing. In the 1989 study comparing primary ("classic") with reactivation-type pleuritis, 12% of the former and 39% of the latter had false-negative skin test results (40). Among 70 patients with tuberculous pleural effusions recently reported, skin testing results were available for 43 cases (43); 40 of the 43 (93%) were reportedly positive. Although the authors concluded that an intermediate-strength skin test was a sensitive test, it is possible that there was a selection bias among the patients reported. I would conclude, rather, that the Mantoux skin test is neither sensitive nor specific for tuberculous pleurisy. A strongly positive reaction increases the probability of a tuberculous etiology, but it is not conclusive. Likewise, a negative test only reduces the probability modestly and does not exclude the diagnosis.

Among patients with undiagnosed pleural effusions who have parenchymal shadows or productive cough, obtaining *sputum for mycobacterial microscopy and culture* is a potentially very useful diagnostic measure. Among patients deemed to have pleuritis in association with reactivation-type tuberculosis, 50% had positive sputum smears, and 63% positive cultures (40). In another series, 88.6% of those with effusions and parenchymal infiltrates had positive sputum cultures (43). For both series cited, patients without pulmonary infiltrates had substantially lower culture yields, 23% and 11.4%, respectively. However, because of its easy availability and complete safety, one would conclude that this study should be performed on all patients with suspected tuberculous pleural disease.

Thoracentesis with pleural fluid analysis should be performed promptly on all patients for whom less invasive measures (particularly sputum for smear) have not yielded a presumptive diagnosis. Although microscopic examination of pleural fluid for mycobacteria is rarely positive, there are other attributes of the fluid that are highly characteristic of tuberculosis (Table 7.4). Although the various patterns of standard pleural fluid tests may be highly suggestive of tuberculosis, many diverse disorders can produce similar abnormalities; a comprehensive review of pleural disorders, including the differential diagnosis of exudative effusions, is available in Sahn's 1988 article (44).

Among the other tests listed in Table 7.4 are a variety of studies that potentially offer greater sensitivity and specificity than the standard tests routinely performed on pleural fluid. The current status of these methods is briefly reviewed below.

The pleural concentration of *adenosine deaminase* (ADA) has enjoyed considerable popularity outside the United States for the diagnosis of tuberculous pleural effusion. The level of ADA has been associated with the population of CD4

TABLE 7.4. *Characteristic findings of tuberculosis pleural effusions*

Appearance	Straw-colored, serous
Cell profile	1,000–6,000 WBCs; 50–90% lymphocytes; rarely >5% eosinophils; few mesothelial cells
Protein	5.0 ± 1 g/dl
pH	Usually in 7.3–7.4 range; occasionally <7.3; never >7.4
Glucose	Typically slightly below the serum concentration; greater disparity with prolonged duration of effusion
LDH	500–1,500 IU/L; increases with prolonged duration
Microscopy	Approximately 10–25% of specimens are positive on smear for mycobacteria
Culture	Positive cultures for mycobacteria found in wide range (roughly 25–75%) in different series; higher yield seen in chronic, reactivation-type disease
Other tests	Adenosine deaminase (ADA) and lysosome concentrations, tuberculostearic acid, cytokines, antibodies, antigen–antibody complexes, and polymerase chain reaction probes (see text)

These ranges are derived from multiple sources and may be seen as broad indicators of the pleural fluid characteristics. Histopathological demonstration of caseating granulomas on biopsy has a strong positive predictive value (see text).

lymphocytes in the pleural space (45); it was assumed to reflect an active cellular immune response. One observer recently questioned whether ADA levels would perform consistently because of the existence of two forms of the enzyme: ADA_1, which he contended was produced via cell necrosis, and ADA_2, which was released from monocyte-macrophages when harboring intracellular parasites (46). This distinction between ADA_1 and ADA_2 levels in parapneumonic and tuberculous effusions was observed by another group (47). Nonetheless, multiple studies have indicated that ADA levels, as measured, performs well in identifying tuberculous effusions (48–53). Among patients with effusions of various etiologies, the ADA sensitivity in these series ranged from 0.69 to 1.0, while the specificity fell between 0.21 to 0.97. The cutoff point to distinguish tuberculous effusions in these series ranged from 45 to 70 IU/L. The greatest number of false-positive results occurred among patients with chronic bacterial empyema. Efforts to enhance the accuracy of the ADA test by adding other markers such as pleural serum lysozyme levels (54), lysozyme and interferon-γ (49), or monoclonal antibodies against a complement complex (53) have not met with success. Thus, ADA appears to have potential utility as a screening test: if the value is very low, it theoretically excludes tuberculosis as the etiology, and if it is very high, it strengthens the case for tuberculosis. However, a report from the Netherlands questioned whether, in a country with a low prevalence of tuberculosis, ADA would perform well in identifying tuberculous effusions (52). In a group of 95 cases, ADA levels were elevated in four of five tuberculosis effusions, four of seven empyemas, and three of seven mesothelioma effusions; notably, it was not increased in neoplastic and various other pleural fluid collections. Unfortunately, insufficient information was provided to determine why they observed the one false-negative test among their few tuberculosis cases. Certainly, it is possible that in patients with tuberculous pleurisy who have additional conditions that generate *transudative* effusions (congestive heart failure, ascites from portal hypertension, or trapped lung), a dilutional effect may reduce the ADA levels. The preponderance of data suggests, though, that ADA activity may be a reasonable means of detecting tuberculous effusions. Like most tests in clinical medicine, its operational performance will depend on the population to which it is applied.

Other parameters examined to identify tuberculosis effusions include *cytokines*. Soluble IL-2 receptor concentrations were significantly elevated in tuberculous effusions in comparison with bacterial and malignant exudates (55). However, a subsequent report indicated that this test lacked sufficient specificity to be clinically useful (56).

Polymerase chain reaction (PCR) or other nucleic acid amplification techniques may prove useful. A study from South Africa of tuberculous pleurisy indicated a sensitivity of 0.81 for PCR, although there were some false positives among persons with malignant effusions (57). A report from France yielded only 0.20 to 0.60 sensitivity for PCR (58). However, a later study from Spain yielded a sensitivity of 81% and specificity of 100% for a PCR assay for pleural tuberculosis (59). On balance, it is difficult to estimate the utility of this test in pleural disease, and it is not currently approved for this use in the United States.

Pleural biopsy has been a highly useful method for the diagnosis of tuberculous pleurisy. Percutaneous techniques employing Cope or Abrams needles have been employed with reasonable safety and yield for nearly four decades. Certainly for patients with exudative effusions for whom the less invasive methods noted above (pleural fluid analysis, sputum studies, and radiography) have not yielded a diagnosis, biopsy is usually indicated. In his review, Sahn notes that the diagnostic yield of closed needle biopsies for tuberculous pleurisy was 245 of 345, or 75% (44): the biopsy offers histological identification of granulomatous inflammation in 50–80% of cases, and cultures of the biopsy are positive in 55–80%. Overall, this analysis indicates that analysis of pleural fluid and needle biopsy can establish the diagnosis in 90–95% of cases. Among the variables in the biopsy are the number of specimens taken at the site (logically, the more specimens the better the yield) and the number of times that biopsies are performed (if the first procedure does not yield a diagnosis, a second percutaneous biopsy will offer a worthwhile probability of diagnosis). Percutaneous biopsies have modest and generally acceptable morbidity: pneumothorax 3–15%, local pain 1–15%, vasovagal reactions 1–5%, hemothorax 2%, and various rare (<1%) complications. Moreover, there have been no fatalities of which I am aware. Perhaps the greatest utility of the biopsy is the high yield on culture. While other means can offer an inferential case strong enough to justify initiation of antituberculosis therapy, but recovery of the tubercle bacillus remains the most definitive means of diagnosis. And, given the rising prevalence of drug resistance (see Chapter 11), exclusion of resistance to standard drugs will be of progressively greater importance. Thoracopic video-guided biopsies may provide a diagnosis when closed techniques have failed (60,61). When preliminary efforts have failed to provide a secure diagnosis, this method should be considered.

The *management of tuberculous pleurisy* is generally straightforward, entailing chemotherapy with conventional agents. The duration of treatment has not been studied in a controlled manner, but given the relative paucity of bacilli in most effusions, 6-month therapy is very likely adequate. In the great majority of cases, one-time removal of the fluid (at the time of the diagnostic procedures) is sufficient (62). Tube thoracostomy drainage of the usual case is not necessary and, due to the potential hazards including superinfection, is generally contra-indicated. Decortication is required only in the rare instances of long-standing, large-volume effusions that have resulted in markedly-thickened pleura and trapped lung with substantial physiological impairment. In such cases, surgical intervention should be deferred until anti-tuberculosis chemotherapy has diminished the mycobacterial burden and reduced the chances of infection at the operation sites probably a matter of 6 to 8 weeks of medication. Steroids may dramatically curtail pleuritic chest pain, the rate of fluid accumulation, and dyspnea associated with tuberculous effusions. A recent randomized, controlled trial compared prednisolone 0.75 mg/kg/day for 2 to 3 months with placebo (63). Symptom duration in the treated group was a mean of 2.4 days versus 9.2 days for the placebo group; complete resolution of the effusion was also faster, 54.5 days versus 123.2 days. However, the development of residual pleural thickening was not influenced by corticosteroids. Similar results were reported in another randomized trial of steroids, with rapid reduction in symptoms but no effect on late fibrosis (62). Thus, I would recommend steroids now primarily for relief of disabling symptoms, an uncommon scenario.

Unusual aspects of tuberculosis of the pleura should be considered briefly. As noted above, gross rupture of a cavitary lesion into the pleural space may result in the rare finding of a chronic pyopneumothorax. Historically, pneumothorax collapse therapy may result decades later in a chronically trapped lung. Long-standing atelectasis and infection of the lung typically result in extensive lung injury and severe pleural thickening with calcification. Figure 7.4 demonstrates a typical chest x-ray and CT scan of a patient with remote pneumothorax treatment. This patient, after decades of quiescence, experienced reactivation of his tuberculosis that was complicated by the development of a secondary bronchopleural fistula (BPF). Through this BPF, bacilli from the chronic tuberculous empyema were expelled in the sputum. Efforts at chemotherapy of this patient and four others with similar findings resulted in transient improvement but subsequent relapse with acquired drug resistance (64). Data from one such case demonstrated poor penetration of antituberculosis medications into the pleural space, resulting in the poor outcome above (65). Aggressive medical management followed by resectional surgery when tolerable appears to be the treatment of choice for such cases.

Other complications of old pneumothorax treatment include tension effusions where, for unexplained reasons, the volume of the chronic fluid debris within the thorax expands, causing increasing dyspnea and blood gas disturbances; in the absence of evidence for active infection within the pleural space, three such patients were managed conservatively with thoracentesis to decompress the process (66). Other complications of prior pneumothorax treatment include pyogenic superinfection, bronchial and esophageal fistulas, and pleural-cutaneous fistulas. Among a series of such patients from Switzerland, conservative management was adequate in 45% of cases (67).

A rare form of collapse therapy was *lucite ball plombage*. Late complications of this procedure include migration with erosion or compression of mediastinal/chest wall structures and tubercu-

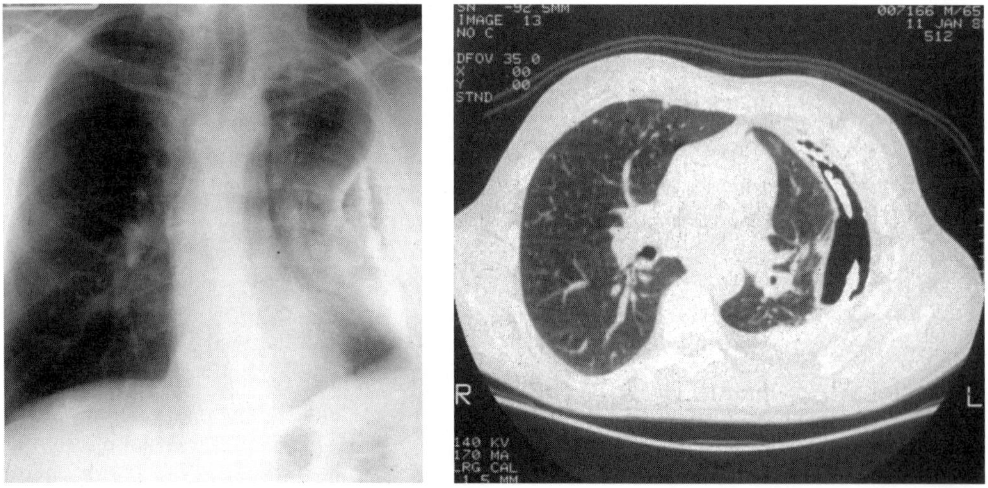

A B

FIG. 7.4. Chest x-ray and computed tomographic views of a chronic, calcific tuberculous empyema and bronchoplasmic fistulas related to remote pneumothorax ("collapse") therapy. This patient had been treated in the 1940s with pneumothorax or collapse therapy, whereby air was deliberately instilled in the left pleural space to promote closure of a cavitary lesion in that lung (see Chapter 1 for details). When he presented now with productive cough, malaise, and weight loss, his chest x-ray **(A)** showed that a thick pleural rind had formed in the left hemithorax. The presence of an air–fluid level in the pleural space was evidence that there was a connection between the bronchial tree and the pleural empyema that had allowed fluid to escape and air to enter, a bronchopleural fistula (BPF). Sputum and pleural fluid were both culture-positive for *M. tuberculosis*. The computed tomographic view of the chest **(B)** showed the pleural rind, both parietal and visceral, to be grossly thickened and densely calcified. Because of the extensive pleural scarring, drug penetration into this fortress was limited, resulting in treatment failure and acquired drug resistance; see text for discussion of management.

lous infection both around and within the (cracked) spheres. Removal of the spheres is generally indicated in these cases, although limited ventilatory capacity makes this complicated and potentially hazardous surgery (68).

Genitourinary Tuberculosis

Genitourinary tuberculosis is consistently among the more common forms of XPTB. Included in this grouping are urological disease of the kidneys, ureters, and bladder. Also, other genital structures, including the fallopian tubes, endometrium, and ovaries of women and the prostate, epididymis, and testes of men may be involved.

Epidemiologically, genitourinary tuberculosis is notably more prevalent among older persons. Children ages 0 to 14 had an adjusted relative odds likelihood of 0.1 for experiencing this form of XPTB, one of the greatest deviations from norm of any group with any form of XPTB in the 1986 CDC survey (5). This surely reflects the long period typically found between the primary infection and genitourinary tuberculosis; a mean of 22 years was estimated to have elapsed in one series of women (69), while the interval was greater than 15 years in 25% of another large series (70). Also remarkable in the CDC survey was the relative vulnerability of Amerinds, women, and foreign-born persons to genitourinary tuberculosis.

Pathogenesis varies, and distinctions should be made between those forms of genitourinary disease that result from infection of the renal cortex during the primary bacillemia and those which represent direct hematogenous seeding of a particular site. During the initial infection with *M. tuberculosis,* the bacilli are apparently filtered out by the glomeruli in the renal cortex. Multiple small granulomatous lesions evolve, then presumably involute with the development of competent immunity. Later, some of these lesions may reactivate, spreading downward into the medullary and calyceal structures where gross cavitary lesions may eventually develop. At this point, large numbers of bacilli and inflammatory debris are dumped into the renal pelvis and thence into the ureter, ultimately reaching the bladder. In this manner, renal disease may spread to involve the lower urinary structures. Among men, there appears to be a significant risk that tuberculosis may spread from the bladder to involve the epididymis, testes, and prostate, although in some instances these organs are diseased without evidence of bladder tuberculosis. By contrast, most authorities feel that genital tuberculosis in women is usually the result of direct hematogenous infection.

Clinically, most cases of genitourinary tuberculosis present with local rather than systemic manifestations. In a series of 102 patients with genitourinary tuberculosis, 37% of whom also had active pulmonary tuberculosis, the most common complaints were dysuria, frequency, nocturia, urgency, pain in the back, flank, or abdomen, tenderness/swelling of the testes or epididymis, and hematuria (69); only 18.6% had constitutional complaints. Another series of 78 patients with genitourinary tuberculosis, 13% of whom had simultaneous pulmonary or miliary disease, revealed similar findings: 71% of patients primarily exhibited features of local organ dysfunction, 20% were detected solely on the basis of abnormal urine sediment, and only 14% were noted to have constitutional symptoms (71). Common presenting complaints in these patients with tuberculosis of the kidneys, ureters, or bladder included dysuria (34%), gross hematuria (27%), and flank pain (10%). Among those men with genital tuberculosis, all nine presented with mass lesions of the testes or epididymis without fever or other systemic complaints. Among the women with genital tuberculosis there were three broad patterns amid the clinical presentations: infertility, pelvic pain, and menstrual disturbances. Physical examination of these 11 women revealed pelvic masses in five, cervical erosions in two, and no abnormalities in four.

Diagnosis of genitourinary tuberculosis classically entails recovery of the microbe from urine or affected tissues. For those suspected of urinary tract disease, early morning urine study has been shown to have a high yield. Confusion may occur, however, because of possible superinfection with other uropathogens. Because of urinary stasis caused by tuberculosis-induced strictures, some patients with underlying urinary system tuberculosis actually come to medical attention for more acute manifestations of a secondary infection. These patients may have traditional pathogens such as *E. coli* in their urine and receive treatment with cephalosporin, penicillin, sulfa, fluoroquinolone, or aminoglycoside antibiotics. It is vital to note that these agents, which are highly concentrated in the urine, may inhibit the growth of *M. tuberculosis*. Therefore, if one is sending urine for mycobacterial culture, it is important that the patient has not received such broad-spectrum antibiotics for at least 48 hours before the specimen is collected.

For men with possible genital tuberculosis, mass lesions should be biopsied for histological and culture studies. If prostatic tuberculosis is suspected, a massage before culture of seminal fluid may enhance the diagnostic yield. Thin-needle biopsy may demonstrate granulomatous inflammation. Women with suspected genital tuberculosis may require formal procedures such as uterine curettage, cervical biopsy, or laparoscopic biopsy to establish the diagnosis.

Evidence to support the diagnosis of genitourinary tuberculosis includes a prior history of active tuberculosis, the tuberculin skin test (which presumably will be falsely negative in some portion of patients), chest x-ray signs of either active or healed tuberculosis, and characteristic findings on radiographic studies. Plain films of the abdomen may reveal calcifications of the renal parenchyma, occasionally outlining the original medullary abscess or a dilated calyx. In long-standing disease of the lower urinary system, calcifications may develop there as well. Contrast urography should be performed in those with proven or suspected urinary tuberculosis. Findings suggestive of renal tuberculosis include damaged papillae, deformities and obstructions within the calyceal-pelvic system, irregular scarring of the cortex, and irregular narrowing of the ureter, notably at preexisting points where the structure is under pressure, such as the pelvic brim or the ureterovesicle junction.

Laboratory findings other than urine analysis and culture are generally not useful. Physical findings are generally related to localized genital tuberculosis with scrotal masses in men and pelvic or adnexal masses in women.

Management of genitourinary tuberculosis centers on adequate chemotherapy. Modern short-course regimens of 6 to 9 months' duration should prove curative for virtually all forms of tuberculosis, presuming drug-susceptible bacilli and compliance with therapy. Because renal tuberculosis is typically unilateral, azotemia is rare except for those with lower urinary tract disease who develop obstructive uropathy. Hypertension secondary to urinary tract tuberculosis appears very rare (72). Patients who shed large amounts of debris from a kidney lesion may develop transient ureteral obstruction with colic. Stasis may result in stone formation, also presenting with colic and/or hematuria. Endoscopic removal of matter within the ureters and dilation with stent placement are rarely required. Previously, nephrectomies were performed commonly for patients with grossly damaged, nonfunctioning kidneys (71); however, because current medical regimens have sufficient sterilizing capacity, resections rarely need to be performed for control of tuberculosis. Reconstructive surgery to relieve strictures may preserve or restore renal function (73). For women who suffer chronic pain from pelvic scarring and adhesions following chemotherapy, extirpative surgery may provide symptomatic relief (74).

Bone and Joint Tuberculosis

Bone and joint (B–J) tuberculosis has apparently been a constant affliction of humans throughout history. In fact, the persistence of tuberculous osseous remains has been the most useful historical indicator of ancient tuberculosis. Most bone and joint tuberculosis is presumed to arise as osteomyelitis from foci in the growth plates of bones where the blood supply is richest. Because these growth plates, or metaphyses, are typically near joints, the infection is believed generally to spread locally into joint spaces, resulting in tuberculous arthritis. In this section, disease of the long bones, flat bones, vertebrae, joints, and disk spaces is reviewed. In addition, such phenomena as noninfectious arthritis associated with tuberculosis (Poncet's syndrome) and carpal tunnel syndrome are discussed.

Epidemiologically, bone and joint disease afflicts all age groups, although the adjusted relative odds analysis indicated that the greatest propensity lies with those 65 years and older. For women with XPTB, bone and joint disease constituted a relatively greater proportion of morbidity than for men. In the period from 1975 to 1990 in the United States, 6,202 cases of bone and joint tuberculosis were reported, comprising 9.4% of the total XPTB morbidity (75). Data from a prior United States survey indicate that vertebral column disease constituted roughly 40%, hip 13%, knee 10%, and other sites the remainder of bone and joint tuberculosis during the period 1969 to 1973 (7). If these proportions remained constant to the present era, one would approximate there to be annually the following numbers of cases in the United States: 155 spinal, 50 hip, and 40 knee.

Clinically, local manifestations typically predominate over constitutional complaints. However, with chronic infection that results in large inflammatory collections, fever and wasting may ensue. Pain is the most common complaint. Soft tissue collections at or near the bone and joint focus, so-called cold abscesses, occur commonly when the condition goes untreated for long periods. Neurological findings such as weakness or numbness from compression of the spinal cord occasionally bring patients to medical attention.

Spinal or vertebral tuberculosis has been known historically as Pott's disease. The infection usually arises in the subchondral cancellous bone with spread to the cortex. Classically, there is more extensive destruction of the ventral portion of the vertebra, which results in anterior wedging as the bone collapses. Eventually, the disk is involved, analogous to the joint involvement with tuberculosis of the peripheral skeleton. The usual patient presents with two vertebrae involved, either contiguous or in a skip fashion with spread beneath the anterior longitudinal ligament. As the inflammation advances, paraspinous collections develop; these have a typical fusiform appearance. Radiographically, tuberculosis causes lytic destruction without sclerotic (new bone formation) reactions. Calcifications within the paraspinous collection or cold abscess are deemed highly suggestive but not pathognomonic of tuberculosis.

A recent review from Spain was singularly useful in comparing the clinical, laboratory, and radiographic manifestations of vertebral osteomyelitis caused by tuberculosis, *Brucella,* and pyogenic organisms (76). Features that were significantly associated with tuberculous etiology included prolonged symptomatic course, absence of fever or chills, spinal angulation, neurological defects, and paraspinous masses. The relative lack of fever, chills, and constitutional symptoms with spinal tuberculosis was dramatically demonstrated in a patient seen recently at National Jewish (Fig. 7.5).

Different anatomical regions of the spine are preferentially involved among different age groups. Among those from childhood through adolescence, the thoracic vertebrae are most commonly diseased; among 25 children from South Africa with spinal disease, 18 had thoracic spine involvement, and seven lumbar (77). Special aspects of thoracic spine tuberculosis include the high risk of neurological compromise and the propensity for development of the gibbus or hunchback deformity. Among adults, disease more commonly involves the lumbar vertebrae. In a group of 19 patients with a mean age of 36.5 years, there were 38 vertebrae with radiographically visible disease; 23 were lumbar, 12 were thoracic, and three were sacral (78). The cervical spine is an uncommon location for tuberculosis, but cases have been reported of osteomyelitis (79–81), paraspinous abscesses (82), and retropharyngeal abscess (83). Involvement of the sacroiliac joint was recently reported in 11 patients (84). Notable among those with sacroiliac disease were a pattern of pain in the buttock, thigh, and low back, an uncomfortable limping gait, tenderness on sacroiliac stress maneuvers, and cold abscesses.

Hip tuberculosis may involve the head of the femur, the joint space, or both. Typically, the patient complains of pain on walking or weightbearing. In long-standing disease, a cold abscess or sinus tract may form. Radiologically, the earliest change usually is swelling of the capsule

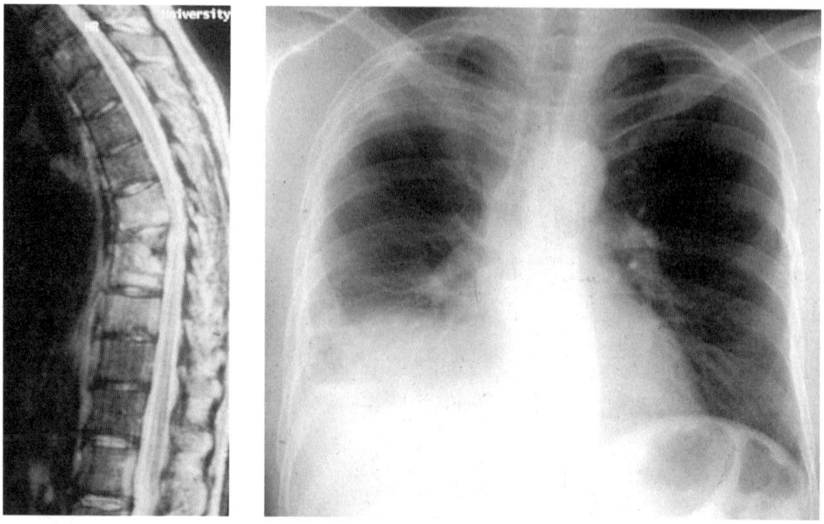

A B

FIG. 7.5. Tuberculous pleural disease following needle biopsy of a paraspinous abscess. A young Asian man had reported severe, progressive back pain for over 15 months. However, he denied any feverishness, chills, sweats, malaise, or weight loss during this period. Eventually, spinal x-rays were done and showed extensive destruction of multiple vertebrae and a large paraspinous abscess; an MRI showed extensive involvement of three consecutive vertebra **(A)**. A needle biopsy of this process was performed, showing caseating granulomas and yielding *M. tuberculosis* on culture. However, within a few weeks of this biopsy, despite initiation of antituberculosis chemotherapy, he developed right-sided pleuritic chest pain, fever, chills, sweats, malaise, and a 15-lb weight loss. Chest x-rays revealed a new right effusion; pleural fluid studies revealed a dense exudate culture positive for tubercle bacilli. Presumably, the needle biopsy traversed the posterior pleural recess near the spine, introducing the infection into the pleural space. Among the more notable aspects of this case was the striking absence of inflammatory signs and symptoms when the infection was confined to the spine/paraspinous space and the abrupt deterioration when the infection was introduced into the pleural space. The patient sequentially underwent pleural decortication for a trapped lung **(B)** (post-decortication chest x-ray) and an anterior spinal fusion because of the structural instability caused by destruction of three contiguous vertebrae.

without visible osseous lesions. Subtle subchondral and metaphyseal erosions, cysts, and osteopenia commonly precede gross destruction; the joint space commonly is narrowed (85). Involvement in hip prostheses, either by local reactivation or by hematogenous spread, has been reported (86).

The knee is involved with approximately the same frequency as the hip. Pain on walking and weight-bearing are typical early signs. Swelling and tenderness along the joint space may be appreciated as an effusion develops. Early radiographic changes are similar to those noted above for the hip.

Miscellaneous other bone and joint sites regularly involved with tuberculosis include the bones of the forearm, wrist, ankle, hand, and the ribs. Lytic, cystic lesions are the most common radiographic abnormalities found at these sites; see Fig. 7.6 for an extreme example of destructive tuberculosis of the bones of the forearm, wrist, and hand. Tuberculosis of the ribs that occurs anteriorly at the costochrondral junctions commonly forms cold abscesses; these collections may present ventrally as chest wall masses and/or protrude into the retrosternal or mediastinal spaces. Computed tomographic findings of tuberculosis of the ribs, chondral cartilage, and sternoclavicular joint were recently described (87). Uncommon presentations of bone and joint disease include multifocal lesions of the ribs (88), long bones, spine, and skull (89), or sternal osteomyelitis following cardiac surgery (90).

A rare articular manifestation of tuberculosis is a noninfectious polyarthritis that accompanies acute tuberculosis, similar in manner to the hypersensitivity phenomena, erythema nodosum or induratum. Referred to as Poncet's syndrome or disease, the disorder presents typically as stiffness of major joints with mild to moderate objective swelling, inflammation, or tenderness (91–94). Poncet's is associated usually with fever and other constitutional symptoms, which likely are reflections of the active tuberculosis at other sites. It is a diagnosis of exclusion: polyarthralgias/polyarthritis without serological markers of connective tissue disease that resolves with therapy of the active tuberculosis.

Another uncommon manifestation of B-J tuberculosis is carpal tunnel syndrome. Compromise of the median nerve as it courses though the flexor compartment of the wrist may lead to weakness and awkwardness of the thumb, pain in the palm and wrist, and paresthesias in the hand in the distribution of the median nerve. Tuberculosis, arising usually in the carpal bones, has been noted as an unusual cause of this syndrome (95). In my experience, *M. tuberculosis* has been a relatively rare cause of carpal tunnel syndrome, but recently we have seen a number of cases in which soft tissue infection with *M. avium* complex or rapid-growing mycobacteria has resulted in this or a similar presentation.

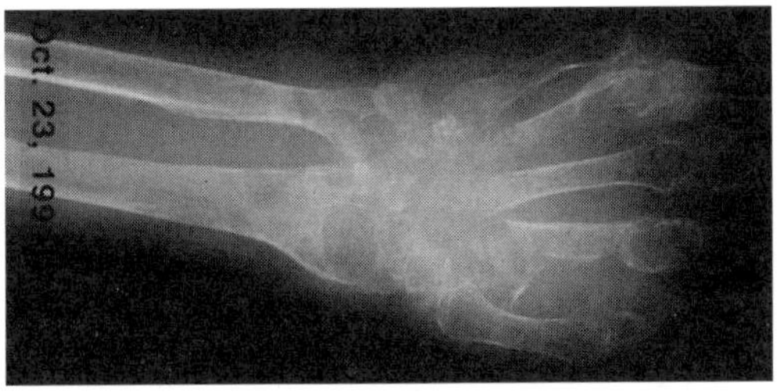

FIG. 7.6. Tuberculosis of the hand, wrist, and forearm. A 68-year-old Asian woman reported tenderness and swelling of her left wrist and hand for many months. Biopsy in her home community had demonstrated granulomas and yielded drug-susceptible *M. tuberculosis.* Her bone x-rays reveal classical destruction of the metacarpal bones and extensive cystic damage to the carpal bones, radius, and ulna. Because of progressive destruction of the bones and joints despite 6 months of chemotherapy, plans were considered to amputate her hand and forearm. However, she was referred to National Jewish for a second opinion. Pharmacokinetic studies revealed negative or negligible levels of drugs following directly observed administration of medication. She was cheeking, then spitting out her drugs despite the proposed amputation of her arm! She was not psychotic; she simply did not believe in Western medications.

Diagnosis of tuberculosis arthritis optimally entails recovery of the pathogen from the suspected site. Basically, the following features should alert the clinician: (a) any monoarticular arthritis, (b) cold abscesses, (c) positive tuberculin skin test, (d) epidemiological risk factors, or (e) chest x-ray abnormalities consistent with healed or active pulmonary tuberculosis. If there is an abscess, this material should be aspirated promptly for stain and culture. If a joint is involved, the synovial fluid should be examined; characteristic findings of tuberculous arthritis include a thick, mucinous, xanthochromic appearance with a high protein concentration, *no other pathogens* demonstrable on smear or culture, and a widely variable white blood cell count. A literature review done in 1976 (96) reported the following: (a) white blood cell counts ranged from 1,000/ml to 136,000/ml, with average counts varying from 16,200 to 28,258; (b) differential counts ranged from 10% to 99% polymorphonuclear leukocytes, with the average PMN counts varying from 51% to 73%; (c) 22 of 27 cases reported polymorphonuclear predominance; (d) synovial fluid glucose was less than 50 mg/dl in 61% of cases, and there was disparity greater than 40 mg between serum and synovial concentrations in 63% of cases; (e) synovial fluid protein concentrations ranged from 3.5 to 6.3 g/dl; (f) only 14 of 74 (19%) of fluids examined were positive on microscopy for acid-fast bacilli; and (g) 91 of 115 (79%) of synovial fluid specimens were positive on culture for tubercle bacilli.

This literature review indicated that open-joint synovial biopsy was the most sensitive method for the diagnosis of tuberculous arthritis. Histological evidence of tuberculosis was noted in 210 of 223 (94%) cases from the eight series analyzed. A recent report, however, cautions that synovial biopsy in tophaceous gout may demonstrate granulomatous changes (97). Culture of synovial tissue obtained at the open biopsies in these eight series was similarly sensitive with 140 of 149 (94%) being positive. Because the synovial fluid findings enumerated above are not specific for tuberculosis (other than positive smears or cultures), biopsy should be done for monoarticular arthritis in which a definitive diagnosis or a circumstantial case sufficiently strong to initiate therapy cannot be promptly made. The choice between open- or closed-needle synovial biopsy technique will depend on locally available expertise and preference. A recent review of infectious arthritis helps frame the differential diagnosis including a helpful discussion of risk factors (98).

The *management of tuberculous arthritis* depends substantially on the extent of inflammation and destruction of the joint. This emphasizes the importance of early diagnosis in order to conserve joint integrity. During the initial phase of chemotherapy, rest with avoidance of weight-bearing is indicated. Drainage with debridement may be performed when there are large collections that inhibit healing and function. If the joint needs to be temporarily immobilized, it should be placed in a position of function. As chemotherapy reduces inflammation and tenderness, graduated range of motion followed by strength exercises should be performed. Fusion of a joint may be required when there is such extensive destruction that return of function is not anticipated; however, the conservative measures noted above should be pursued for several months in most cases. If a major joint such as the hip or knee is irreversibly damaged, consideration should be given to replacement with an artificial joint rather than fusion, particularly for younger persons for whom mobility is a premium issue. Modern chemotherapy is sufficiently sterilizing that placement of a foreign body is feasible, but only after extended drug administration.

Diagnosis of vertebral tuberculosis usually entails a complex of historical, radiographic, and biopsy findings. Epidemiologically, minorities, immigrants, and the elderly are at highest risk. The tuberculin skin test is usually positive but may be falsely negative, particularly among debilitated or older persons. The finding of a cold abscess is highly suggestive; these collections may be found in diverse sites including the back, flank, and the perineal and inguinal areas. Plain radiographs may reveal vertebral collapse with angulation, fusiform paraspinous pus collections, and evidence of active or healed pulmonary tuberculosis. Computed tomography (CT) and magnetic resonance imaging (MRI) have proven highly useful in the differential diagnosis, localization of osseous and soft tissue disease, guidance of biopsies, and directing surgical management (77,99). One group of authors found CT to be the most useful technique in delineating bone destruction but MRI superior in identifying soft tissue disease and characterizing the spinal cord and its compromise (99). A recent series from France provides a helpful comparison of tuberculous and pyogenic vertebral osteomyelitis (100).

Management of vertebral tuberculosis universally entails intensive chemotherapy. Controversy exists, however, about the role of surgery (101). Among a series of patients from Korea, medical therapy without bed rest or splintage resulted in a clinically favorable status at 3 years in 92%, excluding those who presented with advanced neurological impairment (102). Nonetheless, there is disputation of the acceptability of this allegedly favorable status. In an editorial that accompanied this report of medical management, Leong, an orthopedic surgeon, pointed out that severe progressive skeletal deformity occurred in 20% of those treated conservatively in prior MRC trials (103). In the Korean trial, only 44% of the patients demonstrated complete bony fusion, and 16% manifested no fusion at all. Kyphosis or angulation of the spine in the anterior–posterior plane progressed throughout the 3-year period of observation for a substantial proportion of the patients. Beginning with an abnormally high 40° mean angle of kyphosis, 32% to 52% of the patients, depending on their medical regimen, experienced increases in angle from 11° to 30°, and 18% to 23% had increases of 31° or more. Leong points out that among patients in prior MRC trials, those receiving medical treatment alone experienced mean increases of 17.8° with thoracic and thoracolumbar disease and 5.2° with lumbar lesions. By comparison, those treated with radical surgery and anterior spinal fusion experienced a mean decrease in kyphosis of 1.4° and 0.5°, respectively, for thoracic/thoracolumbar and lumbar disease. Leong states that "such severe deterioration of the kyphosis in conservatively treated, although it occurred in only some 20%, is quite unacceptable, and could lead to paraplegia of late onset." A 1996 report from England describes seven patients with severe thoracic scoliosis leading to respiratory insufficiency, another complication of Pott's disease (104).

Paraplegia may be seen at the time of presentation or late in the course of Pott's disease. A series of patients from India who presented with paraplegia were recently described in terms of response to a standard chemotherapy regimen and various surgical interventions (105). Among these cases, the 9-month regimen (2 months of daily INH, RIF, SM, and EMB followed by 7 months of twice-weekly INH and RIF) proved effective in controlling the infection; because of the small numbers in the series, it was not possible to discern the effectiveness of the surgical techniques. This same group described another series of patients who had received prior medical treatment for Pott's disease but subsequently developed paraplegia (106). They identified these factors as predictors for severe delayed kyphosis: (a) age less than 15 years with involvement of three or more thoracic vertebrae, (b) involvement of two or more vertebrae with progression to involve three or four during treatment, and (c) an initial gibbus angle greater than 30°. Dwyer, in an accompanying editorial, emphasized the need for ongoing radiographic and clinical surveillance of previously treated patients (107). A dramatic example of successful surgical treatment of posttreatment Pott's paraplegia included normalization of neurological function (108).

Based on the risk for severe kyphotic angulation and the preexisting narrow tolerance of the thoracic canal for the spinal cord, persons with thoracic and thoracolumbar vertebral tuberculosis should be carefully considered for aggressive debridement and fusion. The case is particularly compelling for younger persons who will have a longer period for kyphotic angulation to develop, who have a relatively greater need for full mobility and strength, and who presumably can withstand the rigors of surgery more readily. Surgery should be contemplated also for those who present with multivertebral disease and neurological signs. Primary surgical management of selected patients with thoracic vertebral tuberculosis was recently reported from California (78). Obviously, this type of intervention is highly demanding and problematic; it should be undertaken only by experienced practitioners.

Disseminated Tuberculosis

Disseminated tuberculosis refers to simultaneous involvement of multiple organs. Such disease has commonly been referred to as miliary because of the appearance in the involved tissues of an immense number of small, 1- to 2-mm, well-defined nodules that reminded an 18th-century French physician of millet seeds (for clinicians without agrarian experience, millet may be found in seed trees sold as a parakeet treat). This miliary pattern may be seen antemortem only on chest radiography. Because a considerable proportion of patients who present with disseminated multiorgan tuberculosis do not have these characteristic findings visible on their chest x-rays, I prefer to use the term disseminated, lest the normal chest film dissuade the clinician from consideration of tuberculosis.

Pathogenetically, there presumably are multiple scenarios associated with the development of disseminated tuberculosis. Among certain vulnerable persons, the bacillemia associated with the primary pulmonary infection may cause progressive disease in multiple organs. This sequence might occur in an infant or an immunocompromised adult such as an AIDS patient or an organ transplant recipient. On the other hand, disseminated disease may develop as a form of reactivation tuberculosis, years or decades remote from the primary infection. In some instances, this may occur due to the abrupt release into the bloodstream of massive numbers of bacilli from eroding lymphatic, pulmonary, osseous, or other lesions. Another potential occurrence is the simultaneous reactivation of multiple sites that had been seeded remotely during the primary bacillemia due to an abrupt decline in immunocompetency.

Before chemotherapy, many died of chronic, destructive pulmonary tuberculosis associated with wasting (consumption). Despite the severe debility and malnutrition that occurred, late miliary spread was not a common occurrence. Thus, one may speculate that dissemination represented either an unusual bacterial event (invasion of a vascular structure with sudden discharge of massive numbers of bacilli) or an uncommon immunological response (immunosuppression from cachexia or infection). In any case, there is a temptation to regard persons who experience disseminated multiorgan tuberculosis as relatively more vulnerable and to treat them somewhat more aggressively (see below).

Epidemiologically, the profile of disseminated tuberculosis in the United States has evolved dramatically in the last half-century. Before drug treatment, miliary disease was most prevalent among infants and children. However, in the 1986 USPHS survey, the adjusted relative odds calculations indicated a bipolar pattern with the highest predisposition among those in the 0 to 14 years or 65 years and above age ranges (5). Notable also in this report was the apparent vulnerability of blacks (ARO 2.1) and Amerinds/Alaskan natives (ARO 3.1) to this form of tuberculosis; conversely, it was relatively rare among the foreign born (ARO 0.5). Gross inspection of the recent epidemiological patterns in comparison to the 1969–1973 data (7) suggests relatively more disseminated disease among young adults, presumably related to HIV/AIDS. Other special risk factors reported in various series of disseminated tuberculosis include alcoholism, steroid therapy, pregnancy or postpartum status, cancer, renal failure, and organ transplantation. In some instances, the primary disease is the risk factor; in others, immunosuppressive therapy may be a central or abetting element. Overall, the CDC recorded 5,599 cases of miliary tuberculosis from 1975 to 1990, or 350 cases per year. This averaged 8.5% of the total XPTB morbidity during this period.

Clinically, the presentations of disseminated tuberculosis are very diverse, depending on the particular organs involved and the prominence of inflammatory manifestations such as fever. Historically, series have identified large numbers of organs typically involved. However, many of these reports relied substantially on autopsies, where obviously the disease was very far advanced. It is important to emphasize that early in the course of most cases, one or two organ systems typically are more prominently involved in the process. Recognition of these leading-edge organs allows us to focus our diagnostic efforts in the most productive manner.

Symptomatically, constitutional complaints including feverishness, weakness or debility, anorexia, and weight loss are found in the majority of patients (109). Fever or feverishness is present in 80–95% of patients in most series. However, among elderly patients febrility may be less prominent than the wasting component, giving rise to the designation, *cryptic.* Commonly, headache is associated with meningeal disease while abdominal pain/swelling typically reflects peritoneal involvement. Dyspnea is usually indicative of fairly extensive pulmonary involvement. Cough is noted in roughly two-thirds of the patients in several large series (110–113).

Chest radiography is obviously a critical element in the recognition of disseminated tuberculosis. In older reported series, a very high proportion of patients, usually 90–100%, were reported to have abnormal chest x-rays consistent with miliary disease. However, these reports did not consistently indicate the status of the radiographs at the time when the patient *first* came to medical attention; my clinical experience indicates that a sizable portion of patients do not have discernible miliary shadows at initial presentation, but the lesions evolve during the days to weeks that often pass during the diagnostic evaluation. Indeed, in a review of 71 cases of disseminated tuberculosis from British Columbia, three blinded chest radiologists noted evidence of miliary disease in only 59% to 69% of chest films (114). Radiographic techniques may influence the visibility of the early lesions; highly penetrated or "hard" films tend to obscure the findings, whereas underpenetrated techniques exaggerate parenchymal shadows but lose specificity. Recent reports have noted that high-resolution computed tomography provides a rather distinctive pattern early in miliary tuberculosis (115–118). Rarely, disseminated tuberculosis presents with diffuse alveolar filling, so-called adult respiratory distress syndrome (see below). Pleural effusions are demonstrable in a modest proportion of cases.

Tuberculin skin-testing among persons with disseminated disease is significantly more likely to yield falsely negative results than with any other form of tuberculosis. Among HIV-negative patients, significant reactions to first or intermediate strength PPD tests were recorded in 43% (119), 48% (120), and 48% (113) of patients presenting with miliary tuberculosis. Hence, a nonreactive tuberculin skin test has very little power in excluding the diagnosis. Some have reported utility in repeat testing with a stronger antigen (110,113); however, second strength or 250 TU tuberculin is not currently available and, if used, would probably lose specificity. Using multiantigen panels to detect anergy would have very little utility in suggesting the diagnosis or in defining the prognosis and is not clinically useful in my opinion.

Other laboratory findings tend to relate to the specific organs involved and/or underlying disease. Hematologic disturbances are relatively common; see Table 7.5 for findings in several series. Anemia, usually mild, is present in roughly half of the patients. Leukopenia and leukocytosis are reported with nearly equal frequency, 15% and 14% in a recent report from South Africa (119); in this series, lymphopenia was the most common abnormality, being recorded in 87% of cases. Among other recent series from South Africa, lymphopenia was found in 100% of 25 patients with tuberculosis involving the bone marrow (121); this series was not really reflective of unselected disseminated tuberculosis, for it focused on cases with proven bone marrow involvement. Leukemoid reactions have been noted infrequently and may cause confusion regarding possible acute leukemia. Platelet counts may vary widely: in the South African series, platelets were elevated in 24% of cases, depressed in 23% (119). Marrow failure or aplastic anemia is quite rare among patients with disseminated tuberculosis. Some contend that it occurs when the marrow is depressed by drugs or by primary hematological disorders (122); others speculate that malnutri-

TABLE 7.5. *Bone marrow and liver biopsy findings in disseminated tuberculosis*

	Liver biopsy			Bone marrow biopsy		
Reference	Granulomata	Caseation	AFB	Granulomata	Caseation	AFB
Prout (138)	12/13	NS	3/13	15/21	NS	5/21
Cucin[a]	21/23	11/21	11/23	13/25	2/13	6/25
Gelb (113)	31/38	14/31	NS	2/2	2/2	2/2
Berger[b]	5/5	NS	NS	4/5	NS	2/5
Heinle[c]	3/4	NS	3/4	5/8	NS	1/8
Alvarez[d]	15/17	10/15	5/17	3/6	2/3	3/6
Maartens (119)	11/11	5/11	5/11	18/22	9/18	3/22
Totals	98/111	40/89	27/68	60/89	15/36	22/89
Averages	88%	45%	40%	67%	42%	25%

Adapted from Maartens et al. (119). Series of patients with miliary tuberculosis in whom both liver and bone marrow biopsies were done consistently. From the different numbers subjected to these procedures in the various series, it is apparent that selection was occurring. Criteria for submitting patients to these tests were generally not defined. AFB, acid-fast bacillus, stain positive.

[a] Cucin R, Coleman M, Eckhardt J, Silver R. The diagnosis of miliary tuberculosis: utility of peripheral blood abnormalities, bone marrow and liver needle biopsy. *J Chronic Dis* 1973;26:355–361.

[b] Berger H, Samortin T. Miliary tuberculosis: diagnostic methods with emphasis on the chest roentgenogram. *Chest* 1970;58:586–589.

[c] Heinle E, Jensen W, Westerman M. Diagnostic usefulness of marrow biopsy in disseminated tuberculosis. *Am Rev Respir Dis* 1965;91:701–705.

[d] Alvarez S, McCabe W. Extrapulmonary tuberculosis revisited: a review of the experience at the Boston City Hospital and other hospitals. *Medicine (Baltimore)* 1984;63:25–55.

tion may be a risk factor for both the miliary tuberculosis and the anemia (121). Amid various contradictory case reports and series, the impression emerges that patients with lymphohematogenous malignancies are at increased risk of disseminated tuberculosis and that patients with miliary tuberculosis have sundry disturbances of their hematopoietic lines, which result in a variety of transient, occasionally severe, cellular abnormalities. Two patients with miliary disease with neutropenia and thrombopenia who initially reversed their hematological abnormalities after antituberculosis treatment, only to later develop well-delineated hematopoietic malignancies, represent another variation on this theme (123).

Liver chemistries are abnormal in variable proportions of disseminated case series. The frequency of derangement of liver chemistry findings in two reports, one from South Africa (119) the other from North Carolina (110) are noted, respectively: (a) alkaline phosphatase 83% and 34%; (b) transaminases 42% and 93%; and (c) bilirubin 15% and 24%. Given the relatively high risk for tuberculosis among chronic alcohol abusers, caution must be taken in interpreting these abnormalities. One case of fatal massive liver failure and probable hepatorenal syndrome associated with miliary tuberculosis has been reported (124).

An unusual subset of disseminated tuberculosis patients with variable combinations of *disseminated intravascular coagulation* (DIC), *acute respiratory distress syndrome* (ARDS), and multiorgan failure have been reported (119,124–137). Given the similarities of these patients to those experiencing gram-negative sepsis, it is reasonable to speculate about excessive release or response to tumor necrosis factor (TNF-α), or other related cytokines.

Diagnosis of disseminated tuberculosis is often a complex and elusive process. Even for patients with a high-risk epidemiological profile and a typically abnormal chest x-ray, it may be difficult to obtain microbiological confirmation. Obviously, diagnostic efforts should be focused on the organs most likely to be involved. This requires knowledge of the prior probabilities based on previous clinical and autopsy series as well as particular evidence for organ involvement in the individual patient. Necropsy series indicate that the most commonly involved organs are the lungs, liver, and spleen, all ranging approximately from 80-100%. The next most consistently involved organ is the kidney, circa 60%, followed by the bone marrow, roughly 25 to 75% (113,130,138). Evidence for specific organ involvement is delineated above.

Confronted with an individual patient in whom disseminated tuberculosis is suspected, one might initiate the evaluation with these variables in mind: (a) Which organs seem involved in this patient, e.g., headache: suspect meningitis; abdominal pain/swelling: suspect peritonitis; abnormal chest x-ray: suspect pulmonary; hematologic abnormalities: suspect bone marrow; and so on. (b) What is the probability of a positive result from a given diagnostic study if that organ is involved, e.g., what is the possibility of a false-negative sampling error from an undirected transbronchial biopsy in a case with subtle retinulonodular shadows on the chest x-ray? (c) What is the potential for morbidity/mortality for the patient from a given procedure, e.g., is there a risk of uncal herniation from a lumbar puncture in a patient with probable papilledema, of respiratory failure due to pneumothorax from a transbronchial biopsy, and so on? (d) What local clinical skills are available, e.g., is there a surgeon competent at thoracoscopic lung biopsy, a gynecologist capable of directed biopsy through a laparoscope, and so on?

Although one might develop a relatively clear set of probabilities in terms of the likely yields of potential procedures, commencing with several of the more benign procedures is prudent, as no single test can be assured of providing the diagnosis. In the natural history of disseminated tuberculosis, there are critical risk periods for the evolution of highly morbid, potentially lethal conditions such as meningitis, pericarditis, disseminated intravascular coagulation (DIC), or adult respiratory distress syndrome (ARDS). Hence, clinicians should pursue the question with alacrity and resolve.

In my estimation, the following tests should be performed on all patients with suspected disseminated tuberculosis: (a) chest radiography—

begin with plain posteroanterior and lateral roentgenograms; if nondiagnostic, proceed to high-resolution computed tomography (see reference above); (b) sputum for mycobacterial smear and culture—induce if patient is unable to spontaneously produce; (c) morning urine for concentrated smear and culture—although it is possible for the urinary system to be contaminated with saprophytic mycobacteria, in a person suspected of miliary tuberculosis, a positive smear would be strong evidence to justify initiating therapy; because the glomeruli filter roughly 20% of the cardiac output, there is a good chance that a culture might yield bacilli even in the absence of abnormal sediment; also, it is cheap and benign; (d) biopsy and culture of new skin lesions or superficial lymph nodes—these are accessible, benign, and potentially very useful in differential diagnosis.

Because of the unique implications for management of meningeal tuberculosis (see section on meningeal tuberculosis above), lumbar puncture should be performed unless clearly contraindicated by high intracranial pressure or a bleeding diathesis. Other procedures such as transbronchial biopsy, bronchoalveolar lavage, open or thoracoscopic lung biopsy, closed-needle biopsy of the liver, bone-marrow biopsy, needle aspirate/biopsy of soft-tissue abscess or osseous lesions, paracentesis, laparoscopic biopsy and aspiration of fluid, thoracentesis, or closed-needle pleural biopsy should be performed according to the indications and tolerances of the individual patient.

Regarding the yields of these various procedures in disseminated tuberculosis, it is critical to note that there have been no systematic, prospective studies in which all or some of these tests have been routinely performed in persons suspected of this disorder. In large measure, clinicians have ordered the study if there were some evidence for involvement of that organ or site. Hence, it is not correct to say, for instance, that sputum culture is positive in a certain percentage of cases of disseminated tuberculosis. Obviously, the probability of a positive finding relates to the likelihood that the site is diseased and the extent of the disease there. For sites such as the meninges, the pleural space, or the peritoneal cavity, the yield would be comparable to that when these sites were involved singly. Hence, the reader is referred to sections related to these organ systems elsewhere in this chapter. The unique aspects of disseminated tuberculosis are miliary disease within the lung and involvement of such sites as the liver or bone marrow. These topics are detailed below.

Reports of the yield of studies of lung tissue or secretions in series of miliary tuberculosis vary widely, probably in part because of the great diversity in cases included in these series. Studies done on sputum, gastric aspirates, transbronchial biopsies, etc., will give vastly different results from a group with early, subtle interstitial shadows and small hard nodulations than from another group with more advanced disease in which there are more extensive soft, nodose shadows indicating that the process has involved the airspaces as well as the interstitium. Also, some series included cases in which the miliary disease evolved from an active pulmonary focus; in these cases, the positive results may well have reflected the parenchymal and not the miliary disease. Nonetheless, as indicated above, all persons with suspected disseminated tuberculosis should have sputum studies because of its benign availability. Overall, roughly 50% of suspected cases from whom sputum was obtained yield positive cultures. If patients are in the hospital and sputum is negative or cannot be obtained, gastric aspirates may be fruitful. If there are abnormalities on the chest radiographs, bronchoscopy with biopsy and washings for smear and culture should be obtained. A recent series from South Africa actually indicated a lower yield of bronchial wash cultures (55%) than for sputum culture (62%) (119). However, there almost certainly was selection bias involved, with the more advanced cases able to provide sputum and the more subtle cases being sent for bronchoscopy. In their experience, 30 of 48 (63%) of transbronchial biopsies revealed granulomata, 20 of these revealed caseation, and 13 of 30 were smear-positive for acid-fast bacilli (AFB).

Two sites likely to be involved and accessible for study are the liver and bone marrow. Maartens and colleagues summarized prior studies and included the results of their investigations of these organs (119); the yields are displayed in Table 7.5. However, they emphasize appropriately that merely finding granulomata in these tissues is not specific. Caseation on histopathology certainly raises the probability of tuberculosis; in addition, there is a substantial yield on culture.

Physical findings among patients with disseminated tuberculosis tend to be related to the specific organs involved and, unfortunately, are often nonspecific and of modest utility in establishing the diagnosis. Febrility has been noted in approximately 85% to 95% of patients in most recent series of miliary disease. One series of cases from South Africa in 1980 reported fever in only 44% of 62 patients (138); however, a later report from the same institution noted fever in 96% of 107 patients (119). Depending on the evolution of the pulmonary component, the lungs may be free of adventitious sounds, or there may be diffuse crackles. Hepatomegaly was found in roughly one-third of patients in the United States series (110,113), although among South African patients 65% (138) and 52% (119) had liver enlargement. Splenomegaly is less frequent, being found in roughly 15–30% of cases. Choroidal tubercles, gray-white lesions located near the optic disk, are somewhat controversial: early reports noted such lesions in 28% of 727 patients with miliary disease (139). However, recent series report this finding far less frequently, with less than 2% of 109 South African patients noted to have choroidal tubercles (119). Lymphadenopathy is found among 15% to 30% of HIV-negative persons with disseminated tuberculosis; however, AIDS patients are vulnerable to a generalized lymphadenopathic form of tuberculosis (see Chapter 8). Children with disseminated tuberculosis are considerably more likely to manifest hepatomegaly, splenomegaly, and/or lymphadenopathy (see Chapter 9).

Prognosis in disseminated tuberculosis inevitably includes considerable mortality in spite of optimal chemotherapy. All series reported have described early deaths, presumably related to the advanced stage of disease at presentation. Death rates during hospitalization have included 21.7% (110), 27.5% (113), 24% (119), and 38% (140). Factors associated with mortality include delayed diagnosis/therapy (which was often related to normal or atypical chest x-rays) and presence of meningitis. One recent series from Canada compared death rates for disseminated tuberculosis patients with abnormal or normal admitting chest x-rays (140). These patients, who were seen throughout Manitoba, Canada from 1979 to 1993, had remarkable diverse outcomes: those with normal chest films had 86% mortality versus only 21% for those whose x-rays were initially abnormal. The authors noted that those with normal chest x-rays were more likely to have identified risk factors for tuberculosis including alcoholism, diabetes mellitus, cancer, or immunosuppressive therapy. They speculated that the unfavorable outcome was largely related to delayed diagnosis and therapy. However, an equally tenable hypothesis is that the patients with normal chest x-rays had them because of failure to mount an immune response (137). Presentation with ARDS, respiratory failure, and/or DIC was associated with a lethal outcome in the great majority of cases (119,124, 137).

Management centers on prompt initiation of effective chemotherapy. Unless clearly contraindicated, four-drug treatment consisting of isoniazid, rifampin, pyrazinamide, and either streptomycin or ethambutol should be started when the preponderance of evidence indicates tuberculosis. Because the only definitive means of diagnosis is cultivation of the tubercle bacillus, and this typically entails a minimum of 3 weeks, nearly all patients with disseminated tuberculosis are begun on treatment on a *presumptive* basis. Indeed, in a substantial portion of cases treatment is begun without microscopic demonstration of mycobacteria because positive smears are so infrequent from the fluids and tissue analyzed.

A variation of this practice is the therapeutic trial in which, typically, a patient with a fever of unknown origin undergoes an evaluation that fails to yield conclusive evidence. In such instances, a clear response with defervescence and clinical improvement is strong presumptive evidence of tuberculosis. For patients in whom there is a low epidemiological probability of drug resistance, the clinician might choose to employ a very narrow-spectrum antimicrobial combination such as isoniazid, pyrazinamide, and ethambutol drugs, which have no activity other than against mycobacteria and relatively minimal activity against mycobacteria other than tuberculosis. Defervescence and clinical improvement in response to these drugs is very likely to indicate tuberculosis.

For patients who are desperately ill with disseminated tuberculosis, treatment with anti-inflammatory agents such as corticosteroids has been a common practice. Except for meningeal tuberculosis (see below), such steroid trials have largely been uncontrolled, anecdotal, and without clear evidence of efficacy. Nonetheless, I believe that most regular practitioners of tuberculosis would use such a modality in a patient who suffers from severe respiratory distress, toxicity, inanition, or ARDS/DIC. Because of the limited success in this anecdotal experience, prospective studies should be performed. Based on its efficacy in inhibiting the action of TNF-α and controlling inflammation in leprosy, consideration also might be given to studies of the agent thalidomide in these devastating forms of tuberculosis (141).

Tuberculosis of the Central Nervous System

Tuberculous meningitis (TBM) is by far the most common form of central nervous system tuberculosis and is the major focus of this section.

Considered to be almost universally fatal before the advent of chemotherapy, meningitis is an uncommon but dramatic form of XPTB. Historically, it was most commonly seen among immunologically vulnerable younger children. However, the epidemiology of TBM has evolved to embrace diverse groups in contemporary medicine.

Pathogenetically, most cases are believed to evolve from a small submeningeal focus that was deposited during the bacillemia of the primary infection. In some cases, TBM appears as a manifestation of disseminated or miliary tuberculosis, whereas in others it is the sole site of active tuberculosis. TBM has also been seen as a consequence of a paraspinous osseous focus that invades the spinal canal or following a skull fracture that presumably damaged the blood–brain barrier (110).

Most cases of TBM involve very few bacilli in cerebrospinal fluid and appear to reflect delayed-type hypersensitivity to the tuberculoprotein antigen that is released into the CSF. A unique study from South Africa measured the levels of proinflammatory cytokines in the cerebrospinal fluid of 30 children with proven or highly probable TBM (142). There were no differences in the levels of TNF-α or IL-1β when the TBM cases were compared to children with regular bacterial meningitis; however, levels of IFN-γ were initially and consistently higher. Curiously, no differences in cytokine levels were seen in relation to stage of disease or receipt of prednisone; see below for further discussion of the role of steroids in TBM. Because this inflammatory response occurs in a closed space that is cased tightly by the skull or spinal canal, pressure-induced ischemic injury may occur quickly. Another cause for therapeutic alacrity is the propensity for vascular endothelial necrosis, which leads to thrombosis and tissue infarction. The same center from South Africa noted that 30% of children with TBM had cerebral infarcts on admission, and another 22% experienced infarction despite initiation of therapy (143). These considerations place a great premium on early diagnosis and control of inflammation (see below).

Epidemiologically, TBM comprised approximately 4.5% of the total XPTB morbidity in the United States between 1969 and 1973 (7). From 1975 through 1990, there were 3,083 cases of TBM reported to the Centers for Disease Control, an average of 193 cases per year; this comprised 4.7% of the total XPTB cases during this 16-year period. However, in 1990 there were 284 cases, constituting 6.2% of the XPTB morbidity. The most likely sources of this increasing number of TBM cases are more central nervous system tuberculosis among HIV/AIDS patients and, because of rising tuberculosis case rates among young minority adults, more tuberculosis among their infants and children.

In the CDC's in-depth analysis of XPTB in the United States in 1986, several salient features of the epidemiology of TBM were noted (5). Children under 15 years of age had adjusted relative odds of nearly 5 for having TBM (see above for details of ARO); essentially, this indicates that a disproportionate amount of the total XPTB morbidity in this age group takes the form of TBM. Hispanic, black, and Amerind minorities had modestly greater propensities for TBM than did whites or Asians. Also, foreign-born persons were significantly *less* likely to develop TBM with an ARO of 0.4.

The *clinical presentations* of TBM generally follow a gradual course. Classically, three stages have been described, but, for the individual patient, transitions may be blurred. A prodromal phase, stage I, lasting for weeks to months has been described, typically consisting of feverishness, malaise, anorexia, irritability, headache, backache, and infrequent vomiting. Indeed, among a small subset of patients with similar symptoms, a pattern of transient meningitis has been described in association with tuberculosis (144). These authors speculated that, either in association with the bacillemia of primary infection or localized inflammation in a parameningeal focus, patients might experience a self-limited episode of meningitis, resolving without drug therapy. This concept is supported by necropsy studies that demonstrated localized foci of tuberculous meningitis among patients dying of consumption (145). These findings should alert us to the potential for a very indolent, almost benign course among persons with early tuberculous involvement of their central nervous system.

Although a rare case may undergo spontaneous involution, the great majority advance on to the next phase, stage II, which is marked by neurological signs. Progressive headache, lethargy, personality changes, disturbed memory, impaired cognition, and confusion are frequent findings. These behavioral features may be so prominent that patients may initially be directed for psychiatric care rather than somatic evaluation. Fever typically is the clue that directs clinicians to consider meningitis. As the basilar arachnoiditis advances, meningismus appears, and cranial nerve defects become manifest, commonly resulting in strabismus from paralysis of the superior oblique ocular muscle from infringement of the fourth (trochlear) nerve. Focal seizures and other localized disturbances of function occur as the TBM devolves.

The final phase, stage III, is marked by progression to stupor–coma. At this juncture, it is common for substantial hydrocephalus, intracranial hypertension, and vascular thrombosis to have developed. Tragically, even if antituberculous chemotherapy, aggressive anti-inflammatory treatment, and surgical decompressive measures are taken at this time, the patients, if they survive, have a substantial likelihood of residual neurological deficits.

Diagnosis of TBM most commonly entails recognition of classic abnormalities of the cerebrospinal fluid, emphasizing the importance of performing a lumbar puncture promptly in a suspected patient. Distinctive details of the CSF analysis are delineated below. Other very helpful elements include histories of recent exposure or prior tuberculosis; membership in a high risk epidemiological group; radiographic or clinical evidence of tuberculosis elsewhere, e.g., miliary shadows on the chest x-ray; or choroidal tubercles on funduscopic examination. Two disorders typically included in the differential diagnosis of patients suspected of TBM include neurocysticercosis and brain abscesses. These topics were subjects of recent excellent reviews (146,147).

Cerebrospinal fluid abnormalities are generally quite useful, but, short of demonstrating AFB on smear, they are not diagnostic because a variety of infections or other disorders can mimic the findings. The range of test results for CSF analysis in TBM are displayed in Table 7.6. In addition to standard laboratory assessment, investigational tests such as immune complex ELISA assays, adenosine deaminase levels, antibody immunoassays, and polymerase chain reaction assays are noted (148–157). Because of the infrequency with which AFB are found on microscopic examination of the fluid and the obvious delays in waiting for culture results, these experimental techniques are of great interest. But, until a rapid method has been perfected that has both high sensitivity and specificity for TBM, clinicians should continue to initiate treatment on a presumptive basis relating to CSF findings as well as clinical and epidemiological features.

TABLE 7.6. *Typical cerebrospinal fluid findings in tuberculosis meningitis*

Test	Results	Comments
Opening pressure	Elevated; extent dependent on severity and location of process.	Beware of ventricular or basilar obstruction with failure to transmit increased pressure.
Appearance	Clear early; opalescent to turbid to cloudy with chronicity.	Rarely xanthochromic.
Cellularity	Number ranges from few to 1,000+; usual range from 100 to 500.	If PMNs high, repeated tap after few days may show shift to mononuclear predominance.
	Differential may be PMN preponderant early; later, up to 95% mononuclear.	
Protein	Majority 100–500 mg/dl; >25% below 100 or normal; rarely over 1,000 mg/dl.	Very high levels with blockage or extreme chronicity.
Glucose	Usual range about 40–50 mg/dl; rarely <20. CSF to blood glucose typically about 50%.	Important to obtain a simultaneous blood glucose for comparison.
Microscopy	Positive for AFB in 20–37%; serial studies may increase yield.	Smear pellicle, which forms when CSF is allowed to stand.
Culture	Positive in 40–80%; increase yield with repeat studies.	Improved yield with larger volumes of CSF.
Polymerase chain reaction (PCR)	Overall, 65% sensitivity; among highly probable cases, 75% sensitivity; false positive in 6 of 51 (12%) of controls (148).	PCR in this trial compared to ELISA; see below. 44% sensitivity.
	80% sensitivity among highly probable and probable tuberculous meningitis (TBM) cases; no control group reported (149).	Reported a 91% positive predictive value.
	Overall 54% sensitivity; among culture-positive cases, 83% sensitivity; false positive in 9% (150).	Combining PCR and ELISA immune complex detection in this study gave 100% sensitivity in culture-positive and 74% in culture-negative but probable cases (see ELISA results below).
	Overall, 80% sensitivity; but 0 of 40 cases were culture-positive; 6.1% false positives in controls (151).	Appears useful, but lack of any positive cultures is somewhat disconcerting regarding the diagnostic criteria.
ELISA	52% sensitivity, 96% specificity (152); 44% sensitivity, 94% specificity (148); 64% sensitivity, 9% false positive (150).	More sensitive than culture but far from ideal.
Immune complex	64% sensitivity overall; positive in only 4 of 6 with culture positive TBM; false positive in 3 of 34 (9%) controls (150).	An IgG immune complex.
	60% sensitivity overall; false positive in only 3 of 101 (3%) controls with diverse CNS disorders or normals (153); was tested against "antimycobacterial antibodies" below.	Note that combining the IgG immune complex with "antimycobacterial antibodies" (below) yielded positive results in 82% of proven or highly probable cases.
ntibody immuno-assays	*M. tuberculosis* (MTB) "soluble extract" 67% sensitive overall, but positive in only one of six cultures positive for TBM; false positive in 4 of 34 (12%) controls (150). "LAM" 58% sensitive overall; false positive in 7 of 34 (21%) controls (150). "38 kDa" 39% sensitive overall; false positive in 3 of 34 (9%) controls (150).	Overall, these three assays were neither sensitive, nor specific; however, two of the three antigens appeared to distinguish TBM from controls.
	"Antimycobacterial antibodies" 55% sensitive; no reported false positives (153).	Appeared to complement the immune complex, assay above.
denosine deaminase (ADA)	Sensitivity of 100% and specificity of 99% in initially reported series by Ribera (154).	Both Donald (155) and Chawla (156) found great overlap between TBM and bacterial meningitis.
	Sensitivity of 50% but specificity low because of high values in CNS *Brucella* and pyogenic numagitis (157).	This report and those of Donald and Chawla above substantially discredit the utility of ADA in diagnosis of TBM.

These data are complied from the references cited in the text. As noted, none of these tests are perfect. These values fer broad guidelines increasing or lessening the likelihood of TBM. PCR, although it appears sensitive in some series, as performed poorly in others, presumably because of the presence of inhibitory factors (see Chapter 2). Because of e potentially profound consequences of delayed or missed diagnosis, presumptive therapy should be initiated early for atients suspected of TBM and for whom alternative diagnoses cannot be established.

Radiographic imaging of the central nervous system can be useful both in the diagnosis and management of TBM (158–161). While not diagnostically specific, computed tomographic views of the brain typically reveal basilar arachnoiditis, meningeal thickening, ventricular dilation, and in advanced cases scattered ischemic areas secondary to arteritis (158). In addition, CT scans may delineate tuberculous brain abscesses that are occasionally part of CNS tuberculosis; in such cases, MRI may be the more sensitive modality (162,163). And, in cases where meningitis has developed because of an osseous/soft tissue focus that abuts the central nervous system (CNS), these imaging techniques may identify the location and extent of these foci. Hydrocephalus may be detected and quantified by CT scans or MRI, offering guidance for the need and method of decompression. Given the potential for the delayed evolution of hydrocephalus or tuberculosis, serial imaging studies are indicated for those patients who do not improve in a timely manner or who experience deterioration.

The *chemotherapy* of TBM is problematic in terms of the ability of various drugs to cross the blood–brain barrier and reach therapeutic levels at the site(s) of infection. Unlike pulmonary tuberculosis, for which well-controlled studies have been conducted delineating the roles for various agents, there are only fragmentary data about the contribution of the drugs in TBM. Early information on the penetration of drugs into the CSF was often contradictory, possibly reflecting variables among the patients studied and the pharmacological assays employed. In general terms, the ability of a medication to cross the meninges is enhanced by small molecular weight, low protein binding, lack of ionization, and lipid solubility (164–166). A recent state-of-the-art review on general antibiotic pharmacodynamics in cerebrospinal fluid provides excellent data regarding medications and the central nervous system (167).

During the acute phase of TBM during which the meninges are highly inflamed and are highly permeable (elevated CSF protein being a marker of permeability), most of the standard antituberculosis medications penetrate the blood–brain barrier sufficiently well to exert a therapeutic effect. However, as the inflammation subsides, concentrations for some drugs fall substantially. Efforts have been made to establish predictable ratios between serum and CSF levels of the various antituberculosis medications. Although these studies have some general utility in helping to estimate the potential utility of these drugs, I believe that these data have limitations that must be appreciated: (a) levels of medications in the CSF derived from a lumbar puncture may well not reflect local concentrations in the cerebral or brainstem meninges, where the inflammation is most intense; (b) there are enough interpatient and intrapatient variations in the results of these studies to suggest that the pharmacokinetic information, favorable or unfavorable, about the different drugs may not be universally applicable to all patients with TBM. With these uncertainties acknowledged, some general observations about the drugs or categories of drugs may be made (Table 7.7). Specific pharmacodynamic data regarding CSF levels are shown in Table 7.8. A recent case that highlights the dis-

TABLE 7.7. *Antituberculosis medications in tuberculous meningitis (TBM): general observations*

Agent	Comments
Isoniazid (INH)	Prompt and complete penetration of CSF; clinical efficacy well documented
Rifampin (RIF)	CSF levels 5–25% of serum; impact on treatment not dramatic. May wish to increase dosage above routine
Pyrazinamide (PZA)	Prompt and complete penetration of CSF; efficacy not proven but considered a first-line agent
Streptomycin (SM)	Modest early activity; useful for TB outside CNS; concern for eighth-nerve toxicity.
Ethambutol (EMB)	Marginal activity in CNS; useful for TB outside CNS; no evidence for increased optic toxicity
Ethionamide (ETA)	Although penetration is good, drug has only modest activity in other sites; poor GI tolerance in adults, better in children
Cycloserine (CSN)	Good CSF penetration, but use in TBM problematic because of potential CNS toxicity including seizures and altered mental status

These are general comments about the utility of these agents. Specific data about the CNS levels of INH, RIF, PZA, and SM are displayed in Table 7.8.

TABLE 7.8. *Drug levels of first-line agents in TB meningitis*

Agent	Dosing by body weight	Serum/CSF levels at times after dosing 2 hr	4 hr	5 hr	6 hr	Comments
Isoniazid	7.5–9.1 mg/kg	4.4 ± 0.5/ 1.9 ± 0.3	2.6 ± 0.8/ 3.2 ± 0.8	2.1 ± 0.6/ 1.8 ± 0.5	1.0 ± 0.3/ 1.8 ± 0.5	Chinese adults (204). Delayed but excellent penetration into CSF.
	20 mg/kg	19.1 ± 4.2/ 8.9 ± 2.7[a]	14.3 ± 4.2/ 11.7 ± 3.1[b]	10.5 ± 3.0/ 12.0 ± 2.3[c]	6.4 ± 4.1/ 10.0 ± 3.5[d]	African children (205). Study also reported on 10 mg/kg dosing and influence of acetylation status.
Pyrazinamide	34–41 mg/kg	52.0/38.6		39.5/44.5	28.4/36.0	Chinese adults (206). Virtually equivalent at all times.
	40 mg/kg	N.R.[e]/18.1	N.R./28.5	N.R./33.5	N.R./38.4	African children (207). Serum levels not done. Values are mean levels.
Rifampin	10–11 mg/kg	11.5 ± 1.0/ 0.39 ± 0.06	10.6 ± 1.4/ 0.38 ± 0.06	10.1 ± 1.1/ 0.78 ± 0.13	4.7 ± 0.6/ 0.47 ± 0.06	Chinese adults (204). High protein-binding ionization and high molecular weight impede access to CSF.
Streptomycin	12.8–14.2 mg/kg	30.5 ± 2.8/ 2.1 ± 0.4	16.4 ± 1.6/ 1.6 ± 0.3		10.6 ± 0.9/ 2.2 ± 0.5	Chinese adults (204). High molecular weight and ionization impede access to CSF.

The values derived from these studies indicate that INH and PZA promptly reach "therapeutic" levels in CSF. Although clinical studies clearly confirm the therapeutic utility of INH, such data do not exist for PZA. These levels of PZA are associated with clinical activity in *pulmonary* tuberculosis, but PZA is believed to be active against only a limited population of tubercle bacilli in pulmonary diseases (see Chapter 10 for more thorough discussion). This population, believed to be defined by local acidic conditions in walls of cavities, may *not* have an analogous counterpart in TBM. Thus, we should be cautious with our expectations of this agent in TBM.

The CSF levels of both RIF and SM are very marginal, barely exceeding usual MIC. These data suggest to me the potential utility of increasing the dosage of these agents early in the treatment of TBM. This may be particularly important for RIFG, which—through autoinduction—may be expected to result in progressively lower serum levels over the initial 3 weeks. One study reported on CSF levels of RIF given at 25 mg/kg (208). The CSF levels as reported were no greater than those seen in another trial following a dose of 10–11 mg/kg (204). However, the serum levels in the high-dose trials were much lower than would be anticipated, suggesting a methodological problem with the study. For SM or the other aminoglycosides, to avert eighth nerve or renal toxicity, the drugs may be given thrice weekly.

Ethambutol would be expected to achieve very low CSF levels because of its higher degree of ionization and molecular weight (204). In six normal subjects, CSF levels done 2 to 4 hours after a single 50 mg/kg dose were all 0 (209). However, among eight patients with TBM, CSF levels reportedly ranged from 0.55 to 4.21 μg/ml at 2 to 6 hours after dosing (210). Thus, the role of EMB is not clearly defined in TBM. Although it should not be counted on to play a major role, it is possible that early on, when the blood–brain barrier is disrupted, intermittent high-dose EMB, e.g., 40 mg/kg thrice weekly, might prove beneficial.

[a] 1–2 hours.
[b] 2–3 hours.
[c] 3–4 hours.
[d] 4–5 hours.
[e] N.R., not recorded.

crepant drug delivery to the central nervous system is presented with Fig. 7.7.

In addition to the pharmacokinetic information provided above, the choice of regimen for TBM ideally should be based on demonstrated efficacy in trials. However, it is important to recognize that treatment studies for TBM have substantially less clear and satisfactory endpoints than do those for pulmonary tuberculosis. Hence, we are left with vaguer criteria of efficacy. Among the conclusions that I believe are justified on the basis of currently available data are these: (a) monotherapy with streptomycin, although of limited success, poses a substantial risk for acquired drug resistance, relapse, and treatment failure; (b) multidrug regimens are associated with higher rates of sterilization and clinical cures; (c) the success of treatment regimens that include at least isoniazid is much more closely related to the patient's stage of disease than to regimen variables; (d) isoniazid and pyrazinamide cross the blood–brain barrier readily with or without meningeal inflammation; other standard agents cross less readily, even in the presence of meningitis (Tables 7.7 and 7.8); (e) increasing the doses of medications to achieve higher CSF levels, albeit logical and supported by fragmentary data, is of unproven utility and may increase the risk of drug toxicity; (f) the optimal duration for treatment has not been established; (g) corticosteroids very probably reduce the morbidity and mortality, especially in advanced TBM; and (h) among those who survive advanced TBM there are substantial risks for serious neurological sequelae. For details, see below.

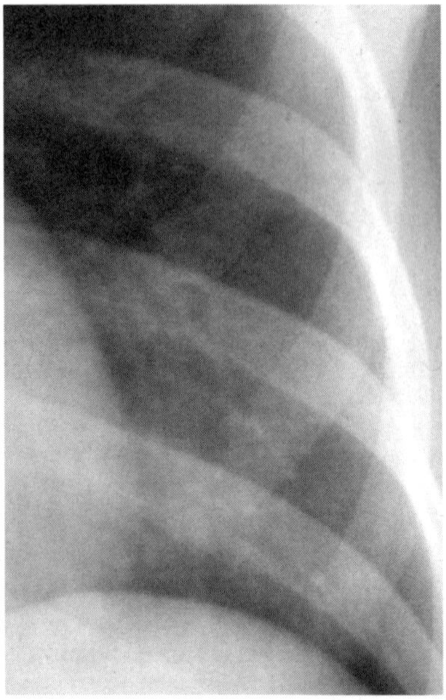

FIG. 7.7. Disseminated tuberculosis including miliary disease in lungs and meningitis. The patient is a 25-year-old Vietnamese immigrant who presented in his home community with feverishness, sweats, malaise, and 15-lb weight loss. This admission chest x-ray showed fine miliary stippling, most prominent in lower zones. A presumptive diagnosis of tuberculosis was made and treatment begun with INH/RIF/PZA/EMB. A disappointing clinical response was noted. At 4 weeks, initial culture and susceptibility results identified the organism as *M. tuberculosis* resistant to isoniazid, rifampin, and streptomycin. Therapy was revised with the addition of ciprofloxacin and cycloserine. On this regimen, the patient experienced virtual clearing of his chest x-ray. However, he had progressively severe headaches, nuchal rigidity, and irritability. Serial lumbar punctures revealed substantial worsening of his CSF parameters including progressive pleiocytosis and increasing protein levels. We interpreted this course to reflect failure of the retreatment drugs to adequately penetrate the blood–brain barrier. Therefore, we placed a cisternal reservoir to directly instill amikacin and levofloxacin. On this regimen, his CSF parameters normalized, and his symptoms abated.

Early trials in which streptomycin was employed alone showed improved survival but suboptimal rates of failure, relapse, and acquired resistance (168–173). While PAS improved the outcome modestly, it was the addition of isoniazid that dramatically improved the response to therapy (174,175). One series noted that the mortality was 70% for streptomycin alone but fell to 30% for those receiving streptomycin and isoniazid (176). In fact, in all series of TBM cases, there has been an overall minimum mortality rate of at least 20% to 30%, suggesting that the addition of additional agents such as rifampin, pyrazinamide, or ethambutol has relatively small impact on the outcome (177–179). Among children in Hong Kong, two variables were central to prognosis: stage (see above for details) and age (179). Those presenting in stage

I enjoyed 96% complete recovery; those in stage II had a 78% complete recovery rate with 12% experiencing moderate to severe sequelae; but of those presenting in stage III, only 21% experienced complete recovery, and death occurred in 17% of cases. Indeed, 41 of 60 (68%) survivors of stage III TBM suffered moderate to severe sequelae. The prognosis in this Hong Kong series was most severe among the younger children as well. In India, there was a similar association between the stage of TBM and prognosis (177); overall in this report, which compared three different 12-month regimens with variable combinations of the five major drugs, 34% of the children enjoyed complete recovery, 27% died, and 39% had sequelae. On long-term follow-up, ten of the survivors died of the neurological sequelae of the TBM (178). Hypopituitarism occurred in 10 of 49 (20.4%) young-adult patients who had been treated for childhood TBM, typically occurring around age 5; endocrine studies suggested hypothalamic dysfunction (180). In the Indian study, the incidence of hepatitis was related to dosage and schedule of the drugs: when isoniazid was given at 20 mg/kg, 39% of the children experienced jaundice; when the dose was reduced to 12 mg/kg, the jaundice occurred in only 16%; and when the rifampin was reduced from 12 mg/kg daily to twice weekly, jaundice was seen in only 5% (177). Two recent series of patients with TBM described very unfavorable outcomes despite treatment (181,182). However, the results were clearly biased by the setting, an ICU (181), and a substantial admixture of persons with AIDS in both groups. Because of significant differences in presentation and management, TBM in AIDS is discussed separately in Chapter 8.

Corticosteroid treatment in the management of TBM has been a disputed issue. Potential favorable effects include reduction of intracranial hypertension, abatement of cerebral edema, diminished arachnoiditis with lessening of risks for hydrocephalus and cranial nerve palsies, and prevention of spinal cord blockage. However, concern has been expressed for deleterious consequences including reducing the permeability of the inflamed meninges for drugs (183). An early study that examined the impact of dexamethasone on cerebrospinal fluid indices in relation to efficacy suggested that although steroids quickly improved such parameters as CSF leukocytosis, protein levels, and glucose concentrations, the sole factor that was associated with improved mortality was reduction of cerebral edema/intracranial hypertension (184). However, it must be noted that the number of patients in this trial, 23, was too small to allow firm conclusions to be drawn. Among a series of patients from China, steroid therapy appeared to reduce the mortality rates among those presenting in stages II or III of TBM (185). Similar findings were recorded in a study from Egypt in which steroid therapy reduced overall mortality, the effect being more dramatic among those who survived for 10 days or more after admission (186). Overall, the data point clearly in the direction of reduced mortality among patients with advanced TBM who receive corticosteroids. A vital issue, yet unanswered, is whether those who receive corticosteroids and survive have diminished neurological sequelae; limited data (186,187) and intuition suggest this should be so.

Neurosurgical intervention may be indicated for complications such as hydrocephalus or, less likely, large local collections. For patients with symptomatic, functionally significant hydrocephalus, early decompression may be associated with improved survival (188). Computed tomography is a sensitive means of monitoring hydrocephalus (158,160,161,189). Emergency relief may be achieved by simple ventriculostomy; more definitive management may entail ventriculoatrial or ventriculoperitoneal shunting (190–193).

A group from South Africa that sees many cases of TBM advocates intracranial pressure monitoring for children with stage II or III disease (189,194). They suggest that in cases with *communicating* hydrocephalus (detected by inserting air during a lumbar puncture with subsequent appearance of air in the ventricles), diuretic therapy employing furosemide and acetazolamide can effectively control intracranial pressure (194). By contrast, they indicate that, for patients with *noncommunicating* hydrocephalus, prompt ventriculoperitoneal shunting is required. Although these methods have not, to my knowledge, been employed in other centers, the experience of this distinguished group commends this method for consideration.

Tuberculomas, other than with AIDS, represent a small subset of CNS tuberculosis. Sophisticated radiographic monitoring of TBM has shown that local tuberculomas occur in a modest proportion of meningitis cases (195–200). Uncontrolled studies suggest, however, that most of these lesions involute with medical treatment and do not need surgical drainage (201). Seven patients who were found to have mass lesions of the CNS caused by *M. tuberculosis* on initial presentation were recently reported from Switzerland (202); three originally were from Africa, and one from India. Notable in their clinical pictures were the prominence of seizures, hemiparesis, and rapid progression of headache. Response to therapy was disappointing, with two deaths and overall slow rates of improvement; outcome was better with less extensive lesions and younger patients. Paradoxical worsening was noted in three of seven patients. A recent series from India reported on the efficacy of short-course chemo-therapy for tuberculosis of the brain (203); very favorable results were described with low morbidity and mortality. However, another group questioned the validity of the diagnostic criteria in this study, suggesting that a substantial number of these patients may have had CNS cysticercosis (204).

The overall management of CNS tuberculosis remains problematic (205–211). Based on an amalgam of clinical treatment studies and the available pharmacokinetic data, I would recommend the following approach. Begin therapy with a four-drug regimen unless there are strong epidemiological factors suggesting drug-susceptible tuberculosis. The regimen should include isoniazid, pyrazinamide, and rifampin. Dosages of these drugs for TBM might reasonably be increased above those used for other forms of tuberculosis; in particular, the dose of rifampin should be increased because of evidence of diminished efficacy with very modest reduction in dosage in clinical trials of pulmonary disease (see Chapter 10). Streptomycin might reasonably be the fourth drug: when used in monotherapy, early beneficial efforts were clearly demonstrable. Regarding the schedule and dosage of streptomycin, I personally would opt for thrice weekly at 22 mg/kg, which in our experience at National Jewish Hospital has resulted in higher serum levels with toxicity comparable to that of the lower daily dose; see Chapter 10 for more extensive discussion of this practice. If ethambutol is given as the fourth drug, it might be started at 25 mg/kg for the first 2 months, then reduced to 15 mg/kg; thrice-weekly dosing at 40 mg/kg could be advantageous. Pediatricians may prefer to employ ethionamide instead of ethambutol; this reflects better gastrointestinal tolerance of this agent by infants and children than adults, better CNS penetration (212) than ethambutol, and inability to monitor for EMB ocular toxicity in infants and young children. If there is major toxicity or demonstrated high-level in vitro resistance to isoniazid, the other four drugs—rifampin, pyrazinamide, streptomycin and the fourth drug of choice—should be employed for the initial 2 to 4 months. At that point, I would recommend that, in distinction to that which typically would be done in tuberculosis located outside the CNS, the three oral drugs, rifampin, pyrazinamide, and ethambutol, be continued for the duration of treatment (the pyrazinamide is continued because of its superior penetration of the progressively less inflamed meninges). The duration of treatment is not well defined, but, based on the potentially immense implications of recrudescent disease, most authorities have advocated periods significantly in excess of the now-standard 6-month regimen. I would suggest a 12-month target with 9 months as the lower limit if drug-intolerance or nonadherence were confounding issues.

Steroids are generally considered appropriate for all cases with stage II (objective neurological findings) or stage III (stupor–coma) disease. Personally, I prefer to employ steroids for all cases of CNS tuberculosis unless clearly contraindicated. There are no data that clearly indicate superior penetration or activity within the CNS of any particular corticosteroid compound.

My practice has been to employ prednisone at a dose of 1 mg/kg for 4 to 8 weeks; however, because of the accelerated catabolism of prednisone from rifampin hepatic induction, higher doses might be employed if a prompt anti-inflammatory effect is not seen. Then, the steroids should be tapered over 2 to 3 weeks, observing for both rebound CNS inflammation and adrenal insufficiency. (In addition to suppression of the hypophyseal–pituitary–adrenal axis by the exogenous steroids, patients with disseminated disease may have tuberculous adrenal involvement.)

As a result of alterations of the sensorium, some patients with TBM will be unable to ingest oral medications. Management options at this point include nasogastric instillation, percutaneous endoscopic gastrostomy, or parenteral administration. Isoniazid, rifampin, streptomycin (and the other aminoglycosides), and fluoroquinolones are currently available in the United States for parenteral use; a parenteral preparation of ethambutol has been employed in Europe and Canada but is not routinely available in the United States.

Abdominal Tuberculosis

Abdominal tuberculosis is comprised largely of peritoneal, ileocecal, anorectal, and mesenteric lymph node infection. In the United States, the great preponderance of disease takes the form of peritonitis. In the 1969–1973 USPHS survey of XPTB, abdominal disease represented only 3.5% of morbidity (7). Similarly, from 1975 to 1990, there were 2,372 notifications of peritoneal tuberculosis, an average of 148 cases per year, constituting 3.6% of the total number of XPTB cases.

Pathogenetically, there are a variety of mechanisms involved with the different forms of abdominal tuberculosis. Peritonitis is sometimes seen in association with genital tuberculosis in women, and it has been speculated that there is retrograde spread of the bacilli from the fallopian tubes into the abdominal cavity. Peritonitis may also be a prominent component of disseminated or miliary tuberculosis in which there is a widespread hematogenous spread of the infection. Diseases of the alimentary canal, ileocecitis or anoproctitis, are seen most commonly in association with chronic pulmonary tuberculosis, and it is believed that chronic ingestion of massive numbers of tubercle bacilli from the sputum results in infection of the distal bowel. In the prechemotherapeutic era, patients with longstanding consumption frequently suffered bowel problems including abdominal pain, obstruction, diarrhea, and *fistulae-in-ano.* In the developing nations where chronic pulmonary tuberculosis is relatively more common, ileocecal and anorectal tuberculosis constitute a larger portion of contemporary abdominal tuberculosis. A potential confounding factor in the higher prevalence of alimentary tract disease in these areas is infection caused by ingestion of *M. bovis* where dairy cattle are not tuberculin tested and milk is not pasteurized.

Epidemiologically, an analysis of the 1986 patterns of XPTB in the United States indicated very high adjusted relative odds for peritoneal tuberculosis among Amerinds, ARO 11.4, and blacks, ARO 2.5 (5). To reemphasize the meaning of the ARO, these findings mean that Amerinds with XPTB are much more likely than other racial/ethnic groups to manifest their disease as peritonitis. Also notable in the analysis was the total lack of tuberculous peritonitis among those ages 0 to 14. From 1970 to 1981 in British Columbia, Canada, 81 cases of abdominal tuberculosis were recorded; 41 were peritoneal, 17 ileocecal, 16 anorectal, and eight mesenteric adenitis (213).

Given the small number of cases in the United States recently, it is difficult to clearly ascertain patterns. However, in earlier reports from the United States (214) and current studies from high-prevalence areas (215), peritonitis appears to have modest predilections for young women in the child-bearing ages and for older men, commonly in association with chronic alcoholism. In the Canadian series cited above, peritonitis was most common among Amerinds, whereas ileocecal disease was more prevalent among Asians (213).

Clinically, peritoneal tuberculosis is typically

an elusive entity, particularly in the men with alcoholism in whom there are coexisting disorders that mimic the signs and symptoms of the tuberculosis, for whom peritoneal fluid analysis may not yield classical findings, and among whom the tuberculin skin test is more likely to be falsely negative (216). Patients manifest extremely diverse findings; signs and symptoms reported in various series are displayed in Table 7.9. Historically, a modest number of patients in all of these series had reported prior tuberculosis. Some patients presented with a subacute, relatively abrupt illness whereas others described a gradual, insidious process that can best be described as cryptic (217,218).

Ileocecal tuberculosis is now an uncommon disease in North America, and that rareness frequently results in delayed or missed diagnosis. The more common signs and symptoms include long-standing abdominal pain, nausea, vomiting, anorexia, diarrhea and/or constipation, postprandial distress, and weight loss; fever appears less prominent than in peritonitis, reported in 31% of one series (219) and 38% of another (220). Mass lesions in the abdomen were recognized in 23% (219), 65% (220), and 35% (213). Frequently, ileocecal tuberculosis is mistaken for Crohn's disease (213,219–221).

Fisulae-in-ano caused by tuberculosis is most often seen in association with chronic pulmonary tuberculosis; it also occurs in association with osseous tuberculosis of the spine or sacroiliac region. Mesenteric adenitis is seen most often in association with active pulmonary tuberculosis; it may present as a mass lesion or peritonitis.

Diagnosis of abdominal tuberculosis is very often problematic because of its protean manifestations, limited accessibility, and an array of other disorders with similar findings. A recent brief report suggests the utility of ultrasound in identifying patients with abdominal tuberculosis (222). Among patients with suspected peritonitis, laparoscopic evaluation with guided biopsy is the diagnostic procedure of choice (223,224). Paracentesis of ascitic fluid may offer highly suggestive clues such as lymphocytic exudate, but positive cultures occur in a clear minority of cases reported, except in the experience in Iran where 1 L of fluid was sent for culture (225). It is unclear whether this reflected an increased likelihood of positive cultures because of the volume studied or whether patients with more extensive disease were apt to have large volumes of ascitic fluid. Laparoscopy provides both access to peritoneal fluid and an opportunity to visually inspect the abdominal cavity and biopsy suspicious areas. Because of the ability to inspect the site of biopsy, laparoscopy should reduce the chance for hemorrhage or inadvertent penetration of viscera attendant to the closed-needle technique. If the patient has a large fluid collection, the closed-needle technique is theoretically somewhat safer because of clearance of the viscera. However, if there is

TABLE 7.9. *Signs and symptoms in tuberculous peritonitis*

	Study (ref.)				
Finding	Singh (217)	Borhanmanesh (225)	Cromartie (218)	Karney (216)	Menzies (215)
Abdominal pain	60%	81%	65%	60%	60%
Abdominal swelling	100%	53%	60%	53%	–
Anorexia/weight loss	76%	90%	65%	50%	61%
Fever	100%	96%	68%	90%	45%
Demonstrable ascites	100%	71%	50%	77%	100%
Abdominal mass(es)	?	53%	23%	3%	?
Positive tuberculin test	100%	100%	75%	30%	52%
Pleural TB, concomitant	32%	28%	20%	83%	23%
Pulmonary TB, concomitant	6%	19%	33%	?	7%

In these five series, a broad clinical picture may be derived. Among the most striking disparities are the inconsistencies in tuberculin reactivity and the coexistence of pulmonary or pleural tuberculosis.

little fluid, and laparoscopy is not available readily, a limited laparotomy is the safest and most likely means to establish the diagnosis (225–227). The tuberculin skin test has substantial risk of false negativity, but the chest x-ray may offer diagnostic guidance in the form of either pulmonary parenchymal or pleural abnormalities; in a recent series of abdominal tuberculosis from Taiwan, 22 of 27 patients (82%) had chest x-ray evidence of pulmonary tuberculosis (226).

Ileocecal tuberculosis commonly masquerades as idiopathic inflammatory bowel disease. Distinguishing tuberculosis from Crohn's disease involves such factors as identifying persons from groups at high risk of tuberculosis, uncovering prior histories of tuberculosis, tuberculin skin testing (if positive, it supports the diagnosis, but a negative skin test does not exclude tuberculosis), and identifying chest radiographic abnormalities suggestive of tuberculosis. Endoscopic examinations may reveal suggestive but not diagnostic morphologic findings (228); histologic demonstration of acid-fast bacilli and/or caseating granuloma would strongly support tuberculous etiology (229,230). A recent brief communication from India describes a colonoscopic technique wherein six to eight biopsies were taken at the same site in the cecum, creating a small well (231). The biopsy specimens were sent for histopathology, stain, and culture. Then a colonoscopic brush was introduced into the well, and brushings were obtained for AFB smear. Although only two of nine biopsies showed characteristics of tuberculosis, eight of nine brushings were smear positive, and *M. tuberculosis* was grown from seven of nine procedures.

A technique that has not been carefully studied but has considerable potential is culture of stool for mycobacteria. Our experience at the National Jewish Center in Denver among patients with active pulmonary tuberculosis has shown that stool cultures closely reflect sputum culture status *(unpublished data).* It therefore seems reasonable to culture stool from persons with ileocecitis. If positive for *M. tuberculosis* (or *M. bovis* in foreign-born persons), it would strongly suggest mycobacterial etiology.

Radiographic studies, including contrast examinations, unfortunately cannot distinguish between idiopathic and tuberculous inflammatory bowel disease (232,233). Among those in whom distinction between Crohn's and tuberculosis cannot be made, laparotomy offers the best chance for obtaining biopsy material with distinguishing histologic features and/or positive cultures (213,219,220). Although this invasive approach obviously entails hazard for the patient, failure to distinguish has considerable potential for morbidity, even mortality: steroids given inadvertently to a patient with tuberculosis may have dire consequences (213). Conversely, fear of tuberculosis may create reluctance to employ steroids suitably in those with idiopathic inflammatory bowel disease.

It should be noted that, in addition to infection localized to the ileum or cecum, tuberculosis may rarely involve other segments of the alimentary canal including the duodenum, ascending colon, and appendix (233).

The *management* of all forms of abdominal tuberculosis hinges on chemotherapy (234,235). Standard regimens should be initiated promptly in proven or highly suspected cases. Perhaps the only particular note of warning would be in patients with ileus/hypomotility, gross disease of the ileum, and/or interstitial fistulas to assure that there is adequate drug absorption (236). Some have recommended corticosteroids in an effort to diminish late fibrotic obstructive sequelae; two reports, one from India (217), the other from Saudi Arabia (237), suggested that corticosteroids reduced morbidity including late adhesions. However, these were nonrandomized series. Overall, this is probably a justifiable practice, but one that likely entails potential risks including masking of serious intra-abdominal pathology. Surgical extirpation of grossly distorted, obstructed bowel segments may be indicated if chemotherapy does not restore normal function (234).

Pericardial Tuberculosis

Pericardial tuberculosis is an uncommon form of XPTB in the United States, but because of the high probability of a complicated, lethal outcome if it is untreated (238,239), it is worth considering in detail.

Pathogenetically, most cases are believed to result from contiguous spread from subcarinal lymph nodes that abut the heart (240); occasionally, pericarditis is felt to arise during miliary dissemination or from direct spread from an adjacent pulmonary focus.

Epidemiologically, the number of cases seen in the United States recently has been so small that it is difficult to discern patterns. However, two of the more recent series noted an apparent predilection among blacks, one citing a 12:1 proportionality (239), the other a 10:1 ratio among a Veterans Administration Hospital population (241). In a region of South Africa, pericardial tuberculosis is seen so commonly that the condition has become known after the area, Transkei heart (242). Most of the patients are members of one of the major black tribes of South Africa, the Xhosa, the predominant population of this region. Curiously, unlike other reports of tuberculous pericarditis, the majority of patients in recent studies from this region (59%) have been women (243). HIV infection was not tested for in these trials; however, it is the impression of one of the participating clinicians that very few, if any, of the patients in these series were coinfected (244).

Clinically, pericardial tuberculosis patients tend to present complaining of the physiological consequences of their disease as well as the constitutional or inflammatory manifestations. Dyspnea is the most consistently reported symptom, around 80% in these series (239,241,245) and 54% in another (246). Other common findings in these reports were cough (38–94%), chest pain (39–76%), orthopnea (39–66%), night sweats (14–58%), and ankle swelling (36–55%). *Physical findings* varied modestly according to the stage of the effusion or constrictive process. The range of signs is displayed in Table 7.10.

Diagnosis may involve direct evidence of pericardial involvement such as bacteriological or histopathological study of pericardial tissue or fluid; alternatively, evidence of active tuberculosis elsewhere in the body strongly supports inference that the pericardial process is tuberculosis. Common laboratory findings include cardiomegaly (70–98%) and pleural effusion (39–71%) on chest x-rays as well as low voltage (19–35%) and T-wave inversion (77–99%) on ECG (239,241,242,247). A combination of electrocardiographic and chest radiographic abnormalities should alert clinicians to the possibility of pericardial tuberculosis. Documentation of pericarditis with effusion or thickening can be done with echocardiography, computed tomography, or magnetic resonance imaging; choice of these tests will be dependent on local facilities and expertise. If a reasonably assured diagnosis can be established by indirect means, it may not be necessary to perform pericardiocentesis unless impaired hemodynamics necessitates. However, in many cases, the diagnosis is elusive, and it is important to appreciate the yield from vari-

TABLE 7.10. *Clinical findings in patients presenting with tuberculous pericarditis*

	Series (ref.)				
Findings	Hageman et al. (241)	Rooney et al. (239)	Fowler (245)	Strang (243)	Strang (247)
Fever	73%	97%	83%	NS	NS
Paradoxical pulse	45%	23%	71%	29%	33%
Pericardial rub	41%	37%	84%	NS	NS
Tachycardia (>100)	68%	94%	83%	56%	73%
Neck vein distension	59%	46%	61%	74%	47%
Hepatomegaly	68%	63%	65%	76%	67%
Edema	64%	49%	39%	39%	24%
Ascites	34%	NS	NS	33%	31%

These series present a fairly consistent picture of pericarditis tuberculosis. However, clinicians must appreciate that only approximately one-third to two-thirds of the patients manifested any one of these individual signs.

ous diagnostic approaches. From the various series cited above, it becomes apparent that applying strict criteria such as recovery of tubercle bacilli from the pericardial fluid or tissue or demonstrating caseating granulomata from the pericardium will almost certainly result in failure to recognize a substantial portion of cases. Among the most important aspects of the two reports from South Africa is the frequency with which resected pericardium from patients eventually deemed to have tuberculosis failed to demonstrate classical findings associated with tuberculosis: only 11 of 32 (34%) and 33 of 47 (70%) specimens taken at admission manifested characteristic lesions, the remainder showing nonspecific pericarditis (243,247). The authors suggest that in the pathogenesis of tuberculous pericarditis, there is an evolutionary sequence with a transition from undistinguished fibrinous pericarditis toward the typical granulomatous pathology; however, they also note that tissue removed during late pericardiectomy for adhesive/constrictive disease or at necropsy also could appear bland. These findings emphasize that, despite appropriate steps, for some patients, no definitive evidence for tuberculous etiology can be obtained and a diagnosis by inference is to be made.

In series for which strict criteria mandated high yields, pericardial cultures were positive in 34 of 44 (77%) of the VA study (241) and 50% of the Brooklyn report (239). In other series, taking a broader approach to diagnosis, approximately 25% of pericardial cultures were reported positive (238,243,248,249). In the 1988 series from South Africa, the authors describe a new methodology that they believe enhanced their yield substantially, with 59% of specimens positive on culture (247). Because of the paucity of organisms, acid-fast bacilli are seen on smear of fluid very rarely. The pericardial fluid, when described, is usually exudative; cellular profiles and other findings such as protein or glucose have not been well described; when obtained by pericardiocentesis, the fluid may be bloody as a result of trauma associated with the procedure.

As noted above, histopathology of the resected pericardium usually, but not always, demonstrates characteristic findings. Among 49 patients whose pericardial fluid yielded *M. tuberculosis,* only 35 (71%) pericardial specimens showed findings classified typical for tuberculosis, while the remainder were nonspecific (247). Acid-fast bacilli were seen in only 2 of 47 admission biopsies in this series.

Obviously, the probability of a patient with pericarditis and nonspecific findings on biopsy having tuberculosis depends greatly on the prevalence of tuberculosis in the population. In South Africa, where tuberculosis is rampant among the black population, the prior probability is very high. By contrast, in a North American, white, upper class, HIV-negative, heavy cigarette smoker, the probabilities would favor neoplastic disease. By employing indirect and epidemiological evidence, a clinician may help overcome the lack of specificity of findings of pericardial fluid and tissue study.

The *management of tuberculous pericarditis* entails prompt initiation of chemotherapy for proven or highly suspicious cases. In the evolution of the pericardial response to tuberculosis, the risk of both acute and chronic complications escalates over time without treatment (241).

Two previously noted studies from South Africa showed significant benefit from early administration of corticosteroids (242,247). In these trials, adults with pericarditis received 20 mg three times daily for 4 weeks, then 10 mg three times daily for the next 4 weeks, then 5 mg three-times daily for weeks 9 and 10, then 5 mg daily for week 11. The first paper described the outcome in patients who presented with an unusual state which the authors termed active tuberculous constrictive pericarditis. These cases were marked by evidence of hemodynamic constrictive compromise but a normal or near-normal heart size on chest x-ray. The echocardiograms showed an amorphous collection in the pericardial space, not a large effusion or thick rind. Treatment with steroids compared to placebo resulted in significantly more rapid improvement of physiological parameters, improved functional status, reduced need for repeated pericardiocentesis, reduced deaths from acute pericarditis (4% versus 11%), and, diminished need for subsequent pericardiectomy (21% versus 30%). By contrast, the second series focused on patients with acute effusive pericarditis with enlarged cardiac silhouette on x-ray, the diagnosis confirmed by pericardiocentesis. The study employed two randomized comparisons: (a) early and complete open surgical drainage of pericardial fluid versus percutaneous pericardiocentesis as needed, and (b) initial prednisolone versus placebo. Steroid therapy was associated with both reduced need for subsequent surgical pericardiectomy, 8% versus 12%, and deaths from acute pericarditis, 3% versus 14%.

In the 1988 study of acute, effusive pericarditis, complete open-surgical drainage was not shown to be advantageous compared to closed pericardiocentesis (247). Although substernal pericardiotomy and suction drainage under general anesthesia did reduce the requirement for subsequent drainage by pericardiocentesis, it did not reduce the need to perform pericardiectomy for subsequent constrictive dysfunction or the risk of death. Because only 9% of the patients in the study required serial pericardiocentesis (in part because of the use of steroids), the authors did not generally advocate the open procedure.

Overall, at the end of 24 months of observation, those receiving steroids had higher rates of favorable status (94% vs. 85% in the 1987 study and 96% vs. 84% in the 1988 report patients who had not undergone open drainage). However, it is important to emphasize that, in spite of prompt chemotherapy and intensive corticosteroid therapy, modest numbers of patients with tuberculous pericarditis will still require pericardiectomy to restore acceptable cardiac function (246). The timing of this surgery is important: done too early, it is difficult to strip away the tuberculous debris efficiently; done too late, the fused pericardium becomes intensely adherent to the myocardium. For patients with subacute fibrocaseous inflammation, as demonstrated by echocardiography or other imaging techniques, one of the authors of the South African studies recommends the following: commence chemotherapy and corticosteroids; if there is no substantial improvement of the cardiac impairment by 4 to 6 weeks, undertake the pericardiectomy (250).

Other Sites

Other sites of extrapulmonary tuberculosis are diverse, but because of their relative infrequency are infrequently seen in the United States. *Upper respiratory tract disease* is most often a complication of pulmonary tuberculosis, the result of bathing these structures in sputum laden with mycobacteria. Laryngeal disease typically occurs during prolonged chronic tuberculosis; prompt and effective treatment of acute pulmonary disease usually prevents laryngeal involvement. Rarely, the larynx may be involved without overt lung disease (251,252). Manifestations of laryngeal tuberculosis include dysphonia, hoarseness, and referred ear pain. Hoarseness and dysphonia in patients with pulmonary tuberculosis has occasionally been reported in association with vocal cord paralysis caused by mediastinal entrapment of the recurrent laryngeal nerve, not laryngitis (253). Morphologically, tuberculous laryngitis may resemble carcinoma (254). Other sites in the upper respiratory tract involved by tuberculosis include the middle ear, mastoids, nasopharynx, nasal turbinates, tonsils, and tongue (255,256). Tuberculous retropharyngeal masses secondary to cervical spine osteomyelitis may also present with pain, swelling, and disturbance of phonation and breathing (80,83).

Ocular tuberculosis, an infrequent occurrence, is seen most commonly in disseminated infection in the form of choroidal tubercles (see above). Tuberculosis may result in localized retinal, uveal, corneal, scleral, or panophthalmic pathology (257). Eales' disease consists of retinal periphlebitis, vitreous hemorrhage, and retinal neovascularization (258,259). It is not clear if this reflects true infection or a remote hypersensitivity effect. External structures including the conjunctiva, lid, and orbit have been noted only rarely to be involved.

The *skin* may be involved in various ways by tuberculosis. Lupus vulgaris is a chronic tuberculous infection of the skin manifested classically by low-grade inflammation, nodules, plaques, and fissures; it is often but not universally seen in association with pulmonary tuberculosis (260). It has been noted to occur as the sole manifestation of, or in relation to, XPTB at other sites (261). Lupus vulgaris is believed to reflect hematogenous implantation and should be distinguished from cold abscesses of the skin caused by contiguous spread from an underlying focus (262). Another form of cutaneous disease is induced by direct inoculation (263). Generalized miliary tuberculosis of the skin has been noted to occur as part of acute disseminated tuberculosis in both children and adults (264). Clinically, it may present with a mixture of papulovesicular, pustular, macular, purpuric, and nodular lesions; rarely do frank abscesses form (265).

In addition to these forms, which entail overt local infections with tubercle bacilli, there are cutaneous "id" reactions such as erythema nodosum, erythema induratum, and erythema annulare centrifugum, which are believed to represent hypersensitivity reactions to the bacillus, not true infection (260,266,267). A recent study from Finland described a diverse array of skin manifestations including both hypersensitivity phenomena and true infections with *M. tuberculosis* and other slow-growing mycobacteria (268).

Glandular involvement by tuberculosis is infrequent and pleomorphic. Although several patients in Addison's original series had tuberculosis of the adrenal glands, such disease is rare in Europe and North America today. Adrenal glands are most commonly involved as part of disseminated disease; however, the involvement rarely results in adrenal insufficiency (130). Chronic inflammation can cause calcification of the glands; acutely, they typically are enlarged in a nondescript manner. Potentially confusing is the observation that rifampin may provoke an Addisonian-like reaction among small numbers of patients being treated with this agent; this is believed to represent induction by rifampin of hepatic cytochrome P450 pathways causing accelerated breakdown of endogenous corticosteroids, thus unmasking borderline adrenal function (see Chapter 10 for details). Invasive disease of the thyroid (269,270), thymus (271), breast (272) and pancreas (273) have been reported recently.

The *liver* is commonly involved as part of miliary or disseminated tuberculosis. Less commonly, localized abscesses of the hepatic parenchyma have been noted, presenting as fever of unknown origin (274,275). Biliary tract compression by tuberculous lymphadenitis of the peri-pancreatic or portal lymph nodes has been recorded (276,277). Granulomatous hepatitis, an illness typically involving cholestatic liver chemistry abnormalities with or without constitutional symptoms is rarely caused by tuberculosis; among 88 patients seen at the Mayo Clinic with this complex, only 3 were due to tuberculosis (278). One case of tuberculous cholecystitis was recently reported (279).

Very rare manifestations of tuberculosis include esophageal involvement with external compression by mediastinal lymph nodes (280) and tracheoesophageal fistula (281). Relief of tuberculous obstruction of the esophagus by a course of corticosteroids (282) and primary esophageal tuberculosis resembling carcinoma (283) have been described. Tuberculous invasion of the aorta with or without aneurysm has been noted to occur due both to bacetermic seeding of the vessel and invasion from abutting structures (284,285). A recent report suggests that tuberculous pyomyositis occurring at a site of trauma in a patient with pulmonary tuberculosis is an example of locus minoris resistentiae (286). Tuberculous myositis of paraspinous muscles, associated with constipation and fever in a 7-year-old child (287) and fever and back pain in a renal transplant recipient (288), have been noted, as well.

CORTICOSTEROID THERAPY FOR XPTB

Contemporary to the discovery of modern antituberculosis medications was the evolving understanding of the physiology of pituitary–adrenal axis. Having recognized the anti-inflammatory effects of both adrenocorticotropic hormone (ACTH) and synthetic analogues to cortisol, researchers began to explore the utility of these agents in tuberculosis. Based on adverse consequences when steroid therapy was used in

TABLE 7.11. *Selected reports of steroid therapy for tuberculous meningitis*

			Observations			
Report	Patients	Steroid therapy	LAB	Acute	Chronic	Comments
Ashby (293)	6 control, 6 treated	Cortisone, 100 mg qd for months, tapered over 12 days	Rapid ↓ in CSF cells	"Striking and early clinical improvement"	Controls: 1 death and 3 sequelae, Treated: no complications	Treated after INH and SM
Voljavec (294)	17 control, 16 treated	Cortisone, 2.3 to 3.2 mg/kg body weight; prednisone in unstated doses; mean duration, 34 days	N.S.	N.S.	Controls: 9/17 died Treated: 3/16 died	Adults and children, all "Negroes"
O'Toole (295)	18 control, 19 treated	Dexamethasone, 9 mg/day for 1 week, then tapered final week.	More rapid return to normal of CSF cells, sugar, and protein.	At day 4, 5 of 5 controls had to ↑ OP; only 1 of 7 treated with ↑ OP	Controls: 9 of 12 died (75%) Treated: 6 of 11 died (55%)	Many early deaths, other 2% to adrenal TBM at presentation
Escobar (292)	36 control, 36 treated	Prednisone, 1 or 10 mg/kg/day, tapered 10 mg/kg dose ↓ over 30 days	N.S.	N.S.	Calculated mortality rates from 99 TBM patients; modest survival advantage for steroids.	Prednisone, 1 mg equal to 10 mg/kg.
Girgis (296)	70 control, 66 treated	Dexamethasone, 8–12 mg/day for 21 days	N.S.	N.S.: early deaths reduced number of observations	Controls: 7 of 28 developed ocular complications (atrophy) Treated: 2 of 27 with optic atrophy.	42 of 70 control subjects (60%) died; 39 of 66 (59%) of treated died.
Girgis (186)	85 control, 75 treated	Adults: dexamethasone, 12 mg/day Children: 8 mg/day, tapered over 6 weeks	More rapid normalization of CSF glucose, protein, and cells	Fatalities greater in controls (59%) than in treated (43%) ($p < 0.04$)	If patients survived first 10 days, saw greater benefit with steroids, deaths in 14% vs. 33%.	Also, saw ↓ sequelae with steroids: 6 vs. 13 patients.
Kumarvelu (187)	23 control, 24 treated	Dexamethasone, 16 mg/day for 7 days; then 8 qd for 21 days.	N.S.	Faster recovery of sensorium and higher mental functions with treatment	No significant differences but a trend toward survival and milder sequelae with treatment	Overall good outcome at 3 mos: controls = 13/21, treated = 15/20

None of these studies had ideal design or methodology. However, in the aggregate, they point toward diminished morbidity and mortality when patients with TBM receive corticosteroids. Because of the critical effects of swelling within the rigid cranial enclosure, I believe that steroids—unless clearly contraindicated—should be administered to patients with proven or suspected TBM.

OP, opening pressure.

animal models of tuberculosis, the American Trudeau Society—predecessor to the American Thoracic Society—sounded a cautionary note in 1952 (289). However, based on some encouraging reports from Europe, Johnson and Davey reviewed the issue in 1954 and concluded that, when steroids were given with streptomycin, beneficial effects were seen without unfavorable sequelae (290).

The most extensive use of steroids initially was for patients with pulmonary disease. An excellent review of this literature was recently published, describing 12 prospective randomized trials (291). Briefly, the authors noted that there were broad and consistent observations of faster defervescence, weight gain, and radiographic clearing among steroid recipients; however, no long-term benefits were seen in terms of preservation of pulmonary function or cure rates.

Therefore, attention turned to the use of steroid therapy for various forms of XPTB. The two forms of tuberculosis in which such adjunctive treatment appears most protective are meningeal/CNS and pericardial disease.

The most compelling case for steroids can be made for meningitis. Dooley, Carpenter, and Rademacher put data from seven trials into tabular form; I have deleted one of these studies for lack of data and added a more recent report. These articles are summarized in Table 7.11. Briefly, because of the relatively small numbers in most of the studies, statistically significant differences were reported in only two (186,292) of the reports (187,292–296). However, as with the pulmonary studies, there were broad and generally consistent favorable trends. Certainly, the studies do not permit one to choose optimal agents, dosages, or durations. However, they do support the utility of steroids in reducing morbidity and mortality with TBM. Although it has been stated that the benefits are seen only in patients with clinical stage II or III disease, I am not persuaded by the reports that this is the case. Hence, I continue to advocate steroids for all cases of TBM.

The other form of XPTB for which steroids appear of utility is pericardial disease. As noted in the text, two large studies from South Africa demonstrated statistically significant efficacy in reducing morbidity with marginal benefits in terms of mortality. An earlier, nonrandomized series from Brooklyn reported a dramatic difference in mortality, with deaths among four of ten who did not receive steroids versus 0 of 18 who did (239).

Pleural tuberculosis may be ameliorated by steroids, as well (see above). As in pulmonary disease, early reduction in fever, dyspnea, and volume of effusion has been reported. However, no consistent long-term benefits in terms of pleural thickening or pulmonary function have been shown. Although one additional recent randomized study did not demonstrate any favorable effects from steroids in reducing pleural fibrosis (62), it should be noted that two earlier reports did indicate lessened pleural thickening (297,298). On balance, this therapy should probably be reserved for patients with large effusions, dyspnea, and/or disabling chest pain. However, I do not believe the available information rigorously excludes potential benefits from steroids.

In summary, there is a considerable body of literature demonstrating the capacity of steroids to ameliorate the inflammatory manifestations of tuberculosis (299). In some forms of XPTB, there appears to be significant curtailment of morbidity and even mortality. In other situations, the benefits appear more palliative or temporary. However, I think it behooves clinicians who see predictable numbers of tuberculous patients to familiarize themselves with this material.

REFERENCES

1. Hirschmann JV. Fever of unknown origin in adults. *Clin Infect Dis* 1997;24:291–302.
2. Arnow PM, Flaherty JP. Fever of unknown origin. *Lancet* 1997;350:575–580.
3. Zumla A, James DG. Granulomatous infections: etiology and classification. *Clin Infect Dis* 1996;23:146–158.
4. Meylan P, Richman DD, Kornbluth RS. Reduced intracellular growth of mycobacteria in human macrophages at physiologic oxygen pressure. *Am Rev Respir Dis* 1992;145:947–953.
5. Rieder HL, Snider DE, Cauthen GM. Extrapulmonary tuberculosis in the United States. *Am Rev Respir Dis* 1990;141:347–351.
6. Cowie RL, Sharpe JW. Extra-pulmonary tuberculosis: a high frequency in the absence of HIV infection. *Int J Tuberc Lung Dis* 1997;1:159–162.

7. Farer LS, Lowell AM, Meador MP. Extrapulmonary tuberculosis in the United States. *Am J Epidemiol* 1979;109:205–217.
8. Baydur A. The spectrum of extrapulmonary tuberculosis. *West J Med* 1977;126:253–262.
9. Weir MR, Thorton GF. Extrapulmonary tuberculosis. Experiences of a community hospital and review of the literature. *Am J Med* 1985;79:467–478.
10. Grzybowski S, Allen EA. History and importance of scrofula. *Lancet* 1995;346:1472–1474.
11. Yew WW, Lee J. Pathogenesis of cervical tuberculous lymphadenitis: pathways to anatomic localization. *Tuberc Lung Dis* 1995;76:275–278.
12. Wolinsky E. Mycobacterial lymphadenitis in children: a prospective study of 105 nontuberculous cases with long-term follow-up. *Clin Infect Dis* 1995;20:954–963.
13. Artenstein AW, Kim JH, Williams WJ, Chung RCY. Isolated peripheral tuberculous lymphadenitis in adults: current clinical and diagnostic issues. *Clin Infect Dis* 1995;20:876–882.
14. Silveric P, Steel SJ. Mediastinal lymphatic gland tuberculosis in Asian and coloured immigrants. *Lancet* 1961;1:1254–1256.
15. Farrow PR, Jones DA, Stanley PJ, Bonley JS, Wales JM, Cookson JB. Thoracic lymphadenopathy in Asians resident in the United Kingdom: role of mediastinoscopy in initial diagnosis. *Thorax* 1985;40: 121–124.
16. Chang SC, Lee PY, Perug RP. Clinical role of bronchoscopy in adults with intrathoracic tuberculous lymphadenopathy. *Chest* 1988;93:314–317.
17. Im JG, Song KS, Kang KS, Park JH, Yeon KM, Han MC. Mediastinal tuberculous lymphadenitis: CT manifestations. *Radiology* 1987;164:115–119.
18. Khan J, Akhtar M, von Sinner WN, Bouchama A, Bazarbashi M. CT-guided fine needle aspiration biopsy in the diagnosis of mediastinal tuberculosis. *Chest* 1994;106:1329–1332.
19. Chin Y-M, Lee P-Y, Su W-J, Perug R-P. Lymph node tuberculosis: 7-year experience in Veterans General Hospital, Taipei, Taiwan. *Tuberc Lung Dis* 1992;73: 368–371.
20. Case records. Case 5-1997. *N Engl J Med* 1997;336: 492–499.
21. McClusky DR, Buckley MRE, McCluggage WG. Night sweats and swollen glands. *Lancet* 1998;351: 722.
22. Weiden PL, Bauermeister DE, Fatta EA. An Asian man with enlarged glands. *Lancet* 1998;351:1098.
23. Peel MM, Palmer GG, Stacpoole AM, Kerr TG. Human lympadenitis due to *Corynebacterium pseudotuberculosis:* report of ten cases from Australia and review. *Clin Infect Dis* 1997;24:185–191.
24. Lai KK, Stottmeier KD, Sherman IH, McCabe WR. Mycobacterial cervical lymphadenopathy. Relationship of etiologic agents to age. *JAMA* 1984;251: 1286–1288.
25. Pang SC. Mycobacterial lymphadenitis in Western Australia. *Tuberc Lung Dis* 1992;73:362–367.
26. Cantrall RW, Hensen JH, Reid D. Diagnosis and management of tuberculous cervical adenitis. *Arch Otolaryngol* 1975;101:53–57.
27. Ord RF, Matz GJ. Tuberculous cervical lymphadenitis. *Arch Otolaryngol* 1974;99:327–329.
28. Hsu K. Atypical mycobacterial infections in children. *Rev Infect Dis* 1981;3:1075–1080.
29. von Reyn CF, Barber TW, Arbeit RD, et al. Evidence of previous infection with *Mycobacterium avium–Mycobacterium intracellulare* complex among healthy subjects: an international study of dominant mycobacterial skin test reactions. *J Infect Dis* 1993;168:1553–1558.
30. Pinder SE, Colville A. Mycobacterial cervical adenitis in children: can histological assessment help differentiate infections caused by non-tuberculois mycobacteria from *Mycobacterium tuberculosis*? *Histopathology* 1993;22:59–64.
31. American Thoracic Society. Treatment of tuberculosis and tuberculosis infection in adults and children. *Am J Respir Crit Care Med* 1994;149:1359–1374.
32. British Thoracic Society Research Committee. Short course chemotherapy for lymph node tuberculosis. Final report at 5 years. *Br J Dis Chest* 1988;82: 282–284.
33. Byrd RB, Bopp RK, Gracey DR, Puritz EM. The role of surgery in tuberculosis lymphadenitis in adults. *Am Rev Respir Dis* 1971;103:816–820.
34. Campbell IA, Dyson AJ. Lymph node tuberculosis: a comparison of various methods of treatment. *Tubercle* 1977;58:171–179.
35. Malik SK, Behera D, Gilhotra R. Tuberculous pleural effusion and lymphadenitis treated with rifampin-containing regimen. *Chest* 1987;92:904–905.
36. Dutt A, Moers D, Stead W. Short-course chemotherapy for extrapulmonary tuberculosis. *Ann Intern Med* 1986;104:7–12.
37. Stead WW, Eichenholz A, Strauss HK. Operative and pathological findings in twenty-four patients with the syndrome of idiopathic pleurisy with effusion presumably tuberculosis. *Am Rev Tuberc* 1955;71: 473–502.
38. Abrams WB, Small MJ. Current concepts of tuberculous pleurisy as derived from pleural biopsy studies. *Scand J Respir Dis* 1960;38:60–65.
39. Centers for Disease Control and Prevention. *Reported tuberculosis in the United States, 1997.* Atlanta: CDC, 1998.
40. Antoniskis D, Amin K, Barnes PF. Pleuritis as a manifestation of reactivation tuberculosis. *Am J Med* 1990;89:447–450.
41. Berger HW, Mejia E. Tuberculous pleurisy. *Chest* 1973;63:88–92.
42. Matthay RA, Neff TA, Iseman MD. Tuberculous pleural effusions developing during chemotherapy in pulmonary tuberculosis. *Am Rev Respir Dis* 1974;109: 469–472.
43. Seibert AF, Haynes J, Middleton R, Bass JB. Tuberculous pleural effusion. Twenty year experience. *Chest* 1991;99:883–886.
44. Sahn SA. State of the art. The pleura. *Am Rev Respir Dis* 1988;138:184–234.
45. Baganha MF, Pego A, Lima MA, Gaspar EV, Cordeiro AR. Serum and pleural adenasive deaminase. Correlation with lymphocyte populations. *Chest* 1990;97: 605–610.
46. Gakis C. Adenosine draminase in pleural effusions (Letter). *Chest* 1995;107:1772–1773.
47. Ungerer JPJ, Oosthuizen HM, Retief JH, Bissbort SH. Significance of adenosine deaminase activity and its

isoenzymes in tuberculous effusions. *Chest* 1994;106: 33–37.
48. Ocana I, Martinez-Vazquez JM, Ribera E, Segura RM, Pascual C. Adenosine deaminase activity in the diagnosis of lymphocytic pleural effusions of tuberculous neoplastic, and lymphomatous origin. *Tubercle* 1986;67:141–145.
49. Valdes L, San Jose E, Alvarez D, et al. Diagnosis of tuberculous pleurisy using the biologic parameters adenosine deaminase, lysozyme, and interferon gamma. *Chest* 1993;103:458–460.
50. Strankinga WFM, Nauta JJP, Straub JP, Stam J. Adenosine deaminase activity in tuberculous pleural effusions: a diagnostic test. *Tubercle* 1987;68: 137–140.
51. Banales JL, Pineda PR, Fitzgerald JM, Rubio H, Selman M, Salazar-Lazama M. Adenosine deaminase in the diagnosis of tuberculous pleural effusions. *Chest* 1991;99:355–357.
52. van Keimpema ARJ, Slaats EH, Wagenaar JPM. Adenosine deaminase activity, not diagnostic for tuberculous pleurisy. *Eur J Respir Dis* 1987;71:15–18.
53. Hara N, Abe M, Inuzuka S, Kawara Y, Shigematsu N. Pleural SC5b-9 in differential diagnosis of tuberculous, malignant, and other effusions. *Chest* 1992; 102:1060–1064.
54. Fontan-Bueso J, Verea Hernando H, Perez Garcia Buela JP, Dominguez-Juncal L, Martin Egana MT, Montero Martinez MC. Diagnostic value of simultaneous determination of pleural adenosine deaminase and pleural lysozyme/serum lysozyme ratio in pleural effusions. *Chest* 1988;93:303–307.
55. Ito M, Kojiro N, Shirosaka T, Moriwaki Y, Tachibana I, Kokubu T. Elevated levels of soluble interleukin-2 receptors in tuberculous pleural effusions. *Chest* 1990;97:1141–1143.
56. Chang S-C, Hsu Y-T, Chen Y-C, Lin C-Y. Usefulness of soluble interleukin 2 receptor in differentiating tuberculous and carcinomatous pleural effusions. *Arch Intern Med* 1994;143:1097–1101.
57. DeWit D, Maartens G, Steyn L. A comparable study of the polymerase chain reaction and conventional procedures for the diagnosis of tuberculous pleural effusions. *Tubercle* 1992;73:262–267.
58. deLassence A, Lecassier D, Pieere C, Cadrenel J, Sttern M, Hance AJ. Detection of mycobacterial DNA in pleural fluid from patients with tuberculous pleurisy by means of polymerase chain reaction: comparison of two protocols. *Thorax* 1992;47:265–269.
59. Querol JM, Mínguez J, García-Sánchez E, Farga MA, Gimeno C, García-de-Lomas J. Rapid diagnosis of pleural tuberculosis by polymerase chain reaction. *Am J Respir Crit Care Med* 1995;152:1977–1981.
60. Harris RJ, Kavuru MS, Rice TW, Kirby TJ. The diagnostic and therapeutic utility of thoracoscopy. A review. *Chest* 1995;108:828–841.
61. Yim AP. Thoracoscopic management of pleural effusions (Letter). *Chest* 1995;108:1765.
62. Wyser C, Walzl G, Smedema JP, Swart F, van Schalkwyk WM, van de Wal BW. Corticosteroids in the treatment of tuberculous pleurisy. A double-blind, placebo-controlled, randomized study. *Chest* 1996;110:333–338.
63. Lee C-H, Wang W-J, Lan R-S, Tsai Y-H, Chiang Y-C. Corticosteroids in the treatment of tuberculous pleurisy. *Chest* 1988;94:1256–1259.
64. Iseman MD, Madsen LA. Chronic tuberculous empyema with bronchopleural fistula resulting in treatment failure and progressive drug resistance. *Chest* 1991;100:124–127.
65. Elliott AM, Berning SE, Iseman MD, Peloquin CA. Failure of drug penetration and acquisition of drug resistance in chronic tuberculous empyema. *Tuberc Lung Dis* 1995;76:463–467.
66. Neff TA, Buchanan BD. Tension pleural effusion. A delayed complication of pneumothorax therapy in tuberculosis. *Am Rev Respir Dis* 1975;14:543–598.
67. Schmid FG, De Halter R. Late exudative complications of collapse therapy for pulmonary tuberculosis. *Chest* 1986;89:822–827.
68. Pomerantz M. Surgery for tuberculosis. In: Pomerantz M, ed. *Challenging pulmonary infections.* Philadelphia: WB Saunders, 1993:723–727.
69. Christensen WI. Genito-urinary tuberculosis: review of 102 cases. *Medicine* 1974;53:377–390.
70. Horne NW. Renal tuberculosis. *BJ Hosp Med* 1975;14:158–169.
71. Simon HB, Weinstein AJ, Pasternak MS, Swartz M, Kunz LF. Genitourinary tuberculosis. Clinical features in a general hospital population. *Am J Med* 1977; 63:410–420.
72. Schwartz DT, Lattimer JK. The incidence of arterial hypertension in 540 patients with renal tuberculosis. *J Urol* 1968;98:651–652.
73. Gow JG. The management of patients suffering from genito-urinary tuberculosis by short course chemotherapy and early surgery. A several year review. *Bull Int Union Against Tuberc* 1979;54:298–299.
74. Sutherland AM. Tuberculosis of the female genital tract. *Tubercle* 1985;66:79–83.
75. Centers for Disease Control. *Tuberculosis statistics in the United States.* Atlanta: CDC, 1992.
76. Colmenero JD, Jiménez-Mejías ME, Sánchez-Lora FJ, et al. Pyogenic, tuberculous, and brucellar vertebral osteomyelitis: a descriptive and comparative study of 219 cases. *Ann Rheum Dis* 1997;56:709–715.
77. Hoffman FB, Crosier JG, Cremin BF. Imaging in children with spinal tuberculosis. *J Bone Joint Surg [Br]* 1993;75-B:233–239.
78. Omari B, Robertson JM, Nelson RF, Chiu LC. Pott's disease. A resurgent challenge to the thoracic surgeon. *Chest* 1989;95:145–150.
79. Marcq M, Sharma OP. Tuberculosis of the spine: A reminder. *Chest* 1973;63:403–408.
80. Wurtz R, Quader Z, Simon D, Langer B. Cervical tuberculous vertebral osteomyelitis: case report and discussion of the literature. *Clin Infect Dis* 1993;16: 806–808.
81. Kennedy N, McKendrick MW, Forster DMC, Douglas DL. Pott's paraplegia today (Letter). *Lancet* 1995; 346:899.
82. Wilkinson IMS, Lascelles RG. An unusual neurological manifestation of tuberculosis. *Br Med J* 1973;2: 697–698.
83. Al Soub H. Retropharyngeal abscess associated with tuberculosis of the cervical spine. *Tuberc Lung Dis* 1996;77:563–565.
84. Pouchot J, Vinceneux P, Barge J, et al. Tuberculosis of the sacroiliac joint: clinical features, outcome, and evaluation of closed needle biopsy in 11 consecutive cases. *Am J Med* 1988;84:622–628.

85. Berney S, Goldstein M, Bishko F. Clinical and diagnostic features of tuberculous arthritis. *Am J Med* 1992;53:36–42.
86. Tokumoto J, Follansbee S, Jacobs R. Prosthetic joint infection due to *Mycobacterium tuberculosis*. Report of three cases. *Clin Infect Dis* 1995;21:134–136.
87. Adler BD, Padley SPG, Mueller NL. Tuberculosis of the chest wall: CT findings. *Comput Assist Tomagr* 1993;17:271–273.
88. Mall JC, Genant HK, Gamsu G. Multifocal tuberculosis of the ribs. *Am Rev Respir Dis* 1976;114:635–637.
89. Ip M, Tsui E, Wong KL, Jones B, Pung CF, Ngan H. Disseminated skeletal tuberculosis with skull involvement. *Tuberc Lung Dis* 1993;74:211–214.
90. Rubinstein EM, Lehman T. Sternal osteomyelitis due to *Mycobacterium tuberculosis* following coronary artery bypass surgery. *Clin Infect Dis* 1996;23: 202–203.
91. Wilkinson AG, Roy S. Two cases of Poncet's disease. *Tubercle* 1984;65:301–303.
92. Dal L, Long L, Stanford J. Poncet's disease: tuberculous rheumatism. *Rev Infect Dis* 1989;11:105–107.
93. Vermani A, Agarwal A, Murali MV, Iyer PU. An unusual manifestation of tuberculous hypersensitivity. *Tubercle* 1989;70:65–67.
94. Perez C, Torroba L, Gonzalez M, Vives R, Guarch R. Unusual presentation of tuberculous rheumatism (Poncet's disease) with oral ulcers and tuberculid. *Clin Infect Dis* 1998;26:1003–1004.
95. Klofkorn RW, Steigerwald JC. Carpal tunnel syndrome as the initial manifestation of tuberculosis. *Am J Med* 1976;60:583–586.
96. Wallace R, Cohen AS. Tuberculous arthritis. A report of two cases with review of biopsy and synovial fluid findings. *Am J Med* 1976;61:277–282.
97. Kostman J, Rush P, Reginato A. Granulomatous tophaceous gout mimicking tuberculous tenosynovitis: report of two cases. *Clin Infect Dis* 1995;21:217–219.
98. Smith JW, Piercy EA. Infectious arthritis. *Clin Infect Dis* 1995;20:225–231.
99. Desai SS. Early diagnosis of spinal tuberculosis by MRI. *J Bone Joint Surg* 1994;76:863–869.
100. Perronne C, Saba J, Behloul Z, et al. Pyogenic and tuberculous spondylodiskitis (vertebral osteomyelitis) in 80 adult patients. *Clin Infect Dis* 1994;19:746–750.
101. Miller JD. Pott's paraplegia today (Comment). *Lancet* 1995;346:264.
102. Twelfth Report of the Medical Research Council Working Party on Tuberculosis of the Spine. Controlled trial of short-course regimens of chemotherapy in the ambulatory treatment of spinal tuberculosis. Results at three years in Korea. *J Bone Joint Surg [Br]* 1992;75-B:240–248.
103. Leong JCY. Tuberculosis of the spine (Editorial). *J Bone Joint Surg [Br]* 1993;75-B:173–175.
104. Smith IE, Laroche CM, Jamieson SA, Shneerson JM. Kyphosis secondary to tuberculosis osteomyelitis as a cause of ventilatory failure. Clinical features, mechanisms, and management. *Chest* 1996;110:1105–1110.
105. Rajeswari R, Balasubramanian R, Venkatesan P, et al. Short-course chemotherapy in the treatment of Pott's paraplegia: report on five year follow-up. *Int J Tuberc Lung Dis* 1997;1:152–158.
106. Rajeswari R, Ranjani R, Santha T, Sriram K, Prabhakar R. Late onset paraplegia—a sequela to Pott's disease. A report on imaging, prevention and management. *Int J Tuberc Lung Dis* 1997;1:468–473.
107. Dwyer AP. Late onset Pott's paraplegia. *Int J Tuberc Lung Dis* 1997;1:387–388.
108. Shaw BA. Pott's disease with paraparesis. *N Engl J Med* 1996;334:958–959.
109. Sahn SA, Neff TA. Miliary tuberculosis. *Am J Med* 1974;56:495–505.
110. Munt PW. Miliary tuberculosis in the chemotherapy era: with a clinical review in 69 American adults. *Medicine* 1972;51:139–155.
111. Biehl JP. Miliary tuberculosis. A review of sixty-eight adult patients admitted to a municipal general hospital. *Am Rev Respir Dis* 1958;77:605.
112. Chapman CB, Whorton CM. Acute generalized miliary tuberculosis in adults. A clinicopathological study based on sixty-three cases diagnosed at autopsy. *N Engl J Med* 1946;235:239.
113. Gelb AF, Leffler C, Brewin A, Mascatello V, Lyons HA. Miliary tuberculosis. *Am Rev Respir Dis* 1973; 108:1327–1333.
114. Kwong JS, Carignan S, Kang E-Y, Müller NL, FitzGerald JM. Miliary tuberculosis. Diagnostic accuracy of chest radiography. *Chest* 1996;110:339–342.
115. Im J-G, Itoh H, Shim Y-S, et al. Pulmonary tuberculosis: CT findings—early active disease and sequential change with antituberculous therapy. *Radiology* 1993;186:653–660.
116. Lee KS, Im J-G. CT in adults with tuberculosis of the chest: characteristic findings and role in management. *Am J Radiol* 1995;164:1361–1367.
117. McGuinness G, Naidich DP, Jagirdar J, Leitman B, McCauley DI. High resolution CT findings in miliary lung disease. *J Comput Assist Tomogr* 1992;16:384–390.
118. Optican RF, Ost A, Ravin CE. High-resolution computed tomography in the diagnosis of miliary tuberculosis. *Chest* 1992;102:941–943.
119. Maartens G, Wilcox PA, Benetar SR. Miliary tuberculosis: rapid diagnosis, hematologic abnormalities and outcome in 109 treated adults. *Am J Med* 1990;89:291–296.
120. Grieco MN, Chmel H. Acute disseminated tuberculosis as a diagnostic problem. A clinical study based on twenty-eight cases. *Am Rev Respir Dis* 1974;109:554–560.
121. Lombard EH, Mansvelt EPG. Haematological changes associated with miliary tuberculosis of the bone marrow. *Tuberc Lung Dis* 1993;74:131–135.
122. Glasser RM, Walker RI, Herion JC. The significance of hematologic abnormalities in patients with tuberculosis. *Arch Intern Med* 1970;125:691–695.
123. Katzen H, Spagnolo SV. Bone marrow necrosis from miliary tuberculosis. *JAMA* 1980;244:2438–2439.
124. Godwin JE, Coleman A, Sahn SA. Miliary tuberculosis presenting as hepatic and renal failure. *Chest* 1991;99:752–754.
125. Goldfine ID, Schacter H, Barclay WR, Kingdom HS. Consumption coagulopathy in miliary tuberculosis. *Ann Intern Med* 1969;71:775–777.
126. Homan W, Harman E, Braun NMT, Felton CP, King TKC, Smith JP. Miliary tuberculosis presenting as acute respiratory failure: treatment by membrane oxygenator and ventricle pump. *Chest* 1975;67:366–369.

127. Huseby J, Hudson LD. Miliary tuberculosis and adult respiratory distress syndrome. *Ann Intern Med* 1976; 85:609–611.
128. Murray HW, Tuazon CU, Kimoni N, Sheagren JN. The adult respiratory distress syndrome associated with miliary tuberculosis. *Chest* 1978;73:37–43.
129. Rosenberg MJ, Rumans LW. Survival of a patient with pancytopenia and disseminated coagulation associated with miliary tuberculosis. *Chest* 1978;73:536–539.
130. Slavin RE, Walsh TJ, Pollock AD. Late generalized tuberculosis: a clinical pathological analysis and comparison of 100 cases in the pre-antibiotic and antibiotic eras. *Medicine* 1980;59:352–366.
131. So SY, Yu D. The adult respiratory distress syndrome associated with miliary tuberculosis. *Tubercle* 1981; 62:49–53.
132. Dyer RA, Chappell WA, Potgieter PD. Adult respiratory distress syndrome associated with miliary tuberculosis. *Crit Care Med* 1985;13:12–15.
133. Piqueras AR, Marruecos L, Artigas A, Rodriquez C. Miliary tuberculosis and adult respiratory distress syndrome. *Intens Care Med* 1987;13:175–182.
134. Lintin SN, Isaac PA. Miliary tuberculosis presenting as adult respiratory distress syndrome. *Intens Care Med* 1988;14:672–674.
135. Heap MJ, Bion JF, Hunter KR. Miliary tuberculosis and the adult respiratory distress syndrome. *Respir Med* 1989;83:153–156.
136. Sydow M, Schauer A, Crozier TA, Burchardi H. Multiple organ failure in generalized disseminated tuberculosis. *Respir Med* 1992;86:517–519.
137. Case Records of the Massachusetts General Hospital. Case 23-1995. *N Engl J Med* 1995;333:241–248.
138. Prout S, Benatar SR. Disseminated tuberculosis. A study of 62 cases. *S Afr Med J* 1980;58:835–842.
139. Illingsworth RS, Wright T. Tubercles of the choroid. *Br Med J* 1948;2:365–368.
140. Long R, O'Connor R, Palayew M, Hershfield E, Manfreda J. Disseminated tuberculosis with and without a miliary pattern on chest radiograph: a clinical–pathologic–radiologic correlation. *Int J Tuberc Lung Dis* 1997;1:52–58.
141. Moreira AL, Sampaio EP, Zmuidzinas A, Frindt P, Smith KA, Kaplan G. Thalidomide exerts its inhibitory action on tumor necrosis factor α by enhancing mRNA degradation. *J Exp Med* 1993;177:1675–1680.
142. Donald PR, Schoeman JF, Beyers N, et al. Concentrations of interferon γ, tumor necrosis factor α, and interleukin-1β in the cerebrospinal fluid of children treated for tuberculous meningitis. *Clin Infect Dis* 1995;21:924–929.
143. Schoeman JF, Van Zyl LE, Laubscher JA, Donald PR. Serial CT scanning in childhood tuberculous meningitis: prognostic features in 198 cases. *J Child Neurol* 1995;10:320–329,
144. Zinneman HH, Hall WH. Transient tuberculosis meningitis. *Am Rev Respir Dis* 1976;114:1185–1188.
145. MacGregor AR, Green CA. Tuberculosis of the central nervous system with special reference to tuberculous meningitis. *J Pathol Bacteriol* 1937;45:613–630.
146. White AC Jr. Neurocysticercosis: a major cause of neurological disease worldwide. *Clin Infect Dis* 1997;24:101–115.
147. Mathisen GE, Johnson JP. Brain abscess. *Clin Infect Dis* 1997;25:763–781.
148. Shankar P, Manjunath N, Mohan K, et al. Rapid diagnosis of tuberculous meningitis by polymerase chain reaction. *Lancet* 1991;337:5–7.
149. Ahuja GK, Mohan KK, Prasad K, Behari M. Diagnostic criteria for tuberculous meningitis and their validation. *Tuberc Lung Dis* 1994;75:149–152.
150. Miörner H, Sjöbring U, Nayak P, Chandramuki A. Diagnosis of tuberculous meningitis: a comparative analysis of 3 immunoassays, an immune complex assay and the polymerase chain reaction. *Tuberc Lung Dis* 1995;76:381–386.
151. Seth P, Ahuja GK, Vijaya Bhanu N, et al. Evaluation of polymerase chain reaction for rapid diagnosis of clinically suspected tuberculous meningitis. *Tuberc Lung Dis* 1996;77:353–357.
152. Watt G, Zaraspe G, Bautista S, Laughlin L. Rapid diagnosis of tuberculous meningitis by using an enzyme-linked immunosorbent assay to detect mycobacterial antigen and antibody in cerebrospinal fluid. *J Infect Dis* 1988;158:681–686.
153. Patil SA, Gourie-Devi M, Anand AR, et al. Significance of mycobacterial immune complexes (IgG) in the diagnosis of tuberculous meningitis. *Tuber Lung Dis* 1996;77:164–167.
154. Ribera E, Martinez-Vazquez JM, Ocana I, Segura RM, Pascual C. Activity of adenosine deaminase in cerebrospinal fluid for the diagnosis and follow-up of tuberculous meningitis in adults. *J Infect Dis* 1987;155: 603–607.
155. Donald P, Malan C, Schoeman J. Adenosine deaminase activity as a diagnostic aid in tuberculous meningitis. *J Infect Dis* 1987;156:1040–1041.
156. Chawla R, Seth R, Raj B, Saini A. Adenosine deaminase levels in cerebrospinal fluid in tuberculous and bacterial meningitis. *Tubercle* 1991;72:190–192.
157. López-Cortés LF, Cruz-Ruiz M, Gómez-Mateos J, et al. Adenosine deaminase activity in the CSF of patients with aseptic meningitis: utility in the diagnosis of tuberculous meningitis or neurobrucellosis. *Clin Infect Dis* 1995;20:525–530.
158. Teoh R, Humphries MJ, Hoare RD, O'Mahoney F. Clinical correlation of CT changes in 64 Chinese patients with tuberculous meningitis. *J Neurol* 1989; 236:48–51.
159. Jinkins JR. Computed tomography of intracranial tuberculosis. *Neuroradiology* 1991;33:126–135.
160. Bullock MR, Welchman JM. Diagnostic and prognostic features of tuberculous meningitis on CT scanning. *J Neural Neurosurg Psychiatry* 1982;45:1098–1101.
161. Bhargava S, Gupta AK, Tandon PN. Tuberculous meningitis—a CT study. *Br J Radiol* 1982;55: 189–196.
162. Chang KH, Han MH, Roh JK, Kim IO, Han MC, Kim CW. Gd-DTPA-enhanced MR imaging of the brain in patients with meningitis: comparison with CT. *Am J Roentgenol* 1990;154:809–816.
163. Schoeman J, Hewlett R, Donald P. MR of childhood tuberculous meningitis. *Neuroradiology* 1988;30:473–477.
164. Brodie BB, Kurze H, Schankar LS. The importance of dissociation constant and lipid solubility in influencing the passage of drugs into the cerebrospinal fluid. *J Pharmacol Exp Ther* 1960;130:20–25.

165. Barling RWA, Selkon JB. Penetration of antibiotics into cerebrospinal fluid and brain tissue. *J Antimicrob Chemother* 1978;4:203–207.
166. Schanker LS. Passage of drugs into and out of the central nervous system. *Antimicrob Agents Chemother* 1965;:1044–1050.
167. Lutsar I, McCracken GH Jr, Friedland IR. Antibiotic pharmacodynamics in cerebrospinal fluid. *Clin Infect Dis* 1998;27:1117–1129.
168. Lincoln EM, Kirmse KW. The diagnosis and treatment of tuberculous meningitis in children. *Am J Med Sci* 1950;219:382–393.
169. Bunn PA. One hundred cases of miliary and meningeal tuberculosis treated with streptomycin. *Am J Med Sci* 1948;216:286–315.
170. Bunn PA. Two-year follow up report of patients with miliary and meningeal tuberculosis treated with streptomycin. *Am J Med Sci* 1950;219:127–132.
171. Illingsworth RS, Lorber J. Results of streptomycin treatment in tuberculous meningitis. *Lancet* 1951;2: 511–516.
172. Perry TL. Treatment of tuberculous meningitis in children. *J Pediatr* 1952;40:687–707.
173. McDermott W, Muschenheim C, Hadley ST, Bunn PA, Gorman RV. Streptomycin in treatment of tuberculosis in humans: meningitis and generalized hematogenous tuberculosis. *Ann Intern Med* 1947;27: 769–822.
174. Clark CM Jr, Elmendorf DF, Cawthon WV, Muschenheim C, McDermott W. Isoniazid (isonicotinic acid hydrazide) in the treatment of miliary and meningeal tuberculosis. *Am Rev Tuberc* 1952;66:391–415.
175. Lanier VS, Russell WF Jr, Heaton A, Robinson A. Concentrations of active isoniazid in serum and cerebrospinal fluid of patients with tuberculosis treated with isoniazid. *Pediatrics* 1958;21:910–915.
176. Wasz-Hockert O. Late prognosis in tuberculous meningitis. *Acta Peadiatr* 1962;51:1–119.
177. Ramachandran P, Duraipandian M, Nagarajan M, Prabhaker R, Ramakrishnan CV, Tripathy SP. Three chemotherapy studies of tuberculous meningitis in children. *Tubercle* 1986;67:17–29.
178. Ramachandran P, Duraipandian M, Reetha AM, Mahalakshmi SM, Prabhaker R. Long-term status of children treated for tuberculous meningitis in South India. *Tubercle* 1989;70:235–239.
179. Humphries MJ, Teoh R, Lau J, Gabriel M. Factors of prognostic significance in Chinese children with tuberculous meningitis. *Tubercle* 1990;71:161–168.
180. Lam KSL, Sham MMK, Tam NG, Ma HTG. Hypopituitarism after tuberculous meningitis in childhood. *Ann Intern Med* 1993;118:701–706.
181. Verdon R, Chevret S, Laissy J-P, Wolff M. Tuberculous meningitis in adults: review of 48 cases. *Clin Infect Dis* 1996;22:982–988.
182. Yechoor VK, Shandera WX, Rodriguez P, Cate TR. Tuberculous meningitis among adults with and without HIV infection. *Arch Intern Med* 1996;156:1710–1716.
183. Parsons M. The treatment of tuberculous meningitis. *Tubercle* 1959;70:79–82.
184. O'Toole RD, Thorton GF, Mukherjee MK, Nath RL. Dexamethasone in tuberculous meningitis. *Ann Intern Med* 1969;70:39–48.
185. Shaw PP, Wang SM, Tung SG, et al. Clinical analysis of 445 adult cases of tuberculous meningitis. *Chin J Tuberc Respir Dis* 1984;3:131–132.
186. Girgis NI, Farid Z, Kilpatrick ME, Sultan Y, Mikhail IA. Dexamethasone adjunctive treatment for tuberculous meningitis. *Pediatr Infect Dis J* 1991;10:179–183.
187. Kumarvelu S, Prasad K, Khosla A, Behari M, Ahuja GK. Randomized controlled trial of dexamethasone in tuberculous meningitis. *Tuberc Lung Dis* 1994;75: 203–207.
188. Peacock WF, Deeny JE. Improving the outcome of tuberculous meningits in childhood. *S Afr Med J* 1984; 66:597–598.
189. Schoeman JF, LeRoux D, Bezuidenhout PB, Donald PR. Intracranial pressure monitoring in tuberculous meningitis: clinical and computerized tomographic correlation. *Dev Med Child Neurol* 1985;27:644–654.
190. Roy TK, Sicar PK, Chandar V. Peritoneal-ventricular shunt in the management of tuberculous meningitis. *Indian J Paediatr* 1979;16:1023–1027.
191. Bullock MR, Van Dellen JR. The role of cerebrospinal fluid shunting in tuberculous meningitis. *Surg Neurol* 1982;18:274–277.
192. Palur R, Rajshekhar V, Chandy MJ, Joseph T, Abraham J. Shunt surgery for hydrocephalus in tuberculous meningitis: a long-term follow-up study. *J Neurosurg* 1991;74:64–69.
193. Murray HW, Brandstetter RD, Lavyne MH. Ventriculo-atrial shunting for hydrocephalus complicating tuberculous meningitis. *Am J Med* 1981;70:895–898.
194. Schoeman J, Donald P, van Zyl L, et al. Tuberculous hydrocephalus: comparison of different treatments with regard to ICP, ventricular size and clinical outcome. *Dev Med Child Neurol* 1991;33:396–405.
195. Loizou LA, Anderson M. Intracranial tuberculomas; correlation of computerized tomography with clinicopathological findings. *Q J Med* 1982;51:104–114.
196. Arrington JA. Meningeal tuberculoma. *Semin Roentgenol* 1987;22:7–8.
197. Chang CM, Chan FL, Yu YL, Huang CY, Woo E. Tuberculous meningitis associated with meningeal tuberculoma. *J R Soc Med* 1986;79:486–487.
198. Lees AJ, Macleod AF, Marshall J. Cerebral tuberculomas developing during treatment of tuberculous meningitis. *Lancet* 1980;1:1208–1211.
199. Teoh R, Humphries MJ, O'Mahoney G. Symptomatic intracranial tuberculoma devloping during treatment of tuberculosis: a report of 10 patients and review of the literature. *Q J Med* 1987;241:449–460.
200. Shepard WE, Field ML, James DH Jr, Tonkin IL. Transient appearance of intracranial tuberculoma during treatment of tuberculous meningitis. *Pediatr Infect Dis* 1986;5:599–601.
201. Tandon PN, Bhargava S. Effect of medical treatment on intracranial tuberculoma—a CT study. *Tubercle* 1985;66:85–97.
202. Labhard N, Nicod L, Zellweger JP. Cerebral tuberculosis in the immunocompetent host: 8 cases observed in Switzerland. *Tuber Lung Dis* 1994;75:454–459.
203. Rajeswari R, Sivasubramanian S, Balambal R, et al. A controlled clinical trial of short-course chemotherapy for tuberculoma of the brain. *Tuber Lung Dis* 1995; 76:311–317.
204. Rajshekhar V, Chandy MJ. Short-course chemotherapy for intracranial tuberculomas. *Tuber Lung Dis* 1996;77:295–296.
205. Ellard GA, Humphries MJ, Allen BJ. Cerebrospinal fluid drug concentrations and the treatment of tubercu-

losis meningitis. *Am Rev Respir Dis* 1993;148:650–655.
206. Donald PR, Gent WL, Seifart HI, Lamprecht JH, Parkin DP. Cerebrospinal fluid isoniazid concentrations in children with tuberculous meningitis: the influence of dosage and acetylation status. *Pediatrics* 1992;89:247–250.
207. Ellard GA, Humphrie MJ, Gabriel M, Teoh R. Penetration of pyrazinamide into the cerebrospinal fluid in patients with tuberculous meningitis. *Br Med J* 1987;294:284–285.
208. Donald PR, Seifart H. Cerebrospinal fluid pyrazinamide concentrations in children with tuberculous meningitis. *Petiatr Infect Dis J* 1988;7:469–471.
209. Sippel JE, Mikhail IA, Girgis NI, Youssef HN. Rifampin concentrations in cerebro-spinal fluid of patients with tuberculous meningitis. *Am Rev Respir Dis* 1974;109:579–580.
210. Place VA, Pyle MM, de la Huerga J. Ethambutol in tuberculous meningitis. *Am Rev Respir Dis* 1969;99: 783–785.
211. Bobrowitz ID. Ethambutol in tuberculous meningitis. *Chest* 1972;61:629–632.
212. Donald PR, Seifart HI. Cerebrospinal fluid concentrations of ethionamide in children with tuberculous meningitis. *J Pediatr* 1989;15:483–486.
213. Jakubowski A, Elwood RK, Enarson DA. Clinical features of abdominal tuberculosis. *J Infect Dis* 1988; 158:687–692.
214. Harrison GN, Chew WH. Tuberculous peritonitis. *S Med J* 1979;72:1561–1588.
215. Menzies RI, Alsen H, Fitzgerald JM, Mohapeloa RG. Tuberculous peritonitis in Lesotho. *Tubercle* 1986; 67:47–54.
216. Karney WW, O'Donoghue JM, Ostrow JH, Holmes KK, Beaty HN. The spectrum of tuberculous peritonitis. *Chest* 1977;72:310–315.
217. Singh MM, Bhargava AN, Jain KP. Tuberculous peritonitis. An evaluation of pathogenetic mechanisms, diagnostic procedures, and therapeutic measures. *N Engl J Med* 1969;281:1091–1094.
218. Cromartie RS III. Tuberculous peritonitis. *Surg Gynecol Obstet* 1977;144:876–878.
219. Schulze K, Warner HA, Murray D. Interstitial tuberculosis. Experience at a Canadian teaching institution. *Am J Med* 1977;63:735–745.
220. Paustian FF, Backus HL. So-called primary ulcerohypertrophic ileocecal tuberculosis. *Am J Med* 1959; 27:509–518.
221. Richards RJ, Hamwi Y, Rodriguez PS. Intestinal tuberculosis with associated coloduodenal fistula. *Clin Infect Dis* 1998;26:761–762.
222. Portielje J, Lohle P, van der Werf S, Puylaert J. Ultrasound and abdominal tuberculosis (Letter). *Lancet* 1995;346:379–380.
223. al-Quorain AA, Facharzt, Satti MB, al-Freihi HM, al-Gindan YM, al-Awad N. Abdominal tuberculosis in Saudi Arabia: a clinicopathological study of 65 cases. *Am J Gastroenterol* 1993;88:75–79.
224. Menzies RI, Fitzgerald JM, Mulpeter K. Laparoscopic diagnosis of ascites in Lesotho. *Br Med J* 1985;291: 473–475.
225. Borhanmanesh F, Hekmat K, Vaezzadeh K, Rezai HR. Tuberculous peritonitis. Prospective study of 32 cases in Iran. *Ann Intern Med* 1972;76:567–572.
226. Chen Y-M, Lee P-Y, Perng R-P. Abdominal tuberculosis in Taiwan: a report from Veterans' General Hospital, Taipei. *Tuberc Lung Dis* 1995;76:35–38.
227. Sheldon CD, Probert CSJ, Cock H, et al. Incidence of abdominal tuberculosis in Bangladeshi migrants in East London. *Tuberc Lung Dis* 1993;74:12–15.
228. Mohal MG, Baker IW, Lautre G, et al. Colonoscopy: 100 examinations. *S Afr J Surg* 1973;2:73.
229. Morgante PE, Gandara MA, Sterle E. The endoscopic diagnosis of colonic tuberculosis. *Gastrointest Endosc* 1989;35:115–118.
230. Watanabe H, Kiwatsaki N, Goto Y. Biopsy under direct vision for the diagnosis of Crohn's disease. *Tohoku J Exp Med* 1979;1:1–8.
231. Bhasin DK, Roy P, Sharma M, et al. Acid-fast bacilli in colonscopic brushings (Letter). *Lancet* 1991; 338:184–185.
232. Shukla HS, Hughes LE. Abdominal tuberculosis in the 1970's: a continuing problem. *Br J Surg* 1978;65: 403–405.
233. Vaidya MG, Sodhi JS. Gastro-intestinal tract tuberculosis: a study of 102 cases including 55 hemicolectomies. *Clin Radiol* 1978;29:189–195.
234. Fitzgerald JM, Menzies RI, Elwood RK. Abdominal tuberculosis: a critical review. *Dig Dis* 1991;9: 269–281.
235. Balasubramanian R, Nagarajan M, Balambal R, et al. Randomised controlled clinical trial of short course chemotherapy in abdominal tuberculosis: a five-year report. *Int J Tuberc Lung Dis* 1997;1:44–51.
236. Ramadan IT, Abdul-Ghaffar NUAMA. Malabsorption syndrome complicating tuberculous peritonitis. *Int J Tuberc Lung Dis* 1997;1:85–86.
237. Alrajhi AA, Halim MA, Al-Hokail A, Alrabiah F, Al-Omran K. Corticosteroid treatment of peritoneal tuberculosis. *Clin Infect Dis* 1998;27:52–56.
238. Harvey AM, Whitehill MR. Tuberculous pericarditis. *Medicine* 1937;16:45–94.
239. Rooney JJ, Crocco JA, Lyons HA. Tuberculous pericarditis. *Ann Intern Med* 1970;72:73–78.
240. Finney JO, Yarbrough R, Scott CW. Tuberculous pericarditis. *South Med J* 1971;64:49–57.
241. Hageman JH, D'Esopo ND, Glenn WWL. Tuberculous pericarditis. A long-term analysis of forty-four proved cases. *N Engl J Med* 1964;270:327–332.
242. Strang JIG. Tuberculous pericarditis in Transkei. *Clin Cardiol* 1984;7:667–670.
243. Strang JIG, Gibson DG, Nunn AJ, Kakoza HHS, Girling DJ, Fox W. Controlled trial of prednisolone as adjuvant in treatment of tuberculous constrictive pericarditis in Transkei. *Lancet* 1987;2:1418–1422.
244. Girling D. *Personal communication,* 1993.
245. Fowler NO, Manitsas GT. Infectious pericarditis. *Prog Cardiovasc* 1973;16:323–336.
246. Sagristá-Sauleda J, Permanyer-Miralda G, Soler-Soler J. Tuberculous pericarditis: ten year experience with a prospective protocol for diagnosis and treatment. *J Am Coll Cardiol* 1988;11:724–728.
247. Strang JIG, Gibson DG, Mitchison DA, et al. Controlled clinical trial of complete open surgical drainage and of prednisolone in treatment of tuberculous pericardial effusion in Transkei. *Lancet* 1988;2:759–763.
248. Stepman TR, Owyong E. Clinically primary tuberculous pericarditis. *Ann Intern Med* 1947;27:914–922.
249. Schrier EV. Experience with pericarditis at Groote Schuur Hospital, Cape Town: an analysis of one hun-

dred and sixty cases studied over a six-year period. *S Afr Med J* 1959;33:810–817.
250. Strang JIG. *Personal communication,* 1991.
251. Horowitz G, Kaslow R, Friedland G. Infectiousness of laryngeal tuberculosis. *Am Rev Respir Dis* 1976;114: 241–244.
252. Kilgore TL, Jenkins DW. Laryngeal tuberculosis. *Chest* 1983;83:139–141.
253. Farmer WC, Fulkerson LL, Stein E. Vocal cord paralysis due to pulmonary tuberculosis. *Am Rev Respir Dis* 1975;112:565–569.
254. Case records of the Massachusetts General Hospital. Case 51-1983. *N Engl J Med* 1983;309:1569–1574.
255. Rohwedder JJ. Upper respiratory tract tuberculosis. Sixteen cases in a general hospital. *Ann Intern Med* 1974;80:708–713.
256. Prada JL, Kindelan JM, Villanueva JL, Jurado R, Sánchez-Guijo P, Torre-Cisneros J. Tuberculosis of the tongue in two immunocompetent patients. *Clin Infect Dis* 1994;19:200–202.
257. Bouza E, Merino P, Munoz P, Sanchez-Carrillo C, Yánez J, Cortés C. Ocular tuberculosis. A prospective study in a general hospital. *Medicine* 1997;76;53–61.
258. Reny JL, Challe G, Geisert P, Aerts J, Ziza JM, Raguin G. Tuberculosis-related retinal vasculitis in an immunocompetent patient. *Clin Infect Dis* 1996;22: 873–874.
259. Case Records of the Massachusetts General Hospital. Case 4-1998. *N Engl J Med* 1998;338:313–319.
260. Horwitz O. Lupus vulgaris in Denmark 1895–1954: its relation to the epidemiology of other forms of tuberculosis. *Acta Tuberc Scand* 1960;49:1–142.
261. Case records of the Massachusetts General Hospital. Case 43-1972. *N Engl J Med* 1972;287:872–878.
262. Chen CH, Shih JF, Wang L-S, Perng RP. Tuberculous subcutaneous abscess: an analysis of seven cases. *Tuberc Lung Dis* 1996;77:184–187.
263. Beyt BE, Ortbals DW, Santa Cruz DJ, Kobayashi GS, Eisen AZ, Medoff G. Cutaneous mycobacteriosis: analysis of 34 cases with new classification of the disease. *Medicine* 1980;60:95–109.
264. Schermer DK, Simpson CG, Haserick JR, Van Ordstrand HS. Tuberculosis cutis miliaris acuta generalisata. *Arch Dermatol* 1969;99:64–69.
265. Valdez LM, Schwab P, Okhuysen PC, Rakita RM. Paradoxical subcutaneous tuberculous abscess (Brief report). *Clin Infect Dis* 1997;24:734.
266. Degitz K, Steidl M, Thomas P, Plewig G, Volkenandt M. Aetiology of tuberculids. *Lancet* 1993;341:239–240.
267. Schneider JW, Geiger DH, Rossouw DJ, Jordaan HF, Victor T, van Helden PD. *Mycobacterium tuberculosis* DNA in erythema induratum of Bazin (Letter). *Lancet* 1993;342:747.
268. Mattila JO, Katila M-L, Vornanen M. Slowly growing mycobacteria and chronic skin disorders. *Clin Infect Dis* 1996;23:1043–1048.
269. Liote HA, Spaulding C, Bazelly B, Milleron BJ, Akoun GM. Thyroid tuberculosis associated with mediastinal lymphadenitis. *Tubercle* 1987;68:229–231.
270. Sachs MK, Dickinson G, Amazon K. Tuberculous adenitis of the thyroid mimicking subacute thyroiditis. *Am J Med* 1988;85:573–575.
271. FitzGerald JM, Mayo JR, Miller RR, Jamieson WRF, Baumgartner F. Tuberculosis of the thymus. *Chest* 1992;102:1604–1605.
272. Wilson JP, Chapman LD. Tuberculosis mastitis. *Chest* 1990;98:1505–1509.
273. Crook LD, Johnson FP Jr. Tuberculosis of the pancreas: a case report. *Tubercle* 1988;69:148–151.
274. Zipser RD, Rau JE, Ricketts RR, Bevans LC. Tuberculous pseudotumors of the liver. *Am J Med* 1976; 61:946–951.
275. Spiegel CT, Tuazon CU. Tuberculous liver abscess. *Tubercle* 1984;65:127–131.
276. Murphy TF, Gray GF. Biliary tract obstruction due to tuberculous adenitis. *Am J Med* 1980;68:452–454.
277. Kohen MD, Altman KA. Jaundice due to a rare cause: tuberculous lymphadentis. *Am J Gastroenterol* 1973; 59:48–52.
278. Sartin JS, Walker RC. Granulomatous hepatitis: a retrospective review of 88 cases at the Mayo Clinic. *Mayo Clin Proc* 1991;66:914–918.
279. Gowrinath K, Ashok S, Thanasekaran V, Rao KR. Tuberculous cholecystitis. *Int J Tuberc Lung Dis* 1997; 1:484–485.
280. Gupta SP, Arora A, Bhargava DK. An unusual presentation of oesophageal tuberculosis. *Tuberc Lung Dis* 1992;73:174–176.
281. Wigley FM, Murray HW, Mann RB, Saba GP, Kashima H, Mann JJ. Unusual manifestation of tuberculosis. *Am J Med* 1976;60:310–314.
282. García-Gasalla M, Yebra-Bango M, García-Lomas MV, Mellor-Pita S. Resolution of symptoms of esophageal compression due to mediastinal tuberculosis after treatment with corticosteroids (Letter). *Clin Infect Dis* 1998;27:234.
283. Wort SJ, Puleston JM, Hill PD, Holdstock GE. Primary tuberculosis of the oesophagus (Brief report). *Lancet* 1997;349:1072.
284. Felson B, Akers PV, Hall GS, Schreiber JT, Greene RE, Pedrosa CS. Mycotic tuberculous aneurysm of the thoracic aorta. *JAMA* 1977;237:1104–1108.
285. Estera AS, Platt MR, Mills LJ, Nikaidoh H. Tuberculous aneurysms of the descending thoracic aorta. Report of a case with fatal rupture. *Chest* 1979;75: 386–388.
286. Bonomo R, Graham R, Makley J, Petersilge C. Tuberculous pyomyositis: an unusual presentation of disseminated *Mycobacterium tuberculosis* infection. *Clin Infect Dis* 1995;20:1576–1577.
287. Stricker T, Willi UV, Pfyffer GE, Nadal D. A schoolgirl with constipation (Case report). *Lancet* 1996; 348:306.
288. Indudhara R, Singh SK, Minz M, Yadav RVS, Chugh KS. Tuberculous pyomyositis in a renal transplant recipient. *Tuberc Lung Dis* 1992;73:239–241.
289. American Trudeau Society. The effect of cortisone and/or corticotropin on tuberculous infection in man. *Am Rev Tuberc* 1952;66:254–256.
290. Johnson JR, Davey WN. Cortisone, corticotropin, and antimicrobial therapy in tuberculosis in animals and man. *Am Rev Tuberc* 1954;70:623–636.
291. Dooley DP, Carpenter JL, Rademacher S. Adjunctive corticosteroid therapy for tuberculosis: a critical reappraisal of the literature. *Clin Infect Dis* 1997;25: 872–887.
292. Escobar JA, Belsey MA, Duenas A, Medina P. Mortality from tuberculous meningitis reduced by steroid therapy. *Pediatrics* 1975;56:1050–1055.
293. Ashby M, Grant H. Tuberculous meningitis treated with cortisone. *Lancet* 1955;1:65–66.

294. Voljavec BF, Corpe RF. The influence of corticosteroid hormones in the treatment of tuberculous meningitis in Negroes. *Am Rev Respir Dis* 1960;81:539–545.
295. O'Toole RD, Thornton GF, Mukherjee MK, Nath RL. Dexamethasone in tuberculous meningitis: relationship of cerebrospinal fluid effects to therapeutic efficacy. *Ann Intern Med* 1969;70:39–48.
296. Girgis NI, Farid Z, Hanna LS, Yassin MW, Wallace CK. The use of dexamethasone in preventing ocular complications in tuberculous meningitis. *Trans R Soc Trop Med Hyg* 1983;77:658–659.
297. Menon NK. Steroid therapy in tuberculous pleural effusion. *Tubercle* 1964;45:17–20.
298. Tani P, Poppius H, Mäkipaja J. Cortisone therapy for exudative tuberculous pleurisy in the light of a follow-up study. *Acta Tuberc Pneum Scand* 1964;44:303–398.
299. Alzeer AH, Fitzgerald JM. Corticosteroids and tuberculosis: risks and use as adjunct therapy. *Tuberc Lung Dis* 1993;74:6–11.

8

Tuberculosis in Relation to Human Immunodeficiency Virus and Acquired Immunodeficiency Syndrome

The human immunodeficiency virus (HIV) is perhaps the most perverse or destructive single element that might be introduced to exacerbate the situation with tuberculosis. Biologically, the HIV attacks the specific cell line primarily responsible for tuberculoimmunity, greatly enhancing the risk of endogenous reactivation of latent tuberculosis infection. Epidemiologically, HIV has primarily afflicted a population, young adults, that is both inherently at high risk for tuberculosis and, because of extended families, likely to spread tuberculosis to many others, including children. Geographically, the first wave of the virus swept over a region, sub-Saharan Africa, that was already rife with tuberculosis. Socioeconomically, these two microbes have demonstrably coinfected similar groups in the industrialized nations, including minorities, the medically underserved, and substance abusers. Therapeutically, HIV-infected acquired immunodeficiency syndrome (AIDS) patients appear to be more susceptible to disease with drug-resistant strains of *M. tuberculosis,* which may be otherwise modestly less virulent than drug-susceptible strains. Thus, it seems probable that treatment and control programs in the future will necessarily entail broader in vitro susceptibility testing, employment of more drugs, and administration of expensive regimens under rigorous oversight for extended periods of time. Similarly, preventive chemotherapy with isoniazid (INH), the most economical drug available, may become compromised.

On the other side of the relationship, tuberculosis has several very significant adverse effects on those infected with HIV. Because of the rapidity with which the mycobacteria proliferate and disseminate, tuberculosis is a major cause of death in HIV-infected persons, particularly in developing nations. In addition, evidence is accumulating that the hosts' immunological responses to active tuberculosis accelerate HIV replication within the virus-infected lymphocytes, monocytes, and other tissues, thereby accelerating the course from HIV infection to AIDS. This process exacerbates the immune dysfunction of persons with AIDS, resulting in death from causes other than tuberculosis.

And, sadly, comorbidity from tuberculosis may stigmatize and create public and professional fears about associating with HIV-infected AIDS patients, undoing previous efforts at public and professional education and reassurance.

Despite immense scientific efforts, mostly on the HIV side of the equation, I am pessimistic about the prospects for practical, affordable modalities that would allow the rapid cure or prevention of either of these infections. And because of financial constraints as well as the frustrating inertia demonstrated in the past by national and supranational health agencies, I am skeptical about the ability to deploy effective treatment or prevention strategies, once developed. Therefore, a massive, lethal, copandemic of these two infections seems almost inevitable over the next two to three decades, with the suffering most prominent in sub-Saharan Africa, the Pacific Rim nations, and Indo-Asia.

Nonetheless, there are things that can and must be done to limit the fear, sickness, and death attendant to these disorders, one among the newest, the other among the oldest in the pantheon of infectious diseases.

BIOLOGICAL RELATIONSHIPS BETWEEN HIV AND TUBERCULOSIS INFECTION AND DISEASE

Tuberculoimmunity is a complex process primarily involving mononuclear phagocytes and lymphocytes. The capacity to limit proliferation of tubercle bacilli within macrophages resides largely with $CD4^+$ T-helper lymphocytes. As HIV infection produces progressive depletion and dysfunction of this lymphocyte population, there is a progressively increased risk of reactivation of latent tuberculosis infection (1). HIV infection has also been shown to impair macrophage function including diminished phagocytic capacity, altered cytokine production, decreased elaboration of intermediate oxygen metabolites, and impaired antigen-presentation capacity (2–4). Observations regarding the influences of these phenomena on the incidence and manifestation of tuberculosis are delineated below.

HIV and Acquisition of New Infection with *M. tuberculosis*

Among persons with HIV infection, particularly in advanced stages, there is evidence of diminished numbers and/or impaired function of alveolar macrophages (2–4). Although it is not possible to definitely prove increased risk for acquisition of *M. tuberculosis,* the remarkably high proportions of persons with HIV infection/AIDS who have developed active tuberculosis following nosocomial exposure to tuberculosis in several outbreaks suggests to me heightened vulnerability. If, as I infer, there is increased risk for acquisition of tuberculosis, several potential explanations come to mind.

Is There a Defective Initial Alveolar Macrophage Response?

Specifically, are there deficiencies of the preimmune, nonspecific inhibitory effects of the alveolar macrophages on mycobacterial proliferation? One potential explanation for the extraordinarily high infection and disease rates seen among HIV-infected persons relates to current assumptions regarding the probability of depositing infectious droplet nuclei in the alveolar spaces. Epidemiologists and investigators have developed an approximation of the likelihood of this occurring based on observations of skin-test conversion rates among normal exposed hosts, assuming that when a droplet nucleus reaches the alveolus of such a host, infection will occur (see Chapter 3 on Transmission). However, it is possible that tubercle bacilli are deposited in alveoli more frequently than tuberculin skin testing—the surrogate marker—would indicate. Stead has recently shown higher frequencies of skin test conversion among similarly exposed blacks than whites (5). Limited information indicates that alveolar macrophages from blacks are more permissive *ex vivo* for replication of tubercle bacilli (6). Analogous to these findings, it is plausible that more mycobacteria-laden droplet nuclei reach the alveoli than has been previously postulated and that the innate, preimmune capacity of the macrophages may in some instances prevent mycobacterial replication to the extent that "infection" or tuberculin conversion does not occur. Thus, in this logic, alveolar macrophage function in advanced HIV infection may be so disrupted that tubercle bacilli that have been delivered to the distal air spaces may survive to replicate and invade such patients.

Does HIV/AIDS Enlarge the Anatomical Area Through Which Tuberculosis Invasion Might Occur?

An alternative hypothesis could entail loci other than alveoli for mycobacterial invasion. Tubercle bacilli could invade some AIDS patients through the bronchial tree as well as the conventional alveolar pathway. The tubercle bacillus is thought to require uptake by a phagocytic cell in order to proliferate and invade (see Chapter 4). Classically, this is thought to involve resident alveolar macrophages. However, recent reports document macrophage distribution and activity within the prealveolar airways (7). Conceivably, in patients with airways inflamed by chronic infection, increased numbers of macrophages traversing the bronchial tree could phagocytize, transport, and serve as breeding sites for mycobacteria deposited in the bronchial tree. A heavy initial inoculum delivered through such a mechanism could also potentially explain the rapid onset and immense mycobacterial burdens seen in some AIDS patients newly infected with tuberculosis.

HIV Infection and Progression to Overt Disease of New Infection with *M. tuberculosis*

As noted in Chapter 4, the likelihood of a new infection with tubercle bacilli rapidly advancing to active disease varies according to the age and immune status of the host. Infants (8) and the elderly (9) are quite susceptible to this phenomenon, with approximately 5% to 10% of the newly infected in both of these groups progressing to overt clinical disease within 6 months. Similarly, individuals with HIV infection who are newly infected with tuberculosis show a striking vulnerability to progressive disease; this is more pronounced with advancing HIV infection (10,11).

In an AIDS residential facility in San Francisco, an explosive epidemic occurred with 11 of 30 exposed persons developing various patterns of pulmonary, pulmonary/extrapulmonary, and extrapulmonary tuberculosis within 120 days following exposure (12).

Multidrug-resistant (MDR) tuberculosis epidemics among HIV-infected persons also are indicative of heightened vulnerability. Among persons with AIDS who were known to have temporally defined exposures to cases of MDR TB in hospitals in New York or Florida, the time from such exposures to overwhelming tuberculosis has been extraordinarily brief (13,14). In these outbreaks, the reported range of time from contact to the index case and manifest tuberculosis ranged from 4 to 16 weeks, periods comparable to the San Francisco data above. Such compressed incubation periods have never been described before in any other exposed groups including infants, oncology patients, organ transplant recipients, or end-stage renal failure patients. The MDR TB epidemics were readily recognized because of the distinctive patterns of drug resistance among the index strains.

In the community at large, molecular epidemiology studies using restriction-fragment length polymorphism (RFLP) also indicate that in San Francisco and portions of the Bronx, New York, 30% to 40% of cases were clustered, suggesting recent exposure and early progression to disease (15,16). In these reports, HIV infection and AIDS were associated with risk for clustering at significant levels.

In summary, these observations indicate that persons with advanced HIV infection and AIDS are supremely vulnerable to rapidly progressive infection following exposure to tuberculosis. The profound clinical and public health implications for this finding are developed later in this chapter.

HIV Infection and the Risk of Reactivation of Remote, Latent *M. tuberculosis* Infection

Most persons who have been infected with *M. tuberculosis* have sufficient immune capacity to cause the primary infection to involute, resulting in an asymptomatic carrier state. This state is denoted clinically in most patients only by the tuberculin skin test; in a minority of cases there remains fibronodular scarring in the apex of the lungs as a vestige of this experience. Among infected persons, there is a lifelong risk of recrudescence of the tuberculosis, so-called "endogenous reactivation." Factors associated with increased risk for reactivation are discussed in Chapters 4 and 5. Of the various risk factors, infection with HIV is the most powerful.

Active tuberculosis develops in a substantial proportion of persons harboring latent tuberculous infection who become HIV infected. It is important to note, however, that most of the studies that report on this phenomenon are at least partially confounded by the fact that there are high rates of transmission of new tuberculosis infection in the communities from which these reports are derived. With this caveat, we may still recognize gross differences in the risk of developing tuberculosis for young adults. Because of numerous variables including race, geography, and environmental tuberculosis exposure, one cannot assign an absolute relative risk for the impact of HIV in promoting reactivation of endogenous tuberculosis. However, three studies comparing groups of tuberculin-reactive patients, some HIV positive, others negative, all indicated that HIV infection conferred relative risks greater than 20-fold: New York City injection drug users, 20.5-fold (17); young women in Zaire, 26-fold (18); urban women in Rwanda, 22-fold (19).

EPIDEMIOLOGICAL RELATIONSHIPS BETWEEN HIV INFECTION AND TUBERCULOSIS

The Impact of HIV on the Prevalence of Tuberculosis

Although the "epidemiological" relationship between HIV/AIDS and tuberculosis flows from their "biological" interplay, quantification of the effects is best described through numerical assessments of the impact of the coepidemics in large populations. The most significant interrelationship between the HIV and the tubercle bacillus is reactivation of latent tuberculosis as a result of impaired immunity from progressive HIV infection; this pattern is shaped by the fact that tuberculosis generally antedates HIV infection in the populations at risk. However, other critical elements of the interplay between these two pathogens include recent tuberculosis transmission to other HIV-infected persons in congregate settings, increased risk for progression to overt disease of the new tuberculosis infection in those already HIV infected, and spread of the tuberculosis by the HIV-infected to their HIV-negative contacts—so-called "horizontal transmission."

Because of the prominence of reactivation tuberculosis, the impact of HIV on tuberculosis in any community is now closely related to the preexisting prevalence of latent tuberculosis in the population experiencing epidemic HIV infection.

Global Tuberculosis and HIV: Epidemiological Patterns

The World Health Organization (WHO) estimates that, as of 1997, approximately 31 million persons have been infected with HIV since the onset of the pandemic (20), and it may be calculated that today nearly 12 million of these persons are coinfected with tuberculosis (21). WHO estimates that by the year 2000, over 40 million could have been infected by HIV. The distribution of the numbers of HIV infected and the proportion of those persons coinfected with *M. tuberculosis* are displayed in Tables 8.1 to 8.3, broken down by continent or region. As may be seen, the greatest impact of HIV TB currently is centered in sub-Saharan Africa, where 20.8 million HIV-infected people are estimated, and 6 to 7 million may be coinfected. With only 10% of

TABLE 8.1. *Persons living with HIV infection/AIDS, worldwide, 1997*

Region	Number HIV/AIDS	
North America	860,000	Western Hemisphere, 2.5 M
Central America	310,000	
South America	1,300,000	
Europe	530,000	Euro/Russia, 0.7 M
Russia "plus"	150,000	
Eastern Mediterranean	210,000	Africa, 21 M
Sub-Saharan Africa	20,800,000	
East Asia (China, Japan+)	440,000	Asia/India/ Oceania, 6.5 M
S. Asia/Indian subcontinent	6,000,000	
Australia/West Pac	12,000	
Total		World, 30.5 M

UNAIDS and WHO estimated that, by the end of 1997, roughly 30.5 million persons would be living with HIV infection or AIDS. Of these, more than 40% are women, more than half are aged 15–24, and approximately 16,000 new infections occur daily—mainly via heterosexual transmission. Russia "plus" includes most of the former republics. Data from UNAIDS/WHO (20).

TABLE 8.2. *Worldwide prevalence of tuberculosis infection, 1990*

WHO region	Prevalence of tuberculosis infection	Number infected
Africa (north and south)	34%	171 M
Americas (except United States and Canada)	26%	117 M
SE Asia	34%	426 M
West Pacific	44%	195 M
China	34%	379 M
Eastern Mediterranean	19%	52 M
Industrialized nations (Europe, United States, Canada, Japan, Australia/NZ)	32%	382 M
Total	33%	1.722 B

The numbers are estimates based on various direct (e.g., tuberculin surveys) and indirect (e.g., annual risk of infection surveys) sources (21). Although I believe they may modestly overestimate the prevalence(s) of infection, they presumably offer valid insights into the relative prevalence of tuberculous infections in these regions. Table 8.3 represents the estimated prevalence of coinfection with tuberculosis and HIV among the most sexually active population, ages 15 to 49 years.

the world's population, sub-Saharan Africa harbors 65% of the world's HIV-infected (22); over 50% of adult patients admitted to the hospital in this region are HIV-positive. Case rates for tuberculosis in this region had been falling at an average rate of 1.6% per year before 1985 but rose at a rate of 7.7% per year in subsequent years (23). A recent review quantified the problem, noted that well-organized national tuberculosis programs were able to impact the spread of tuberculosis, and proposed various remediations (24).

The next largest aggregation is in Asia, where 6.0 million HIV infections are estimated and over 2 million may be coinfected. Although the near-term impact will be most profound in Africa, the ultimate morbidity and mortality from this coepidemic may be most extensive in Southeast Asia. The situation in Asia is potentially so dire for the following reasons: (a) the prevalence of latent tuberculosis in Asia is modestly higher than in Africa, roughly 40% to 42% versus 30%; (b) a greater percentage of the Asian population lives in crowded urban environments, where tuberculosis transmission is facilitated; and (c) the prevalence of drug-resistant tuberculosis is substantially higher in the South-Southeast Asian nations, where ineffectual treatment programs and ungoverned dispensing of tuberculosis medications have bred high levels of resistance including multidrug resistance (25–28); and (d) WHO projections indicate a dramatic surge in HIV infection in this region over the next decade. Indeed, 4 million cases of HIV infection occurred in Southeast Asia between 1990 and 1995, and authorities calculate that by the end of this millennium there will be more new cases annually in Asia and the Pacific Rim than in Africa (21). Although HIV infection rates among young men in Thailand fell after a large public health initiative (29), explosive increases have been noted elsewhere (30,31).

TABLE 8.3. *Worldwide estimation of coinfection, TB and HIV, ages 15–49 years, 1997*

WHO region	Number of HIV-infected[a]	Prevalence of TB infection (by age)[b]	Number coinfected
Africa	18.7 M	48%	9 M
Americas	1.3 M	30%	0.4 M
SE Asia, West Pacific, and China	5.9 M	40%	2.4 M
Eastern Mediterranean	0.18 M	23%	0.04 M
Europe, United States/Canada, Japan, Australia/NZ	1.35 M	11%	0.15 M
Total			12 M

These data represent extrapolations from 1990 WHO estimates[b] of the prevalence of tuberculous infections in the population ages 15–49 years in these regions (21) and 1997 UNAIDS/WHO estimates (20) of the numbers of persons with HIV/AIDS.[a] I have calculated that approximately 90% of the HIV infections/AIDS cases in these regions occur among those in this age range.

United States Tuberculosis and HIV Epidemiological Patterns

In the United States, the District of Columbia, Puerto Rico, and the U.S. territories, approximately 574,000 cases of AIDS among persons at least 13 years of age have been reported to the Centers for Disease Control through 1996 (32). The crest of reported new cases occurred in 1993, when the case definition was expanded. In that year, nearly 105,000 cases were reported. Subsequently, there were approximately 79,000 AIDS cases in 1994, 73,000 in 1995, and 68,000 in 1996. By 1996, cases had risen disproportionately among non-Hispanic blacks, blacks, and women; in 1996, non-Hispanic blacks comprised 41% and women accounted for 20% of adults with AIDS. Among U.S. women with AIDS in 1995, rates were highest among blacks and those living in large metropolitan areas (33); notably, the highest rates of increase for women from 1991 to 1995 occurred in the South among heterosexual contacts. Despite reductions in HIV incidence among young (20–25 years) homosexual white males, the overall incidence fell only 14% between 1988 and 1993 because of stable rates in blacks and Hispanic men and rising rates among women (34).

Unlike sub-Saharan Africa or South-Southeast Asia, where the prevalence of latent tuberculosis infection is very high throughout the entire population, the prevalence of tuberculosis infection in the United States varies widely according to economic, racial, and national origin factors. Overall, the CDC has estimated that 4% of Americans, 10,000,000 persons, are infected with tuberculosis (CDC, *unpublished data*). However, among the HIV-infected persons, very wide ranges of latent tuberculosis infection would be expected based on race, age, route of (HIV) transmission, and geographical region. Within the Pulmonary Complications of HIV Infection Study Group, there was considerable disparity between tuberculosis risks for homosexual men versus injection drug users (risk ratios 0.5 vs. 1.7), whites versus blacks or Hispanics (risk ratios 0.4 vs. 1.5 and 1.7), and persons from the West/Midwest versus those from the East (risk ratios 0.4/0.2 vs. 2.0), presumably in large part because of the prior probabilities of previous infection with the tubercle bacillus (35).

Thus, the rising number of tuberculosis cases in the United States has largely been concentrated in geographic areas and demographic groups in which these infections are coincident. Overall, in the United States between 1985 and 1994, roughly 70,000 excess cases of tuberculosis were recorded above the numbers projected based on stable trends from 1953 to 1984 (36); based on this model, nearly 40% of the cases in 1994 were in excess of that predicted. Recent CDC analyses have ascribed approximately 30% of the total excess to the effects of HIV infection (37) and 29% of the increase to the effects of immigration (38).

In the aggregate, recent CDC analyses (32,39) suggest that approximately 40% of new tuberculosis cases among persons aged 15 to 44 in the United States now occur among persons with HIV infection or AIDS. This might be regarded as "direct" HIV-related TB morbidity. Because many such cases develop among young adults of child-bearing ages, an additional portion of cases has occurred from spread of infection to their spouses, children, or other close contacts, "indirect" HIV-related TB morbidity. For details on the impact of HIV infection on tuberculosis in these groups, see Chapter 5.

The Incidence of Tuberculosis in Relationship to the Stage of HIV Infection

Among the various opportunistic infections (OIs) that afflict persons with HIV, *M. tuberculosis,* by virtue of its demonstrated pathogenicity in normal hosts, is the most inherently virulent microbe. *Pneumocystis carinii,* cytomegalovirus, *Candida,* and *M. avium* complex have shown clear propensities for individuals with diminished immune capacity or other abnormal host defenses. Hence, it is logical that tuberculosis would be among the earliest if not the initial opportunistic infection to appear in HIV-infected persons. Multiple series do, in fact, demonstrate that many HIV-infected patients who develop active tuberculosis may do so with $CD4^+$ lymphocyte counts considerably higher than those associated with other OIs and before the appearance of other AIDS-defining illnesses. Median CD4 counts were 326 in a series of HIV-infected patients from San Francisco (40), 240 in a series from France (41), and 316.5 among patients from Zaire (42).

However, among the series cited above, meaningful numbers of HIV-infected persons presented with tuberculosis with very low CD4 counts and following other AIDS-defining diagnoses. Also, other reports of tuberculosis in HIV-infected persons demonstrated lower ranges of CD4 counts at presentation (11, 43–45). There are no consistent explanations for this wide distribution of CD4 counts and other manifestations of immunosuppression in relation to tuberculosis. Potential variables include exogenous infection or reinfection, which might occur throughout the course of HIV progression, the relative "virulence" of the strain of *M. tuberculosis,* the number and viability of tubercle bacilli in the "latently infected" persons, or functional alterations of cellular immunity that do not correspond directly with CD4 numbers.

I believe that the initial factor above, exogenous infection or reinfection, is the most significant element in this phenomenon for the following reasons: (a) the aggregate data noted above suggest that there is a bipolar pattern of tuberculosis in relation to CD4 counts with clusters between 200 and 300 and below 50 $CD4^+$ cells; (b) epidemiologically, patients with diminishing CD4 counts and clinical AIDS are more likely to visit facilities where tuberculosis transmission is likely to occur, such as hospitals, clinics, pentamidine aerosol units, and special residencies or hospices; (c) AIDS patients very often present with the so-called "primary complex" pattern on chest x-ray, lower zone infiltrate with pleural effusions and hilar adenopathy, a finding consistent with recent exogenous infection; and (d) recent molecular epidemiology studies using restriction-length fragment polymorphism (RFLP) techniques have shown that nearly 40% of the new cases of tuberculosis in San Francisco and portions of the Bronx, New York are clustered by strain (15,16). These and other reports have shown that HIV infection is a highly significant risk factor for clustering, giving the implication of recent transmission (see Chapter 5).

CLINICAL PRESENTATIONS OF TUBERCULOSIS IN RELATION TO HIV INFECTION

As described in Chapter 4, the pathogenesis of the illness "tuberculosis" is intrinsically involved with the host's responses to the microorganisms, most notably involving the phenomenon known as delayed-type hypersensitivity (DTH). Because this phenomenon is largely an expression of T-lymphocyte activity, the host's immune response and thereby the clinical manifestations of tuberculosis are substantially altered as progressive HIV infection depletes and alters the functions of the $CD4^+$ lymphocyte and blood monocyte populations.

The typical features of tuberculosis occurring early and late in the course of HIV infection are displayed in Table 8.4. Although these generalizations are supported by numerous reports (11,42–48), there is considerable variation at both ends of the spectrum. Because of this unpredictability, it is vital that clinicians consider tuberculosis with virtually any inflammatory or febrile illness occurring in HIV-infected persons, particularly if their current or prior epidemiological profile indicates risk of exposure.

Patients with AIDS who develop active tuberculosis are more likely to manifest anergy, prominent fever and weight loss, multifocal extrapulmonary disease, and atypical chest x-ray patterns (see below).

Pulmonary Tuberculosis in HIV Infection

Early reports commented on the frequency of the so-called "primary complex pattern" of tuberculosis unilateral infiltrate, pleural effusion and hilar adenopathy in patients with advanced AIDS. However, these commonly were attributed to reactivation (49). But it has become apparent that many of these persons have been newly infected in their communities or in nosocomial settings; reference the above-cited molecular epidemiology studies, which document clear patterns of recent transmission among these vulnerable subjects (15,16).

As noted in Table 8.4, chest x-ray findings in persons with HIV infection or AIDS may vary significantly from those seen in comparable in-

TABLE 8.4. *Features of clinical tuberculosis in relation to HIV infection and immune suppression*

Clinical features	HIV-negative	Early HIV	Advanced AIDS	Comments
Tuberculin skin test (TST)	75–80% positive, ≥10 mm	40–70% positive, ≥ 10 mm	10–30% positive, ≥ 10 mm	As the percentage of reactors falls, the size of the reactions has been said to diminish; thus, 5 mm is regarded as a "significant" TST reaction.
Chest x-ray (CXR)	50–70% typical upper lobe, fib-nod; ~50% cavities	Mixed typical and atypical (see AIDS)	↑ Adenopathy, effusions, lower zone and miliary; ↓ cavitation	Although there is a clear trend toward atypical features with falling CD4 counts, these features may cross among the various HIV groups; see Table 8.5 for more detailed descriptions.
Sites involved	Pulm, 80%	Intermediate	Pulm, 20–30%	↑ XP in blacks regardless of HIV status
	XP, 16%		XP, 20–50%	Bacteremia with advanced AIDS
	Both, 4%		Both, 30–70%	↑ Lymphadenitis, pleural and pericardial disease with AIDS.
Sputum smear positivity (in culture-positive cases)	70–80%	± 50%	30–40%	See text. The lessened sensitivity of positive smears makes diagnosis more difficult.

↑, increased; ↓, decreased; pulm, pulmonary; XP, extrapulmonary

With diminishing numbers of CD4 lymphocytes, both cellular immunity and delayed-type hypersensitivity are compromised. This results in more widespread disease and exotic or atypical presentations of tuberculosis.

dividuals without HIV/AIDS. In reviewing the reported findings in various series, it is important to keep in mind that, among persons of differing racial and age groups, pulmonary tuberculosis has typically resulted in quite disparate findings: in African adults, extensive cavitation, intrathoracic lymphadenopathy, and relatively large pleural effusions are probably more common than among white adults. Hence, to appreciate the effects of HIV/AIDS on radiographic findings, it is most useful to compare with contemporary race- and age-adjusted groups. Also, one must consider the impact of advancing immunodeficiency on these results. Virtually every report that incorporates a contemporary control group notes significant differences between the HIV-positive and -negative patients (42–55). The most carefully studied quantitative analysis is represented in two articles from Tanzania and Burundi (54,55). Despite large numbers of patients and excellent methodology, this system was predictive of HIV serological status in only 68% to 75% of cases, dependent on operator-curve characteristics. See below for a more complete discussion.

Among patients with sputum culture-positive pulmonary tuberculosis, negative sputum smears are more likely to be found in HIV-positive persons. In series in which there were HIV-negative controls, there were generally more smear-negative/culture-positive cases among those with AIDS than those without HIV infection: 55% versus 19% (56), 37% versus 18% (57), 34% versus 21% (47), 43% versus 24%

(58), 23% versus 10% (59), and 49% versus 36% (59). The wide variations in yields presumably reflect variable laboratory techniques. Overall, the data indicate a modestly increased likelihood for negative sputum smear results. Fewer bacilli in sputum are arguably a result of failure of patients with advanced HIV infection to generate sufficient tissue-damaging immunity to form cavities. As noted in Chapter 4, the cavitary environment is highly conducive to mycobacterial growth and to delivery of the bacilli to the airways. The extraordinary proliferation of tubercle bacilli in the tissues and monocytes of HIV-infected AIDS patients suggests that the total mycobacterial burden in such patients may be even higher than in normal hosts with extensive cavitation. But, in view of the relative paucity of bacilli in sputum, alternative means of prompt diagnosis are of great importance. Bronchoscopy, blood cultures, biopsy, and other techniques are discussed below.

A comprehensive discussion of the differential diagnosis of pulmonary disease in persons with HIV/AIDS is beyond the scope of this chapter. It is obvious, however, to emphasize that although virtually any clinical presentation in these patients may be tuberculosis, there is an immense array of infection, neoplastic, or idiopathic disorders that may masquerade in TB-like raiment. Depending on the population observed, various mycobacteria (60–62), *Nocardia* (62, 63), other fungi (64), pneumococci (65–67), *Pneumocystis carinii* (68–71), *Salmonella* (66), lymphoma or Kaposi's sarcoma (68), lymphocytic interstitial pneumonitis (68), and numerous other microorganisms and disorders may invade these vulnerable lungs.

Extrapulmonary Tuberculosis in AIDS

Extrapulmonary tuberculosis (XPTB) has been an AIDS-defining illness in the United States since 1987 (72). In a CDC survey, XPTB was noted in 2.5% of all persons with AIDS reported from October, 1987 through March, 1989 (73). The prevalence of XPTB among AIDS patients varied considerably with nation of origin: United States born, 2.3%; Mexican born, 7.6%; and Haitian born = 12.7%. Race was also a significant variable for XBTB among males with AIDS: whites = 1.3%, blacks = 4.3%, and Hispanic = 2.8%. The risk of XPTB was also clearly related to the means by which HIV infection had been acquired: the highest rates of XPTB were seen among male intravenous drug users (IVDUs), 4.6%, with lower rates seen among others. The prevalence was lowest among homo/bisexuals, 1.5%; but, because this group constituted the bulk of AIDS cases, it yielded the greatest absolute number of XPTB cases.

The largest published series of patients with HIV infection and XPTB offers valuable insights into the nature of this co-infection (74). Between 1983 and 1988, 199 patients with positive serology or other indicators of HIV infection and tuberculosis involving extrapulmonary sites were seen at State University of New York Medical Center in Brooklyn; 158 HIV-negative contemporary patients with XPTB were used for comparison. Notable aspects of this series include the following: (a) due to the demographics of the community, 86% of the HIV infected patients were black, 11% were Hispanic, 54% were Haitian; (b) IVDU was the risk factor for HIV in 59% of the cases; (c) the HIV patients were more likely to have disseminated, mediastinal, intra-abdominal, and concurrent pulmonary tuberculosis; (d) the HIV patients presented with more prominent constitutional, respiratory, and gastrointestinal symptoms; (e) 95% of HIV patients with XPTB presented with fever, contrasted to 66% of those not infected with HIV; indeed, the median maximum temperature for the HIV patients was 40.0° versus 38.7° C for the HIV negative groups, and (f) tuberculin anergy was seen in 76% of HIV-infected cases versus 37% of HIV-negative.

Of particular interest, HIV-infected persons with XPTB were more likely to manifest generalized lymphadenopathy, hepatosplenomegaly, anemia, leukopenia, elevated liver enzymes, hyponatremia, and miliary infiltrates than the HIV-negative XPTB patients.

Positive sputum smears were the most common means by which the diagnosis of tuberculosis was initially indicated in this series of patients with AIDS and extrapulmonary tuberculosis. However, smears were positive in only 40% of patients despite the fact that sputum cultures were positive in 91% of cases. Similarly, urine cultures were positive in 61 of 79 (77%) of patients on whom specimens were submitted. The authors concluded that genitourinary disease was common despite the fact that symptoms typical of tuberculosis of the kidneys or bladder were uncommon and only 40% of these patients had significant hematuria or pyuria. Rather, I suspect that many of these positive sputum and urine cultures reflected mycobacteremia (blood cultures were positive in 56% of the cases) rather than gross structural disease of the lungs or GU tract.

Biopsies of various organs were commonly performed in this series of patients and are worthy of comment. The lesions from both the HIV positive and negative patients demonstrated granulomatous pathology. However, distinctive features of the lesions in HIV-infected persons included focal areas of necrosis laden with acid-fast bacilli; surrounding inflammation, if present, consisted of polymorphonuclear leukocytes and macrophages, not the classical cellular components of granulomas. Similar findings have been noted in other series of HIV-infected persons with disseminated tuberculosis (75).

A series of 97 HIV-infected patients from Los Angeles with all forms of tuberculosis was analyzed, relating clinical presentations to CD4 cell counts (43). An inverse relationship was observed between the CD4 counts and overt XPTB (Fig. 8.1). The patients with low CD4 counts were similarly prone to have intrathoracic lymphadenopathy on chest X-ray.

In summary, as the immunodeficiency worsens, a rising percentage of patients with tuberculosis manifest the infection at extrapulmonary sites. Furthermore, among those most severely compromised, increasingly exotic sites and presentations are involved including massive abdominal lymphadenopathy and solid organ abscesses (73–77), skin and soft tissues (73,74, 78–81), hemophagocytic syndrome (82), bronchoeso-phageal fistulae (83), multiple osseous foci (84), brain abscesses (85,86) and even a clinical illness mindful of septic shock associated with widely disseminated tuberculosis (87–91).

Consistent with the suggestion that extrapulmonary tuberculosis may be a manifestation of advanced immunosuppression, two reports showed that, among HIV-infected persons, XPTB was associated with shorter survival than with pulmonary tuberculosis. Among 126 HIV-positive patients from Tanzania with XPTB,

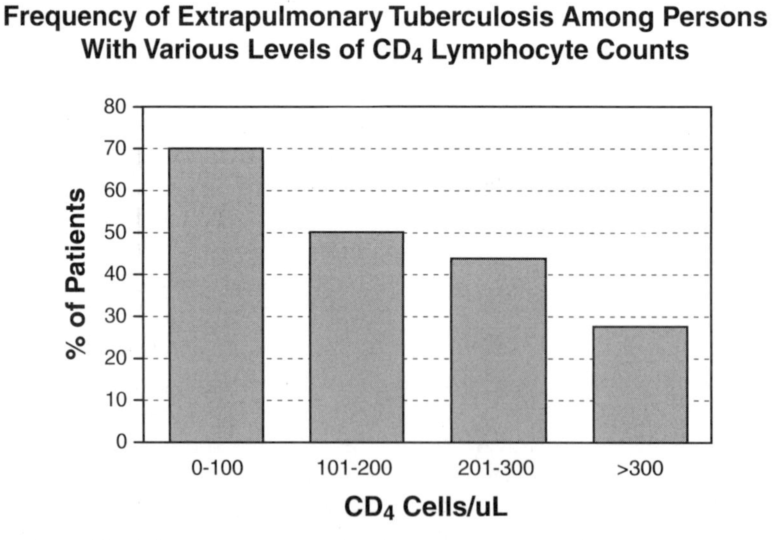

FIG. 8.1. Among HIV-infected persons who developed active tuberculosis, the percentage of those with manifest disease at extrapulmonary sites was progressively higher among those with advanced lymphocyte depletion.

29.7% had disseminated disease (92). Within 12 months of initiating treatment, there was a 22% case fatality rate; independent risk factors for death included peripheral lymphadenitis, lymphopenia, and mycobacteremia. Similarly, among 112 HIV-positive patients with tuberculosis from the U.S., 40% died during follow-up (93). Median survival for those with pulmonary tuberculosis was 30.4 months, extrapulmonary was only 15.6 months, and pulmonary plus XPTB, e.g., disseminated, was merely 8.4 months.

Specific Diagnostic Tests in HIV-Infected Persons Suspected of Tuberculosis

Tuberculosis may be an elusive disease, even in normal hosts. However, given the numerous effects of HIV infection on the manifestations of tuberculosis, it is even more difficult to recognize in this setting. Below, the standard tools employed in diagnosis will be reviewed.

Tuberculin Skin Testing

In normal hosts with newly diagnosed pulmonary tuberculosis, 15 to 25% do not manifest a significant reaction to 5-TU intermediate strength PPD testing (94–96). By comparison, among tuberculosis patients with advanced HIV infection, lymphopenia and inanition, there is a steady reduction in the proportion of those reacting to tuberculin. Among persons early in the course of HIV infection who have not developed other opportunistic infections, lymphopenia, and cachexia, 50 to 90% react to tuberculin; but, among those with AIDS and advanced debility, as few as 0 to 20% may be reactive (43,47,49). Among IDUs in Baltimore there was evidence that the amount of reactive induration diminished as the CD4 count fell (97); the authors attributed this to the increased prevalence of anergy among those with low CD4 numbers. Similarly, a national survey compared HIV-seropositive persons, homosexual males, IDUs, and females infected via heterosexual contact with seronegative controls for these groups (98); they observed that tuberculin reactivity overall was 4-fold lower among HIV-infected, 2.7% versus 10%.

Some have suggested using a panel of other delayed-type hypersensitivity antigens to identify anergic patients and clarify the meaning of negative tuberculin skin test results (97–100). However, in view of the inconsistent and ambiguous results of such anergy testing, this strategy must be regarded with skepticism. One recent study documented considerable fluctuation in DTH reactivity over time among HIV-positive subjects including both the development of and reversion from anergy (101). Another study of HIV-infected persons in the U.S. also found fluctuating skin-test reactivity and anergy to tuberculin despite retained DTH to mumps antigen (102). Among HIV-infected persons in Thailand, tuberculin reactivity was considerably depressed, but similar to the above report there was discordance between reactivity to mumps and Candida antigens and tuberculosis reactivity (103).

To overcome the limitations of skin testing in HIV-infected persons, some have advocated that the cut-point for significance be reduced from 5 mm to 2 mm induration (104). Two groups have suggested as an alternative that persons with either tuberculin reactivity or anergy should receive preventive chemotherapy; these recommendations were based on roughly comparable rates of tuberculosis among patients with tuberculin reactivity or anergy (105,106). However, these studies were done in countries with relatively high prevalences of tuberculosis. In two United States studies, anergy has *not* been predictive of subsequent tuberculosis risk (35,107). Reversing earlier recommendations, the 1997 USPHS/IDSA guidelines did not advocate anergy panel testing for HIV-infected persons (108).

At this time, it is difficult to describe a simple system for the detection of latent or new infection with tuberculosis among persons with HIV infection or AIDS. Tuberculin testing will continue to be performed since it is the only test for this purpose. However, the interpretation of such tests remains controversial. Current ATS/CDC guidelines state that 5 mm induration is significant, but there are frequent instances in which I believe epidemiological factors should supervene. For example, in close contacts to cases in which large numbers of other contacts have been newly infected or in persons from populations in which there is an extremely high prior probability of tuberculosis infection, e.g., Haitians or East Coast, inner-city, minority injecting drug users, preventive therapy might be given regardless of tuberculin reactivity (109).

Chest X-Ray

Most persons with HIV infection/AIDS who develop tuberculosis demonstrate abnormal findings on chest radiographic studies. However, as noted above, these findings often deviate far from the classical abnormalities associated with tuberculosis. Thus, given the immense array of other infectious or neoplastic conditions that involve the lungs of AIDS patients, there is great risk for confusion and delayed diagnosis (110–113) . Classic findings in the normal adult host with pulmonary tuberculosis include upper lobe, posterior segment, cavitary, fibronodular shadowing without hilar adenopathy or pleural effusions. While some HIV-infected patients with tuberculosis have x-rays similar to this, the pulmonary manifestations of tuberculosis in these patients are many and varied. Reports include confluent pneumonia, lower zone infiltrates, hilar/paratracheal adenopathy, pleural effusions and miliary shadowing (42–55); comparative chest x-ray findings among patients without HIV, with early HIV, and with AIDS are shown in Table 8.5 (114–117). Some patients with positive sputum cultures have been reported to have normal chest x-rays, presumably reflecting either endobronchial disease or "filtration" of bacilli by the pulmonary capillary bed during mycobacteremia. The nonspecificity of these findings reinforces the need to be ever alert to the possibility of tuberculosis in individuals known to be HIV infected or among persons with significant risk factors for HIV exposure. Failure to obtain sputum and other suitable studies is associated with delayed or failed diagnosis and risks for continued transmission of infection and death (110,118).

Sputum Smears and Cultures

Patients with HIV infection or AIDS are slightly less likely to have positive sputum smears than other persons with pulmonary tuberculosis. Among various series of HIV-infected tuberculosis patients with sputum culture-proven disease, positive smears were reported in 31% (119), 45% (56), 57% (58), 66% (120), 60% (121), 54% (11), and 83% (52) of cases. The likelihood of positive smears in HIV-infected persons generally relates to the extent of pulmonary involvement as reflected by the chest x-ray. Among those with cavitary disease, smears are typically positive, whereas among those with early interstitial or lymphadenopathic disease, the likelihood of positive smears was diminished, as would be the case in HIV-negative patients. However, among those with far-advanced disseminated disease and confluent, acinar shadowing, over 90% may be smear positive (121).

Other Diagnostic Aids

Because cultures of the sputum were used to define the pulmonary cases noted above, the test was *de facto* sensitive. However, commensurate with the reduced number of bacilli seen on smears, cultures were often sparse and, thus, slower to be recognized in the laboratory. Hence, the clinician is confronted with a distinct management problem in dealing with an HIV-positive patient with symptoms and radiographic findings compatible with tuberculosis but with negative initial sputum smears. If the evaluation fails to yield a plausible diagnosis, options include the following: (a) *Sputum induction* may be useful in persons who do not spontaneously produce lower respiratory secretions. Obviously, caution should be taken to perform such procedures in a controlled environment to reduce the likelihood of transmission. (b) *Gastric aspirates* might be useful, particularly in a hospitalized patient for whom an early morning procedure can be performed before peristalsis carries away the overnight accumulation of secretions. Although gastric matter is potentially vulnerable to contamination by environmental mycobacteria, a positive smear in the appropriate setting should, I believe, be regarded as presumptive evidence of tuberculosis. (c) *Bronchoscopy* has yielded variable results. Two studies indicated that fiberoptic bronchoscopy with transbronchial biopsy was useful in early diagnosis of sputum smear-nega-

TABLE 8.5. *Chest x-ray findings in pulmonary tuberculosis among HIV-infected: variations in relation to CD4 depletion*

Series	Dates	HIV-negative controls	Early HIV ≥200 CD4	Advanced HIV, HIV/AIDS
South Africa (114)	1989–1994	N.A.	18/150 "Typical" 32/150+ effusions	136/150= low or midzone, adenopathy, interstitial
Côte D'Ivoire (115)	1990–1992	56% cavitary 42% noncavitary 2% hilar adenopathy 2% miliary 4% effusions	53% cavitary 39% noncavitary 8% hilar adenopathy 3% miliary 8% effusions	29% cavitary 58% noncavitary 20% hilar adenopathy 9% miliary 11% effusions
U.S. (116)	1993–1995	N.A.	20% cavitary 7% hilar adenopathy 17% interstitial pattern 10% effusions 3% "normal"	7% cavitary 30% hilar adenopathy 27% interstitial pattern 7% effusions 9% "normal"
U.S. (43)	1990–1991	N.A.	27% upper lobe, cavities too rare to be analyzed 13% hilar adenopathy 27% effusions	26% upper lobe, cavities too rare to be analyzed 36% hilar adenopathy 10% effusions
			"HIV without AIDS"	"HIV/AIDS"
Rwanda (46)	1988–1989	91% cavitary 55% upper lobe 0% hilar adenopathy 9% miliary 9% effusions	69% cavitary 30% upper lobe 7% hilar adenopathy 23% miliary 46% effusions	28% cavitary 16% upper lobe 40% hilar adenopathy 26% miliary 42% effusions
			HIV-infected, not stratified	
Uganda (117)	1992–1993	57% cavitary 26% pneumonic 6% adenopathy 11% effusions 0% miliary	18% 46% 26% 23% 7%	
			"Non-AIDS"	"AIDS"
Haiti (47)	1988–1989	87% cavitary 13% noncavitary 8% adenopathy 12% effusions <1% normal	76% cavitary 21% noncavitary 23% adenopathy 11% effusions 5% normal	33% cavitary −40% noncavitary −60% adenopathy 0% effusions −20% normal

Between these series of patients with pulmonary tuberculosis, there are wide variations among described abnormalities. The origins of these inconsistencies are not readily apparent. However, within each of these series there is a very clear and predictable gradient toward higher rates of "atypical" radiographic findings with diminishing CD4 counts and progressive immunosuppression.

tive tuberculosis despite the fact that nonspecific inflammation, rather than classic caseating granulomata, were often seen (122,123). [Indeed, a careful study of the histopathology of the lungs of persons with HIV infection and tuberculosis found there to be a progression toward less well-formed granulomas and increasing numbers of bacilli with advancing CD4 depletion (124). As noted by Horsburgh, this tuberculosis without tubercles reflects profound changes in the biology of tuberculosis (125).] In contrast to the two studies cited above, another report, which did not address exactly the same types of patients, suggested that transbronchial biopsy did not contribute significantly above sputum studies and bronchial washings or bronchoalveolar lavage (126). Similarly, among 95 HIV-infected patients hospitalized for pulmonary disease in Tanzania, fiberoptic bronchoscopy with BAL was the sole source of diagnosis in only 8% of cases (67). By contrast, among 111 patients with AIDS from Rwanda, who had pulmonary disease of unknown etiology, bronchoscopy yielded a diagnosis in 84% of cases including 25 patients with tuberculosis (111). Of note, transbronchial biopsy had a substantially greater yield (82%) than bronchoalveolar lavage (26%) among these patients. Transbronchial needle aspiration of mediastinal lymph nodes was shown to have unique diagnostic utility among a series of patients with sputum smears negative intrathoracic tuberculosis (127). Also, bronchoscopy may be central to the diagnosis of endobronchial disease due to *M. tuberculosis, M. avium* complex, *Pneumocystis carinii,* or various other disorders seen in patients with AIDS (128,129). (d) *Computed tomographic scans of intrathoracic lymphadenopathy.* Highly suggestive CT findings were noted on 20 of 25 (80%) AIDS patients with proven tuberculosis (130). Typically, there were massive, heterogeneous soft tissue lesions with very low density centers. Although the authors did not regard this finding as pathognomonic, they did deem it sufficient to begin presumptive treatment for tuberculosis. As noted above (67), this group has recently employed TBNA for diagnosis in this setting.

In *summary*, in cases with suspected tuberculosis, clinicians have an array of diagnostic approaches. Although empirical therapy may well be initiated based on an amalgam of nonspecific clinical, laboratory, and epidemiological features, aggressive efforts should be made to obtain positive cultures to verify the diagnosis. This is critical in cases where there is an equivocal response to empirical treatment, the most important issue to address being the possibility of drug resistance. Obviously, in view of the frequency with which there is extrapulmonary involvement in HIV/AIDS patients, cultures of blood, urine, peripheral lymph nodes, and other involved sites should be obtained when the diagnosis is in question (43,74, 131,132).

Pediatric Tuberculosis and HIV Infection

HIV has influenced pediatric tuberculosis by three broad avenues: (a) household spread of tuberculosis from HIV-infected parents, (b) congenital transmission of HIV infection, and (c) blood-borne transmission of HIV to children, particularly to those with inherited clotting disorders. Clearly, the dominant factor has been (a); as noted in Chapter 5, childhood tuberculosis rates soar from the "trickle-down" effect.

The actual direct impact of HIV-infected children has been more difficult to discern, largely because of the relative paucity of these infections. Please see Chapter 9 for a more extensive review of the influence of HIV infection on the clinical presentation, treatment, and prevention of tuberculosis in children.

TREATMENT OF TUBERCULOSIS IN HIV-INFECTED PERSONS

There are numerous issues that potentially might distinguish the treatment of patients with tuberculosis who are coinfected with HIV from those without HIV. Some of the more salient questions are discussed below. Although many of these questions lack sufficient data for resolution, I will attempt to delineate the issues involved and offer what I deem to be practical responses to these problems.

How Does HIV Infection Influence the Choice and Duration of Tuberculosis Chemotherapy?

Numerous reports have suggested that the initial response to therapy is comparable among HIV-positive and -negative populations (48,53, 133–138). These series generally demonstrate that among "surviving" patients, the bacteriological, clinical, and radiographic responses are similar between the two groups. However, there are consistent indications of higher rates of early (first month) deaths from tuberculosis as well as excessive deaths from other causes during the course of treatment in the above-noted series (see Table 8.6 for details). In a large sense, these deaths appear related to the ad-

TABLE 8.6. *Treatment of tuberculosis in persons with HIV infection: results from selected studies*

Studies					Results				
Site first author (ref.)	Dates of trial (date of report)	Regimen(s) employed	No. of patients	Post-Rx follow-up	Mortality	Failures	Recurrence	Adverse reactions (ARs)	Comments
Zaire, Perriëns[a]	1987–1989 (1991)	2 IThS/4 ITh	170	24 mo	47/150 (31%)	13/82 (16%)	8/58 (14%)	18/66 (27%)	Relapses in HIV (+) > than HIV(−)
San Francisco, Small (133)	1981–1988 (1991)	2 IR ± E/7 IR 2 IRP ± E/4 IR	132	>20 mo	58/132 (44%)	1/125 (1%)	3/58 (5%)	23/125 (18%)	
Kenya, Nunn[b]	1989–1990 (1992)	(a) 1 IThS/11 ITh (b) 2 IRP(S)/6 ITh	91 16	NA	22/91 (24%) 0/16 (0%)	NA	NA	NA	(S), SM given 1 month
Kenya, Hawken (139)	1989–1991 (1993)	(a) 1 IThS/11 ITh (b) 2 IRP(S)/6 ITh	58	15 mo	10/58 (17%) (see comments)	NA	10/58 (17%)	(a) 18/93 (19%) (b) 4/18 (22%)	9 of 10 deaths in regimen (a). Recurrence associated with ARs.
Europe, Euro. TB Study Group[c]	(1992)	(a) 9 IRP (b) 2 IRPE(S)/7 IRP	137 125	NA	38/138 (28%) 32/125 (26%)	7/137 (5%) 11/125 (9%)	NA	18/137 (13%) 20/125 (16%)	Low primary resistance; thus, EMB of no benefit.
Zaire, Mukadi[d]	1989–1991 (1992)	(a) 2 IRPE/4 I_2R_2 (b) 2 IRPE/10 I_2Th_2	107 107	NA	22/107 (21%) 22/107 (21%)	8/107 (7%) 7/107 (6%)	8/107 (7%) 7/107 (6%)	NA	

continues

TABLE 8.6. *Continued.*

Studies					Results				
Site first author (ref.)	Dates of trial (dateof report)	Regimen(s) employed	No. of patients	Post-Rx follow-up	Mortality	Failures	Recurrence	Adverse reactions (ARs)	Comments
Uganda, Okwera[e]	1990–1991 (1994)	(a) 2 IThS/10 ITh (b) 2 IRP/7 IR	90 101	16 mo	(35%) (28%) (see comments)	NA	NA	(a) 12/90 (13%) (b) 1/101 (1%)	Numbers not reported; only percentage of deaths
Los Angeles, Jones[f]	1990–1992 (1994)	(a) 2 IRP/7 IR (b) 2 IRP/7 I_2R_2	50 32	17–22 mo	29/66 (44%)	5/89 (6%)	0/66 (0%)	5/89 (6%)	Regimen (b) involved DOT for noncompliant patients
Zambia, Elliott[g] Elliott (181)	1989–1993 (1995)	(a) 2 IRPS Th/10 ITh (b) 2 IThS/10 ITh	65 108	14 mo	74/103 (43%)	NA	(a) 8/26 (31%) (b) 7/77 (19%)	26/174 (17%)	More non-compliance with regimen (a) because of travel required to get SM shots.
Zaire, Perriëns (140)	1989–1991	(a) 2 IRPE/4 I_2R_2 (b) 2 IRPE/10 I_2R_2	124 123	24 mo	15/119 (13%) 19/121 (16%)	"3.8%"	(a) 9/119 ("9%") (b) 1/121 ("1.9%")	NA	Deaths mostly early in course. Failures not given per regimen. Recurrences based on survivors
USA, El-Sadr (142)	1993–1995 (1998)	2 IRPE ± LQN (a) 4 I_2R_2 (b) 7 I_2R_2	(a) 51 (b) 50	Median, 24 mo	21/50 (41%) 26/50 (52%)	NA	(a) 2/50 (4%) (b) 1/50 (2%)	Initial phase ARs = 7–21% ARs in (a) arm = 8% ARs in (b) arm = 10%	• LQN randomized; no effects upon regimen efficiency. • Only 1 death due to TB. • 2 relapses with RIF monoresistance.

Haiti, Chaisson (138)	1990–1992 (1996)	2 $I_3R_3P_3E_3$/4 I_3R_3	159	28 mo	9% during Rx; 34% at 1.5 years follow	3/159 (2%)	7/129 (5.4%)	Rash 3% Arthralgia 2% Abnl LFTS 3–12%	Low CD4# was risk factor for death
Côte D'Ivoire, Kassim[b]	1992–1993 (1995)	2 IRP/4 IR	410	24 mo	Mos 0–6, 12% Mos 7–24, 21%	"2%"	HIV-1: 3/106 (3%) HIV-1 and -2: 9/138 (7%)	"4%"	Included patients with HIV-1 or HIV-1 and -2 infection. Authors felt data were "minimum estimates" of failure/ relapse rates

[a] Perriëns JH, Colebunders RL, Karahunda C. Increased mortality and tuberculosis treatment failure rate among human immunodeficiency virus (HIV)-seropositive compared with HIV-seronegative patients with pulmonary tuberculosis treated with "standard" chemotherapy in Kinshasa, Zaire. *Am Rev Respir Dis* 1991;144:750–755.

[b] Nunn P, Brindle R, Carpenter L. Cohort study of HIV infection in tuberculosis patients, Nairobi, Kenya: analysis of early (6-months) mortality. *Am Rev Respir Dis* 1992;146:849–854.

[c] European Tuberculosis Study Group. *Tuberculosis in HIV-infected patients: a multicentric randomized comparative study of a three- versus a four-drug regimen.* Paper presented at the VIII International Conference on AIDS/III STD World Congress, Amsterdam, 1992.

[d] Mukadi Y, Perriëns J, St. Louis M. *Immunological evaluation of HIV-1-positive patients with pulmonary tuberculosis in Kinshasa, Zaire.* Paper presented at the VIII International Conference on AIDS III STD World Congress, Amsterdam, 1992. Mukadi Y, St. Louis M, Perriëns J. *Maintenance chemotherapy after short-course treatment of tuberculosis in HIV-infected persons: is it needed and it is effective?* Paper presented at the VIII International Conference on AIDS/III STD World Congress, Amsterdam, 1992.

[e] Okwera A, Whalen C, Byekwaso F, et al. Randomised trial of thiacetazone and rifampicin-containing regimens for pulmonary tuberculosis in HIV-infected Ugandans. *Lancet* 1994;344:1323–1328.

[f] Jones BE, Otaya M, Antoniskis D, et al. A prospective evaluation of antituberculosis therapy in patients with human immunodeficiency virus infection. *Am J Respir Crit Care Med* 1994;150:1499–1502.

[g] Elliott AM, Halwiindi B, Hayes RJ, et al. The impact of human immunodeficiency virus on mortality in patients treated for tuberculosis: two-year follow-up of cohort in Lusaka, Zambia. *Trans R Soc Trop Med Hyg* 1995;89:75–82.

[h] Kassim S, Sassan-Morokro M, Ackah A, et al. Two-year follow-up of persons with HIV-1- and HIV-2–associated pulmonary tuberculosis treated with short-course chemotherapy in West Africa. *AIDS* 1995;9:1185–1191.

vanced stage of tuberculosis at diagnosis as well as the debilitating and underlying diseases from which the patients suffer and not primarily the drug regimens with which they are treated. However, several of the reports from Africa suggested increased early mortality in those who received the less-potent traditional isoniazid, thiacetazone, and streptomycin regimens than the modern short-course regimens featuring isoniazid, rifampin, and pyrazinamide (135,137,139). Excess mortality was seen also among a subset of patients with AIDS and tuberculosis in Uganda receiving a thiacetazone regimen in comparison to those receiving a rifampin regimen; there was both excess mortality and higher rates of drug reactions sequestered among those patients who had elevated levels of neopterin and other markers of cellular immune activation (135).

Furthermore, several series have shown a modestly greater risk for relapse or recurrence posttreatment for persons with AIDS that does seem related to the *duration* of therapy. Perriens and colleagues in a study from Zaire compared the outcome of HIV-positive patients treated with 6-month regimen (2-IRPE daily followed by 4-IR twice weekly) and a 12-month regimen (2-IRPE daily followed by 10-IR twice weekly) (140). Relapse rates were significantly higher among those receiving the 6-month regimen (9%) than 12 months of treatment (1.9%) ($p <$ .01). Pulido and colleagues in Spain observed in a nonrandomized series that, among patients with AIDS and tuberculosis, 10 of 41 (24%) patients who received less than 9 months of chemotherapy relapsed, whereas only 5 of 148 (3.4%) receiving 9 months or more did so (141). Multivariant analysis identified duration of therapy as a major element in the disparate relapse rates, with a relative hazard of 9.2 for the shorter-duration therapy. Most recently, a multicenter national trial in the United States compared 6 months and 9 months of treatment for HIV-infected adults with pansusceptible tuberculosis (142). Relapse rates were 3.9%, two patients, for the 6-month regimen, and 2%, one patient, for the 9-month regimen; because of the limited numbers, this was not a statistically significant difference.

Several other studies contrasted relapse or cure rates among HIV-infected and uninfected persons treated simultaneously with identical 6-month regimens. They universally showed somewhat worse outcomes among those with HIV infection. Hawkens and colleagues described an increased risk of recurrent tuberculosis in a group of patients from Kenya (139). This report documented that 10 of 58 (17%) HIV-positive patients available for follow-up had recurrence, contrasted with 1 of 138 HIV-negative patients, a 34-fold apparent relative risk. However, seven of the ten who experienced recurrence had major cutaneous drug reactions, interrupting therapy and confounding the issue. But, Elliott in Zambia noted a marked disparity in relapse rates without the confusing association between relapses and drug reactions: HIV-positive patients relapsed at a rate of 22/100 patient years of observation versus 6/100 patient years among HIV-negatives (137). A recent Johns Hopkins study in Haiti found lower cure rates (69% vs. 79%) and slightly higher relapse rates (5.4% vs. 2.8%, $p = .36$) among HIV-infected individuals receiving a 6-month regimen (138).

The studies cited above do not provide unassailable evidence of the need for extended therapy for HIV-infected persons with tuberculosis. Indeed, despite the significantly higher risk of relapse among the HIV-positive patients from Zaire, the authors concluded that for various operational reasons the 6-month regimen was still the better option (140). The CDC/American Thoracic Society Guidelines of 1994 endorse the 6-month regimen with the caveat that treatment should be prolonged if patients are slow to respond (143).

However, I would argue that the available information does indicate that there is a biologically meaningful, greater likelihood of recurrent tuberculosis in HIV-infected persons *regardless* of the duration or drugs employed. The size of this disparity tends to be diminished by early deaths during and after tuberculosis therapy from other complications. However, among populations receiving antiretroviral therapy and/or better prevention and treatment of opportunistic infections, prolonged survival will afford more time for tuberculosis relapses to occur.

Although one may propose that in resource-poor nations a shorter regimen may be more cost-effective (140), I would suggest that for the industrialized nations strong consideration should be given to the use of 9-month regimens (134,144). In addition to protecting the individual patient at risk, the prevention of relapses should protect family members or other contacts (including many who may be HIV-infected and very susceptible to tuberculosis).

Another option might be to complete a 6-month regimen, then put the patients on lifetime "preventive therapy" with INH (145,146). This might prevent both endogenous reactivation as well as exogenous reinfection. This approach might not be suitable for generalized application, but for selected populations or highly motivated individuals, this strategy seems quite defensible to me.

Are Twice- and Thrice-Weekly Regimens Adequate?

Intermittent chemotherapy is a vital tactic in facilitating directly observed therapy. There has been some reluctance to apply intermittent regimens in HIV-infected persons out of concern that less frequent drug administration might weaken the chemotherapy. However, among HIV-negative patients there is abundant evidence that regimens that are entirely intermittent or begin with 0.5 to 1 month of daily and continue with 5.5 to 5.0 months of intermittent therapy are fully the equal of daily regimens of comparable duration (see Chapter 10). Notably, in the study from Zaire cited above (140), results for a 6-month regimen (2 months of IRPE daily followed by 4 months of IR twice weekly) were quite similar for HIV-positive or -negative patients: failure rates 3.8% versus 2.7% and relapse rates 9% versus 5.3%. The Haitian study cited above, which employed an entirely intermittent, thrice-weekly regimen, resulted in a relapse rate, 5.4%, that was not significantly different from that of HIV-negative persons, 2.8% (138). Similarly, HIV-infected patients in Los Angeles (134), Denver (147), New York (148), and a national trial (142) have been treated with regimens employing intermittency in the continuation phase with excellent response and relapse rates. Hence, we should anticipate that thrice- or twice-weekly regimens would be comparable in efficacy to daily schedules if they are comprised of highly effective drugs such as isoniazid, rifampin, and pyrazinamide. The major caveat which should be noted is the potential deleterious effect of malabsorption on the effectiveness of intermittent regimens. Given fewer doses, particularly for the rifamycins which typically are not administered in higher than daily amounts when given intermittently, malabsorption could potentially have a more disruptive effect in this setting (see below).

Does the High Prevalence of Extrapulmonary Tuberculosis, Including CNS Disease, Require Special Consideration in Chemotherapy?

Tuberculosis specialists commonly believe that even HIV-negative patients with disseminated or CNS disease should receive extended duration of treatment (143,149). Although not well founded in controlled studies, higher doses of standard drugs also have been advocated for CNS disease because of considerations of poor penetration of the blood–brain barrier (150). Therefore, it is logical to project these concerns onto HIV-infected persons with such forms of tuberculosis. In the absence of controlled trials, one cannot offer firm recommendations in these situations. However, it seems prudent with HIV-infected cases to be aggressive in treatment including extending treatment to a minimum of 9 months, measuring serum levels of the antituberculosis drugs, and if these levels are low or even in the "low normal" range, increasing the dosage (see below for discussion of suboptimal absorption of drugs in AIDS patients). Regarding CNS tuberculosis, it is important to stress that the one drug that predictably crosses the blood–brain barrier is isoniazid (150) and that CNS tuberculosis with INH-resistant tuberculosis requires particularly thoughtful management (see Chapter 7 on chemotherapy of tuberculous meningitis).

Does the Risk of Drug-Resistant Tuberculosis in HIV-Infected Persons Merit Special Consideration in Initial Therapy?

Recent outbreaks of MDR TB among AIDS patients in New York and Florida have focused attention on this issue (13,14). Notable aspects of these epidemics included rapid progression and high lethality of MDR TB in this population. A recent multicenter survey from AIDS trial centers around the United States documented that persons with AIDS are at significantly higher risk to have drug-resistant tuberculosis than contemporary HIV-negative controls in those communities (151). In the New York City area, the differences were dramatic: overall, 37% versus 19%, and MDR TB, 19% versus 6%. The preponderance of MDR TB cases among HIV-infected persons can be ascribed to massive numbers of nosocomially transmitted cases in 11 hospitals in the New York City area during this period (152). Outside the New York City area in this survey, there was no greater likelihood of drug resistance among HIV-infected persons save for a modestly higher rate of rifampin resistance. Recent reports from Argentina (153), Spain (154,155), and France (156) confirm outbreaks of MDR TB in association with HIV/AIDS.

In an ongoing surveillance project in San Francisco, an apparent increase in acquired drug resistance cases was noted between 1990 and 1994 (157); these cases were associated with AIDS, noncompliance with antituberculosis therapy, and gastrointestinal symptoms. This series from San Francisco was remarkable for the frequency with which monoresistance to rifampin was involved: 6 of 14 cases. This selective or early acquired resistance to rifamycins has been very rarely seen before, but several other reports have confirmed the phenomenon (158–160).

Although some cases appeared to be related to previous rifabutin prophylaxis against *M. avium* complex, most cases involved acquired rifamycin resistance while receiving multidrug regimens for tuberculosis. Features associated in a CDC study with risk for acquired resistance included diarrhea and antifungal therapy (161). By comparison, a retrospective analysis of all patients with monoresistance to rifampin in New York City in 1993–1994 found that 76 of 96 were known HIV-positive (162). In terms of choosing an initial regimen, it is important to note that 48 (50%) of these cases entailed primary rifampin resistance. Multivariant analysis of this group indicated that sputum-smear positivity, advanced immunosuppression, and nonadherence to therapy were associated with acquired rifampin resistance. These observations strongly suggest that persons with AIDS and tuberculosis are at some increased risk for both primary and acquired rifamycin resistance.

The actual mechanism(s) of rifampin monoresistance are not well understood. Malabsorption or other mechanisms that result in diminished bioavailability are discussed below and in Chapter 11. Noncompliance with erratic drug ingestion also is considered in detail below and in Chapters 10 and 11. Although these elements certainly are associated with acquired resistance, they do not specifically address rifamycin monoresistance. As reviewed in Chapter 10, the concept of subpopulations of tubercle bacilli that are acted on by some but not all of the medications in a regimen may be important here. If persons with advanced AIDS have a particularly large compartment of rapidly multiplying bacilli on which rifamycin antibiotics have a uniquely bactericidal role, this could result in de facto monotherapy, thus spawning such resistance (163,164).

The impact of these findings on choice of treatment for an individual patient is not yet clear. My inferences at this time would be as follows: (a) all AIDS patients with previously treated TB who have relapsed should be managed on the assumption of at least rifampin resistance; (b) all patients with AIDS and *any* indication of rapid transit, malabsorption, or potential pharmacokinetic interference should have pharmacokinetic confirmation of adequate drug levels *or* treatment with high-range rifampin dosage such as 600 mg rather than 450 mg for those weighing less than 50 kg and 750 mg rather than 600 mg for those over 50 kg body weight.

Because the drug susceptibility patterns of tuberculosis among AIDS patients generally reflects the indigenous prevalence of resistance in the communities or populations from which the patients come, it is essential to take meticulous histories of travel and personal and institutional exposure to determine the possibility of exposure to MDR TB. And, if one cannot be reasonably sure in excluding the likelihood of drug resistance, initial therapy should include a sufficient number of drugs to anticipate the probable pattern(s) of resistance. This would be particularly true in patients with advanced HIV infection, debility, and other markers of high risk for mortality including multisite disease, anergy, anemia, lymphopenia, and prolonged diarrhea (137). For example, in New York City, where MDR TB had proved rapidly lethal among AIDS patients despite treatment with standard regimens, initial treatment for patients deemed at risk of MDR TB has included second-line drugs to which resistance was uncommon. This approach has significantly improved response rates and survival (165,166). Obviously, such polypharmacy potentially entails considerable medication side effects, potential toxicity, and expense. In light of these findings, it is imperative that rapid susceptibility testing be performed promptly to resolve the question of drug resistance (see Chapter 2 for review of these techniques).

Does the Risk of Malabsorption of Antituberculosis Medications Influence the Dosage of Medications Administered?

A brief case history may help frame the potential significance of this problem (167).

Case

A 35-year-old white male HIV-infected health care worker from New York City was referred to National Jewish for treatment of relapsing tuberculosis presumed secondary to drug resistance. His present illness had begun in May 1991 with fever, wasting, and generalized lymphadenopathy. An axillary node biopsy was positive on smear for AFB, but the culture yielded no growth. He had been started empirically on four-drug therapy with isoniazid, rifampin, pyrazinamide, and ethambutol, resulting in defervescence, involution of the adenopathy, and weight gain. However, 10 months later, while still receiving these drugs, fever, adenopathy, and weight loss recurred. Repeat node biopsy was smear positive for AFB, and while cultures and susceptibility were pending, he was referred to Denver. On admission, he recalled a long history of 3 to 5 loose bowel movements per day but denied diarrhea or unusual stool characteristics. However, fecal fat was 23.4 g per 24 hours, normal being 0–7 g. Pharmacokinetic studies of his medications revealed the data in Table 8.7.

Susceptibility studies of his culture returned at this time, indicating resistance only to isoniazid and streptomycin. Dosage of the rifampin and pyrazinamide were increased to 1,200 mg and 2,000 mg twice daily, respectively, and ethambutol plus capreomycin were incorporated in the regimen. He enjoyed a prompt clinical response and remained free of signs and symptoms of tuberculosis 18 months later.

We inferred that this patient had experienced recrudescent tuberculosis caused by progressive malabsorption related to some type of enteropathy (stools were negative for ova and parasites as well as bacterial pathogens). These observations led to the collection of the data on larger numbers of persons with HIV infection and mycobacterial diseases noted below (168).

Prospective studies of the prevalence of malabsorption of antituberculosis medications among persons with AIDS have been limited. However, early anecdotal data indicated that there may be highly significant reductions in the amounts of medications absorbed (169). More recently, a report from Canada analyzed absorption of INH, rifampin, and pyrazinamide

TABLE 8.7. *Pharmacokinetic data on antituberculosis drugs, case report*

Drug	Dose (mg)	2-Hour level (μg/ml)	6-Hour level (μg/ml)	Normal range (μg/ml)
Isoniazid	300	0.84	0.13	3–5
Rifampin	600	1.1	2.6	8–24
	900	7.1	3.2	
	1,200	13.0	9.1	
Pyrazinamide	1,500	41.0	22	60–70
	2,000	50.0	42	

(PZA), comparing levels in 12 normal subjects with those in three groups with 12 each of HIV-infected persons—those with CD4 = 200 and no symptoms, those with CD4 = 200 and symptoms but no loose stools, and those with CD4 = 200 and three or more loose stools daily (170). They found significant malabsorption in none of the normals, but in 33%, 50%, and 67% of the three groups. Another study from the United States examined serum levels in 26 patients with AIDS and tuberculosis (168). They observed low 2-hour concentrations commonly, most notably for rifampin and ethambutol. In addition, they described apparent interactions between pyrazinamide and zidovudine resulting in lower PZA levels, and between pyrazinamide and rifampin resulting in lower RIF levels. By contrast with these observations, a study from South Africa did not demonstrate malabsorption of INH, rifampin, or pyrazinamide among 13 patients with tuberculosis and AIDS (171). Rather, they showed that, although the timing of drug uptake might be delayed, the persons with AIDS, some of whom had clinical indications of enteropathy, had comparable AUC and C_{max} median values to 14 controls.

Despite these conflicting data from South Africa, I believe that it behooves clinicians to consider the possibility that malabsorption may interfere with the chemotherapy of tuberculosis in persons with AIDS. Markers or risk factors for malabsorption may include histories indicative of rapid bowel transit. Diarrhea was a prominent predictor of mortality among AIDS patients treated for tuberculosis in Zambia (137) and was present in one of two patients with AIDS who acquired drug resistance in association with malabsorption (172). Because the potential implications of malabsorption are so profound, including treatment failure, continued transmission of tuberculosis, acquired drug resistance, and death, I would suggest that persons with AIDS (or other conditions with high risks of malabsorption) undergo early therapeutic drug monitoring. Based on the observation of delayed uptake in the South African study, however, a single 2-hour postadministration assay may not be adequate.

Should the Risk of Adverse Drug Reactions Influence the Choice of Antituberculosis Medications?

Adverse drug reactions (ADRs) to antituberculosis medications have been noted to occur more frequently among HIV-infected persons. In San Francisco, ADRs requiring cessation of therapy occurred in 18% of 125 patients on treatment with modern agents (133). Reactions included rash in 13 patients and hepatitis in six; these findings were attributed mostly to rifampin and pyrazinamide. Similarly, among 65 Zambian children with HIV infection, seven (11%) developed cutaneous reactions within 8 weeks of commencing regimens without thiacetazone (173); two cases of fatal Stevens-Johnson syndrome were reported. This propensity is not unique to antituberculosis agents: an increased prevalence of cutaneous drug reactions was noted among 125 of 684 (18.3%) HIV-infected persons in Boston taking other medications; as in the African thiacetazone patients discussed below, these reactions tended to occur more frequently among patients later in the course of HIV infection (174).

In addition to cutaneous ADRs, a recent report from Florida demonstrated that HIV infection also predisposed patients to antituberculosis drug-induced hepatitis (175). In this study, it was shown that HIV infection increased fourfold the likelihood of perturbations of liver chemistries, viral hepatitis C infection increased the risk fivefold, and that coinfection with HIV and hepatitis C increased the risk 14-fold.

Overall, however, these observations do not change the use of standard medications including INH, the rifamycins, pyrazinamide, ethambutol, or streptomycin. Nonetheless, patients and clinic staff should be informed of the relatively greater likelihood of cutaneous ADRs, particularly among high-risk individuals as described below.

The one major drug toxicity unassailably linked to HIV infection is major dermatitis associated with thiacetazone administration. In Africa, where thiacetazone, because of its affordability, has been a standard component of regimens, cutaneous hypersensitivity reactions among HIV-infected patients have been noted in

20% of Kenyan patients in one report (176), 32% of patients in another Kenyan study (48), 11% of a series from Uganda (135), and 12% of yet another series from Kenya (139). Notably, among these patients with dermatologic reactions, there were three cases of fatal toxic epidermal necrolysis (176), two cases of "exfoliative dermatitis" and one case of Stevens-Johnson syndrome (48). Curiously, there was a significantly higher risk of tuberculosis relapse among patients in one series who had cutaneous reactions to thiacetazone despite replacing the drug with ethambutol, an ostensibly "stronger" agent (139); the authors speculate on the potential explanations for this phenomenon including gaps in therapy and the use of steroids in the treatment of the cutaneous reaction.

The debate regarding continued use of thiacetazone in populations with differing prevalences of HIV infection has been associated with considerable passion. Fundamentally, the arguments against thiacetazone (THA) include the following: (a) regimens employing THA are less effective in promoting cures than traditional 6-month regimens, (b) regimens that do not include medications such as rifampin and pyrazinamide with potent early bactericidal activity result in prolonged T-cell activation and faster progression of HIV infection, resulting in excessive mortality (177), (c) the increased rates of major dermatologic complications from THA result directly in excessive early mortality, (d) the grisly spectre of suffering and death from exfoliation is disruptive and demoralizing for patents and health care workers, very likely resulting in diminished adherence to treatment and increased transmission of tuberculosis (173).

The counterarguments for continued use of THA include these issues: (a) the incidence of major dermatological reactions may be lower than has been reported in some series (178); (b) other drugs are associated with fatal toxicity, yet we still use them; (c) the increased costs of non-THA regimens could not be met by many developing nations and would result in patients going untreated; and (d) the International Union Against Tuberculosis and Lung Disease (IUATLD) and the World Health Organization have recently declined to withdraw THA from the Essential Drugs List (179).

Reading these conflicting reports and opinions, I am persuaded strongly that we must begin the process of abandoning THA. The clear preponderance of evidence indicates that poorer response rates, the need for extended therapy, increased rates of abandonment of treatment, excessive mortality from both tuberculosis and HIV-related causes, and clinically relevant risks of toxic reactions and death are associated with the use of THA in such populations.

Alternatively, van Gorkom and Kibuga published an analysis that describes three different strategies for the use of THA: (a) continued use of THA coupled with education regarding skin reactions among populations with low-prevalence HIV infection; (b) routine HIV testing and avoidance of THA in seropositive subjects for populations with midrange prevalence; and (c) replacement of THA with ethambutol among populations with high-prevalence HIV infections (180). They based their decision analysis on the cost-effectiveness of the expenditures per-death-averted, but, as argued persuasively by Elliott and Foster, the more appropriate measure would have been cost per-patient-cured (181). Furthermore, Elliott and Foster, who have extensive field experience in Africa, argue that the continued use of THA, even under the scenarios outlined by van Gorkom and Kibuga, would have numerous other subtle, but not inconsequential, deleterious effects upon TB programs including erosion of trust and confidence in care-givers.

Regarding Rieder and Enarson's comment that both the IUATLD and WHO continue to list THA as an essential drug, this is somewhat disingenuous since these two individuals have been instrumental in determining IUATLD practices and were the major advocates at the WHO meeting in 1995 for retention of THA on this list (179). As a coparticipant in this program, I would note that there was considerable sentiment in favor of the abandonment of THA, countered only in the end by the argument that the developing nations could not afford to do so. These authors' argument that other drugs such as

INH and rifampin also cause fatal toxic reactions but remain in use is specious. These two drugs are the backbone of modern therapy; there are no alternatives to their use. And, finally, their implication that to argue against the use of THA represents an irrational or emotional response to the situation represents to me the major shortcoming of the mathematical or financial-model of decision analysis. This process, which holds so much influence in contemporary health care, blithely ignores the verity that illness and healing are laced with powerful emotions. I would hope that physicians, nurses, and other health workers would never become so inured to iatrogenic suffering and death that they would accept a strategy that, based on very marginal financial advantage (173), would result in predictable misery and deaths directly related to treatment.

A recent report from the Case Western Reserve program in Uganda suggested that the risk of allergic drug toxicity was associated with a state of "immune activation" and that there were markers that could prospectively identify such patients (177). In this series of patients, markers of activation included levels of neopterin $\geq$14 ng/ml, TNF-α receptors $\geq$6.5 ng/ml, and anergy; these were associated with both heightened overall mortality and drug toxicity. Notably, patients who received an INH–RIF–PZA regimen experienced falling levels of these markers, whereas those getting INH–SM–THA had rising levels during the initial 2 months. An additional report from this group noted that 13 of 90 patients assigned to a thiacetazone regimen experienced an ADR (182); 11 of these were cutaneous hypersensitivity, including a case of fatal Stevens-Johnson syndrome. Risk factors for these ADRs were anergy and lymphocytopenia with absolute lymphocyte counts less than 2,000/mm^3. These more readily available markers might identify individuals at special risk for such ADRs.

Certainly, the onslaught of tuberculosis and HIV will result in immense morbidity and mortality in the decades to come. In the next few years, the truly impoverished nations of Africa may have no alternatives to the use of THA. However, we should not accept this as an inevitable state of affairs and should work arduously to see that more resources are made available to support national programs, that the costs of medications are lowered to the tolerable limits of the pharmaceutical industries, and that all parties are made aware of the "unacceptability" of the status quo. It is time to emphasize the potentially great benefits of doing things "the right way."

Should the Potential for Drug–Drug Interactions Influence the Choice of Antituberculosis Chemotherapy? What Should Take Precedence: Highly Active Antiretroviral Therapy or Optimal Antituberculosis Chemotherapy?

Rifampin is one of the most potent medications currently in use in terms of altering the metabolism of other medications and hormones: see Chapter 10 for a comprehensive discussion of this topic. The most potentially important interactions for HIV-infected persons are clinically relevant reductions in the serum levels of protease inhibitors; less important but still clinically relevant are interactions with ketoconazole, itraconazole, methadone, glucocorticoids, both endogenous and exogenous, and other antiretroviral compounds including zidovudine.

HIV-1 protease inhibitors are the most encouraging, apparently efficacious agents for controlling the progression and manifestations of HIV infection to date (183). By inhibiting the cleavage of the large intracellular polyprotein that is produced when the HIV virus has been integrated into the lymphocyte (or other host cell) genome, the HIV protease inhibitors substantially curtail viral replication. In this or other yet unrecognized manner(s), these agents with varying efficacy have been shown to reduce serum viral load, to increase CD4 lymphocyte numbers, to diminish constitutional symptoms, to slow clinical progression, and to reduce mortality (184–187). Thus, they have become the central element in the current management of persons with HIV/AIDS (188,189). Contemporary experience indicates that these agents should not be used in monotherapy but in combination with nucleoside analogue retroviral agents or other protease inhibitors. Because of the risk of acquired viral resistance to these drugs, great concern has been directed toward assuring compliance/regular administration and adequate serum levels of the protease inhibitors—principles identical to those of antituberculosis chemotherapy.

Unfortunately, rifampin, the most important single drug in short-course therapy, may be incompatible with simultaneous use of HIV protease inhibitors. By accelerating the hepatic cytochrome P450 pathway, RIF results in dangerously low levels of these antiviral agents. Thus, the CDC in 1996 issued a notice proposing various strategies to deal with the problem of drug–drug interactions (190). Although these options were carefully structured, they are, in my assessment, based on some dubious premises and are potentially hazardous. These guidelines include the options of: (a) deferring highly active antiretroviral therapy (HAART) until standard tuberculosis therapy is completed; (b) discontinuing HAART and treating with a standard short-course regimen; (c) using a standard four-drug regimen for 2 months, then introducing HAART and using an extended nonrifamycin continuation therapy such as INH and ethambutol; or (d) continuing protease inhibitor therapy with indinavir, 800 mg every 8 hours and employing a 9-month tuberculosis regimen substituting rifabutin, 150 mg daily, a relatively low dose, for rifampin. The last option represented an effort to balance drug–drug interactions in the hope that rifabutine will not induce the cytochrome pathway to the extent that the protease inhibitor will be compromised, and the protease inhibitor, which impairs the cytochrome pathway, will result in adequate levels of the rifabutin. This option is particularly troublesome to me. If these interactions do not play out according to this scenario, the option could result in acquired resistance to both protease inhibitors and rifamycins!

My current assessment is that the most critical element of management for persons with progressive HIV infection is HAART. Reviewing Table 8.6, one must be struck by the high numbers of tuberculosis patients who die within a matter of months despite receiving optimal antituberculosis therapy. Thus, for motivated individuals in the appropriate clinical settings, I would suggest that consideration be given to the early initiation of HAART and the use of a nonrifamycin antituberculosis regimen (see Chapter 10 for a review of this topic). Among the drawbacks of this model are the risks for paradoxical worsening of the tuberculosis as the immune system is reconstituted (see below) and the need for an extended tuberculosis regimen including the potential use of prolonged parenteral therapy. Regarding the former issue, paradoxical worsening, one might consider using a brief course of corticosteroids to lessen the inflammation (see below). Regarding the problems of prolonged parenteral therapy, the use of such indwelling devices as PICC-lines and thrice- or twice-weekly regimens can minimize the inconvenience and risks of toxicity.

Certainly, this approach is not suitable for all persons with AIDS and tuberculosis, but I suspect it would result in optimal survival statistics. Alternatively, one might employ option (c) above, use a standard rifampin-containing regimen for 2 months, then drop rifampin and commence HAART. This has two obvious advantages—lessening the risk of paradoxical reactions and not overwhelming patients with simultaneous four-drug tuberculosis therapy and three-drug HAART regimens.

Aside from interactions with protease inhibitors, rifampin may result in potentially important interactions with other medications commonly used for persons with HIV/AIDS. For this reason, one might consider use of rifabutin rather than rifampin because of its lesser effects accelerating the cytochrome P450 system (191). Although these two rifamycins have similar in vitro activity (192,193) and reportedly comparable efficacy in the treatment of pulmonary tuberculosis (194), my personal experience and anecdotal clinical reports suggest that neutropenia and thrombopenia are modestly more frequent with rifabutin use. In view of the frequency with which these events occur in persons with AIDS receiving polypharmacy, this might constitute a clinical problem.

For an excellent review of the various drug interactions seen with medicaments commonly employed for persons with HIV/AIDS, see recent commentary from the National Institutes of Health (195).

How Does Highly Active Antiretroviral Therapy Influence the Manifestations of Tuberculosis? Does It Produce Paradoxical Worsening?

As noted in detail in Chapter 4, many of the clinical features of tuberculosis—fever, serositis, and tissue destruction—are modulated by the hosts' response to the tubercle bacilli rather than by any inherent toxic properties of the bacilli. Thus, among patients with advanced HIV infection, who have depletion of lymphocytes and attentuation of immune/hypersensitivity responses, the clinical presentations of TB may be blunted (see above). Therefore, if highly active antiretroviral therapy (HAART) would reconstitute the number and function of lymphocytes, one might expect intensification of these inflammatory phenomena. [It should be noted that paradoxical worsening of tuberculosis (196–198) or MAC disease (199) may occur simply with the introduction of antimycobacterial therapy. This may be related to diminishing the immunosuppressive effects of the uncontrolled infection; see Chapter 4.]

Indeed, in three recent reports, patients with AIDS and tuberculosis experienced a paradoxical worsening of the tuberculosis in association with the introduction of HAART (200–202). Elements of this process include recrudescent fever, worsened chest x-rays, enlarging lymphadenitis, increased pleural fluid accumulations, and expansion of intracranial tuberculomas. Such reactions begin approximately 1 to 2 weeks after initiation of HAART and persist for 2 to 8 weeks. No severe or life-threatening events occurred, but some patients experienced considerable discomfort or distress. Analogously, institution of indinavir resulted in the appearance of lymphadenitis caused by *M. avium* in five AIDS patients (203); this was believed to be secondary to uncovering subclinical infection by the reconstitution of immunity.

Indeed, Sepkowitz's editorial that accompanied the report of paradoxical worsening of the *M. avium* complex (MAC) lymphadenitis (204) documented other situations in which HAART resulted in clinical problems including CMV retinitis (205). In response, correspondents noted similar complications including tuberculosis, Herpes simplex myelitis and/or encephalitis, cutaneous H. zoster, and molluscum contagiosum (206).

However, Sepkowitz noted multiple reports in which protease inhibitors or HAART resulted in substantial improvements of a variety of infectious complications. Also, a 1998 report from Brazil documented spontaneous clearance of MAC bacteremia following HAART (207), while DePerri and colleagues from Italy described two cases in which HAART was associated with paradoxical reaction in MAC disease but on balance resulted in favorable outcomes (208).

Overall, I believe the data clearly document that initiation of HAART can result in transient paradoxical worsening of tuberculous and other infectious lesions. However, this process tends to be self-limited and to be overbalanced by the salutary effects of such treatment. In the case of tuberculosis, there are certain types of disease, however, in which this paradoxical inflammation might prove highly problematic, e.g., central nervous system, miliary, pericardial, or endobronchial disease. In these settings, acute swelling or inflammation might prove life-threatening. Thus, management options here might include deferral of HAART and/or the simultaneous use of an anti-inflammatory course of corticosteroids.

Does Accelerated Mortality from Tuberculosis Lower the Threshold for Empirical Chemotherapy?

Tuberculosis in HIV-infected persons is associated with considerably greater mortality than among HIV-negative patients. Much of the mortality that is ascribed directly to tuberculosis occurs in the first weeks or month after diagnosis (53,136,137,173). The mortality in several clusters of MDR TB occurring in AIDS patients was consistently greater than 50% (13); these deaths generally occurred within 4 to 16 weeks following exposure and infection. Although most of these victims of tuberculosis were in advanced stages of AIDS, the singular rapidity with which the tuberculosis progressed is a compelling indication to commence therapy whenever a reasonable balance of information suggests active tuberculosis.

Early administration of chemotherapy is indicated for patients with suspected tuberculosis, particularly among those with inanition, lymphopenia, and anergy, in whom the diagnosis of tuberculosis may be obscured by atypical findings and for whom untreated tuberculosis poses a great risk of lethality. Certainly aggressive efforts should be made to obtain diagnostic material to refute or confirm the diagnosis and to facilitate susceptibility testing, but early empirical treatment may well be life-saving among selected patients.

Does Tuberculosis Accelerate the Course of HIV Infection/AIDS? If So, Is It Appropriate to Attempt to Modulate the Immune Response to Tuberculosis?

As noted, the near-term mortality associated with tuberculosis in AIDS patients is strikingly high (Table 8.6). Some of these deaths are caused directly by tuberculosis, particularly in patients in Africa who receive weaker, thiacetazone-based regimens. However, many of the deaths are due to other AIDS-associated conditions including various opportunistic infections, malignancies, and wasting disorders. The clinical features of the patients most likely to die early indicate an advanced stage of HIV infection with inanition, anergy, and disseminated tuberculosis (11,137). However, mortality also occurs with tuberculosis in persons who are relatively early in the course of HIV infection with CD4 counts in excess of 200 and no antecedent AIDS-defining illnesses. This suggests that tuberculosis infection may well serve to accelerate the course of the HIV infection, thereby promoting premature mortality. One cohort study from New York indicated 1-year survival rates among tuberculosis patients with AIDS of only 70% to 80% compared to nearly 100% among HIV-negative persons similar in age and race (209). More recently, a multicenter, retrospective cohort study from the United States compared survival for 106 HIV-infected tuberculosis cases with 106 HIV-infected persons with comparable CD4 counts, age, sex, race, prior opportunistic infections and use of retroviral therapy (210). In this analysis, tuberculosis was associated with higher rates of subsequent AIDS-defining OIs, 4.0 infections per 100 person-months versus 2.8 among controls. Survival rates were significantly reduced among the tuberculosis cases: one year survival for the HIV-infected controls was 90%, for patients with pulmonary tuberculosis it was 83%, and for those with extrapulmonary tuberculosis it was 49% (Fig. 8.2). Six of the 45 deaths among the tuberculosis cases occurred within one month and were ascribed directly to tuberculosis. But, even when these cases were excluded from the analysis, death rates were significantly greater among the tuberculosis patients. The authors concluded that active tuberculosis might well act as an accelerating cofactor, although they could not exclude the possibility of it being a marker, independent of CD4 counts and other risk factors, for advanced immunosuppression.

If tuberculosis does act as an accelerant, how might it exert this effect? Studying HIV-infected persons with pulmonary tuberculosis, a group at Belleview Hospital in New York found greatly increased levels of HIV p24 in lung lavagates from regions with tuberculosis compared to lung regions without apparent tuberculosis (211). Reasoning that this might reflect local enhancement of HIV replication, they also studied in vitro cell cultures, confirming that both intact *M. tuberculosis* and lipoarabinomannan (LAM) were potent inducers of HIV-1 replication. These effects appeared to be mediated, at least in part, by the primary cytokines of the granulomatous response, IL-1 and TNF-α. These observations were consistent with multiple studies that have shown enhancement of HIV replication by these cytokines (212–214). More recently, two groups have shown directly that *M. tuberculosis* increases HIV replication in the whole lung (215) and isolated monocytes (216). Fauci and colleagues have shown that HIV replication in this setting is governed by a balance of pro- and anti-inflammatory cytokines (217).

It should be stressed that the accelerated progression of HIV phenomena is not specific to tuberculosis. Disseminated infection with *M. avium* complex (MAC) has been noted to result in substantial reductions in survival for persons with AIDS (14). As noted, cytokines elaborated

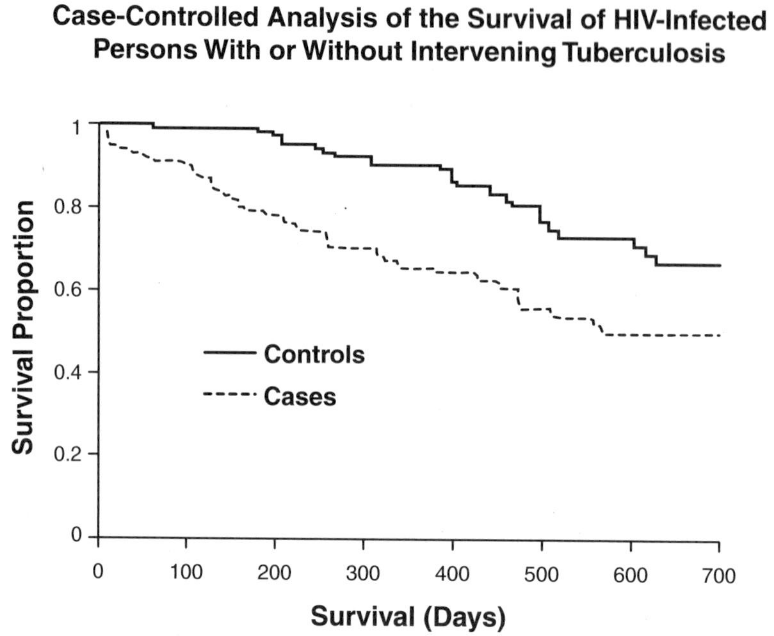

FIG. 8.2. In this case-controlled retrospective analysis, the controls were chosen from the same centers in which the tuberculosis cases were found. They were chosen on the bases of comparable CD4 lymphocyte counts, age, sex, race, prior OIs, and antiretroviral therapy. Survival among the tuberculosis cases was significantly shorter than among control subjects ($p = .03$, generalized Wilcoxson's test). Modified from Whalen et al. (210).

in the immune response to *M. avium* have been demonstrated *ex vivo* to cause activation and rapid proliferation of dormant HIV within human bronchoalveolar macrophages (218) and mononuclear cells (219). However, recent reports of persons with AIDS who developed MAC bacteremia found in one series only modest increases in HIV RNA plasma levels (220) and, in the other, no increases despite rising levels of IL-6, a proinflammatory cytokine (221). Amplified HIV-1 viral expression following immunization has been reported with the recall antigen of tetanus toxoid (222), hepatitis-B vaccinations (223) or pneumococcal vaccine (224). These data collectively support the concept that the cellular milieu of *activated* CD4 lymphocytes is a favorable environment—a "safe haven"—for the attachment, invasion, replication, and export of the HIV-1 virus (225). Because of the sustained inflammatory status associated with tuberculosis, even when treated, it stands to reason that this infection may very well be a highly powerful promoter of the transition of HIV infection from a contained disorder with relatively minimal manifestations and generally intact host defenses to the devastating systemic illness we recognize as AIDS (226). Indirect data in support of this hypothesis include the observations from Haiti that administering INH-preventive therapy to HIV-infected persons not only reduced the risk for tuberculosis but delayed progression of asymptomatic HIV infection to disease and death among PPD-positive patients (227). More direct evidence for the role of tuberculosis in accelerating the pathogenetic pathways to AIDS is derived from Wallis' report of excessive mortality among HIV-infected Ugandan patients with high levels of neopterin, TNF-α, and anergy (177). Similar findings were noted in a study from Zambia in which prolonged elevation of neopterin levels during antituberculosis therapy was associated with increased risk for reactivation tuberculosis or other adverse events including inanition and anemia (228).

If tuberculosis does act as an accelerant for HIV/AIDS, can measures be taken to ameliorate this process? As described in Chapter 4, tuberculosis damages hosts' tissues not by direct toxic products of the mycobacteria but largely through the elaboration of inflammatory cytokines integral to the hosts' defenses. In settings like tuberculous meningitis or pericarditis, clinical studies have suggested that administration of anti-inflammatory doses of glucocorticoids palliates the potentially lethal CNS or serous inflammation without adversely affecting the antimicrobial chemotherapy (see Chapter 7 for a more thorough review). Based on this loose analogy, it is reasonable to inquire whether glucocorticoids or other anti-inflammatory agents might diminish the facilitation of HIV proliferation without compromising the efficacy of antimycobacterial chemotherapy.

Prednisolone was administered in a nonrandomized study to HIV-infected tuberculosis patients in Zambia with these indications: pericardial effusions, pleural effusions, or cutaneous drug eruptions (229). Favorable effects included significant reduction in generalized lymphadenopathy and cough at 2 months; undesirable observations included herpes zoster (13%) and Kaposi's sarcoma (6%) among those receiving steroids. Overall, there was no difference in survival at one year among those receiving prednisolone and the other patients. However, these groups were not comparable with respect to sites of involvement. There was a modest improvement in 1-year survival of patients with pleural effusions who received prednisolone (17 of 19; 89%) versus those who did not (19 of 30; 63%); however, this difference was not statistically significant. In another study of HIV-infected tuberculosis patients in Zambia, the mortality ratio of those treated with prednisolone to those not receiving this drug was 0.78; statistically, this difference was not significant (95% CI 0.46–1.32, $p = .36$, adjusted for age, sex, and site of disease) (137). Analogously, pentoxifylline, an inhibitor of TNF-α production, was studied in a double-blind, placebo-controlled series of 107 patients from Uganda (230). Among these patients with tuberculosis and AIDS, pentoxyphylline treatment resulted in reduced plasma HIV RNA, lowered serum β_2-microglobulin, and in patients with moderate anemia improved red cell mass. However, no benefits were seen in terms of survival, CD4 counts, performance scores, or body mass. Thalidomide also inhibits the production of TNF-α and has been given to patients with tuberculosis, with or without HIV infection, resulting in improved weight gain (231). Subsequently, the drug was administered to HIV-infected persons without tuberculosis in an effort to reduce inflammation and wasting (232); unfortunately, this trial noted considerable side effects and toxicity from the thalidomide.

Thus, to date, the data do not support the use of steroids, pentoxifylline, or thalidomide either in terms of reducing tuberculosis morbidity/mortality directly or influencing survival due to slowing of HIV progression. However, this is a potentially fruitful avenue for future investigation. Certainly, the observation that, in contrast to women with AIDS, African women with asymptomatic HIV infection have high levels of circulating antagonists to the inflammatory cytokines IL-1β and TNF-α should encourage this area of study (233).

Are the Risks of and Consequences from Nonadherence to TB Chemotherapy Greater among HIV-Infected Persons? Do These Patients Merit Special Consideration for DOT?

Nonadherence to treatment is arguably the most significant programmatic problem in tuberculosis control. Despite the fact that modern regimens require no more than 6 to 9 months to "cure" the great majority of active cases, completion results are abysmal in many cities or regions (234). The profound consequences of nonadherence are several: treatment failure, acquired drug resistance, and higher rates of relapse (235,236).

HIV infection per se obviously does not directly promote nonadherence except through such medical sequelae as AIDS dementia or profound debility which would pose problems for clinic attendance and refilling of prescriptions. However, circumstances associated with the acquisition of HIV infection in certain populations, such as injection drug abuse, homelessness, poverty, minority status and alienation, mark these persons as extremely high risk for failure to comply with treatment (237–239).

Although it is said that it is difficult to predict who will be compliant, it is not as difficult to recognize those likely to be noncompliant. There are predictably different risks for patients in Arkansas, where the great majority of patients successfully completed 9 months of largely self-administered treatment (240), and the Harlem area in New York, where only 11% of nearly 200 patients completed 6- to 9-month regimens over two years (241)! Notably, in this latter study, HIV/AIDS or HIV-risk factors were present in the majority of subjects. Similarly, in other reports of urban, substance-abusing, homeless or in other ways disadvantaged persons, spontaneous adherence to therapy is quite uncommon (237–239,242). Of note, this phenomenon is not unique to the United States; reports from Thailand (243), South Africa (244), and Uganda (245) confirm higher rates of noncompliance among HIV-infected patients than contemporary tuberculosis patients without HIV. Certainly, in some well-organized programs adequate treatment results may be achieved without DOT (133). However, in view of the potentially morbid or lethal consequences for a person with AIDS whose tuberculosis goes untreated, particular attention should be given to such persons (239). Also, given the high likelihood that a person with HIV/AIDS and tuberculosis will come into contact with other HIV-infected persons in social, residential, or health-care settings, the potentially immense consequences of wholesale transmission of disease makes a very powerful case for the practice of DOT (10,12–14,44,148,241,246–248). Moreover, DOT will predictably help curtail drug resistance, much of which is derived originally from erratic drug ingestion (235,236) but is then transmitted wholesale to HIV-infected persons (152).

Thus, I would argue that HIV-infected persons be given special consideration for DOT. While we have argued in a simple programmatic sense for the cost-effectiveness and appropriateness of universal DOT (248), we would endorse a practice wherein each HIV-infected patient with tuberculosis would be considered for DOT. If the clinician is satisfied with the prospects for self-administered therapy, exemption from DOT might be granted. In such a model, the clinician—not the patient—would bear the onus for interrupted, failed treatment. Granted, DOT alone cannot assure therapy in all cases (249), but it is arguably the best single tactic.

Lest we believe, though, that DOT/DOTS alone will be sufficient to curtail the AIDS-driven tuberculosis resurgence, we should be aware of the recent experience in Botswana, a small nation on the northern border of South Africa (250). Having operated a highly regarded national tuberculosis program since 1975 and having utilized components of the DOTS strategy since 1985, Botswana nonetheless finds itself in the midst of soaring case rates: from 1989 to 1996 the annual incidence nearly doubled, reaching nearly 450/100,000. Recently, nearly one-half of these patients have been HIV infected. The good news, if it can be so characterized, is that the DOTS program has limited the proportion of primary drug resistance to less than 4%. The inability of DOTs to control tuberculosis in this real laboratory is an excellent segue to the section on prevention.

Is the Risk for Recurrent Tuberculosis High Enough to Warrant Special Posttreatment Management?

Recent ATS/CDC Guidelines on tuberculosis chemotherapy indicated that, once patients had received a satisfactory course of medical treatment, they should be discharged from clinic to return only if symptoms recurred (143). This was predicated on the demonstrated low relapse rates, usually in the range of 2% to 5% for the period up to 5 years after treatment reported from various studies and field programs. However, animal model studies and anecdotal human experiences indicate that even with modern, highly potent regimens, competent "host" immunity is required in addition to the chemotherapy to assure enduring "cures." Because of these concerns, recommendations for extended multidrug therapy (see above under 5.1) or prolonged posttreatment single drug "prophylaxis" (145,146) have been offered. However, the utility of these approaches has not been demonstrated. Current ATS/CDC Guidelines advocate standard 6-month therapy for HIV-infected patients unless there is a "slow response" to treatment (143).

Among HIV-positive patients treated in Africa with less potent regimens, such as INH and thiacetazone, the risk of relapse has been shown to be substantially and significantly increased over that of HIV-negative persons. However, among those treated with intensive short-course regimens, the relapse rates were only modestly increased. Confounding these data is the fact that there were high mortality rates during and following tuberculosis treatment (see Table 8.6 for relapse and death rates). As stated previously, improved care of HIV-infected persons has resulted in progressively extended survival periods; thus, the time of vulnerability for tuberculosis recurrence has been increased (179,251). Also, the possibility of exogenous reinfection from high-risk community, domiciliary, or institutional exposures must be kept in mind (12,15,16,252–254). Therefore, until persuasive data to the contrary are available, I would suggest that, when feasible, clinicians consider either lifetime chemotherapy or continuous posttreatment surveillance for HIV-infected persons who have been treated for tuberculosis. Chemotherapy might consist of isoniazid alone, continuous "preventive therapy"; this should provide protection against both endogenous reactivation and exogenous reinfection.

PREVENTION OF TUBERCULOSIS IN HIV-INFECTED PERSONS

Prevention of tuberculosis has multiple dimensions. (a) Screening programs to detect those with "dormant" or latent tuberculous infection in order to provide preventive chemotherapy are potentially major components of prevention programs for persons with HIV infection. (b) Vaccination with BCG to prevent tuberculosis among general populations is of controversial utility; hence, the role of BCG among HIV-infected persons is even more difficult to assess. (c) Preventing the acquisition of new infections is a component that has several elements: (i) prompt, effective treatment for active cases to diminish sources of infection, (ii) environmental and administrative control programs in congregate settings where transmission is likely to occur, and (iii) "prophylactic" administration of antituberculosis drugs to kill inhaled tubercle bacilli before infection can be established. The first component above, (i), prompt and effective therapy of new cases, is self-evident and the keystone to *any* tuberculosis control program. In programs with limited resources, it should be the first objective and, until satisfactory performance is achieved in this component, no other endeavors should be systematically undertaken. However, as noted above, the experience in Botswana tells us that good treatment programs, while necessary, are not sufficient (250).

Screening Programs for HIV-Infected Persons

Because of the uniquely high risk for reactivation tuberculosis among HIV-infected persons, careful attention must be given to programs that identify latent tuberculosis infection. Although there is higher risk of tuberculosis among minorities, immigrants, and substance abusers, *all* persons with HIV infection should receive evaluation. Sites particularly appropriate for formal screening programs include AIDS clinics, substance abuse clinics, shelters, correctional facilities, residential institutions, and other congregate settings. Persons receiving private health care with documented HIV infection or significant risk factors should have tuberculosis screening as part of their baseline assessment.

Significant components of screening include: *tuberculin skin testing*, *assessment of risk by epidemiologic factors*, and *evaluation to exclude active disease*.

Tuberculin Skin Testing

Tuberculin skin testing (TST) remains the primary tool to detect persons harboring latent infection with *M. tuberculosis*. However, as described above, the test is lacking in sensitivity. Among HIV-negative persons with *active* pulmonary tuberculosis, false negatives with PPD testing using the intradermal Mantoux technique range from 15 to 25% (94–96). Among HIV-infected persons, false-negative results in active tuberculosis range from 30% to 90% (40,47,74, 255–257). Failure to react to tuberculin, anergy, was associated in several U.S. surveys with lower CD4 counts and the presence of other opportunistic infections, Kaposi's sarcoma, and white race (97,98,100).

The *validity of the TST to detect latent infection* in either HIV-negative or -positive persons is more difficult to ascertain because the TST is the means by which infected status is usually determined. The utility of the TST in identifying persons with HIV infection as appropriate candidates for preventive chemotherapy is discussed below.

The 1991 CDC guidelines called for anergy panel testing to assist with the identification of HIV infected at risk of tuberculosis (97). However, the clinical utility of this strategy was largely unproven. Tuberculin reactivity and anergy were studied in a large multicenter cohort of HIV-positive patients without AIDS; results were compared to a smaller number of HIV-negative persons with similar risk factors, male homosexuality, and intravenous drug abuse (98). Broadly speaking, this study showed the following: (a) tuberculin reactivity was significantly associated with injection drug use, black race, and previous tuberculin reactivity or BCG vaccination; (b) anergy increased progressively with CD4 lymphocyte counts less than 600/ml among IDU persons regardless of HIV status; (c) anergy panel testing did not substantially help to validate TST results because there was discordance between responses to PPD and DTH antigens including mumps and *Candida;* (d) if the cut-point for deeming a tuberculin reactive to be significant were reduced to = 1 mm induration in HIV-infected persons with CD4 counts = 400, the reactivity prevalence was similar to that seen among the HIV-negative, epidemiologically similar controls; however, among persons with CD4 counts less than 400, the tuberculin reactivity rates fell steadily despite a lower threshold for significance; and (e) if the TST is to be used to identify candidates for preventive therapy, it should be given early in the course of HIV infection because of the rising risk of anergy as CD4 counts fall.

Results from two other reports in 1993, however, raised broader questions about the validity and utility of the TST in HIV-infected persons from countries with high prevalence of tuberculosis. Among 374 HIV-infected patients from Madrid, Spain, 29% had positive reactions, ≥5 mm induration, to the 2-TU dose of RT-23 tuberculin, 30% were anergic to tuberculin and other antigens, and 41% were unreactive to tuberculin but responsive to other antigens (105). Curiously, the subsequent rates of active tuberculosis among these groups were for tuberculin reactors 10.4 cases per 100 patient-years, for the anergic 12.4 cases, and among the tuberculin-negative but not anergic, 5.4 cases. Similarly, among a smaller group of 144 HIV-infected persons in Brazil, active tuberculosis developed within one year among 16.7% of tuberculin reactors and 10.2% of nonreactors (258). In the Brazilian report, anergy testing was not done; therefore, among their nonreactors, presumably there were both anergic and "true negative" persons. Among Rwandan women of child-bearing age, HIV positives were 60% less likely than HIV negatives to have a reactive TST but 22-fold more apt to develop tuberculosis within 2 years (19). These studies suggest strongly that in countries with high levels of endemic tuberculosis, particularly among high-risk populations, the risk of tuberculosis is sufficiently great to warrant preventive chemotherapy regardless of tuberculin reactivity, even when such testing is reinforced by anergy testing. Among approximately 2,000 subjects with HIV infection in Italy (a country with a lower prevalence of tuberculosis), incidence rates for active tuberculosis for tuberculin reactors was 5.42 per 100 person-years, for anergic subjects 3.00, and for tuberculin negative but not anergic persons, 0.45 (106). Of interest, a recent, very sophisticated decision analysis from Italy found that INH PT given to tuberculin-positive, HIV-infected persons both increased life expectancy and reduced medical costs (259). Regarding the use of INH

PT in anergic subjects, the model was less robust, but, it was still favorable if the underlying rate of latent tuberculosis infection was 15% or greater and compliance with preventive therapy was high.

From the above data one might infer that anergy has some clinical utility in identifying subjects at risk for subsequent tuberculosis. However, as noted by the "Pulmonary Complications of HIV Infection" Group in the United States, there was considerable discordance in response to the various DTH antigens employed in their survey, including PPD, mumps, *Candida,* and trichophyton (98). A subsequent survey of DTH-anergy among a group of HIV-infected IDUs and a control group of HIV-negative IDUs from Baltimore indicated that although anergy was more common among the HIV seropositives, 36% versus 14%, there were high rates of change in both directions, reactive-to-anergic and anergic-to-reactive, in both groups (101). In this report, two consecutive anergy panels were predictive of CD4 counts usually less than 350.

What then is the role for anergy testing in HIV-positive persons? Such testing is not negligible in terms of its costs, including application and reading, and the procedure requires return visits at 48 hours to have the tests read, a predictable inconvenience for the patients. Hence, in 1997 the earlier CDC guidelines were reversed, and anergy testing was no longer advocated for HIV-infected persons (108). It therefore seems appropriate that the following logic be incorporated into decisions regarding tuberculin skin testing, anergy panels, and the administration of INH-preventive therapy (IPT). (a) Apply TSTs as early as possible when CD4 numbers are higher and the results are more likely valid. (b) Search aggressively for prior tuberculin status among previous medical records. (c) If the individual is tuberculin-negative at a time when the CD4 count is ≥400 and no specific risks for anergy such as opportunistic infections or Kaposi's sarcoma are present, consider them to be not infected. Recent data from Uganda indicate that two-step testing will "boost" a modest number of HIV-infected persons with CD4 counts of 200 to 500; those who do not react to the first and second tests may reasonably be deemed uninfected (260). Follow such persons with serial TSTs to identify recent infection until the CD4 count falls below 200 and/or other factors substantially invalidate the positive or negative predictive value of the test, and (d) use anergy panel testing only among tuberculin-negative individuals from groups known through epidemiological risk factors to be at significant risk of tuberculosis—selected minorities or immigrants, residents of high-prevalence urban areas, known case contacts, IDUs, crack-cocaine users, or health care workers. In this situation, identification of anergy allows one to stratify the subsequent risk of tuberculosis. If such high-risk persons are anergic, they might consider INH PT, although this strategy is being debated.

Is there clinical utility of anergy testing regardless of tuberculosis risk assessment? Certainly, evidence has been reported that DTH anergy is associated with relatively rapid progression to AIDS among HIV-infected persons (98). In this group of U.S. Air Force personnel or dependents, the mean CD4 counts were lower among anergic persons, the DTH-reactors. However, among subjects with CD4 numbers ≥400, anergy also was associated with increased risk of progression to Walter Reed Stage 6 (AIDS-defining OIs). At 3 years follow-up, nearly 40% of anergic subjects had progressed while less than 10% of those who had originally reacted to two or more antigens had progressed; the difference in rates of progression was even more pronounced among those with initial CD4 counts <400. In an editorial accompanying the above article, Kornbluth and McCracken speculated that DTH-anergy may reflect alterations of lymphocyte function that operate somewhat independently of CD4 numbers, possibly a shift from Th-1 to Th-2 pathways (261). However, they stopped short of indicating that anergy was suitable for staging HIV infection. In a subsequent series of USAF patients with HIV infection, more comprehensive testing of T-cell function, DTH-reactivity/anergy and CD4 enumeration and subset typing were compared with regard to predictive value for progression to AIDS (262). All three of these elements were significantly associated with predictive values for progression, including multivariant proportion analysis, with the greatest power related to DTH-anergy. The authors conclude that both in vitro tests of T-cell function and skin testing were of independent prognostic utility.

Is there a role for two-step tuberculin testing in HIV-infected persons? Among 709 patients tested in a CPCRA program, 18 individuals (2.7%) had an increase from < 5 mm induration to ≥ 5 mm on closely spaced sequential TSTs (263). This response was seen in 2.1% of anergic and 4.5% of nonanergic subjects and was deemed overall to be of little value. By contrast, among 58 persons in Uganda, 29% had a boosted response (260); these occurred mainly among those with high CD4 counts and better conserved body mass.

Assessment of Risk by Epidemiological Features

In populations with HIV infection, it is possible to identify persons at substantially greater risk of developing tuberculosis by virtue of readily accessible features other than tuberculin reactivity. Among the more powerfully predictive markers are national origin, community of residence, injection drug use, race, socioeconomic status, time spent in correctional facilities, and other institutional exposures including health care facilities where tuberculosis transmission has been documented. Thus, clinicians should decide about preventive chemotherapy for HIV-infected persons based on a variable amalgam of these historical features as well as laboratory observations including the TST, CD4 counts, and chest x-rays. (An obvious and powerful risk factor for tuberculosis among HIV-infected persons would be fibronodular apical shadows on the chest x-ray; although I have not seen an analysis of this variable among HIV-positive patients, I would regard it as a compelling indication for preventive therapy.)

Persons with HIV infection who were born in and/or spent considerable periods of their lives in countries where tuberculosis remains endemic should probably receive preventive chemotherapy unless there is a clear contraindication (particular problems would include major toxicity associated with the appropriate agents or active viral hepatitis with impaired liver function which could substantially amplify the morbidity from drug-induced hepatitis). Countries or regions which should be included under this high-risk rubric would be sub-Saharan Africa, the Indian subcontinent, mainland China, the Pacific Rim nations (excluding Japan and Taiwan), Latin America and the less affluent Caribbean islands such as Haiti and the Dominican Republic. If such persons have additional risk factors such as histories of IDU, crack cocaine use, or periods spent in correctional facilities, I think the case for tuberculosis prevention is compelling.

Evaluation to Preclude Active Tuberculosis

There are two potential major hazards from preventive therapy in HIV-infected persons: drug toxicity (which will be discussed subsequently) and inadvertently giving preventive monotherapy to a patient with cryptic, active tuberculosis. Due to the atypical features of tuberculosis in persons with advanced HIV infection, a simple screening chest x-ray to rule out active pulmonary tuberculosis is not sufficient. A careful physical examination and systems review focusing on the more common manifestations of HIV-associated tuberculosis such as unexplained fever, lymphadenopathy, cutaneous abscesses, or recent weight loss are essential before commencing preventive therapy. If single or even two-drug preventive treatment is begun in the presence of active tuberculosis with a large burden of tubercle bacilli, there is a substantial and unacceptable risk of treatment failure and acquired drug resistance. If the above clinical findings are noted, the clinician should either defer antituberculosis therapy until diagnostic studies have been completed or embark on empirical multidrug therapy for presumed active tuberculosis (see the above section on highly active anti-retroviral therapy (HAART) and its influence on tuberculosis).

Preventive Chemotherapy for HIV-Infected Persons

As described in Chapter 12, isoniazid (INH) has been proven highly effective among HIV-negative persons at curtailing the progression from latent infection to clinically active tuberculosis. In two large randomized, placebo-controlled series, INH PT given for 6 to 12 months afforded 60% to 90% protection (264,265). In the subjects followed for the longest period after INH PT, the protection persisted through 19 years (266).

All of the subjects in these trials were deemed to have latent tuberculosis infection based on combinations of tuberculin skin test reactivity, abnormal chest x-rays, and epidemiological features. The basic premise of this tactic was that the INH killed the mycobacteria that had been sporadically replicating at various sites in the body, thereby reducing the likelihood of subsequent "reactivation" tuberculosis. INH PT appeared to protect against pulmonary and extrapulmonary forms of tuberculosis.

There have been a modest number of trials of preventive chemotherapy for persons with HIV infection or AIDS; data from recent studies are displayed in Table 8.8. In the study from Haiti in Table 8.8, 12 months of INH PT was compared to placebo (pyridoxine) in 118 HIV-positive persons, 63 of whom had tuberculin reactions of at least 5 mm induration (224). Overall, in the mix of tuberculin-reactive and nonreactive individuals, INH PT was significantly protective: 11 cases in the placebo group and four cases in the INH PT group for a relative risk of 3.4 (95% CI 1.1–10.6). In the subset of tuberculin reactors, there also was significant protection with a relative risk of 5.8 (CI 1.2–27.8). Particularly notable in this study was the apparent protection against the development of other AIDS-defining illnesses or symptomatic HIV infection among the persons given INH PT: 12 placebo versus two INH PT patients developed AIDS during the observation period (RR 5.8; CI 1.5–24.5). INH PT was associated with delay in time to symptomatic HIV infection (32 versus 19 months, $p < .05$).

In an early study from Zambia reported in 1990, HIV-positive subjects were randomized to 6 months of INH PT or pyridoxine placebo (267). In this trial, INH PT conferred 60% reduction in tuberculosis. In a subsequent trial from Zambia included in Table 8.8, 544 HIV-positive persons were randomized to 6 months of INH or pyridoxine (268). Among those receiving INH, there were three cases in 273 person-years of observation; in those on placebo, there were 20 cases in 262 person-years. The annual incidence of tuberculosis in these groups was 1.0% and 7.6%, respectively.

Whalen and colleagues studied three different preventive regimens in a placebo-controlled trial seen in Table 8.8: 6 months of INH (6-INH), 3 months of INH and rifampin (3-I/R), and 3 months of INH, rifampin, and pyrazinamide (3-I/R/P) (269). The relative risk for tuberculosis compared to the placebo group was 0.33 for 6-INH, 0.40 for 3-I/R and 0.51 for 3-I/R/P, which was confounded in part by poor tolerance. Similarly, among 121 HIV-infected persons from Spain who were tuberculin reactors, 9 to 12 months of INH PT substantially reduced the relative risk of subsequent tuberculosis, 1.6 cases per 100 patient-years versus 9.9 for those who did not receive INH for a R.R. of 6.5 (270). Receipt of INH PT was also associated with reduced death rates and prolonged survival; unfortunately, this study was neither randomized nor placebo-controlled but based on refusal, contraindication or intolerance of treatment.

Three other recent reports included in Table 8.8 offer different insights into the prevention of tuberculosis in HIV-infected persons. Hawken and colleagues in Kenya described generally disappointing results in a randomized, placebo-controlled trial among 684 HIV-seropositive adults (271). Overall, there was an inexplicably higher risk of tuberculosis among INH recipients, 4.29 per 100 person-years, than among placebo recipients, 3.86. Notably, among the patients who were tuberculin reactors, there *was* a beneficial effect in terms of both tuberculosis case rates and mortality rates. Halsey and colleagues in Haiti demonstrated comparability in the efficacy of 6 months of twice-weekly, high-dose INH and 2 months of twice-weekly rifampin and pyrazinamide (272). And, in a multicenter trial in tuberculin-reactive HIV-positive persons, 12 months of daily INH and 2 months of daily rifampin and pyrazinamide were comparable (273).

In addition to these studies, Selwyn's anecdotal experience among HIV-positive IDUs in

TABLE 8.8. *Preventive chemotherapy of tuberculosis in HIV-infected persons: recent reports*

Site, first author (ref.)	Regimen(s) employed	Admission criteria	Patients	TB morbidity: Cases, %, events/100 patient-years (PY)	Relative risk	Comments
Haiti, Pape (227)	(a) 12 mo INH	Either PPD -positive or -negative; randomized	(a) 58	(a) PPD^+, 2/38 (5%), 1.7/100 PY; PPD^-, 2/20 (10%), 3.2/100 PY	0.17	Overall, INH + PT, 83% efficacy; also, delayed TB and onset AIDS
	(b) 12 mo B_6		(b) 60	(b) PPD^+, 6/25 (24%), 10.0/100 PY; PPD^-, 5/35 (14%), 5.7/100 PY	0.56	
Zambia, Wadhawan (268)	(a) 6 mo INH (b) 6 mo B_6	PPD not reported	(a) 273 (b) 271	(a) 3/273 PY or 1.0/100 PY (b) 20/262 PY or 7.6/100 PY	0.13	Randomized
Spain, Moreno (270)	(a) 9–12 mo INH (b) No therapy	PPD-positive; not randomized	(a) 29 (b) 92	(a) 3/29 (10%), 1.6/100 PY (b) 43/92 (47%), 9.4/100 PY	0.15	Retrospective cohort study
Kenya, Hawken (271)	(a) 6 mo INH	Either PPD-positive or -negative	(a) 342	(a) 25/342 (7.3%) i. PPD^+, 5.6/100 PY; ii. PPD^-, 3.3/100 PY	0.7 vs. (b) i 1.2 vs. (b) ii	Randomized, double-blind
	(b) 6 mo placebo		(b) 342	(b) 23/242 (6.7%) i. PPD^+, 8.0/100 PY; ii. PPD^-, 2.7/100 PY		
United States, Gordin (107)	(a) 6 mo INH (b) 6 mo placebo	Anergic subjects only	(a) 260 (b) 257	(a) 3/260 (1.2%), 0.4/100 PY (b) 6/257 (2.3%), 0.9/100 PY	0.48	Randomized, double-blind
Uganda, Whalen (269)	(a) 6 mo INH (PPD^+) (b) 6 mo INH (anergy) (c) 3 mo INH & RIF (d) 3 mo INH/RIF/PZA (e) 6 mo placebo	All PPD-positive except those in (b); a placebo group was also used in anergic patients.	(a) 536 (b) 323 (c) 556 (d) 462 (e) 464	N.S. N.S. N.S. N.S. N.S.	(a) 0.33 (b) 0.83 (c) 0.40 (d) 0.51 (e) 1.0	Separate placebo group among anergics was basis of comparison for (b); higher rate of ADRs seen in arm (d).
Haiti, Halsey (272)	(a) 6 mo INH, biw (b) 6 mo RIF and PZA, biw	PPD^+	(a) 370 (b) 380	(a) 14/370 (3.8%), 1.7/100 PY (b) 19/380 (5.0%), 1.8/100 PY	1.0 1.3	Randomized, no differences in ADRs. All needs given twice a week, first dose only by DOT
Multi-site, Gordin (273)	(a) 12 mo INH (b) 2 mo RIF and PZA	PPD^+	(a) 792 (b) 791	(a) 27/792 (3.4%), 1.2/100 PY (b) 27/791 (3.4%), 1.2/100 PY	(a) 1.0 (b) 1.0	Both regimens well tolerated

Overall, these studies show significant protection from tuberculosis with preventive chemotherapy. The data are more robust for persons with HIV infection and tuberculin skin test reactivity. Failure to demonstrate protection is most puzzling in the 1997 report from Kenya; if only the TST-positive subjects are considered, there is still only a 30% reduction in morbidity, not a significant difference. The relatively high rates of tuberculosis in all groups raise questions regarding unusually high risk for ongoing exogenous infection. PT for anergic subjects remains of uncertain utility. Anergy has generally been associated with high risks for subsequent tuberculosis. Indeed, in the 1997 Ugandan study, anergic subjects did have tuberculosis rates almost equal to those of tuberculin reactors; however, INH-PT simply was not highly protective in this group. These trials do not provide a clear answer regarding the benefits of extending INH PT to 12 months.

New York was suggestive of efficacy: 13 of the 49 seropositive tuberculin reactors had received prior INH PT; none of these 13 developed tuberculosis, but 8 of the 36 who had not received INH did develop tuberculosis (17). Also, in Baltimore a program of twice-weekly, high dose (10 to 15 mg/kg), directly-observed INH PT was created for 2,960 IDUs, 942 of whom were HIV-positive (274). This was not a randomized trial, but observations were compared with historical data from this population and community. Candidates for the DO-IPT were identified by tuberculin reactivity: ≥5 mm for HIV-positive, ≥10 mm induration for the HIV-negative subjects. Duration of INH PT varied: efforts were made to achieve at least 6 months of treatment with 12 months given to willing and compliant individuals. Among the HIV-positive persons, eight cases of tuberculosis were seen, while *none* were seen among the individuals who had received INH for at least 26 weeks. Overall, among the whole population of IDUs, cases of tuberculosis fell 83% from the peak levels in 1990–1991. Inferential data that also suggest the utility of preventive chemotherapy to protect HIV-positive persons from tuberculosis were derived from a trial comparing oral dapsone/pyrimethamine to inhaled pentamidine as prophylaxis versus *Pneumocystis carinii* (275). Of 501 participants, 274 received the dapsone/pyrimethamine at 200/75 mg once weekly; the others received aerosolized pentamidine. The authors described six cases of "tuberculosis" in the results, but only five were caused by *M. tuberculosis.* The other was associated with *M. africanum,* an organism that belongs taxonomically to the tuberculosis complex but is less susceptible to chemotherapy than is *M. tuberculosis.* Five of the cases were among the pentamidine recipients, 5 of 227, while only one occurred in those receiving dapsone/ pyrimethamine, a compound which, based on in vitro activity and clinical effects in leprosy, might be expected to have only modest antituberculosis efficacy.

The question of the implications of anergy in persons HIV infected was addressed in one of the above studies (269) and in another recent report (107). In neither study did INH PT appear significantly beneficial; in the former report from Uganda, anergy was associated with an increased risk of tuberculosis, but INH PT did not appear protective. However, in the study from the United States, anergy was not associated with a substantially increased risk of tuberculosis; thus, INH PT could not yield much benefit. Although the meaning of these data is not clear, the results of these studies do somewhat lessen enthusiasm for preventive therapy in anergic persons.

Assessment and Summary

There are several arguable truths at this time. (a) Persons with HIV infection are at very high risk for tuberculosis. (b) Tuberculosis, even when detected, treated, and cured, is associated with accelerated morbidity and mortality in this population. (c) Isoniazid and other preventive therapy appears to significantly reduce the risk for tuberculosis *and,* very probably, other morbidity and mortality not directly attributable to tuberculosis.

In the industrialized nations with well-established health-care infrastructures and adequate resources, preventive therapy clearly should be offered to individuals deemed at risk for tuberculosis by tuberculin reactivity or epidemiological markers. Although no studies have compared duration of treatment, the current guidelines of 12 months appear suitable. However, in populations in which there is an ongoing, substantial risk of new infection or reinfection with tuberculosis, a case might be made for lifetime INH PT, the continued therapy acting as true primary prophylaxis to prevent exogenous reinfection from occurring.

Far more contentious is the question of whether preventive therapy can and should be employed in the less affluent, developing nations. Following the success reported from Haiti, others commented about the apparent utility and practicality of the practice (276,277). Individuals representing the Global Programme on AIDS and the Tuberculosis Programme of the World Health Organization mentioned INH PT prominently among the strategies to be considered (78). Others, however, warn that in most developing nations the effort to deliver INH PT would be fraught with many hazards including acquired drug resistance due to failure to recognize patients with active tuberculosis or erratic drug ingestion. And, most importantly, there is concern that such a program would divert resources from the more critical task of assuring effective therapy of persons with active, communicable disease (279,280). However, others who are experienced with HIV and tuberculosis programming in sub-Saharan Africa point out that prevention of tuberculosis may well have substantial financial advantages over the longer term and that, instead of casually dismissing this concept, we should be investigating efficient means of utilizing the tactic (281).

At the risk of appearing to have an unrealistic, "Ivory Tower" approach to the situation, I think it is not simply a potential option but an essential component in the struggle against these coepidemic infections. Tuberculosis is a major cause of suffering and death among HIV victims in the developing nations. These individuals, before their deaths, spread tuberculosis to their families and communities, resulting in "horizontal" morbidity and mortality. And, I believe that preventing tuberculosis would do more to improve the quality and extend the duration of life than any other affordable combination of antiretroviral therapy or preventive treatment of other opportunistic infections (282)!

Perhaps the best tactic will not be 6 or 12 months of INH PT but a shorter, rifamycin-containing regimen. However, although this might be equally or more effective against endogenous reactivation tuberculosis, it would not prevent exogenous reinfection and would potentially cost more. Perhaps the better policy might entail unselective, community-based INH PT such as that practiced in Alaska in the midst of epidemic tuberculosis (266). In any case, not to make programs of preventive therapy a high priority for future control efforts is to resign ourselves to an extreme burden of disease and death.

Bacillus Calmette-Guérin and HIV-Related Tuberculosis

Bacillus Calmette-Guérin (BCG) is a living mycobacterial vaccine derived from an attenuated but viable strain of *M. bovis,* a member of the tuberculosis complex that is closely related to the human tubercle bacillus. BCG is given subcutaneously or intradermally to persons without prior infection with *M. tuberculosis.* It is believed to work by conferring sufficient immunity so that an accelerated host defense response would subsequently limit local invasion and dissemination if vaccinees inhaled tubercle bacilli into their lungs. Although widely employed throughout the world over the past four decades, the protective utility of the vaccine is disputed (see Chapter 13 for an extensive review of this topic).

The central issues in regard to BCG and the HIV epidemic are: (a) How effective is BCG in preventing tuberculosis in HIV-infected persons? (b) How safe is the vaccine in this population? (c) Who should receive the vaccine? (d) When should they be vaccinated? (e) Which vaccine should be employed? These topics are addressed below.

There are no meaningful data about the capacity of BCG to prevent tuberculosis in persons with HIV infection. Among HIV-negative patients, relatively greater protection with BCG has been demonstrated in children and adolescents (283). Recent large BCG trials in general populations in India and Africa without HIV infection have failed to demonstrate overall protection among patients of diverse ages (284,285). Yet, a recent meta-analysis that focused on 26 BCG trials that were judged the most sound methodologically concluded that, based only on these studies, "BCG vaccination" conferred roughly 50% protection against tuberculosis (286). However, this analysis indicated unfortunately that vaccination worked *significantly less well in tropical regions* (such as sub-Saharan Africa and equatorial Asia and Latin America) (287). Indeed, independent analyses by Springett and Sutherland (288) and Fine (289) confirmed that BCG vaccination has performed quite poorly in tropical and subtropical climates. Hence, until there are systematic reports on the protection against tuberculosis among HIV-infected persons from BCG, the impact of this tactic remains conjectural.

The safety of BCG in HIV-infected persons also remains uncertain. BCG given to children with various preexisting immunological disorders other than HIV infection has been noted to cause generalized mycobacteriosis and osteomyelitis (290). Recent reports have documented infrequent infectious complications among HIV-infected individuals: prolonged local ulcerations, regional lymphadenitis, and dissemination (291,292); most of these complications occurred shortly after BCG was given to patients already infected with HIV. However, several cases with apparent late reactivation of BCG infection have been reported including localized lymphadenitis (293), disseminated infection (294), both occurring 30 years after vaccination, and meningitis occurring 12 years after vaccination (295). The likelihood of these complications probably is related to the inherent virulence of the BCG strains employed and the severity of the immunodeficiency. No prospective quantitative data are currently available to predict the frequency of untoward responses. Although some reports suggest the risk of adenitis is not significantly greater, 9% versus 5%, in HIV-infected than normal children (296), it is counter-intuitive not to anticipate some increase in iatrogenic morbidity from this practice.

Apart from local abscesses or disseminated BCG-osis, another major question regarding the safety of BCG in HIV-infected persons was raised by the results of the BCG trial in Karonga, Malawi (297). In this study, persons with prior BCG scars were randomized to receive a second BCG vaccination or placebo. Among those getting the BCG vaccine, an excess rate of active tuberculosis was noted, 69% greater than placebo (298). Notably, this excess was wholly due to tuberculosis among those HIV-infected. The mechanism of this apparent disparity was unclear, but it was speculated that the living bacillary vaccination may have resulted in a prolonged state of immune activation with deleterious effects upon the course of the HIV/AIDS (297) (for more information, see the previous section on HAART and its influence on manifestations of tuberculosis).

In the absence of definitive information about the efficacy or safety of BCG in the setting of HIV infection, it is very difficult to identify candidates for the vaccine. At this time, authorities still continue to endorse the use of BCG among all infants and children in countries or communities where there is an unavoidable high risk of exposure to tuberculosis and limited access to health services (278). In the absence of programs for early detection of disease in adults, contact investigation, and preventive therapy, BCG vaccination is a clearly appropriate decision. Regarding the time at which the BCG should be given, a group from Zambia proposed that the vaccination be deferred until one year of age in order to identify infants at risk of HIV infection and disseminated BCG (299). However, other practitioners from this region argued strongly against the practice, indicating that more harm than good would come due to loss of early protection and missed vaccinations (300–302).

The choice of vaccine strain, if employed, remains unclear. In the above noted meta-analysis, the investigators were unable to identify strain variation as a source for the disparate protection observed (303). Yet, other authorities suggest this is a factor (283,304). For a more complete review of the utility and complications associated with BCG, see Chapter 13.

In summary, BCG appears quite unlikely, in my estimation, to confer significant protection to persons with current or future HIV infection. There is anticipatable morbidity from the vaccines. Auxotrophic vaccines (mutant BCG strains that require exotic amino acids for growth and are thereby limited in pathogenic potential), while of potential efficacy (305) are decades away from proof of effectiveness and safety. BCG, even in comprehensive community programs, is unlikely to have a significant impact on the transmission and epidemiology of tuberculosis among populations with substantial rates of HIV infection. Although the World Health Organization and the International Union Against Tuberculosis have long relied upon BCG as the primary means to control tuberculosis, I believe that the current epidemiological dynamics of tuberculosis indicate that there are potentially greater benefits from preventive chemotherapy.

Administrative Practices, Environmental Systems, and Personal Respiratory Protective Devices in Health Care Facilities

Preventing the transmission of tuberculosis is unequivocally the most important component of a tuberculosis control program: far better to keep a person from becoming infected than to rely upon vaccines of disputable merit or screening/preventive chemotherapy programs with all of their attendant problems. This proposition is particularly true in regards to populations in which HIV infection is prevalent.

Guidelines from the Centers for Disease Control (306) currently advocate the following approaches to limit the spread of tuberculosis in health care facilities: (a) administrative practices that are directed toward early recognition of potentially infectious cases of tuberculosis, leading to their prompt isolation and treatment, (b) environmental systems that control the direction of flow of air containing the aerosolized bacilli, dilute the concentration of bacilli by introduction of fresh air, and/or reduce the numbers of infectious particles by filtration or germicidal ultraviolet irradiation, and (c) personal protection by use of devices that are designed to lessen the likelihood of inhaling infectious particles by filtering the inhaled air.

These issues are discussed more fully in Chapter 14. Briefly, improved infection control measures are a compelling need since most of the facilities in the industrialized nations that house health care programs employ recirculating air systems with low levels of fresh ventilation in order to conserve energy, e.g., not to waste heated or cooled air. And, in the developing nations, large numbers of individuals, many of whom harbor either tuberculosis or HIV-infection, will share air-space as a consequence of over-burdened health facilities.

Administrative measures are universally agreed upon. Who can argue against the utility of prompt diagnosis and physical sequestration of untreated, potentially infectious cases of pulmonary tuberculosis? However, considerable disagreement exists in the areas of environmental practices and the role of personal protection devices. Ultraviolet germicidal irradiation has proven efficacy in killing *M. tuberculosis* on brief exposure and, in my estimation, is the most effective, efficient, and practical intervention that might be employed (307). Employing economical and feasible precautions, the theoretical health hazards of UVGI can be avoided. There is near unanimity that potentially infectious patients ideally should be kept in negative pressure rooms, but the number of air changes per hour and potential inhomogeneities of air movement make this strategy problematic as well as expensive. Personal respiratory protective devices are most appropriate, I believe, in unavoidable, very high-risk situations such as bronchoscopy or tracheal intubation. Personal respiratory protective devices should not be projected as a routine measure due to their discomfort, impedimentary effects on communication, unpredictable fitting, expense, and unenforcability. If, however, a Health Care Worker must spend time in proximity to a patient with untreated, potentially highly infectious tuberculosis in spaces without adequate ventilation, filtration or UVGI, personal respiratory protective devices should be worn (see Chapter 14).

These issues clearly are of considerable importance for all facilities in which persons with tuberculosis might be seen or housed. But, given the rapid progression from infection to life-threatening disease and extremely high levels of transmission among exposed persons with AIDS, these tactics and strategies have risen to the level of compelling priority in contemporary health care.

SUMMARY

The coepidemic of HIV infection and tuberculosis poses major challenges for global health. The following salient issues must be considered in this regard:

- HIV infection is the most powerful agent known to promote reactivation of latent tuberculosis infection
- The effects of HIV on pulmonary defenses and the immune system *may* make HIV-infected persons at greater risk of acquiring new tuberculosis infections
- Persons with AIDS, when newly infected with tuberculosis, may progress to life-threatening disease in a matter of weeks to months

- Tuberculosis is a leading source of morbidity and mortality for young adults with HIV infection in the developing nations
- Tuberculosis is spreading within the households to the children of young adults in those countries and in the industrialized nations
- Among patients with AIDS, tuberculosis presents with various atypical manifestations that elude the standard diagnostic test of third-world countries, the sputum smear; new, more sensitive and rapid diagnostic tests are essential
- Prompt, potent chemotherapy is essential to lessen early mortality associated with tuberculosis
- Because of marginal efficacy and increased rates of major toxicity, the continued use of thiacetazone—the cheapest drug in our current armamentarium—has become unacceptable, further burdening health budgets in the developing nations
- Rising rates of resistance to INH have placed a premium on preserving the effectiveness of rifampin; to do this, large programs of directly observed therapy will be required, further taxing global assets
- BCG vaccination will probably prove inadequate to control the burgeoning case rates among HIV-infected; to do this, large-scale preventive chemotherapy programs must be considered
- Nosocomial transmission of tuberculosis has become an increasing hazard as HIV-related illnesses funnel large numbers of vulnerable subjects together. Systems to control ventilation and/or reduce infectious particles via ultraviolet germicidal irradiation will be required to stem this tide

If the above inventory of needs is broadly correct, immense burdens will be placed on the nations in which the coepidemic is active. Resourceful utilization of current assets, "coping," will be required in the near term (308). But, if we are to make significant progress against these intertwined infections and not allow them to progress to their dreadful Malthusian ends, great moneys and energies must be brought to bear (309). Priorities and procedures of the involved nations and supernational agencies like WHO, The World Bank, and the IUATLD must be reconsidered. Ironically, the tuberculosis program of the Centers for Disease Control initiated a program in the mid-1980s to eliminate tuberculosis in the United States by 2010 (310), only to be greeted by the upsurge in cases from 1985 to 1993. Fortunately, this elimination plan has helped to identify the critical elements needed to bolster control programs. Adequate if not optimal tools are available; what is at question immediately is our resolve to find the means to take the appropriate measures (311). Looking ahead to the 21st century, a compelling research agenda has been identified (312). Indifference or inaction before these needs is not acceptable.

ADDENDUM: THE 1998 CDC REVISED RECOMMENDATIONS ON THE PREVENTION AND TREATMENT OF TUBERCULOSIS AMONG THE HIV-INFECTED

After this chapter was completed in October 1998, these recommendations were published in the *MMWR* (313). Rather than attempt to interdigitate them into the chapter, I have elected to discuss them separately, attempting to delineate when, where, and why differences exist. Broadly speaking, I believe the recommended practices in this document are concordant with the positions advocated earlier in this chapter. Particular areas of agreement that merit notice include the following: (a) early diagnosis and effective therapy of tuberculosis in HIV-infected persons are vital to high rates of cure, minimizing the adverse effects of tuberculosis on the course of HIV and reducing transmission of tuberculosis; (b) screening to detect latent infection with *M. tuberculosis* and to administer preventive chemotherapy should be done in all persons with HIV infection; and (c) consideration should be given to the use of antiretroviral therapy in all patients with tuberculosis.

Differences in emphasis of the CDC document include a more favorable attitude toward the substitution of rifabutine for rifampin in order to simultaneously administer antiretroviral therapy, and a less favorable view of extending the duration of chemotherapy given for active disease.

Material of particular interest and utility from the new Recommendations are included in tabular form. Table 8.9 reveals that strains of *M. tuberculosis* recovered from persons with HIV infection were significantly more likely to manifest drug resistance. In addition, there is highly useful information reported in the CDC document on the drug–drug interactions between rifampin or rifabutin and the protease inhibitors (Table 8.10) and nonnucleoside reverse transcriptase inhibitors (Table 8.11). As shown, there are substantial variations depending both on the rifamycin agent and the various drugs in these two categories. And, the feasibility of using various antiretroviral drugs with rifabutine is commented upon (Table 8.12).

Also, their recommended management strategies for persons with HIV infection and tuberculosis are delineated in a flow diagram (Fig. 8.3). This algorithm embraces the situations wherein a patient already receiving antiretroviral therapy develops active tuberculosis and the case when the HIV infection is detected following the diagnosis of tuberculosis. If antiretroviral treatment is to include protease inhibitors (PIs) and/or non-nucleoside reverse transcriptase inhibitors (NNRTIs), the patients are to be assigned either to a rifabutin-based regimen or a regimen that does not include a rifamycin but does include an injectable agent such as streptomycin. If, on the other hand, both the clinician and the patient agree not to start antiretroviral therapy or the patient is started on a regimen without PIs or NNRTIs, a traditional rifampin-based regimen should be employed. The document advocates that if a patient is not to be started on antiretroviral therapy, his condition should be periodically monitored with HIV RNA levels, CD4 counts, and assessment of the HIV-related syndromes to help determine the appropriate time to commence such treatment.

The recommended treatment options for HIV-infected persons with drug-susceptible tuberculosis include these salient points:

- DOT and other strategies that promote adherence to therapy should be used for all patients
- for patients receiving PIs and/or NNRTIs, initial therapy should include isoniazid, rifabutine, pyrazinamide, and ethambutol

TABLE 8.9. *Percentage of tuberculosis (TB) patients[a] with drug-resistant isolates[b] by drug and human immunodeficiency virus (HIV) serostatus, United States, 1993–1996*

	HIV serostatus (%)		
Drug[c]	HIV positive (n = 5,112)	HIV negative (n = 3,754)	HIV status unknown (n = 7,186)
Isoniazid	11.3	5.5	6.8
Rifampin	8.9	1.6	2.5
Pyrazinamide	5.1	1.8	2.2
Streptomycin	6.7	4.1	5.0
Ethambutol	3.9	1.5	2.0
Isoniazid and rifampin	6.2	1.3	1.5
Rifampin only[d]	2.4	0.2	0.8

These data complement the information in the text. For a variety of known and unknown reasons, persons with HIV infection/AIDS in the United States have modestly but significantly higher levels of drug-resistant tuberculosis, the greatest disparity being with rifampin monoresistance.

[a] Patients were born in the United States, were aged 22–44 years, and were not known to have had a previous episode of TB. All TB cases reported from California are included in the HIV-unknown category.

[b] The patient's *Mycobacterium tuberculosis* isolate had resistance to at least the specified drug but may have had resistance to other drugs as well.

[c] The differences in drug-resistance rates among patients with TB known to be HIV-seropositive, compared with those known to be HIV-seronegative or of unknown status, are statistically significant (χ^2 test statistic, $p < 0.05$).

[d] These figures were calculated for patients with *M. tuberculosis* isolates tested for isoniazid and rifampin always and streptomycin sometimes. Monoresistant isolates were resistant to rifampin but susceptible to the other first-line drugs tested.

From CDC, National Tuberculosis Surveillance System.

TABLE 8.10. *Effects of coadministering rifamycins and protease inhibitors (PIs) on the systemic exposure (area under the concentration–time curve of each drug)*[a]

	Rifampin (RIF)		Rifabutin (RFB)	
PI and source	RIF's effect on PI	PI's effect on RIF	RFB's effect on PI	PI's effect on RFB
Saquinavir[a] Sahai et al., 1996 (85)	80% decrease	Data not reported	45% decrease	Data not reported
Ritonavir Cato et al., 1996 (86); Abbot Laboratories, 1997 (87)	35% decrease	Unchanged[c]	Data not reported	293% increase
Indinavir Indinavir (MK 639) Pharmacokinetic Study Group, 1996 (88)	92% decrease	Data not reported	34% decrease	173% increase
Nelfinavir Kerr et al., 1997 (89)	82% decrease	Data not reported	32% decrease	200% increase
Amprenavir Polk et al., 1998 (90); Sadler et al., 1998 (91)	81% decrease	Unchanged	14% decrease	200% increase[d]

Rifampin induction of the CyP450 hepatic pathways results in major reductions in the bioavalability of all of these PIs; this effect would probably result in treatment failure and acquired resistance to the antiviral agents. By comparison, rifabutin has considerably less effect on the catabolism of these agents. Hence, it is estimated that rifabutin would not significantly interfere with the clinical utility of these agents (see Table 8.12). However, because ritonavir results in extremely high concentrations of rifabutine, their simultaneous use is contraindicated.

[a] Effects are expressed as a percentage change in AUC of the concomitant treatment relative to that of the drug-alone treatment. No data are available regarding the magnitude of these bidirectional interactions when rifamycins are administered two or three times a week instead of daily.

[b] Hard-gel formulation (Invirase).

[c] Data from only two subjects.

[d] Percentages reflect increases in minimum concentrations; values for the AUC are not reported.

TABLE 8.11. *Known and predicted effects of coadministering rifamycins and nonnucleoside reverse transcriptase inhibitors (NNRTIs) on the systemic exposure (area under the concentration time curve) of each drug*[a]

	Rifampin (RIF)		Rifabutin (RFB)	
NNRTI and source	RIF's effect on NNRTI	NNRTI's effect on RIF	RFB's effect on NNRTI	NNRTI's effect on RFB
Nevirapine Roxane Laboratories, 1997 (92)	37% decrease	Unchanged[b]	16% decrease	Decrease[b]
Delavirdine Borin et al., 1997 (93); Borin et al., 1997 (94); Cox et al., 1998 (95)	96% decrease	Unchanged[b]	80% decrease	342% increase[b]
Efavirenz Benedek et al., 1998 (96)	13% decrease	Unchanged[b]	Decrease	Decrease[b]

Rifampin has a moderately greater effect than rifabutin in accelerating the elimination of this category of antiviral agents. The CDC and its panel of consultants recommended that rifabutin could be used with nevirapine, probably with efavirenz, but not with delavirdine (see Table 8.12).

[a] Effects are expressed as a percentage change in AUC of the concomitant treatment relative to that of the drug-alone treatment. No data are available regarding the magnitude of these bidirectional interactions when rifamycins are administered two or three times a week instead of daily.

[b] Predicted effect based on knowledge of metabolic pathways for the two drugs.

TABLE 8.12. *Feasibility of using different antiretroviral drugs and rifabutin*

Antiretroviral agent	Can be used in combination with rifabutin?	Comments
Saquinavir (soft-gel formulation)	Probably	Use of the soft-gel formulation Fortovase in higher-than-usual doses might allow adequate serum concentrations of this drug despite concurrent use of rifabutin.[a] However, the pharmacokinetic data for this combination are limited in comparison with other protease inhibitors. Because of the expected low bioavailability of the hard-gel formulation (invirase) the concurrent use of this agent with rifabutin is not recommended.
Ritonavir	No	Ritonavir increases concentrations of rifabutin 35-fold and results in increased rates of toxicity (arthralgia, uveitis, skin discoloration, and leukopenia). These adverse events have been noted in studies of high-dose rifabutin therapy, when rifabutin is administered with clarithromycin (another Cy450 inhibitor) — an indication that these events might result from high serum concentrations of rifabutin.
Indinavir	Yes	Data from drug interaction studies (*unpublished report*, Merck Research Laboratories, West Point, PA, 1998) suggest that the dose of indinavir should be increased from 800 mg every 8 hours to 1,200 mg every 8 hours if used in combination with rifabutin.[a]
Nelfinavir	Yes	Some clinical experts suggest that the dose of nalfinavir should be increased from 750 mg three times a day to 1,000 mg three times a day if used in combination with rifabutin.[a]
Amprenavir	Probably	The drug interactions between amprenavir and rifabutin (and thus potential for rifabutin toxicity) are reported to be similar to those of ritonavir with rifabutin. However, potential advantages of using this combination are that(s) rifabutin has a minimal effect on reducing the levels of amprenavir and (b) even though it has not been studied, rifabutin toxicity is not expected if the daily dose of rifabutin is reduced when used in combination with amprenavir.
NRTIs[b]	Yes	Not expected to have clinically significant interaction.
Nevirapine	Yes	Not known whether nevirapine or rifabutin dose adjustments are necessary when these drugs are used together.[a]
Delavirdine	No	Not recommended on the basis of marked decreases in concentrations of delavirdine when administered with rifamycins.
Efavirenz	Probably	Newly approved agent. Preliminary drug interaction studies suggest that when rifabutin is used concurrently with efavirenz, the dose of rifabutin for both daily and twice weekly administration should be increased from 300 mg to 450 mg.

The CDC staff and expert panel made these assessments based on limited clinical and pharmacokinetic data. The biggest fear that I harbor is the concern that simultaneous use of a rifamycin and PIs and/or NNRTIs entails potential double jeopardy: (a) the rifamycin results in suboptimal levels of the antiretroviral agents, leading to treatment failure and acquired resistance to these antiviral agents, and (b) the anticipated increase in the concentration of the rifamycin does not occur, resulting in treatment failure and acquired resistance to the antimycobacterial drugs. Ideally, I believe, pharmacokinetic studies should be done to assure adequate and safe levels of these interacting drugs. However, the practices advocated in the CDC document are reasonable and prudent. Nonetheless, careful scrutiny should be applied to patients receiving such simultaneous therapy.

[a] Daily dose of rifabutin should be reduced from 300 mg to 150 mg if used in combination with amprenavir, nelfinavir, or indinavir. It is unknown whether the dose of rifabutin should be reduced if used in combination with sequinavir (Fortovase) or nevirapine.

[b] Nucleoside reverse transcriptase inhibitiors, including zidovudine, didanosine, zalcitabine, stavudine, and lamivudine.

- for patients in whom rifamycins are contraindicated or not tolerated, initial therapy should consist of isoniazid, streptomycin (or, alternatively, amikacin, kanamycin, or capreomycin), and pyrazinamide (specific regimen options are spelled out in the Appendix)
- The minimum duration of a rifamycin-containing regimen is to be 6 months, but the final decision on the duration of therapy should consider the patient's response to treatment. For patients with delayed response to treatment by the end of 2 months of therapy, the

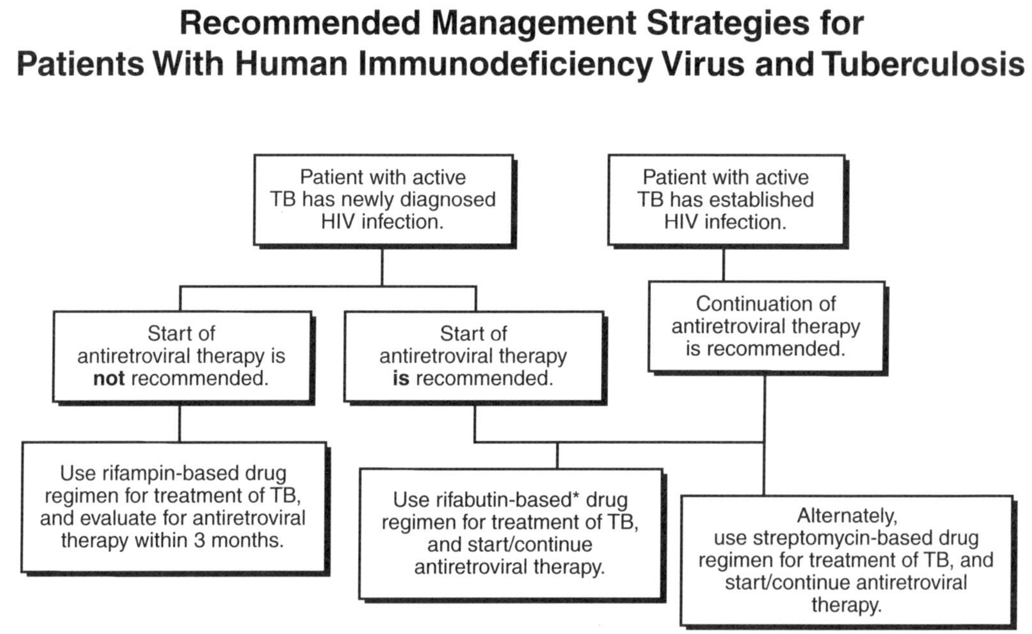

FIG. 8.3. As noted in the text, this algorithm includes the care of patients already receiving antiretroviral therapy or those newly found to be HIV-infected. The decision not to begin antiretroviral therapy (the far-left pathway) involves multiple considerations including the patient's capacity to initiate two complicated multidrug regimens at once and the potential for major complications from paradoxical worsening (see text). Coadministration of rifabutin with ritonavir, saquinavir (Invirase), or delavirdine is not recommended.

patient either remains culture positive for *M. tuberculosis* or has persistent signs and symptoms or clinical worsening that is ascribed to tuberculosis

- Monitoring patients on tuberculosis chemotherapy should include particular attention to the risk of peripheral neuropathy from pyridoxine deficiency (all patients are to receive supplemental B_6), dermatological reactions, and, if on PIs or NNRTIs, with rifabutin to be alert to adverse reactions from high levels of this drug secondary to inhibited catabolism (uveitus, leukopenia, red skin, arthralgias, lupus reactions)
- Also, clinicians are alerted to the risk of paradoxical reactions when PIs and/or NNRTIs reconstitute immune competency and inflammatory capacity

Overall, this is a detailed document with thoughtful analyses and recommendations. It should be reviewed in detail by all practitioners who regularly see patients coinfected with HIV and tuberculosis.

REFERENCES

1. Mocroft AJ, Johnson MA, Sabin CA, et al. Staging system for clinical AIDS patients. *Lancet* 1995;346:12–17.
2. Agostini C, Trentin L, Zambello R, Semenzato G. HIV-1 and the lung. Infectivity, pathogenic mechanisms, and cellular immune responses taking place in the lower respiratory tract. *Am Rev Respir Dis* 1993; 147:1038–1049.
3. Beck JM, Shellito J. Effects of human immunodeficiency virus on pulmonary host defences. *Sem Respir Infect* 1989;4:75–84.
4. Clarke JR, Robinson DS, Coker RJ, Miller RF, Mitchell DM. AIDS and the lung: update 1995. Role of the human immunodeficiency virus within the lung. *Thorax* 1995;50:567–576.
5. Stead W, Senner J, Reddick W, Lofgren J. Racial differences in susceptibility to infection by *Mycobacterium tuberculosis. N Engl J Med* 1990;322:422–427.
6. Crowle A, Elkins N. Relative permissiveness of macrophages from black and white people for virulent tubercle bacilli. *Infect Immun* 1990;58:632–638.
7. Rankin JA, Marcy T, Rochester CL, et al. Human airway macrophages. A technique for their retrieval and a

descriptive comparison with alveolar macrophages. *Am Rev Respir Dis* 1992;145:928–933.
8. Wallgren A. The time-table of tuberculosis. *Tubercle* 1948;29:245–251.
9. Stead W, Lofgren J, Warren E, Thomas C. Tuberculosis: an endemic and nosocomial infection among the elderly in nursing homes. *N Engl J Med* 1985;312: 1483–1487.
10. DiPerri G, Cruciani M, Danzi MC, et al. Nosocomial epidemic of active tuberculosis among HIV-infected patients. *Lancet* 1989;2:1502–1504.
11. Alpert PL, Munsiff SS, Gourevitch MN, Greenberg B, Klein RS. A prospective study of tuberculosis and human immunodeficiency virus infection: clinical manifestations and factors associated with survival. *Clin Infect Dis* 1997;24:661–668.
12. Daley CL, Small PM, Schecter GF, et al. An outbreak of tuberculosis with accelerated progression among persons infected with the human immunodeficiency virus. An analysis using restriction-fragment-length polymorphisms. *N Engl J Med* 1992;326:231–235.
13. Centers for Disease Control. Nosocomial transmission of multidrug-resistant tuberculosis among HIV-infected persons—Florida and New York, 1988–1991. *MMWR* 1991;40:585–591.
14. Fischl MA, Uttamchandani RB, Daikos GL, et al. An outbreak of tuberculosis caused by multiple-drug-resistant tubercle bacilli among patients with HIV infection. *Ann Intern Med* 1992;117:177–183.
15. Small PM, Hopewell PC, Singh SP, et al. The epidemiology of tuberculosis in San Francisco. A population-based study using conventional and molecular methods. *N Engl J Med* 1994;330:1703–1709.
16. Alland D, Kalkut GE, Moss AR, et al. Transmission of tuberculosis in New York City. An analysis by DNA fingerprinting and conventional epidemiologic methods. *N Engl J Med* 1994;330:1710–1716.
17. Selwyn PA, Hartel D, Lewis VA, et al. A prospective study of the risk of tuberculosis among intravenous drug users with human immunodefiency virus infection. *N Engl J Med* 1989;320:545–550.
18. Brown MM, Badi N, Ryder RW, et al. Retrospective cohort study of the risk of tuberculosis among women of childbearing age with HIV infection in Zaire. *Am Rev Respir Dis* 1991;143:501–504.
19. Allen S, Batungwanayo J, Kerlikowske K, et al. Two-year incidence of tuberculosis in cohorts of HIV-infected and uninfected urban Rwandan women. *Am Rev Respir Dis* 1992;146:1439–1444.
20. UNAIDS/WHO. Report on the global HIV/AIDS epidemic. *Lancet* 1997;350:1683.
21. Sudre P, ten Dam G, Chan C, Kochi A. Tuberculosis in the present time: a global overview of the tuberculosis situation. *WHO/TUB* 1991;158:1–47.
22. Msamanga GI, Fawzi WW. The double burden of HIV infection and tuberculosis in sub-Saharan Africa. *Lancet* 1997;337:849–851.
23. Cantwell MF, Binkin NJ. Tuberculosis in sub-Saharan Africa: a regional assessment of the impact of the human immunodeficiency virus and National Tuberculosis Control Program quality. *Tuberc Lung Dis* 1996; 77:220–225.
24. Raviglione MC, Harries AD, Msiska R, Wilkinson D, Nunn P. Tuberculosis and HIV: current status in Africa. *AIDS* 1997;11:S115–S123.
25. Pio A, Chaulet P. Standardization of district-based packages of care for the management of tuberculosis and other respiratory diseases among youth and adults. *Global Tuberc Programme* 1997;97:232.
26. Manalo F, Tan F, Sbarbaro JA, Iseman MD. Community based short-course treatment of pulmonary tuberculosis in a developing nation. Initial report of an eight-month, largely intermittent regimen in a population with high prevalence of drug resistance. *Am Rev Respir Dis* 1990;142:1301–1305.
27. Paramasivan CN, Chandrasekaran V, Santha T, Sudarsanam NM, Prabhakar R. Bacteriological investigations for short-course chemotherapy under the tuberculosis programme in two districts of India. *Tuberc Lung Dis* 1993;74:23–27.
28. Kim SJ, Hong YP. Drug resistance of *Mycobacterium tuberculosis* in Korea. *Tuberc Lung Dis* 1992;73: 219–224.
29. Nelson KE, Celentano DD, Eiumtrakol S, et al. Changes in sexual behavior and a decline in HIV infection among young men in Thailand. *N Engl J Med* 1996;335:297–303.
30. Müller O, Ungchusak K, Leng HB, Chung A, Tadiar F. HIV and AIDS in Southeast Asia (Letter). *Lancet* 1997;350:288.
31. Ryan CA, Vathiny OV, Gorbach PM, et al. Explosive spread of HIV-1 and sexually transmitted diseases in Cambodia (Letter). *Lancet* 1998;351:1175.
32. Centers for Disease Control. Update: trends in AIDS incidence, deaths, and prevalence—United States, 1996. *MMWR* 1997;46:165–172.
33. Wortley PM, Fleming PL. AIDS in women in the United States. *JAMA* 1997;278:911–916.
34. Rosenberg PS, Biggar RJ. Trends in HIV incidence among young adults in the United States. *JAMA* 1998; 279:1894–1899.
35. Markowitz N, Hansen NI, Hopewell PC, et al. Incidence of tuberculosis in the United States among HIV-infected persons. *Ann Intern Med* 1997;126: 123–132.
36. McCray E, Weinbaum CM, Braden CR, Onorato IM. The epidemiology of tuberculosis in the United States. In: Iseman MD, Huitt GA, eds. *Clinics in chest medicine.* Philadelphia: WB Saunders, 1997:99–113.
37. Burwen DR, Bloch AB, Griffin LD, Ciesielski CA, Stern HA, Onorato IM. National trends in the concurrence of tuberculosis and acquired immunodeficiency syndrome. *Arch Intern Med* 1995;155:1281–1286.
38. McKenna MT, McCray E, Onorato I. The epidemiology of tuberculosis among foreign-born persons in the United States, 1986–93. *N Engl J Med* 1995;332: 1071–1076.
39. Rosenblum LS, Castro KG, Dooley S, Morgan M. Effect of HIV infection and tuberculosis on hospitalizations and cost of care for young adults in the United States, 1985 to 1990. *Ann Intern Med* 1994;121: 786–792.
40. Theuer CP, Hopewell PC, Elias D, Schecter GF, Rutherford GW, Chaisson RE. Human immunodeficiency virus infection in tuberculosis patients. *J Infect Dis* 1990;102:8–12.
41. Perrone C, Ghoubontini A, Leport C, Salmon-Ceron D, Bricaire F, Vilde JL. Should pulmonary tuberculosis be an AIDS-defining diagnosis in patients infected with HIV? *Tubercle Lung Dis* 1992;73:39–44.

42. Mukadi Y, Perriens JH, St Louis ME, et al. Spectrum of immunodeficiency in HIV-1-infected patients with pulmonary tuberculosis in Zaire. *Lancet* 1993;342: 143–146.
43. Jones BE, Young SMM, Antoniskis D, Davidson PT, Kramer F, Barnes PF. Relationship of the manifestations of tuberculosis to CD4 cell counts in patients with human immunodeficiency virus infection. *Am Rev Respir Dis* 1993;148:1292–1297.
44. Fischl MA, Daikos GL, Uttamchandani RB, et al. Clinical presentation and outcome of patients with HIV infection and tuberculosis caused by multiple-drug-resistant bacilli. *Ann Intern Med* 1992;117:184–190.
45. Keiper MD, Beumont M, Elshami A, Langlotz CP, Miller WT Jr. CD4 T lymphocyte count and the radiographic presentation of pulmonary tuberculosis. A study of the relationship between these factors in patients with human immunodeficiency virus infection. *Chest* 1995;107:74–80.
46. Batungwanayo J, Taelman H, Dhote R, Bogaerts J, Allen S, van de Perre P. Pulmonary tuberculosis in Kigali, Rwanda. Impact of human immunodeficiency virus infection on clinical and radiographic presentation. *Am Rev Respir Dis* 1992;146:53–56.
47. Long R, Scalcini M, Manfreda J. Impact of human immunodeficiency virus type 1 on tuberculosis in rural Haiti. *Am Rev Respir Dis* 1991;143:69–73.
48. Eriki PP, Okwera A, Aisu T, Morrissey AB, Ellner JJ, Daniel TM. The influence of human immunodeficiency virus infection on tuberculosis in Kampala, Uganda. *Am Rev Respir Dis* 1991;143:185–187.
49. Long R, Maycher B, Scalcini M, Manfreda J. The chest roentgenogram in pulmonary tuberculosis patients seropositive for human immunodeficiency virus type 1. *Chest* 1991;99:123–127.
50. Given MJ, Khan MA, Reichman LB. Tuberculosis among patients with AIDS and a control group in an inner-city community. *Arch Intern Med* 1994;154: 640–645.
51. Pozniak AL, MacLeod GA, Ndlovu D, Ross E, Mahari M, Weinberg J. Clinical and chest radiographic features of tuberculosis associated with human immunodeficiency virus in Zimbabwe. *Am J Respir Crit Care Med* 1995;152:1558–1561.
52. Modilevsky T, Sattler FR, Barnes PF. Mycobacterial disease in patients with human immunodeficiency virus infection. *Arch Intern Med* 1989;149:2201–2205.
53. Chaisson RE, Schecter GF, Theuer CP, Rutherford GW, Echenberg DF, Hopewell PC. Tuberculosis in patients with the acquired immunodeficiency syndrome. Clinical features, response to therapy, and survival. *Am Rev Respir Dis* 1987;136:570–574.
54. Mlika-Cabanne N, Brauner M, Mugusi F, et al. Radiographic abnormalities in tuberculosis and risk of coexisting human immunodeficiency virus infection. Results from Dar-es-Salaam, Tanzania, and scoring system. *Am J Respir Crit Care Med* 1995;152: 786–793.
55. Mlika-Cabanne N, Brauner M, Kamanfu G, et al. Radiographic abnormalities in tuberculosis and risk of coexisting human immunodeficiency virus infection. Methods and preliminary results from Bujumbura, Burundi. *Am J Respir Crit Care Med* 1995;152:794–799.
56. Klein WC, Duncanson FP, Lenox TH III, Pitta A, Cohen SC, Wormser GP. Use of mycobacterial smears in the diagnosis of pulmonary tuberculosis in AIDS/ ARC patients. *Chest* 1989;95:1190–1192.
57. Elliott AM, Luo N, Tembo G, et al. Impact of HIV on tuberculosis in Zambia: a cross sectional study. *Br Med J* 1990;301:412–415.
58. Elliott AM, Namaambo K, Allen BW, et al. Negative sputum smear results in HIV-positive patients with pulmonary tuberculosis in Lusaka, Zambia. *Tubercle Lung Dis* 1993;74:191–194.
59. Nunn P, Mungai M, Nyamwaya J, et al. The effect of human immunodeficiency virus type-1 on the infectiousness of tuberculosis. *Tuberc Lung Dis* 1994;75: 25–32.
60. Montessori V, Phillips P, Montaner J, et al. Species distribution in human immurelated mycobacterial infections: implications for selection of initial treatment. *Clin Infect Dis* 1996;22:989–992.
61. Campo RE, Campo CE. *Mycobacterium kansasii* disease in patients infected with human immunodeficiency virus. *Clin Infect Dis* 1997;24:1233–1238.
62. Gallant JE, Ko AH. Cavitary pulmonary lesions in patients infected with human immunodeficiency virus. *Clin Infect Dis* 1996;22:671–682.
63. Lucas SB, Hounnou A, Peacock C, Beaumel A, Kadio A, De Cock KM. Nocardiosis in HIV-positive patients: an autopsy study in West Africa. *Tuberc Lung Dis* 1994;75:301–307.
64. American Thoracic Society. Fungal infection in HIV-infected persons. *Am J Respir Crit Care Med* 1995; 152:816–822.
65. Gilks CF, Ojoo SA, Ojoo JC, et al. Invasive pneumococcal disease in a cohort of predominantly HIV-1 infected female sex-workers in Nairobi, Kenya. *Lancet* 1996;347:718–723.
66. Kamanfu G, Mlika-Cabanne N, Girard P-M, et al. Pulmonary complications of human immunodeficiency virus infection in Bujumbura, Burundi. *Am Rev Respir Dis* 1993;147:658–663.
67. Daley CL, Mugusi F, Chen LL, et al. Pulmonary complications of HIV infection in Dar es Salaam, Tanzania. Role of bronchoscopy and bronchoalveolar lavage. *Am J Respir Crit Care Med* 1996;154:105–110.
68. Miller R. HIV-associated respiratory diseases. *Lancet* 1996;348:307–312.
69. Case Records of the Massachusetts General Hospital. Case 27-1997. *N Engl J Med* 1997;337:619–627.
70. Malin AS, Gwanzura LKZ, Klein S, Robertson VJ, Musvaire P, Mason PR. *Pneumocystis carinii* pneumonia in Zimbabwe. *Lancet* 1995;346:1258–1261.
71. Barnes PF, Steele MA, Young SMM, Vachon LA. Tuberculosis in patients with human immunodeficiency virus infection. How often does it mimic *Pneumocystis carinii* pneumonia? *Chest* 1992;102:428–432.
72. Centers for Disease Control. Revison of the CDC surveillance case definition for acquired immunodeficiency syndrome. *MMWR* 1987;36:3–9.
73. Braun MM, Byers RH, Heyward WL, et al. Acquired immunodeficiency syndrome and extrapulmonary tuberculosis in the United States. *Arch Intern Med* 1990;150:1913–1916.
74. Shafer RW, Kim DS, Weiss JP, Quale JM. Extrapulmonary tuberculosis in patients with human immunodeficiency virus infection. *Medicine* 1991;70:348–397.
75. Hill AR, Premkuman S, Brustein S, et al. Disseminated tuberculosis in the acquired immunodeficiency

syndrome era. *Am Rev Respir Dis* 1991;144: 1164–1170.
76. Jaber B, Gleckman R. Tuberculous pancreatic abscess as an initial AIDS-defining disorder in a patient infected with the human immunodeficiency virus: case report and review. *Clin Infect Dis* 1995;20:890–894.
77. Fee MJ, Oo MM, Gabayan AE, Radin DR, Barnes PF. Abdominal tuberculosis in patients infected with the human immunodeficiency virus. *Clin Infect Dis* 1995; 20:938–944.
78. Libraty DH, Byrd TF. Cutaneous miliary tuberculosis in the AIDS era: case report and review. *Clin Infect Dis* 1996;23:706–710.
79. Hudson CP, Wood R, O'Keefe EA. Cutaneous miliary tuberculosis in the AIDS era (Letter). *Clin Infect Dis* 1997;25:1484.
80. Antinori S, Bini T, Galimberti L, Meroni L, Esposito R. Cutaneous miliary tuberculosis in a patient infected with human immunodeficiency virus. *Clin Infect Dis* 1997;25:1484–1485.
81. Daikos GL, Uttamchandani RB, Tuda C, et al. Disseminated miliary tuberculosis of the skin in patients with AIDS: report of four cases. *Clin Infect Dis* 1998; 27:205–208.
82. Baraldés MA, Domingo P, González MJ, Aventin A, Coll P. Tuberculosis-associated hemophagocytic syndrome in patients with acquired immunodeficiency syndrome. *Arch Intern Med* 1998;158:194–195.
83. Porter JC, Friedland JS, Freedman AR. Tuberculous bronchoesophageal fistulae in patients infected with the human immunodeficiency virus: three case reports and review. *Clin Infect Dis* 1994;19:954–957.
84. Huth RG, Acebo R, Matthew EB. Osteitis cystica tuberculosa multiplex in a patient infected with human immunodeficiency virus. *Clin Infect Dis* 1994;18: 260–261.
85. Farrar DJ, Flanigan TP, Gordon NM, Gold RL, Rich JD. Tuberculous brain abscess in a patient with HIV infection: case report and review. *Am J Med* 1997;102: 297–301.
86. de la Fuente-Aguado J, Bordón J, Moreno JA, Sopena B, Rodriguez A, Martínez-Vázquez C. Parkinsonism in an HIV-infected patient with hypodense cerebral lesion. *Tuberc Lung Dis* 1996;77:191–192.
87. Gachot B, Wolff M, Clair B, Regnier B. Severe tuberculosis in patients with human immunodeficiency virus infection. *Inten Care Med* 1990;16:487–488.
88. Ahuja SS, Ahuja SK, Phelps KR, Thelmo W, Hill AR. Hemodynamic confirmation of septic shock in disseminated tuberculosis. *Crit Care Med* 1992;20:901–903.
89. Vadillo M, Corbella X, Carratala J. AIDS presenting as septic shock caused by *Mycobacterium tuberculosis. Scand J Infect Dis* 1994;26:105–106.
90. George S, Papa L, Sheils L, Magnussen CR. Septic shock due to disseminated tuberculosis. *Clin Infect Dis* 1996;22:188–189.
91. Clark TM, Burman WJ, Cohn DL, Mehler PS. Septic shock from *Mycobacterium tuberculosis* after therapy for *Pneumocystis carinii. Arch Intern Med* 1998;158: 1033–1035.
92. Richter C, Koelemay MJW, Swai ABM, Perenboom R, Mwakyusa DH, Oosting J. Predictive markers of survival in HIV-seropositive and HIV-seronegative Tanzanian patients with extrapulmonary tuberculosis. *Tuberc Lung Dis* 1995;76:510–517.
93. Whalen C, Horsburgh CR Jr, Hom D, Lahart C, Simberkoff M, Ellner J. Site of disease and opportunistic associated tuberculosis. *AIDS* 1997;11:455–460.
94. Holden M, Dubin MR, Diamond PH. Frequency of negative intermediate-strength tuberculin sensitivity in patients with active tuberculosis. *N Engl J Med* 1971;285:1506–1509.
95. Rooney JJ, Crocco JA, Kramer S, Lyons HA. Further observations on tuberculin reactions in tuberculosis. *Am J Med* 1976;60:517–522.
96. Nash DK, Douglass JE. A comparison between positive and negative reactors and an evaluation of 5-TU and 250-TU skin test doses. *Chest* 1980;77:32–37.
97. Graham NMH, Nelson KE, Solomon L, et al. Prevalence of tuberculin positivity and skin test anergy in HIV-1–seropositive and -seronegative intravenous drug users. *JAMA* 1992;267:369–373.
98. Markowitz N, Hansen NI, Wilcosky TC, et al. Tuberculin and anergy testing in HIV-seropositive and HIV-seronegative persons. *Ann Intern Med* 1993;119: 185–193.
99. Centers for Disease Control. Purified protein derivative (PPD)–tuberculin anergy and HIV infection: guidelines for anergy testing and management of anergic persons at risk of tuberculosis. *MMWR* 1991;40: 27–33.
100. Huebner RE, Schein MF, Hall CA, Barnes SA. Delayed-type hypersensitivity anergy in human immunodeficiency virus-infected persons screened for infection with *Mycobacterium tuberculosis. Clin Infect Dis* 1994;19:26–32.
101. Caiaffa WT, Graham NMH, Galai N, Rizzo RT, Nelson KE, Vlahov D. Instability of delayed-type hypersensitivity skin test anergy in human immunodeficiency virus infection. *Arch Intern Med* 1995;155: 2111–2117.
102. Chin DP, Osmond D, Page-Shafer K, et al. Reliability of anergy skin testing in persons with HIV infection. *Am J Respir Crit Care Med* 1996;153:1982–1984.
103. Yanai H, Uthaivoravit W, Mastro TD, et al. Utility of tuberculin and anergy skin testing in predicting tuberculosis infection in human immunodeficiency virus-infected persons in Thailand. *Int J Tuberc Lung Dis* 1997;1:427–434.
104. Johnson MP, Coberly JS, Clermont HC, et al. Tuberculin skin test reactivity among adults infected with human immunodeficiency virus. *J Infect Dis* 1992; 166:194–198.
105. Moreno S, Bavaia-Etxabury J, Bouza E, et al. Risk for developing tuberculosis among anergic patients infected with HIV. *Ann Intern Med* 1993;119:194–198.
106. Antonucci G, Girardi E, Raviglione MC, Ippolito G. Risk factors for tuberculosis in HIV-infected persons. A prospective cohort study. *JAMA* 1995;274:143–148.
107. Gordin FM, Matts JP, Miller C, et al. A controlled trial of isoniazid in persons with anergy and human immunodeficiency virus infection who are at high risk for tuberculosis. *N Engl J Med* 1997;37:315–320.
108. Centers for Disease Control and Prevention. 1997 USPHS/IDSA guidelines for the prevention of opportunistic infections in persons infected with human immunodeficiency virus. *MMWR* 1997;46:10–12.
109. Jordan TJ, Levit EM, Montgomery EL, Reichman LB. Isoniazid as preventive therapy in HIV-infected intravenous drug abusers: a decision analysis. *JAMA* 1991; 265:2987–2991.

110. Kramer F, Modilesky T, Waliany AR, Leedom JM, Barnes PF. Delayed diagnosis of tuberculosis in patients with human immodeficiency virus infection. *Am J Med* 1990;89:451–456.
111. Murray JF, Mills J. Pulmonary infectious complications of human immunodeficiency virus infection. Part I. *Am Rev Respir Dis* 1990;141:1356–1372.
112. Martínez-Marcos FJ, Viciana P, Canas E, Martín-Juan J, Moreno I, Pachón J. Etiology of solitary pulmonary nodules in patients with human immunodeficiency virus infection. *Clin Infect Dis* 1997;24:908–913.
113. Nelson JE, Forman M. Hemoptysis in HIV-infected patients. *Chest* 1996;110:737–743.
114. Post FA, Wood R, Pillay GP. Pulmonary tuberculosis in HIV infection: radiographic appearance is related to $CD4^+$ T-lymphocyte count. *Tuberc Lung Dis* 1995;76: 518–521.
115. Abouya L, Coulibaly IM, Coulibaly D, et al. Radiologic manifestations of pulmonary tuberculosis in HIV-1–and HIV–2-infected patients in Abidjan, Cote d'Ivoire. *Tuberc Lung Dis* 1995;76:436–440.
116. Perlman DC, El-Sadr WM, Nelson ET, et al. Variation of chest radiographic patterns in pulmonary tuberculosis by degree of human immunodeficiency virus-related immunosuppression. *Clin Infect Dis* 1997;25: 242–246.
117. Awil PO, Bowlin SJ, Daniel TM. Radiology of pulmonary tuberculosis and human immunodeficiency virus infection in Gulu, Uganda. *Eur Respir J* 1997;10: 615–618.
118. Pablos-Méndez A, Sterling TR, Frieden TR. The relationship between delayed or incomplete treatment and all-cause mortality in patients with tuberculosis. *JAMA* 1996;276:1223–1228.
119. Louis E, Rice LB, Holzman RS. Tuberculosis in non-Haitian patients with acquired immunodeficiency syndrome. *Chest* 1986;90:542–545.
120. Long R, Scalcini M, Manfreda J, Jean-Baptiste M, Hershfield E. The impact of HIV on the usefulness of sputum smears for the diagnosis of tuberculosis. *Am J Public Health* 1991;81:1326–1328.
121. Smith RL, Yew K, Berkowitz KA, Aranda CP. Factors affecting the yield of acid-fast sputum smears in patients with HIV and tuberculosis. *Chest* 1994;106: 684–686.
122. Salzman SH, Schindel ML, Aranda CP, Smith RL, Lewis ML. The role of bronchoscopy in the diagnosis of pulmonary tuberculosis in patients at risk for HIV infection. *Chest* 1992;102:143–146.
123. Kennedy DJ, Lewis WP, Barnes PF. Yield of bronchoscopy for the diagnosis of tuberculosis in patients with human immunodeficiency virus infection. *Chest* 1992;102:1040–1044.
124. DiPerri G, Cazzadori A, Vento S, et al. Comparative histopathological study of pulmonary tuberculosis in human immunodeficiency virus-infected and non-infected patients. *Tuberc Lung Dis* 1996;77:244–249.
125. Horsburg CR Jr. Tuberculosis without tubercles. *Tuberc Lung Dis* 1996;77:197–198.
126. Miro AM, Gibilara E, Powell S, Kamhols SL. The role of fiberoptic bronchoscopy for diagnosis of pulmonary tuberculosis in patients at risk for AIDS. *Chest* 1992;101:1211–1214.
127. Harkin TJ, Ciotoli C, Addrizzo-Harris DJ, Naidich DP, Jagirdar J, Rom WN. Transbronchial needle aspiration (TBNA) in patients infected with HIV. *Am J Respir Crit Care Med* 1998;157:1913–1918.
128. Judson MA, Sahn SA. Endobronchial lesions in HIV-infected individuals. *Chest* 1994;105:1314–1323.
129. Wasser LS, Shaw GW, Talavera W. Endobronchial tuberculosis in the acquired immunodeficiency syndrome. *Chest* 1988;94:1240–1244.
130. Pastores SM, Naidich DP, Aranda CP, McGuiness G, Rom WN. Intrathoracic adenopathy associated with pulmonary tuberculosis in patients with human immunodeficiency virus infection. *Chest* 1993;103: 1433–1437.
131. Shafer RW, Goldberg R, Sierra M, Glatt AE. Frequency of *Mycobacterium tuberculosis* bacteremia in patients with tuberculosis in an area endemic for AIDS. *Am Rev Respir Dis* 1989;140:1611–1613.
132. Pithie AD, Chicksen B. Fine-needle extrathoracic lymph-node aspiration in HIV-associated sputum-negative tuberculosis. *Lancet* 1992;340:1504–1505.
133. Small PM, Schecter GF, Goodman PC, Sande MA, Chaisson RE, Hopewell PC. Treatment of tuberculosis in patients with advanced human immunodeficiency virus infection. *N Engl J Med* 1991;324:289–294.
134. Jones BE, Otaya M, Antoniskis D, et al. A prospective evaluation of antituberculosis therapy in patients with human immunodeficiency virus infection. *Am J Respir Crit Care Med* 1994;150:1499–1502.
135. Okwera A, Whalen C, Byekwaso F, et al. Randomised trial of thiacetazone and rifampicin-containing regimens for pulmonary tuberculosis in HIV-infected Ugandans. *Lancet* 1994;344:1323–1328.
136. Ackah AN, Coulibaly D, Digbeu H, et al. Response to treatment, mortality, and CD4 lymphocyte counts in HIV-infected persons with tuberculosis in Abidjan, Cote d'Ivoire. *Lancet* 1995;345:607–610.
137. Elliott AM, Halwiindi B, Hayes RJ, et al. The impact of human immunodeficiency virus on mortality in patients treated for tuberculosis: two-year follow-up of cohort in Lusaka, Zambia. *Trans R Soc Trop Med Hyg* 1995;89:75–82.
138. Chaisson RE, Clermont HC, Holt EA, et al. Six-month supervised intermittent tuberculosis therapy in Haitian patients with and without HIV infection. *Am J Respir Crit Care Med* 1996;154:1034–1038.
139. Hawken M, Nunn P, Gathua S, et al. Increased recurrence of tuberculosis in HIV-1-infected patients in Kenya. *Lancet* 1993;342:332–337.
140. Perriëns JH, St Louis ME, Mukadi YB, et al. Pulmonary tuberculosis in HIV-infected patients in Zaire. A controlled trial of treatment for either 6 or 12 months. *N Engl J Med* 1995;332:779–784.
141. Pulido F, Pena J-M, Rubio R, et al. Relapse of tuberculosis after treatment in human immunodeficiency virus-infected patients. *Arch Intern Med* 1997;157: 227–232.
142. El-Sadr WM, Perlman DC, Matts JP, et al. Evaluation of an intensive intermittent-induction regimen and duration of short-course treatment for human immunodeficiency virus-related pulmonary tuberculosis. *Clin Infect Dis* 1998;26:1148–1158.
143. American Thoracic Society. Treatment of tuberculosis and tuberculosis infection in adults and children. *Am J Respir Crit Care Med* 1994;149:1359–1374.
144. Pulido F, Pena JM, Rubio R. Treatment of tuberculosis in HIV-infected patients in Zaire. *N Engl J Med* 1995; 333:519.

145. Iseman MD. Is standard chemotherapy adequate in tuberculosis patients infected with the HIV? (Editorial) *Am Rev Respir Dis* 1987;136:1326.
146. Shuter J, Bellin E. Secondary prophylaxis for tuberculosis in patients infected with human immunodeficiency virus. *Clin Infect Dis* 1996;22:398–399.
147. Cohn D, Reeves R. *Unpublished data.*
148. Frieden TR, Fujiwara PI, Washko RM, Hamburg MA. Tuberculosis in New York City—turning the tide. *N Engl J Med* 1995;333:229–233.
149. Barnes PFD, Barrows SA. Tuberculosis in the 1990's. *Ann Intern Med* 1993;119:400–410.
150. Ellard GA, Humphries MJ, Allen BJ. Cerebrospinal fluid drug concentrations and the treatment of tuberculosis meningitis. *Am Rev Respir Dis* 1993;148: 650–655.
151. Gordin FM, Nelson ET, Matts JP, et al. The impact of human immunodeficiency virus infection on drug-resistant tuberculosis. *Am J Respir Crit Care Med* 1996; 154:1478–1483.
152. Frieden TR, Sherman LF, Maw KL, et al. A multi-institutional outbreak of highly drug-resistant tuberculosis. Epidemiology and clinical outcomes. *JAMA* 1996;276:1229–1235.
153. Ritacco V, Di Lonardo M, Reniero A, et al. Nosocomial spread of human immunodeficiency virus-related multidrug-resistant tuberculosis in Buenos Aires. *J Infect Dis* 1997;176:637–642.
154. Guerrero A, Cobo J, Fortún J, et al. Nosocomial transmission of *Mycobacterium bovis* resistant to 11 drugs in people with advanced HIV-1 infection. *Lancet* 1997;350:1738–1742.
155. Gutiérrez MC, Bouvet E, Blazquez J, Vincent V. Identification as *Mycobacterium tuberculosis* of previously described *M. bovis* multidrug-resistant strains. *Lancet* 1998;351:758.
156. Schwoebel V, Decludt B, de Benoist A-C, et al. Multidrug resistant tuberculosis in France 1992-4: two case-control studies. *BMJ* 1998;317:630–631.
157. Bradford WZ, Martin JN, Reingold AL, Schecter GF, Hopewell PC, Small PM. The changing epidemiology of acquired drug-resistant tuberculosis in San Francisco, USA. *Lancet* 1996;348:928–931.
158. Nolan CM, Williams DL, Cave MD, et al. Evolution of rifampin resistance in human immunodeficiency virus-associated tuberculosis. *Am J Respir Crit Care Med* 1995;152:1067–1071.
159. Lutfey M, Della-Latta P, Kapur V, et al. Independent origin of non-rifampin–resistant *Mycobacterium tuberculosis* in patients with AIDS. *Am J Respir Crit Care Med* 1996;153:837–840.
160. Bishai WR, Graham NMH, Harrington S, et al. Brief report: rifampin-resistant tuberculosis in a patient receiving rifabutin prophylaxis. *N Engl J Med* 1996; 334:1573–1575.
161. Ridzon R. *Rifampin-resistant tuberculosis: a review.* Paper presented at the Annual Meeting, American Thoracic Society, San Francisco, CA, 1997.
162. Munsiff S, Joseph S, Ebrahimzadeh A, Frieden T. Rifampin-monoresistant tuberculosis in New York City, 1993–1994. *Clin Infect Dis* 1997;25:1465–1467.
163. March F, Garriga X, Rodríquez P, et al. Acquired drug resistance in *Mycobacterium tuberculosis* isolates recovered from compliant patients with human immunodeficiency virus-associated tuberculosis. *Clin Infect Dis* 1997;25:1044–1047.
164. DiPerri G, Bonora S, Vento S, Allegranzi B, Concia E. *M. tuberculosis* drug resistance in AIDS (Letter). *Lancet* 1997;349:60–61.
165. Turett GS, Telzak EE, Torian LV. Improved outcomes for patients with multidrug-resistant tuberculosis. *Clin Infect Dis* 1995;21:1238–1244.
166. Salomon N, Perlman DC, Friedmann P, Buchstein S, Kreiswirth BN, Mildvan D. Predictors and outcome of multidrug-resistant tuberculosis. *Clin Infect Dis* 1995; 21:1245–1252.
167. Berning SE, Huitt G, Iseman MD, Peloquin CA. Malabsorption of antituberculosis medications by a patient with AIDS (Letter). *N Engl J Med* 1992;327: 1817–1818.
168. Peloquin CA, Nitta AT, Burman WJ, et al. Low antituberculosis drug concentrations in patients with AIDS. *Ann Pharmacother* 1996;30:919–925.
169. Peloquin CA, MacPhee AA, Berning SE. Malabsorption of antimycobacterial medications (Letter). *N Engl J Med* 1993;329:1122–1123.
170. Sahai J, Swick L, Tailor S, et al. *Reduced oral absorption of tuberculosis drugs in HIV infection.* Paper presented at the meeting of the American Society for Clinical Pharmacology and Therapeutics, Lake Buena Vista, FL, 1996.
171. Taylor B, Smith PJ. Does AIDS impair the absorption of antituberculosis agents? *Int J Tuberc Lung Dis* 1998;2:670–675.
172. Patel KB, Belmonte R, Crowe HM. Drug malabsorption and resistant tuberculosis in HIV-infected patients. *N Engl J Med* 1995;332:336–337.
173. Luo C, Chintu C, Bhat G, et al. Human immunodeficiency virus type-1 infection in Zambian children with tuberculosis: changing seroprevalance and evaluation of a thioacetazone-free regimen. *Tuberc Lung Dis* 1994;75:110–115.
174. Coopman SA, Johnson RA, Platt R, Steven RS. Cutaneous disease and drug reactions in HIV infection. *N Engl J Med* 1993;328:1670–1674.
175. Ungo JR, Jones D, Ashkin D, et al. Antituberculosis drug-induced hepatotoxicity . The role of hepatitis C virus and the human immunodeficiency virus. *Am J Respir Crit Care Med* 1998;157:1871–1876.
176. Nunn P, Kubuga D, Gathnua S, et al. Cutaneous hypersensitivity reactions due to thiacetazone in HIV-1 seropositive patients treated for tuberculosis. *Lancet* 1991;337:627–630.
177. Wallis RS, Helfand MS, Whalen CC, et al. Immune activation, allergic drug toxicity and mortality in HIV-positive tuberculosis. *Tuberc Lung Dis* 1996;77:516–523.
178. Ipuge YAI, Rieder HL, Enarson DA. Adverse cutaneous reactions to thiacetazone for tuberculosis treatment in Tanzania. *Lancet* 1995;346:657–660.
179. Rieder HL, Enarson DA. Rebuttal: time to call a halt to emotions in the assessment of thioacetazone. *Tuberc Lung Dis* 1996;77:109–111.
180. van Gorkom J, Kibuga DK. Cost-effectiveness and total costs of three alternative strategies for the prevention and management of severe skin reactions attributable to thiacetazone in the treatment of human immunodeficiency virus positive patients with tuberculosis in Kenya. *Tuberc Lung Dis* 1996;77:30–36.
181. Elliott AM, Foster SD. Thiacetazone: time to call a halt? Considerations on the use of thiacetazone in African populations with a high prevalence of human

immunodeficiency virus infection. *Tuberc Lung Dis* 1996;77:27–29.

182. Okwera A, Johnson JL, Vjecha MJ, et al. Risk factors for adverse drug reactions during thiacetazone treatment of pulmonary tuberculosis in human immunodeficiency virus infected adults. *Int J Tuberc Lung Dis* 1997;1:441–445.
183. Deeks SG, Smith M, Holodniy M, Kahn JO. HIV-1 protease inhibitors. A review for clinicians. *JAMA* 1997;277:145–153.
184. Li TS, Tubiana R, Katlama C, Calvez V, Mohand HA, Autran B. Long-lasting recovery in CD4 T-cell function and viral-load reduction after highly active antiretroviral therapy in advanced HIV-1 disease. *Lancet* 1998;351:1682–1686.
185. Palella FJ, Delaney KM, Moorman AC, et al. Declining morbidity and mortality among patients with advanced human immunodeficiency virus infection. *N Engl J Med* 1998;338:853–860.
186. Hogg RS, Heath KV, Yip B, et al. Improved survival among HIV-infected individuals following initiation of antiretroviral therapy. *JAMA* 1998;279:450–454.
187. Powderly WG, Landay A, Lederman MM. Recovery of the immune system with antiretroviral therapy. The end of opportunism? *JAMA* 1998;280:72–77.
188. Carpenter CCJ, Fischl MA, Hammer SM, et al. Antiretroviral therapy for HIV infection in 1998. Updated recommendations of the International AIDS Society-USA Panel. *JAMA* 1998;280:78–86.
189. Feinberg MB, Carpenter C, Fauci AS, et al. Report of the NIH panel to define principles of therapy and HIV infection and guidelines for the use of antiretroviral agents in HIV-infected adults and adolescents. *Ann Intern Med* 1998;128:1057–1100.
190. Centers for Disease Control. Clinical update: impact of HIV protease inhibitors on the treatment of HIV-infected tuberculosis patients with rifampin. *MMWR* 1996;45:921–925.
191. Blaschke TF, Skinner MH. The clinical pharmacokinetics of rifabutin. *Clin Infect Dis* 1996;22(Suppl 1): S15–S22.
192. Heifets LB, Lindholm-Levy PJ, Iseman MD. Rifabutine: minimal inhibitory and bactericidal concentrations for *Mycobacterium tuberculosis. Am Rev Respir Dis* 1988;137:719–721.
193. Grassi C, Peona V. Use of rifabutin in the treatment of pulmonary tuberculosis. *Clin Infect Dis* 1996;22: S50–S54.
194. MacGregor AR, Green CA. Tuberculosis of the central nervous system with special reference to tuberculous meningitis. *J Pathol Bacteriol* 1937;45:613–630.
195. Piscitelli SC, Flexner C, Minor JR, Polis MA, Masur H. Drug interactions in patients infected with human immunodeficiency virus. *Clin Infect Dis* 1996;23: 685–693.
196. Teoh R, Humphries MJ, O'Mahoney G. Symptomatic intracranial tuberculoma developing during treatment of tuberculosis: a report of 10 patients and review of the literature. *Q J Med* 1987;241:449–460.
197. Smith H. Paradoxical responses during the chemotherapy of tuberculosis. *J Infect* 1987;15:1–3.
198. Berg J, Leonard A, Clancy CJ, Nguyen MH. Subcutaneous abscesses due to *Mycobacterium tuberculosis:* paradoxical expansion of disease during therapy for miliary tuberculosis. *Clin Infect Dis* 1998;26:231–232.
199. Koster F. Paradoxical local response to therapy for *Mycobacterium avium* complex infection in four patients with AIDS. *Clin Infect Dis* 1998;26:1231–1232.
200. Narita M, Ashkin D, Hollender ES, Pitchenik AE. Paradoxical worsening of tuberculosis following antiretroviral therapy in patients with AIDS. *Am J Respir Crit Care Med* 1998;158:157–161.
201. Crump JA, Tyrer MJ, Lloyd-Owen SJ, Han LY, Lipman MC, Johnson MA. Miliary tuberculosis with paradoxical expansion of intracranial tuberculomas complicating human immunodeficiency virus infection in a patient receiving highly active antiretroviral therapy. *Clin Infect Dis* 1998;26:1008–1009.
202. Chien JW, Johnson JL. Paradoxical reactions in HIV and pulmonary TB. *Chest* 1998;114:933–936.
203. Race EM, Adelson-Mitty J, Kriegel GR, et al. Focal mycobacterial lymphadenitis following initiation of protease-inhibitor therapy in patients with advanced HIV-1 disease. *Lancet* 1998;351:252–255.
204. Sepkowitz KA. Effect of HAART on natural history of AIDS-related opportunistic disorders. *Lancet* 1998; 351:228–239.
205. Jacobson MA, Zegans M, Pavan PR, et al. Cytomegalovirus retinitis after initiation of highly active antiretroviral therapy. *Lancet* 1997;349:1443–1445.
206. French M, Lenzo N, John M, Mallal S, Price P. Highly active antiretroviral therapy (Letter). *Lancet* 1998; 351:1056–1057.
207. Hadad DJ, Lewi DS, Pignatari ACC, Martins MC, Vitti W Jr, Arbeit RD. Resolution of *Mycobacterium avium* complex bacteremia following highly active antiretroviral therapy. *Clin Infect Dis* 1998;26:758–759.
208. DiPerri G, Bonora S, Vento S, Allegranzi B, Concia E. Highly active antiretroviral therapy (Letter). *Lancet* 1998;351:1056.
209. Stoneburner R, Laroche E, Prevots R, et al. Survival in a cohort of human immunodeficiency virus-infected tuberculosis patients in New York City. *Arch Intern Med* 1992;152:2033–2037.
210. Whalen C, Horsburgh CR, Hom D, Lahart C, Simberkoff M, Ellner J. Accelerated course of human immunodeficiency virus infection after tuberculosis. *Am J Respir Crit Care Med* 1995;151:129–135.
211. Zhang Y, Nakata K, Weiden M, Rom WN. Mycobacterium tuberculosis enhances human immunodeficiency virus-1 replication by transcriptional activation at the long terminal repeat. *J Clin Invest* 1995;95: 2324–2331.
212. Folks TM, Justement J, Kinter A. Cytokine-induced expression of HIV-1 in a chronically infected promonocyte cell line. *Science* 1987;238:800–802.
213. Osborn L, Kunkel S, Nabel GJ. Tumor necrosis factor and interleukin-1 stimulate the human immunodeficiency virus enhancer by activation of the nuclear factor kB. *Proc Natl Acad Sci USA* 1989;36:2336–2340.
214. Lederman MM, Georges D, Zeichner SL, Alwine JC, Toossi Z. *Mycobacterium tuberculosis* and its purified protein derivative activates expression of the human immunodeficiency virus. *J AIDS* 1994;7:727–733.
215. Nakata K, Rom WN, Honda Y, et al. *Mycobacterium tuberculosis* enhances human immunodeficiency virus-1 replication in the lung. *Am J Respir Crit Care Med* 1997;155:996–1003.
216. Mancino G, Placido R, Bach S, et al. Infection of human monocytes with *Mycobacterium tuberculosis* en-

hances human immunodeficiency virus type 1 replication and transmission to T cells. *J Infect Dis* 1997; 175:1531–1535.
217. Goletti D, Weissman D, Jackson RW, Collins F, Kinter A, Fauci AS. The in vitro induction of human immunodeficiency virus (HIV) replication in purified protein derivative-positive HIV-infected persons by recall antigen response to *Mycobacterium tuberculosis* is the result of a balance of the effects of endogenous interleukin-2 and proinflammatory and antiinflammatory cytokines. *J Infect Dis* 1998;177:1332–1338.
218. Denis M, Ghadirian E. Interaction between *Mycobacterium avium* and human immunodeficiency virus type 1 (HIV-1) in bronchoalveolar macrophages of normal and HIV-1-infected subjects. *Am J Respir Cell Mol Biol* 1994;11:487–495.
219. Ghassemi M, Andersen BR, Reddy VM, Gangadharam PRJ, Spear GT, Novak RM. Human immunodeficiency virus and *Mycobacterium avium* complex coinfection of monocytoid cells results in reciprocal enhancement of multiplication. *J Infect Dis* 1995;171: 68–73.
220. Havlir DV, Haubrich R, Hwang J, et al. Human immunodeficiency virus replication in AIDS patients with *Mycobacterium avium* complex bacteremia: a case control study. *J Infect Dis* 1998;177:595–599.
221. Haas DW, Lederman MM, Clough LA, Wallis RS, Chernoff D, Crampton SL. Proinflammatory cytokine and human immunodeficiency virus RNA levels during early *Mycobacterium avium* complex bacteremia in advanced AIDS. *J Infect Dis* 1998;177:1746–1749.
222. Stanley SK, Ostrowski MA, Justement JS, et al. Effect of immunization with a common recall antigen on viral expression in patients infected with human immunodeficiency virus type 1. *N Engl J Med* 1996;334: 1222–1230.
223. Cheeseman SH, Davaro RE, Ellison RT III. Hepatitis B vaccination and plasma HIV-1 RNA. *N Engl J Med* 1996;334:1272.
224. Brichacek B, Swindells S, Janoff EN, Pirrucccello S, Stevenson M. Increased plasma human immunodeficiency virus type 1 burden following antigenic challenge with pneumococcal vaccine. *J Infect Dis* 1996; 174:1191–1199.
225. Greene WC. Denying HIV safe haven. *N Engl J Med* 1996;334:1264–1265.
226. Donaldson YK, Bell JE, Ironside JW, et al. Redistribution of HIV outside the lymphoid system with onset of AIDS. *Lancet* 1994;343:382–385.
227. Pape JW, Jean SS, Ho JL, Hafner A, Johnson WD Jr. Effect of isoniazid prophylaxis on incidence of active tuberculosis and progression of HIV infection. *Lancet* 1993;342:268–272.
228. Hosp M, Elliott A, Rayner JG, et al. Neopterin, B2–microglobulin, and acute phase proteins in HIV-1 seropositive and seronegative Zambian patients with tuberculosis. *Lung* 1997;175:265–275.
229. Elliott AM, Halwiindi B, Bagshawe A, et al. Use of prednisolone in the treatment of HIV-positive tuberculosis patients. *Qtr J Med* 1992;85:855–860.
230. Wallis RS, Nsubuga P, Whalen C, et al. Pentoxifylline therapy in human immunodeficiency virus–seropositive persons with tuberculosis: a randomized, controlled trial. *J Infect Dis* 1996;174:727–733.
231. Tramontana JM, Utaipat U, Molloy A, et al. Thalidomide treatment reduces tumor necrosis factor α production and enhances weight gain in patients with pulmonary tuberculosis. *Mol Med* 1995;1:384–397.
232. Haslett P, Tramontana J, Burroughs M, Hempstead M, Kaplan G. Adverse reactions to thalidomide in patients infected with human immunodeficiency virus. *Clin Infect Dis* 1997;24:1223–1227.
233. Thea DM, Porat R, Nagimbi K, et al. Plasma cytokines, cytokine antagonists, and disease progression in African women infected with HIV-1. *Ann Intern Med* 1996;124:757–762.
234. Sbarbaro JA. Compliance: inducements and enforcements. *Chest* 1979;76S:750S–756S.
235. Goble M, Iseman MD, Madsen LA, Waite D, Ackerson L, Horsburgh CR Jr. Treatment of 171 patients with pulmonary tuberculosis resistant to isoniazid and rifampin. *N Engl J Med* 1993;328:527–532.
236. Mahmoudi A, Iseman MD. Pitfalls in the care of patients with tuberculosis. Common errors and their association with the acquisition of drug resistance. *JAMA* 1993;270:65–68.
237. Pablos-Méndoz A, Knirsch CA, Barr RG, Lerner BH, Frieden TR. Nonadherence in tuberculosis treatment: predictors and consequences in New York City. *Am J Med* 1997;102:164–170.
238. Perlman DC, Salomon N, Perkins MP, Yancovita S, Paone D, Des Jarlais DC. Tuberculosis in drug users. *Clin Infect Dis* 1995;21:1253–1264.
239. Alwood K, Keruly J, Moore-Rice K, Stanton DL, Chaulk CP, Chaisson RE. Effectiveness of supervised, intermittent therapy for tuberculosis in HIV-infected patients. *AIDS* 1994;8:1103–1108.
240. Dutt AK, Moers D, Stead WW. Short-course chemotherapy for tuberculosis with mainly twice-weekly isoniazid and rifampin. Community physicians' seven-year experience with mainly outpatients. *Am J Med* 1984;77:233–242.
241. Brudney K, Dobkin J. Resurgent tuberculosis in New York City. Human immunodeficiency virus, homelessness, and the decline of tuberculosis control programs. *Am Rev Respir Dis* 1991;144:745–749.
242. Weltman AC, Rose DN. Tuberculosis susceptibility patterns, predictors of multidrug resistance, and implications for initial therapeutic regimens at a New York City hospital. *Arch Intern Med* 1994;154:2161–2167.
243. Hongthiamthong P, Riantawan P, Subhannachart P, Fuangtong P. Clinical aspects and treatment outcome in HIV-associated pulmonary tuberculosis: an experience from a Thai referral centre. *J Med Assoc Thai* 1994;77:520–525.
244. Wilkinson D, Moore DA. HIV-related tuberculosis in South Africa—clinical features and outcome. *S Afr Med J* 1996;86:64–67.
245. Johnson JL, Okwera A, Vjecha MJ, et al. Risk factors for relapse in human immunodeficiency virus type 1 infected adults with pulmonary tuberculosis. *Int J Tuberc Lung Dis* 1997;1:446–453.
246. Fineberg HV, Wilson ME. Social vulnerability and death by infection. *N Engl J Med* 1996;334:859–860.
247. Richards SB, St. Louis ME, Nieburg P, et al. Impact of the HIV epidemic on trends in tuberculosis in Abidjan, Cote d'Ivoire. *Tuberc Lung Dis* 1995;76:11–16.

248. Iseman MD, Cohn DL, Sbarbaro JA. Directly observed treatment of tuberculosis. We can't afford not to try it. *N Engl J Med* 1993;328:576–578.
249. Concato J, Rom WN. Endemic tuberculosis among homeless men in New York City. *Arch Intern Med* 1994;154:2069–2073.
250. Kenyon TA, Mwasekaga MJ, Huebner R, Rumisha D, Binkin N, Maganu E. Low levels of drug resistance amidst rapidly increasing tuberculosis and human immunodeficiency virus co-epidemics in Botswana. *Int J Tuberc Lung Dis* 1999;3:4–11.
251. Hoover DR, Saah AJ, Bacellar H, et al. Clinical manifestations of AIDS in the era of *Pneumocystis* prophylaxis. *N Engl J Med* 1993;329:1922–1926.
252. Shafer RW, Singh SP, Larkin C, Small PM. Exogenous reinfection with multidrug-resistant *Mycobacterium tuberculosis* in an immunocompetent patient. *Tubercle and Lung Disease* 1995;76:575–577.
253. Barnes PF, El-Hajj H, Preston-Martin S, et al. Transmission of tuberculosis among the urban homeless. *JAMA* 1996;275:305–307.
254. Godfrey-Faussett P, Githui W, Batchelor B, et al. Recurrence of HIV-related tuberculosis in an endemic area may be due to relapse or reinfection. *Tuberc Lung Dis* 1994;75:199–202.
255. Shafer RW, Chirgwin KD, Glatt AE, Dahdouh MA, Landesman SH, Suster B. HIV prevalence, immunosuppression, and drug resistance in patients with tuberculosis in an area endemic for AIDS. *AIDS* 1991; 5:399–405.
256. Rieder HL, Cauthen GM, Bloch AB. Tuberculosis and acquired immunodeficiency syndrome—Florida. *Arch Intern Med* 1989;149:1268–1273.
257. Pitchenik AE, Burr J, Suarez M, Fertel D, Gonzalez G, Moas C. Human T-cell lymphotropic virus-III (HTLV-III) seropositivity and related disease among 71 consecutive patients in whom tuberculosis was diagnosed. A prospective study. *Am Rev Respir Dis* 1987;135: 875–879.
258. Zajdenverg R, Valle S, Silva D, et al. Reactivity to purified protein derivative and the risk of tuberculosis in HIV-infected Brazilian patients (Letter). *Chest* 1993; 104:646.
259. Sawert H, Girardi E, Antonucci G, Raviglione MC, Viale P, Ippolito G. Preventive therapy for tuberculosis in HIV-infected persons. Analysis of policy options based on tuberculin status and $CD4^+$ cell count. *Arch Intern Med* 1998;158:2112–2121.
260. Hecker MT, Johnson JL, Whalen CC, Nyole S, Mugerwa RD, Ellner JJ. Two-step tuberculin skin testing in HIV-infected persons in Uganda. *Am J Respir Crit Care Med* 1997;155:81–86.
261. Kornbluth RS, McCutchan JA. Skin test responses as predictors of tuberculous infection and of progression in HIV-infected persons. *Ann Intern Med* 1993; 119:241–242.
262. Dolan MJ, Clerici M, Blatt SP, et al. In vitro T cell function, delayed-type hypersensitivity skin testing, and $CD4^+$ T cell subset phenotyping independently predict survival time in patients infected with human immunodeficiency virus. *J Infect Dis* 1995; 172:79–87.
263. Webster CT, Gordin FM, Matts JP, et al. Two-stage tuberculin skin testing in individuals with human immunodeficiency virus infection. *Am J Respir Crit Care Med* 1995;151:805–808.
264. Ferebee SH, Mount FW, Murray FJ, Livesay VT. A controlled trial of isoniazid prophylaxis in mental institutions. *Am Rev Respir Dis* 1963;88:161–175.
265. Krebs A, Farer LS, Snider WE, Thompson NJ. Five years of follow-up of the IUAT trial of isoniazid prophylaxis in fibrotic lesions. *Bull Int Union Against Tuberc* 1979;54:65–69.
266. Comstock GW, Ferebee-Woolpert S, Baum C. Isoniazid prophylaxis among Alaskan Eskimos: a progress report. *Am Rev Respir Dis* 1974;110:195–197.
267. Wadhawan D, Hira S, Mwansa N, Tembo G, Perine PL. *Isoniazid prophylaxis among patients with HIV-infection.* Paper presented at the VI International Conference on AIDS, University of California, San Francisco, 1990:249.
268. Wadhawan D, Hira SK, Mwansa N. *Preventive tuberculosis chemotherapy with isoniazid among persons infected by human immunodeficiency virus.* Paper presented at the VII International Conference on AIDS, Florence, Italy, 1991:247.
269. Whalen CC, Johnson JL, Okwera A, et al. A trial of three regimens to prevent tuberculosis in Ugandan adults infected with the human immunodeficiency virus. *N Engl J Med* 1997;337:801–808.
270. Moreno S, Miralles P, Diaz M, et al. Isoniazid preventive therapy in human immunodeficiency virus-infected persons. Long-term effect on development of tuberculosis and survival. *Arch Intern Med* 1997;157: 1729–1734.
271. Hawken MP, Meme HK, Elliott LC, et al. Isoniazid preventive therapy for tuberculosis in HIV-1–infected adults: results of a randomized controlled trial. *AIDS* 1997;11:875–882.
272. Halsey NA, Coberly JS, Desormeaux J, et al. Randomised trial of isoniazid versus rifampicin and pyrazinamide for prevention of tuberculosis in HIV-1 patients. *Lancet* 1998;351:786–792.
273. Gordin F, Chaisson R, Matts J, et al. A randomized trial of 2 months of rifampin (RIF) and pyrazinamide (PZA) versus 12 months of isoniazid (INH) for the prevention of tuberculosis (TB) in HIV-positive (+), PPD^+ patients (Abstract). Fifth Conference on Retroviruses and Opportunistic Infections, 1998.
274. Graham NMH, Galai N, Nelson KE, et al. Effect of isoniazid chemoprophylaxis on HIV-related mycobacterial disease. *Arch Intern Med* 1996;156:889–894.
275. Opravil M, Pechére M, Lazzarin A, et al. Dapsone/pyrimethamine may prevent mycobacterial disease in immunosuppressed patients infected with the human immunodeficiency virus. *Clin Infect Dis* 1995;20:244–249.
276. Malone JL, Paparello SF, Malone JD, Hill HE, Myers JW, Weiss P. Tuberculosis and HIV infection (Letter). *Lancet* 1993;342:677.
277. Bevilacqua N, Marasca G, Moscati A, Fantoni M, Ricci F, Ortona L. Tuberculosis and HIV infection. *Lancet* 1993;342:677.
278. Narain JP, Raviglione MC, Kochi A. HIV-associated tuberculosis in developing countries: epidemiology and strategies for prevention. *Tuberc Lung Dis* 1992; 73:311–321.
279. Reeve PA. Tuberculosis and HIV infection. *Lancet* 1993;342:676.

280. FitzGerald JM. The downside of isoniazid chemoprophylaxis. *Lancet* 1995;345:404.
281. Godfrey-Faussett P, Mwinga A, Raviglione M, et al. Tuberculosis and HIV infection. *Lancet* 1993;342: 1368–1369.
282. UK NGO AIDS Consortium Working Group on Access to Treatment for HIV in Developing Countries. Access to treatment for HIV in developing countries: statement from international seminar on access to treatment for HIV in developing countries, London, June 5 and 6, 1998. *Lancet* 1998;352:1379–1380.
283. Bjartveit K, Waaler H. Some evidence of the efficacy of mass BCG vaccination. *Bull WHO* 1965;33: 289–319.
284. Tripathy SP. Fifteen-year follow-up of the Indian BCG prevention trial. *Bull Int Union Tuberc Lung Dis* 1987;62:69–72.
285. Pönnighaus JM, Fine PEM, Sterne JAC, et al. Efficacy of BCG vaccine against leprosy and tuberculosis in northern Malawi. *Lancet* 1992;339:636–639.
286. Colditz GA, Brewer TF, Berkey CS, et al. Efficacy of BCG vaccine in the prevention of tuberculosis. Meta-analysis of the published literature. *JAMA* 1994; 271:298–702.
287. Wilson ME, Fineberg HV, Colditz GA. Geographic latitude and the efficacy of Bacillus Calmette-Guérin vaccine. *Clin Infect Dis* 1995;20:982–991.
288. Springett VH, Sutherland I. A re-examination of the variations in the efficacy of BCG vaccination against tuberculosis in clinical trials. *Tuberc Lung Dis* 1994; 75:227–233.
289. Fine PEM. Bacille Calmette-Guérin vaccines: a rough guide. *Clin Infect Dis* 1995;20:11–14.
290. Casanova J-L, Jouanguy E, Lamhamedi S, Blanche S, Fischer A. Immunological conditions of children with BCG disseminated infection. *Lancet* 1995;346:581.
291. Weltman AC, Rose DN. The safety of Bacille Calmette–Guérin vaccination in HIV infection and AIDS. *AIDS* 1993;7:149–157.
292. Talbot EA, Perkins MD, Silva SFM, Frothingham R. Disseminated Bacille Calmette-Guérin disease after vaccination: case report and review. *Clin Infect Dis* 1997;24:1139–1146.
293. Reynes J, Perez C, Lamaury I, Janbon F, Bertrand A. Bacille Calmette-Guérin adenitis 30 years after immunization in a patient with AIDS. *J Infect Dis* 1989;160: 727.
294. Armbruster C, Junker W, Vetter N, Jaksch G. Disseminated Bacille Calmette-Guérin infection in an AIDS patient 30 years after BCG vaccination. *J Infect Dis* 1990;162:1216–1218.
295. van Deutekom H, Smulders YM, Roozendaal KJ, van Soolingen D. Bacille Calmette-Guérin (BCG) meningitis in an AIDS patient 12 years after vaccination with BCG. *Clin Infect Dis* 1996;22:870–871.
296. Mvula M, Ryder R, Manzilla T, et al. *Response to childhood vaccinations in African children with HIV infection.* Paper presented at IV International Conference on AIDS, Stockholm, 1988:341.
297. Rieder HL. Repercussions of the Karonga prevention trial for tuberculosis control. *Lancet* 1996;348:4.
298. Karonga Prevention Trial Group. Randomised controlled trial of single BCG, repeated BCG, or combined BCG, and killed *Mycobacterium leprae* vaccine for prevention of leprosy and tuberculosis in Malawi. *Lancet* 1996;348:17–24.
299. Athale UH, Luo-Mutti C, Chintu C. How safe is BCG vaccination in children born to HIV-positive mothers? *Lancet* 1992;340:434–435.
300. Green SDR, Nganga A, Cutting WAM, Davies AG. BCG vaccination in children born to HIV-positive mothers. *Lancet* 1992;340:799.
301. Lepage P, van de Perre P, Msellati P, Dabis F. BCG vaccination in children born to HIV-positive mothers. *Lancet* 1992;340:799–800.
302. Matondo P. BCG vaccination in children born to HIV-positive mothers (Letter). *Lancet* 1992;340:800.
303. Brewer TF, Colditz GA. Relationship between Bacille Calmette-Guérin (BCG) strains and the efficacy of BCG vaccine in the prevention of tuberculosis. *Clin Infect Dis* 1995;20:126–135.
304. Comstock GW. Field trials of tuberculosis vaccines: how could we have done them better? *Control Clin Trials* 1994;15:247–276.
305. Guleria I, Teitelbaum R, McAdam RA, Kalpana G, Jacobs WR Jr, Bloom BR. Auxotrophic vaccines for tuberculosis. *Nature Med* 1996;2:334–337.
306. Centers for Disease Control. Guidelines for preventing the transmission of *Mycobacterium* tuberculosis in health-care facilities, 1994. *MMWR* 1994;43: 1–132.
307. Iseman MD. A leap of faith—what can we do to curtail intrainstitutional transmission of tuberculosis? [Editorial]. *Ann Intern Med* 1992;117:251.
308. Gilks CF, Haran D. Impact of HIV in sub-Saharan Africa. *Lancet* 1995;346:187.
309. World Health Organization. *Groups at risk. WHO report on the tuberculosis epidemic—1996.* Geneva: WHO Global Tuberculosis Programme, 1996.
310. Centers for Disease Control. A strategic plan for the elimination of tuberculosis in the United States. *MMWR* 1989;38:1–25.
311. Reichman LB. Tuberculosis elimination—what's to stop us? *Int J Tuberc Lung Dis* 1996;1:3–11.
312. De Cock KM, Binkin NJ, Zuber PLF, Tappero JW, Castro KG. Research issues involving HIV-associated tuberculosis in resource-poor countries. *JAMA* 1996; 276:1502–1507.
313. Centers for Disease Control and Prevention. Prevention and treatment of tuberculosis among patients infected with human immunodeficiency virus: principles of therapy and revised recommendations. *MMWR* 1998;47:1–58.

9
Pediatric Tuberculosis

Pediatric tuberculosis is a sentinel public health event (1). Between 1985–1992, tuberculosis cases among children in the United States rose 36.1% among those 0 to 4 years of age and 34.1% among those 5 to 14 years of age (2).

Tuberculosis in children is regarded as particularly meaningful for several reasons. Because of a compressed time period for the development of highly morbid, potentially lethal forms of tuberculosis in persons 0 to 4 years of age, there is great urgency about prompt diagnosis and therapy. The specter of a lifetime of disability or deformity resulting from dilatory care of children with emerging central nervous system or spinal disease is highly compelling. And, because each instance of pediatric tuberculosis reflects recent transmission from an adult, most commonly a parent, these cases signal failure of contemporary tuberculosis control programs.

EPIDEMIOLOGY

Globally, pediatric disease constitutes a greater proportion of the tuberculosis morbidity than it does in the United States. This is due mainly to much higher rates in the developing nations of pulmonary disease in adults of child-bearing age, which results in transmission of infection to their families. Recently, the World Health Organization (WHO) estimated that there were 1,300,000 cases and 450,000 deaths annually among individuals younger than 15 years in the developing nations (3). Pediatric disease in the United States had declined steadily in the modern era, reaching a low of 1,177 cases in 1987 (4). However, between the 1987 nadir and 1992, the number of cases rose to 1,707, a 45% increase (2). Notably, this upsurge in pediatric cases lagged several years behind that seen in adults; given the vertical pattern of transmission, parent-to-child, this pattern would be expected.

Given comparable levels of exposure, there are no apparent differences in the likelihood of infection occurring in relation to the age or sex of exposed children. However, race may be a significant factor. Among adults in nursing homes and prisons, blacks were apparently twice as likely to become infected—as manifested by converting their tuberculin skin tests—as were whites (5); similar predisposition to infection has not been documented among black children. However, one may speculate that this could be one of several factors in the very disparate morbidity in African-American children.

Once infected, age plays a highly significant role in the risk of developing active disease. Figure 9.1 demonstrates the age-related risk of disease for the United States; striking is the pattern of high risk to children 0 to 4 years of age, the markedly diminished rates among those ages 5 to 10 years, and the upturn in cases as the youngsters enter puberty. The period of years of age through puberty has been referred to as the "golden" or "favored" age of childhood; although not understood in terms of immune function, the phenomenon is consistently seen among diverse populations. In the pubertal age groups, there is a slightly higher risk of active tuberculosis among girls.

Commensurate with the greatly increased rates of disease among blacks and Hispanics of child-bearing ages, the offspring of these groups experience the great preponderance of pediatric

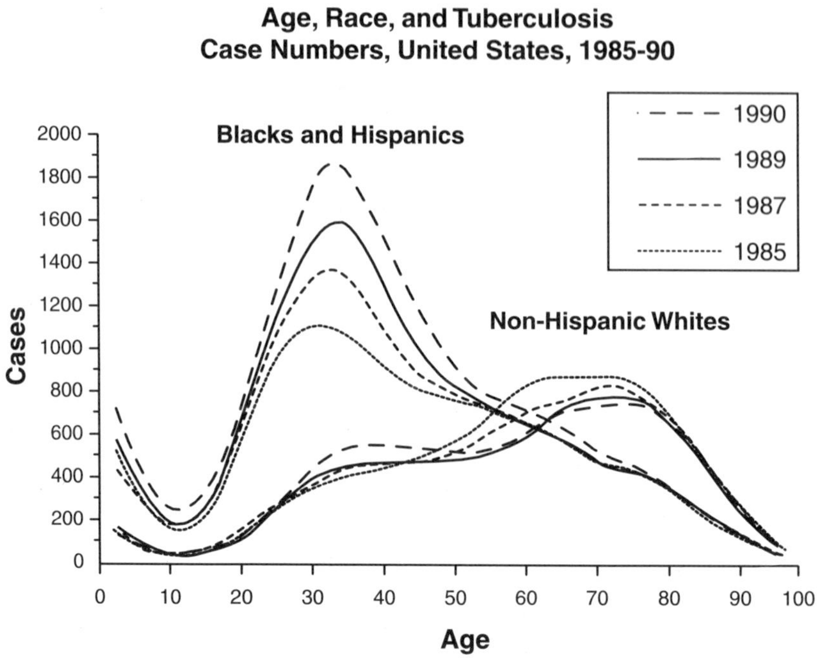

FIG. 9.1. From ref. 1, with permission.

tuberculosis in the United States. Between 1985 and 1992, the number of cases of tuberculosis among children 0 to 14 years of age rose over 35%, almost exclusively among blacks and Hispanics (2). In addition to these indigenous high-risk groups, children of immigrants—many of whom have come largely from areas of high prevalence—constitute a growing component of pediatric tuberculosis. In fact, 2,630 (20%) of the 11,442 cases of tuberculosis in the age group of 15 years of age or younger, between 1986 and 1993, occurred among immigrant children (6). The American Academy of Pediatrics recently identified groups deemed to be at particular risk for tuberculosis infection (Table 9.1).

PATHOGENESIS

As with adults, most children acquire infection with *Mycobacterium tuberculosis* through airborne inhalation of bacilli expelled by another person with active pulmonary disease. Rarely, there are cases wherein there is transplacental infection associated with maternal bacillemia (7–12). Tuberculous invasion of the bloodstream sufficient to infect the placenta and fetus is most likely to occur either during primary infection in a normal host or with any form of tuberculosis in a woman with advanced acquired immunodeficiency syndrome (AIDS). Infections attributable to aspiration of contaminated amniotic fluid or other means of direct inocula-

TABLE 9.1. *Infants, children, and adolescents at high risk for tuberculous infection*

- Contacts of adults with infectious tuberculosis
- Those who are from, or have parents who are from, regions of the world with high prevalence of tuberculosis
- Those with abnormalities on chest roentgenogram suggestive of tuberculosis
- Those with clinical evidence of tuberculosis
- HIV-seropositive children
- Those with immunosuppressive conditions
- Those with other medical risk factors: Hodgkin's disease, lymphoma, diabetes mellitus, chronic renal failure, malnutrition
- Incarcerated adolescents
- Children frequently exposed to the following adults: HIV-infected individuals, homeless persons, users of intravenous and other street drugs, poor and medically indigent city dwellers, residents of nursing homes, migrant farm workers

HIV, human immunodeficiency virus.

From American Academy of Pediatrics Committee on Infectious Diseases. Screening for tuberculosis in infants and children. *Pediatrics* 1994;93:131–134, with permission.

tion from an infected birth canal have been alleged but not well documented.

Following the primary introduction of infection, there devolves a bacillemic dissemination that results in implantation of microbes in many tissues throughout the body (see Chapter 4 for a more comprehensive review of pathogenesis). Over a period of several weeks to months, host immune responses develop that typically result in involution of these microscopic foci. Central to this response is collaboration between T lymphocytes and mononuclear phagocytes. This results in substantial curtailment of mycobacterial proliferation within the macro-phages, as well as the capacity to lyse the permissive macrophages that still support replication of the tubercle bacilli. Nomenclature about these phenomena has been confusing and inconsistent. Most commonly, they have been referred to as cell-mediated immunity (CMI) and delayed-type hypersensitivity (DTH) respectively. The evolution of tissue-damaging immune response or DTH is associated with the appearance of hypersensitivity to mycobacterial proteins, manifested clinically as a reactive tuberculin skin test. The inflammatory response in the lung parenchyma in the region of the implantation of the inhaled initial infection, coupled with an exuberant enlargement of the hilar/paratracheal lymph nodes that subserve this lung region, comprises the typical "primary complex" lesion seen on the chest x-ray of newly infected infants and children (see below).

The tubercle bacilli that have been delivered to remote sites in the body usually are walled off and killed or substantially inhibited by the granulomatous response of the competent host. However, in subjects who are relatively more vulnerable by virtue of age-related, genetically determined, or acquired defects of immunity, severe forms of extrapulmonary tuberculosis may appear within one to 12 months of the primary infection.

Among infants and children who do not develop overt, clinical forms of tuberculosis within the months and early years following primary infection, there usually develops a state of latent infection, which is distinguishable by a significant tuberculin skin test reaction. Since the tuberculin skin test is used to define latent infection, it is problematic to speculate whether persons can have infection with false-negative skin test results. However, it is important to stress that it may take up to 16 weeks after infection for the tuberculin skin test result to become reactive, longer than may be required for the evolution of life-threatening forms of tuberculosis (13). Residual shadows of the primary lesion (the Ghon focus), the primary complex coupled with the regional hilar lymph node (the Ranke complex), or apical, fibronodular scarring (Simon foci) attributable to transitory inflammation in the upper lobes following the primary bacillemia may be seen on the chest x-rays of some of these persons; see Figure 9.2 for schematic illustration of these lesions. Persons with latent tuberculosis infections are at risk of delayed reactivation disease throughout the entire course of their lives, sometimes 70 years or more remote from the primary infection.

CLINICAL PRESENTATIONS

As noted above, the primary site of infection is the lung, but systemic dissemination of bacilli results in seeding of multiple organs. Hence, tuberculosis in children may entail variable combinations of pulmonary and extrapulmonary manifestations. The likelihood of these presentations differs significantly according to the ages of the patients, particularly the age at the time of primary infection. The various types of disease referred to in contemporary pediatric tuberculosis are described below.

Asymptomatic Primary Pulmonary Disease

Among 110 cases of pediatric tuberculosis recently reported from Houston, Texas, there were 62 who were without symptoms (14). A parenchymal infiltrate coupled with hilar/paratracheal lymphadenopathy caused by a pathogen like *M. tuberculosis* might nominally be considered "disease." However, the natural history of these findings in a majority of asymptomatic children is to undergo spontaneous resolution. Indeed, the first U.S. Public Health Service (USPHS) preventive therapy trial consisted of giving 12-months of isoniazid (INH) monotherapy to infants and children with asymptomatic primary tuberculosis (see Chapter 12 for details) (15).

Chest X-ray Residuals of Primary Infection

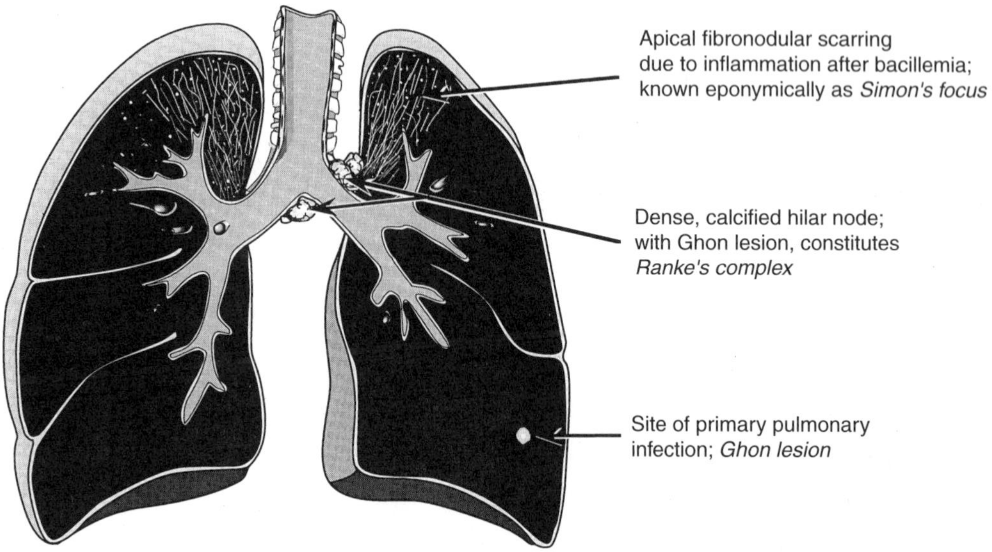

FIG. 9.2. Schematic of lesion.

While emphasis has been given to the protection afforded by INH, only 3% of the children—41 of 1,356—experienced subsequent pulmonary or extrapulmonary disease over 5 years of observation, indicating the generally benign course of this condition. It is important to note that the relatively benign prognosis observed in this trial relates *only* to those without constitutional or respiratory tract symptoms, and it should not be applied to infants who are at greater risk for major morbidity.

Complicated Primary Pulmonary Tuberculosis

Some children do not fare as well with the initial infection. A report of 202 cases of intrathoracic tuberculosis among children aged 0 to 15 years from British Columbia found that 40% had symptoms, most commonly cough (25 of 48) and fever (14 of 48); disease was severe enough to hospitalize 32 patients (16). Chest x-rays revealed various combinations of hilar, mediastinal, and/or paratracheal lymphadenopathy in 93.5% of cases; consolidation of lung parenchyma was noted in 76%; rarely seen were pleural effusions (4%) or cavitation (1.1%). Among a series recently reported from South Africa (17) of 38 children less than 3 months old with culture-proven tuberculosis, the following findings were noted: cough (57%), tachypnea with respirations more than or equal to 50/minute (82%), hepatomegaly (66%), splenomegaly (53%), crepitations (45%), wheezing (40%), and weight below the third centile (42%). Noteworthy is the fact that only 8 of 31 (26%) who were skin-tested reacted significantly to a Mantoux or tine test, probably reflecting both very recent exposure and overwhelming disease. Chest radiographic findings included hilar and/or paratracheal adenopathy in 89% and miliary shadowing in 26%.

The most dramatic pulmonary complications in this setting relate to massive enlargement of peribronchial lymph nodes. Among the consequences are major airway obstruction marked by hyperaeration of the distal lung accompanied often by localized wheezing and sublobar pneumonic disease attributable to erosion of the inflamed lymph node into the bronchial lumen. In the series from South Africa noted above, airway compromise was detected by taking overpenetrated chest x-rays, which allowed improved delineation of the bronchial tree. Because of the short- and long-term sequelae of this situation, including bronchial stenosis and postobstructive bronchiectasis, special therapy directed at relief of this peribronchial obstruction is probably indicated (see below).

Progressive Primary Pulmonary Tuberculosis

Rarely, the initial infection focus does not stabilize or involute, but develops into an intense, localized pneumonia which may undergo central necrosis and/or form pneumatocoeles, thin-walled tension cysts within the pneumonic process. These patients usually experience profound respiratory and systemic symptoms. This sequence in the absence of chemotherapy is associated with a grim prognosis including bronchopleural fistulae and chronic empyema.

Reactivation (Adult-Type) Pulmonary Tuberculosis

The delayed appearance of disease at the site of seeding of the lung apices that occurred during the primary bacillemia is seen almost exclusively in adolescence. This pattern can be distinguished from progressive primary disease by a clearly identifiable period of latency following the primary infection. Although the pathoimmune mechanism(s) that distinguish these clinical events are not well understood, the radiographic localization of disease, propensity for cavitary lesions, and likelihood of positive sputum smears are significantly different from the other forms of "pediatric" tuberculosis; hence, this presentation has been referred to as "adult" or "chronic" pulmonary tuberculosis.

The most common sites involved with this form of disease are the posterior/apical segments of the upper lobes, right more than left, and superior segments of the lower lobes. The propensity for involvement of these areas is believed to be associated with high local oxygen tension, diminished lymphatic flow, and impaired macrophage function in these regions (see Chapter 6 for details). Radiographically, the lesions are characteristically a mixture of nodular and linear shadows associated with regional volume loss; old, healed lesions tend to be dense and clearly marginated while acute, inflamed foci tend to be soft or fluffy in quality with indistinct margins. As the tuberculosis advances, nodular zones tend to coalesce and intensify, ultimately undergoing central necrosis and the formation of a cavity. The appearance of a cavity is of both clinical and epidemiological significance, indicating unfavorable prognosis (in the prechemotherapy era) and marking persons at high risk of having sputum smear–positive, potentially contagious tuberculosis (see Chapter 3 for details).

Tuberculous Pleural Effusions

Radiographically detectable effusions are quite rare among children ages 0 to 4 years, being seen in less than 10% of cases (18). However, among young adolescents who are recently infected, pleural involvement occurs in roughly 25% (19). This may take the form of acute painful pleuritis or asymptomatic fluid accumulations detected only on chest x-ray. Although tubercle bacilli may be recovered from the pleural fluid in a minority of cases, the mechanism of the effusion is mediated substantially through DTH to mycobacterial antigens associated with small numbers of viable mycobacteria. Rarely, this may be associated with classic empyema of the pleural space in which bacilli are readily demonstrable.

Extrapulmonary Tuberculosis

Involvement of organs other than the lungs occurs in a relatively higher percentage of children than adults with tuberculosis. In a USPHS 1986 survey, extrapulmonary tuberculosis (XPTB) made up 25.2% of all tuberculosis in the age group 0 to 14 years, but less than 17.5% in the overall population (18). Particularly common in this age group were lymphatic and meningeal disease; strikingly rare were pleural, genitourinary tract, and peritoneal tuberculosis (see Chapter 7 for a detailed description of these various extrapulmonary syndromes). Among the age group 0 to 4 years, there is a special proclivity for meningeal tuberculosis. In a recent series from South Africa among cases of tuberculous meningitis occurring in those 14 years or younger, 79.8% was reported in children 4 years of age or less; age-specific rates for cases of tuberculosis meningitis were as follows: 0 to 1 year, 31.5; 1 to 4 years, 17.1; 5 to 9 years, 4.8; and 10 to 14 years, 8.7 cases per 100,000 annually (19).

Miliary tuberculosis also is relatively more prominent among very young children, typically occurring within a few months of the original infection. *Miliary* refers to diffuse, tiny nodulations, similar in size to millet seeds, seen on chest x-ray. Such findings were noted in 26% of South African children less than 3 months of age with active tuberculosis (17); however, this was a highly selective series that was biased toward highly symptomatic subjects. More realistically, in the 110 children from Houston with various forms of tuberculosis, only 3 (2.7%) had miliary disease (14).

Tuberculosis in Infants and Children with Human Immunodeficiency Virus Infection

The relation between human immunodeficiency virus (HIV) infection/AIDS and pediatric tuberculosis in the United States appears to involve two mechanisms: (a) increased rates of pulmonary tuberculosis among young adults with AIDS, which results in high rates of tuberculosis transmission to their children, and (b) increased risk for tuberculosis for infants or children with congenital HIV infection (20); in this Centers for Disease Control and Prevention (CDC) analysis in 1992, the former was regarded as the predominant factor. Similarly, in a 1994 report from the Bronx, New York, a demographic or ecological survey indicated that poverty and crowding appeared to play a larger role than HIV in pediatric tuberculosis risk (21). However, a 1994 report from the Pediatric AIDS Clinical Trial Group suggested that the HIV-infected children appeared to be at a very high risk for tuberculosis including a 20% recovery of multidrug-resistant tuberculosis (MDR-TB) isolates from these children (22).

A 1996 report from South Africa compared the clinical, radiographic, and tuberculin skin test responses in 40 children with tuberculosis and HIV infection (TB/HIV) with 40 children solely with tuberculosis (20). Of note, the authors observed that there were no differences in the chest x-ray findings nor of the proportion or types of extrapulmonary disease. They did observe the following differences, however, among the TB/HIV children: (a) more extensive constitutional and pulmonary signs and symptoms, (b) more tuberculin anergy, (c) less clinical improvement with therapy, (d) failure to improve or worsened chest x-rays despite therapy, and (e) higher rates of death within the year of diagnosis. The authors conceded that, because of potential misdiagnosis of tuberculosis (only 7 of 67 cases tested had positive cultures [3 in the HIV-infected children and 4 in the uninfected children]), their results were not definitive. However, in another series from the United States, 7 of 75 children with TB/HIV failed to respond to therapy or relapsed (21).

Other documented differences in this age group include higher rates of cutaneous drug reactions, most notably to thiacetazone (see Chapter 8 for details). Whether infants and children with HIV infection have a greater risk for adverse drug reactions to the medications used in the industrialized nations is not proven.

DIAGNOSIS

Unlike adults, who most commonly manifest distinctly symptomatic pulmonary disease that is associated with positive sputum smears and cultures, children with tuberculosis have more subtle and nondescript clinical syndromes. Also, they typically have paucibacillary forms of disease, which are far less likely to yield positive bacteriological findings. Hence, diagnosis of pediatric tuberculosis usually entails more inferential considerations and more reliance upon invasive procedures.

Epidemiological Factors and Diagnosis

Since young children tend to develop overt tuberculosis within months of exposure/infection, and because children are unlikely to develop communicable forms of tuberculosis that can infect a sibling, an adult with active pulmonary tuberculosis usually can be found in the immediate environment of pediatric cases. In the 1989 report from Houston, an adult source case was found in 70% of the cases (14). Indeed, many children with tuberculosis are detected when contact investigation of new adult cases is performed. Thus, for a child with an illness consistent with or suggestive of tuberculosis, careful questioning regarding possible tuberculosis among adult family members or other regular contacts may provide vital information (23).

Another variable that is very meaningful in identification of children with tuberculosis is race and associated socioeconomic factors. As seen in Figure 9.1, white non-Hispanic children under the age of 10 years had very little morbidity; there were fewer than 100 cases at any age through 10 years. By contrast, among blacks and Hispanics, there were as many as 700 and no fewer than 200 cases at any year of age. Similarly, among the 202 cases of pediatric tuberculosis in British Columbia from 1979 to 1988, 37% were in Amerinds or Inuits and 30% were in Asians (16).

Tuberculin Skin Test

An indurated reaction at 48 to 96 hours following intradermal injection of tuberculoprotein is helpful in identifying persons who have been infected with *M. tuberculosis*. However, it is vital to note that this type of test is neither wholly sensitive nor specific: (a) a variable but clinically relevant number of infants and children with active tuberculosis do not mount significant reactions to tuberculin skin tests (so-called false-negative results), and (b) among those who do have substantial reactions to the test, there are potentially confusing numbers of persons who are not infected with *M. tuberculosis* but with other mycobacteria, thus giving rise to "false-positive" results. Among a large group of children with culture-proven lymphadenitis attributable to mycobacteria other than tuberculosis (MOTT), Wolinsky (24) noted that 42% reacted to a tuberculin skin test with greater than 10 mm induration (Fig. 9.3).

The epidemiological probability of tuberculosis can play a central role in the decision to deem

Tuberculin Reactions (PPD-S or T) of 91 Children with MOTT Lymphadenitis

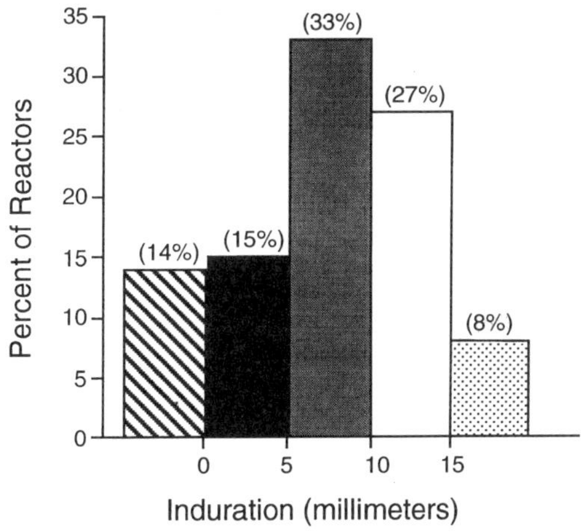

FIG. 9.3. Adapted from ref. 24, with permission.

a child infected or diseased with tuberculosis. Given *identical* clinical, radiographic, biopsy, and tuberculin skin test results, a clinician might judge one child from a low-risk group/community *not* to have tuberculosis, but a nontuberculous mycobacterial condition, while for another child from a high-risk group and setting, a presumptive diagnosis of tuberculosis would be made. Prior vaccination with bacille Calmette Guérin (BCG) is another possible source of "false-positive" tuberculin skin test results, albeit uncommon among those born in North America where this vaccine is rarely employed.

Functionally, tuberculin skin testing is employed in three fairly distinct ways: as a diagnostic aid in establishing whether an individual has active tuberculosis disease, to determine whether an individual has latent tuberculosis infection for the purpose of administering preventive therapy, and—in large populations—for epidemiological assessment of the prevalence of infection within groups or regions. The tuberculin skin test is *most problematic* in the first role, identification of persons with tuberculous disease, largely because of the phenomenon of false-negative test results. Authorities generally cite roughly 10% false nonreactivity among "normal" children with active disease (14); however, in a series of South African infants less than 3 months of age with active tuberculosis, only 8 of 31 (26%) were reported to have significant tuberculin skin test reactions (17). In addition, an ill child with a significant reaction is not necessarily suffering from active tuberculosis; the skin test might be reflecting only latent infection or prior exposure to nontuberculous mycobacteria. Hence, tuberculin skin testing for diagnosis of active disease plays a modest, largely circumstantial role. However, it remains the major tool for contact investigation or screening groups to identify latent infection (see "Preventive Chemotherapy" below).

Because the tuberculin skin test performs differently in various populations, it has a Beyesian operator curve. The impact of some of the common, contemporary variables on defining a "positive" reaction are delineated in Table 9.2. For example, 5 mm of induration is likely to indicate tuberculous infection if that 5-year-old child were a contact of an adult with infectious tuberculosis. By comparison, 5 mm of induration detected on a screening program in a youngster without risk factors would not be regarded as significant; in that case, only a reaction of 15 mm or more would be viewed as indicative of likely infection with *M. tuberculosis.*

TABLE 9.2. *Definition of positive Mantoux skin test result (5 TU-PPD) in children*[a]

Reaction ≥5 mm
Children in close contact with known or suspected infectious cases of tuberculosis
Households with active or previously active cases if treatment cannot be verified as adequate before exposure was initiated after period of child's contact, or reactivation is suspected
Children suspected to have tuberculous disease
Chest roentgenogram consistent with active or previously active tuberculosis
Clinical evidence of tuberculosis
Children with immunosuppressive conditions[b] or HIV infection
Reaction ≥10 mm
Children at increased risk of dissemination from:
Young age: <4 y
Other medical risk factors, including Hodgkin's disease, lymphoma, diabetes mellitus, chronic renal failure, malnutrition
Children with increased environmental exposure
Born in or whose parents were born in high-prevalence regions of the world
Frequently exposed to adults who are HIV infected, homeless, users of intravenous and other street drugs, poor and medically indigent city dwellers, residents of nursing homes, incarcerated or institutionalized persons, and migrant farm workers
Reaction ≥15 mm
Children ≥4 y without any risk factors

[a] The recommendations should be considered regardless of previous Bacillus Calmette-Guérin (BCG) administration

[b] Including immunosuppressive doses of corticosteroids

TU-PPD, tuberculin units of purified protein derivative; HIV, human immunodeficiency virus.

From AAP Committee on Infectious Diseases. Screening for tuberculosis in infants and children. *Pediatrics* 1994;93:131–134, with permission.

Chest X-Ray

Since the portal of entry is almost universally pulmonary, the chest x-ray plays a highly significant role in the assessment of infants and children with possible tuberculosis disease or infection. As noted above, the primary complex findings typically consist of a localized parenchymal infiltrate coupled with prominent lymphadenopathy in the hilar or paratracheal nodes. The various pulmonary syndromes associated with complicated or progressive lung disease are also described above. In addition, it is important to note that the intrathoracic radiographic abnormalities typically persist for long periods—up to a year—even in asymptomatic individuals. This has great importance in a child with extrathoracic disease which *might* be tuberculous in origin (e.g., superficial lymphadenitis, meningitis, or osseous disease). In such cases, the finding of vestigial radiographic abnormalities suggestive of primary tuberculosis may be sufficient grounds to embark upon more aggressive diagnostic evaluation and presumptive tuberculosis chemotherapy. However, it should be stressed that children may have intrathoracic disease attributable to MOTT with similar pathophysiology and radiographic abnormalities (25).

Bacteriological Methods

Certainly, the most conclusive means of diagnosis is identification of tubercle bacilli by culture of sputum or other tissues or body fluids.

However, there are major biological and behavioral impediments to this process.

Sputum

If available, sputum should be sent for smear and culture. However, most children produce minimal respiratory tract secretions in comparison to adults with cavitary disease, and—among infants and younger children—it is very difficult to elicit cooperation with the collection of such specimens.

Gastric Aspirates

Given the limited direct access to respiratory tract secretions, gastric aspiration (GA) has proven very useful. The technique is based on the principle that respiratory tract mucous is being continually propelled upward out of the lungs by bronchial ciliary activity. Such matter is reflexively swallowed as it is deposited in the hypopharynx. Thus, overnight, a considerable volume of lower respiratory tract secretions may accumulate in the stomach. Ideally, GA is performed early in the morning on awakening, before peristalsis is initiated by the actual or anticipated ingestion of food or liquids. However, later-morning GA performed before eating or drinking may still be useful. Among an early series of cases of pulmonary tuberculosis from Texas, GA yielded positive cultures in 39% of children (14). Among a subsequent report from this group, GA was positive in 70% of a reported series (23). In infants from South Africa with extensive complicated disease, GA was positive in 35 of 38 (92%) of subjects (17); however, this high yield reflects the study design which required positive cultures for inclusion. The yield of GA was recently compared with that of bronchoscopy with lavage in children suspected of pulmonary tuberculosis (26). Results of three sequential early-morning GAs were compared to bronchoscopy with lavage on the first day; bronchial lavage was positive in only 2 of 20 patients, both of whom had positive GA. An additional 8 of 18 patients had a positive GA with negative bronchoscopy. While this report may well be a valid comparison, in most cases three early-morning GAs are not feasible if the child is not hospitalized. Comparing the results of the bronchoscopy with lavage only with the final GA, the lavage was positive in one case with a negative GA and one case with a positive GA; the GA was positive in five cases with negative bronchoscopy. Similar findings were reported in a series from India (27). Among 50 children with suspected tuberculosis, the yield was 32% for GA and 12% for bronchoalveolar lavage; among the six patients with positive BAL cultures, five also had positive GAs. Thus, if one were most rigorously trying to obtain a positive culture from the child (perhaps to clarify the issue of drug resistance), one might perform both procedures. However, if forced to choose between them, GA would appear to have a higher yield. In actual practice, many cases of pediatric tuberculosis are diagnosed and treated without confirmation by culture; sputa or GA are positive in less than 50% of cases deemed to be active pulmonary tuberculosis by skilled pediatric practitioners (28).

Bronchoscopy

As noted above, bronchoscopy with lavage probably has a lower yield on culture than does GA. However, pediatric tuberculosis entails a significant likelihood of airway abnormalities including extrinsic compression by exuberant lymphadenitis or actual endobronchial tuberculous inflammation. In such cases, bronchoscopy may provide useful information for both diagnosis and potential management of airway obstruction (28).

Serological Methods

Diagnosis of tuberculosis by serological means has been avidly pursued throughout the 20th century with generally limited and disappointing results. Somewhat analogous to the tuberculin skin test, problems with serological studies have included low sensitivity attributable to false-negative results and lack of specificity attributable to inability to distinguish active disease from latent infection or infection caused by *M. tuberculosis* from that caused by environmental nontuberculous mycobacteria or vaccination with BCG.

For a review of general application of serodiagnosis, see Chapter 2. Pediatric application has been of special interest because of the elusiveness of diagnosis in this population. However, a recent study demonstrated well the conundrum of the methodology: if the sensitivity of the assay were increased by lowering the titer required for diagnosis, the method would lose specificity, and vice versa (29). Certainly, this approach has great inherent appeal; however, given the current state of the art, serodiagnosis probably has little or no role in the health system of a resource-rich country (30).

Molecular Biological Techniques

Amplification of mycobacterial genetic material by polymerase chain reaction or similar methods may be of considerable importance, particularly in tuberculous meningitis where positive cultures are quite uncommon. A more comprehensive review of nucleic acid amplification techniques is given in Chapter 2.

MANAGEMENT OF DISEASE

Modern chemotherapy results in rapid clinical and bacteriological responses in the great majority of cases of tuberculosis caused by bacilli that are susceptible to the standard agents. Particular considerations in treating individual patients include selecting medications with an awareness of the rising prevalence of drug resistance, employing optimal dosages, anticipating and coping with nonadherence, monitoring for drug toxicity, and recognizing the indications for adjunctive use of corticosteroids to reduce inflammatory sequelae.

Choice of Chemotherapeutic Agents

As delineated in Chapter 10, multiple drug treatment of disease is indicated both to prevent the emergence of drug resistance and to accelerate the bacteriological response. Data on the efficacy of regimens in pediatric tuberculosis are less well standardized than those for adult pulmonary tuberculosis because of the inaccessibility of an objective marker of success such as sputum cultures. Hence, the usual practice is to extrapolate from adult pulmonary trials and to use indirect or surrogate markers for efficacy in pediatric studies. Recent published experience in children has confirmed the utility of 6-month regimens comprised of INH and rifampin with an introductory 2-month phase of pyrazinamide for most forms of pulmonary and extrapulmonary disease (30). The 1992 recommendations by the American Academy of Pediatrics for treatment regimens are displayed in Table 9.3; pharmacological data about the individual medications are shown in Table 9.4 (31). Concern has been expressed regarding the adequacy of a 6-month regimen for meningitis or miliary or vertebral tuberculosis. Thus, the above guidelines and the 1994 American Thoracic Society/CDC/American Academy of Pediatrics recommendations call for 12 months of therapy for cases of miliary, meningeal, and bone-joint disease in infants and children (32). The concerns regarding failure or relapses associated with spinal or meningeal tuberculosis reflect both anxiety about the potentially profound sequelae of such unfavorable outcomes and, presumably, concerns that patients who have meningeal or miliary disease may be less competent hosts. In either case, it is prudent—where feasible and affordable—to overtreat rather than undertreat such cases.

Among cases of proven or suspected drug-resistant tuberculosis, it may be necessary to use drugs other than the above-noted agents. Based on the rising prevalence of drug resistance domestically (33), the more recent recommendations have called for initial treatment of most cases with four drugs, typically adding ethambutol until susceptibility has been confirmed (32). This practice, however, has not yet been universally embraced by pediatricians in the United States. Four-drug initial therapy, while certainly appropriate in communities in which the prevalence of drug resistance is known to be high, may not be necessary for other populations. However, given the potential implications for inadequate therapy (34), it would be judicious to use an additional drug in most areas until drug

TABLE 9.3. *Recommended treatment regimens for tuberculosis in infants, children, and adolescents*

Tuberculous infection disease	Regimens	Remarks
Asymptomatic infection (positive skin test result, no disease)	INH susceptible: 9 mo of INH INH resistant: 9 mo of RIF	• At least 6 consecutive mo of therapy with good compliance should be given. • If daily therapy is not possible, twice-weekly therapy may be used for 9 mo.
Pulmonary	**1.** 6 mo (standard): 2 mo INH, RIF, and PZA daily, followed by 4 mo of INH and RIF daily *or* 2 mo of INH, RIF, and PZA daily, followed by 4 mo of INH and RIF twice weekly, directly observed **2.** 9 mo (alternative): 9 mo of INH and RIF daily *or* 1 mo of INH and RIF daily followed by 8 mo of INH and RIF twice weekly, directly observed	• If drug resistance is possible, especially for the 9-mo regimen, an additional drug (ethambutol or streptomycin) should be added to initial therapy until drug susceptibility is determined. • Drugs can be given 2 or 3 times per week under direct observation in the initial phase in noncompliance
Hilar adenopathy	Same as pulmonary	• See "Pulmonary." • 6 mo of INF and RIF has been successful in areas where drug resistance is rare.
Meningitis, disseminated (miliary) and bone/joint	2 mo of INH, RIF, PZA and SM daily, followed by 10 mo of INH and RIF daily *or* 2 mo of INH, RIF, PZA, and SM daily, followed by 10 mo of INH and RIF twice weekly, directly observed	• Streptomycin is used in initial therapy until drug susceptibility is known. • For patients who may have acquired tuberculosis in geographic locales where resistance to streptomycin is common, capreomycin (15–30 mg/kg/d) or kanamycin (15–30 mg/kg/d) may be used instead of streptomycin.
Extrapulmonary other than meningitis, disseminated (miliary) or bone/joint	Same as "Pulmonary"	• See "Pulmonary."

INH, isoniazid; RIF, rifampin; PZA, pyrazinamide; SM, streptomycin.
From ref. 31, with permission.

susceptibility or a satisfactory initial response has been demonstrated. Although there has been some reluctance to use ethambutol in children in whom ophthalmological monitoring is problematic, there is sufficient experience to merit recommendation by an expert panel of pediatricians of the use of this drug under selected circumstances (32).

Special Aspects of Administering Drugs

Some children have difficulty in swallowing pills or tablets. Syrup preparations of INH and rifampin are available, but questions have been raised about the stability of these preparations (31). At National Jewish Medical and Research Center, we have had success with grinding up pills or blending the contents of capsules into applesauce as a means of coping with difficulty ingesting the drugs. However, this approach is not without potential problems and should only be taken after consulting with experienced pharmacists or pharmacologists, who may recommend other means of improvised preparation.

The use of other antituberculosis agents such as para-aminosalicylate (PAS), ethionamide, cycloserine, amikacin, kanamycin, capreomycin, clofazimine, ofloxacin, or ciprofloxacin should

TABLE 9.4. *Commonly used drugs for the treatment of tuberculosis in infants, children, and adolescents*

Drugs	Dosage forms	Daily dose (mg/kg/d)	Twice-weekly dose (mg/kg/d)	Maximum dose	Adverse reactions
Isoniazid[a] (INH)	Scored tablets: 100 and 300 mg Syrup: 10 mg/mL[c]	10–15[b]	20–40	Daily: 300 mg Twice weekly: 900 mg	Mild hepatic enzyme elevation, hepatitis, peripheral neuritis, hypersensitivity
Rifampin[a] (RIF)	Capsules: 150 and 300 mg Syrup: Formulated in syrup capsules[d]	10–20	10–20	600 mg	Orange discoloration of secretions/urine, staining contact lenses, vomiting, hepatitis, flulike reaction, thrombocytopenia, may render birth-control pills ineffective
Pyrazinamide (PZA)	Scored tablets: 500 mg	20–40	50–70	2 g	Hepatotoxicity, hypersensitivity
Streptomycin (SM)	Vials: 1 and 4 g	20–40 (i.m.)	20–40 (i.m.)	1 g	Ototoxicity, nephrotoxicity, skin rash
Ethambutol (EMB)[e]	Tablets: 100 and 400 mg	15–25	50	2.5 g	Optic neuritis (reversible), decreased visual acuity, decreased red/green discrimination, gastrointestinal tract disturbance, hypersensitivity/rash

[a] Rifamate is a capsule containing 150 mg of isoniazid and 300 mg of rifampin. Two capsules provide the usual adult (>50 kg) daily doses of each drug.

[b] When isoniazid is used in combination with rifampin, the incidence of hepatotoxicity increases if the isoniazid dose exceeds 10 mg/kd/d.

[c] Many experts recommend not using isoniazid syrup because it is unstable and is associated with frequent gastrointestinal tract complaints, especially diarrhea.

[d] Some experts recommend not using rifampin syrup because of instability.

[e] Ethambutol is probably safe in young children, but should be used with caution when monitoring visual capacity or color discrimination is difficult.

i. m., intramuscular.

From ref. 31, with permission.

be limited to cases in which there is well-documented resistance to first-line medications or a very high likelihood of such based on epidemiological factors (household or other intimate exposure to a multidrug-resistant case). Management of these cases is a highly complicated matter and should only be undertaken by specialists (see Chapter 11 for more complete discussion).

Dealing with Nonadherence to Therapy

By far, the most common element leading to treatment failure is irregular or incomplete administration of medications. It cannot be overemphasized how important it is for clinicians to deal with this perverse phenomenon. If a patient is to receive treatment at home by a member of the family, it is essential that education be performed regarding the importance of therapy and medication side effects and that there be clear delineation of responsibility. Monitoring in the form of pill counts, surveillance of urinary drug metabolites, and—if available—serum drug levels should be performed. If there is evidence of nonadherence or even a strong likelihood based on a chaotic or unpredictable home situation, directly observed or supervised treatment may be the only means to ensure treatment and protect the child.

To conduct directly observed treatment, intermittent therapy (less than daily) is very useful. There is abundant evidence from adults with extensive, cavitary tuberculosis that medication given thrice or even twice weekly is of comparable efficacy to that given daily (see Chapter 10 for details). Effectiveness of a twice-weekly, 6-month regimen has been shown in pediatric series, as well (23). For patients who are hospitalized, treatment might begin with a daily regimen, switching to intermittency on discharge. Or, if the child does not require an initial hospital phase of care, therapy might commence with a thrice-weekly program. The great advantage of these intermittent regimens is the enhanced opportunity they present to arrange for regular visits by the patient to clinics or by community health workers to the patient's home or school.

Monitoring for Drug Toxicity

Pediatric tuberculosis specialists stress that children generally are subjectively more tolerant and manifest fewer toxic reactions to most antimycobacterial drugs than adults (31); biochemical surveillance is not routinely advocated. Nonetheless, it is appropriate to clinically assess the patients periodically for evidence of hepatic, renal, hematological, neurological or other more common untoward reactions (see Table 9.4 for a listing of the more frequent toxic reactions and the recommended monitoring routines).

Role of Corticosteroids in Treatment

Corticosteroids have demonstrated utility in reducing the morbidity and mortality of tuberculous meningitis (35–37). The benefits are most clearly demonstrable for patients in stage II or III meningitis (see Chapter 7). However, I believe that the rapid reductions in intercranial pressure, accelerated improvement of cerebrospinal fluid abnormalities, and relief of fever merit such treatment in all stages. Usual doses of corticosteroids would be the equivalent of prednisone 1 to 2 mg/kg body weight given for 4 to 8 weeks; because of accelerated degradation of prednisone by patients receiving rifampin, higher doses may be required. During the acute phases, the doses may be split to effect continuous antiinflammatory activity, or a longer-acting agent like dexamethasone may be employed. Usually, the steroid dose is tapered over 2 to 3 weeks before discontinuation; withdrawal of the corticosteroids may result in rebound inflammation, and careful monitoring for possible reinstitution is required.

The utility of corticosteroids for reducing bronchial compression attributable to peribronchial or endobronchial tuberculous lymphadenitis has been demonstrated in only one controlled study (38). In a more recent, smaller series of 29 pediatric cases with primary tuberculosis and bronchial obstruction, randomization to prednisone was associated with favorable responses by both radiographic and bronchoscopic appearance (39). The dose of prednisolone was 2 mg/kg for 15 days followed by a gradual wean over 2.5 to 3.0 months. The study was not ideal in design or execution, but lends support to the practice.

Thus, when confronted with protracted and postobstructive inflammation, an attempt to reduce the endobronchitis and lymphadenitis with corticosteroids is usually warranted. Corticosteroids have been shown efficacious in acute pericarditis in controlled adult studies (see Chapter 7 for details); anecdotal experience has been favorable also with this disorder, which is uncommon in children. Corticosteroids may also provide relief in the infrequent case of large pleural effusions that are associated with dyspnea and high fevers (40).

PREVENTIVE CHEMOTHERAPY

Infants and children are at high risk for the development of disease if infected with tubercle bacilli. Hence, they are very-high-priority candidates for preventive chemotherapy. The means by which most infected youngsters are identified is through contact investigations stemming from parents or other adults in the household with active tuberculosis. In communities or regions with substantial tuberculosis case rates in young adults, prompt and thorough contact investigation is required to prevent serious tuberculous morbidity in infants and children. Children who are deemed to be at higher risk for tuberculous infection in this era are noted in Table 9.1.

The efficacy of INH preventive therapy was clearly shown in a USPHS trial involving children with asymptomatic primary complex tuberculosis (see Chapter 12 for detailed discussion). In this USPHS study, isoniazid preventive therapy (IPT) was given daily for 12 months and resulted in a 75% reduction of morbidity during the years of treatment and 54% reduction during the subsequent year when compared with a randomized control group that received placebo (15). Although the efficacy of IPT is not disputed, several issues remain under active consideration at this time: (a) how long should IPT be given? (b) how should monitoring for INH-associated drug toxicity be performed? and (c) what can be done for those who are intolerant to INH or have been infected with INH-resistant tuberculosis? These issues are discussed below.

At present, IPT for most adults is given for 6 months; exceptions are patients with HIV infection or those with upper-lung zone fibronodular shadowing thought to represent "inactive" tuberculosis; in these cases, 12 months of IPT are advocated (32). The decision to shorten adult IPT to 6 months reflects both evidence of acceptable efficacy with the shorter regimen and a cost-effectiveness analysis that took into account diminishing adherence over time (41). However, because most infants and children for whom IPT is recommended have immature immune systems, pediatric authorities have advocated 9 months of IPT (Table 9.3) (31). This may, however, create confusion in the situation where a parent with active disease is treated and "cured" in 6 months while the healthy child contact requires 9 months of "preventive therapy."

An option that should be studied is multidrug, intermittent, directly observed preventive therapy, given to the children for 6 months or less while the parents are being treated; see Chapter 12 for details. This practice should be seen in the context of contemporary pediatric guidelines, which have regarded children with pulmonary radiographic abnormalities, even in the absence of symptoms, as having "disease" and therefore to be treated with a 6-month multidrug regimen (31). Although children with "asymptomatic primary tuberculosis" responded well to monotherapy with INH in the older study cited above, intensive, multidrug, short-duration therapy is now deemed standard practice.

One controversial element in current tuberculosis control is whether there should be routine screening of pediatric populations for INH preventive chemotherapy. Although it may appear tempting to do so, empirical observations indicate that the yield from such projects is too low to justify diversion of limited resources. A decision analysis, however, indicated that—for a community like Santa Clara, California, which has a large foreign-born population—selected screening of children born in countries with high-prevalence tuberculosis would probably be cost-effective (42). In fact, as pointed out by Starke (43) in an accompanying editorial, the assumption in this analysis may have been overly optimistic, particularly with regard to the likelihood of IPT being completed among the children identified with infection (43). On balance, I believe that public health programs should conserve their assets to perform prompt and thorough contact investigations, and not be distracted by these relatively-low-yield exercises.

The American Academy of Pediatrics 1992 guidelines indicate that routine biochemical monitoring is not indicated for infants or children receiving chemotherapy (31). Rather, clinical assessment for adverse reactions on a monthly basis is advocated. However, INH-related hepatitis does occur among children, but in multiple series this consisted almost exclusively of asymptomatic, minor elevations of serum transaminase values (44–48). Rarely, though, lethal liver failure has been reported among young adolescents receiving INH. In a collection of 20 cases of death from apparent INH-related hepatitis, 3 occurred among persons less than 20 years old (49); in a national retrospective survey performed by the CDC, 14 of 153 deaths occurred among persons less than 20 years old (50); and in a series of 8 cases of INH-related hepatitis referred to liver transplantation programs in New York and Pennsylvania, 3 occurred among individuals less than 20 years of age (51). Hence, if the patient is receiving treatment through a parent or other adult at home, it is prudent to inform that person, in writing, of the likely signs and symptoms of INH toxicity including hepatic and central nervous system disturbances, with explicit instructions to withhold the medications and bring the patient promptly to professional attention.

For children who are intolerant of INH or exposed to cases with INH resistance, rifampin given for 9 months is advocated for preventive therapy (Table 9.3). Most data suggest that rifampin should be comparable to or better than INH in this role and that the risk of hepatitis would be similar or lower. The major drawback of rifampin is its cost, being manyfold greater that than of INH. For children who are exposed to and presumably infected by patients with tuberculosis resistant to both INH and rifampin, there are very limited treatment options (see Chapter 11).

VACCINATION TO PREVENT TUBERCULOSIS

The Bacillus of Calmette and Guérin (BCG) is a live mycobacterial vaccine that has been administered to several billion persons in the past 50 years in the effort to control tuberculosis. BCG is an attenuated strain of *Mycobacterium bovis,* an organism that is very closely related to *M. tuberculosis.* In the decades of the vaccine's use, multiple different substrains have been developed, making it difficult to refer to one standard vaccine when analyzing the efficacy of BCG.

BCG has never been employed widely in the United States, largely because of USPHS analyses which indicated that the vast preponderance of new cases emerged from the pool of Americans who were remotely infected and would not profit from vaccination (see Chapter 12). Rather, tuberculosis control in the United States has relied upon giving IPT to persons with latent infection who were identified by contact investigation and screening of high-risk groups.

In addition, considerable controversy exists regarding the efficacy of BCG. Trials conducted around the world, including several studies in the United States from the 1930s to the 1950s, have yielded widely disparate indications of protection. Efficacy has ranged from an 80% reduction in tuberculous morbidity to slightly higher case rates following BCG. A recent meta-analysis of these studies indicated an overall protective effect of approximately 50% (52). However, there is a sufficient number of confounding variables to raise questions about the overall utility of the BCG strategy (see Chapter 13 for detailed review of BCG).

Recent case-control studies suggested that BCG reduces the risk for such morbid events as miliary, meningeal, and osseous tuberculosis when given to newborns who are subsequently exposed to or infected with tuberculosis during years 0 to 4 (53,54). Such vaccination is clearly unsuitable for all infants in the United States, but some authorities have suggested that it be applied to selected high-risk groups as is done in Great Britain. Most U.S. authorities, however, contend that—because of uncertain vaccine efficacy, the confounding effects on skin testing and preventive chemotherapy, and the sociopolitical controversy surrounding a program that would discriminate along racial, ethnic, and economic lines—such a selective approach is not acceptable today. Perhaps the scenario that would be most likely to justify BCG would involve an infant who, through circumstances beyond control, would be at ongoing high risk of exposure to communicable tuberculosis case(s). Elements of these situations might include transborder travel, members of the household with unresponsive MDR-TB, or other patients with communicable disease who defy efforts to administer therapy or quarantine.

REFERENCES

1. Starke JR, Jacobs RF, Jereb J. Resurgence of tuberculosis in children. *J Pediatr* 1992;120:839–855.
2. Centers for Disease Control and Prevention. Tuberculosis morbidity: United States, 1992. *MMWR* 1993;42: 696–704.
3. Kochi A. The global tuberculosis situation and the new control strategy of the World Health Organization. *Tuberc Lung Dis* 1991;72:1–4.
4. Centers for Disease Control and Prevention. Tuberculosis final data United States 1986. *MMWR* 1988;36:817–820.
5. Stead W, Senner J, Reddick W, Lofgren J. Racial differences in susceptibility to infection by *Mycobacterium tuberculosis*. *N Engl J Med* 1990;322:422–427.
6. McKenna MT, McCray E, Onorato I. The epidemiology of tuberculosis among foreign-born persons in the United States: 1986–93. *N Engl J Med* 1995;332:1071–1076.
7. Foo AL, Tan KK, Chay OM. Congenital tuberculosis. *Tuberc Lung Dis* 1993;74:59–61.
8. Snider DE Jr, Bloch AB. Congenital tuberculosis. *Tubercle* 1984;65:81–82.
9. Cantwell MF, Shehab ZM, Costello AM, et al. Brief report: congenital tuberculosis. *N Engl J Med* 1994;330: 1051–1054.
10. Vucicevic Z, Suskovic T, Ferencic Z. A female patient with tuberculous polyserositis, and congenital tuberculosis in her new-born child. *Tuberc Lung Dis* 1995;76: 460–462.
11. Agrawal RL, Rehman H. Congenital miliary tuberculosis with intestinal perforations. *Tuberc Lung Dis* 1995; 76:468–469.
12. Lee LH, LeVea CM, Graman PS. Congenital tuberculosis in a neonatal intensive care unit: case report, epidemiological investigation, and management of exposures. *Clin Infect Dis* 1998;27:474–477.
13. Riley RL, Moodie AS. Infectivity of patients with pulmonary tuberculosis in inner city homes. *Am Rev Respir Dis* 1974;110:810–812.
14. Starke JR, Taylor-Watts KT. Tuberculosis in the pediatric population of Houston, Texas. *Pediatrics* 1989;84: 28–35.
15. Mount FW, Ferebee SH. Preventive effects of isoniazid in the treatment of primary tuberculosis in children. *N Engl J Med* 1961;265:713–721.
16. Pineda PR, Leung A, Muller NL, Allen EA, Black WA, Fitzgerald JM. Intrathoracic paediatric tuberculosis: a report of 202 cases. *Tuberc Lung Dis* 1993;74:261–266.
17. Schaaf HS, Gie RP, Beyers N, Smuts N, Donald PR. Tuberculosis in infants less than 3 months of age. *Arch Dis Child* 1993;69:371–374.
18. Rieder HL, Snider DE, Cauthen GM. Extrapulmonary tuberculosis in the United States. *Am Rev Respir Dis* 1990;141:347–351.
19. Berman S, Kibel MA, Fourie PB, Strebel PM. Childhood tuberculosis and tuberculous meningitis: high incidence rates in the Western Cape of South Africa. *Tuberc Lung Dis* 1992;73:349–355.
20. Braun MM, Cauthen G. Relationship of the human immunodeficiency virus epidemic to pediatric tuberculosis and Bacillus Calmette-Guérin immunization. *Pediatr Infect Dis J* 1992;11:220–227.
21. Drucker E, Alcabes P, Bosworth W, Sckell B. Childhood tuberculosis in the Bronx, New York. *Lancet* 1994;343:1482–1485.
22. Gutman LT, Moye J, Zimmer B, Tian C. Tuberculosis in human immunodeficiency virus-exposed or -infected United States children. *Pediatr Infect Dis J* 1994;13: 963–968.
23. Vallejo JG, Ong LT, Starke JR. Clinical features, diagnosis, and treatment of tuberculosis in infants. *Pediatrics* 1994;94:1–7.
24. Wolinsky E. Mycobacterial lymphadenitis in children: a prospective study of 105 nontuberculous cases with long-term follow-up. *Clin Infect Dis* 1995;20:954–963.
25. Fergie JE, Milligan TW, Henderson BM, Stafford WW. Intrathoracic *Mycobacterium avium* complex infection in immunocompetent children: case report and review. *Clin Infect Dis* 1997;24:250–253.
26. Abadco DL, Steiner P. Gastric lavage is better than bronchoalveolar lavage for isolation of *Mycobacterium tuberculosis* in childhood pulmonary tuberculosis. *Pediatr Infec Dis J* 1992;11:735–738.
27. Somu N, Swaminathan S, Paramasivan CN, et al. Value of bronchoalveolar lavage and gastric lavage in the diagnosis of pulmonary tuberculosis in children. *Tuberc Lung Dis* 1995;76:295–299.
28. de Blic J, Azevedo I, Burren CP, LeBourgeois M, Lallemand D, Scheinmann P. The value of flexible bronchoscopy in childhood pulmonary tuberculosis. *Chest* 1991;100:688–692.
29. Delacourt C, Gobin J, Gaillard J-L, deBlic J, Veron M, Scheinmann P. Value of ELISA using antigen 60 for the diagnosis of tuberculosis in children. *Chest* 1993;104: 393–398.
30. Starke JR. Childhood tuberculosis: a diagnostic dilemma [editorial]. *Chest* 1993;104:329–330.
31. American Academy of Pediatrics. Chemotherapy of tuberculosis. *Pediatrics* 1992;89:161–165.
32. American Thoracic Society. Treatment of tuberculosis and tuberculosis infection in adults and children. *Am J Respir Crit Care Med* 1994;149:1359–1374.
33. Bloch AB, Cauthen GM, Onorato IM, et al. Nationwide survey of drug-resistant tuberculosis in the United States. *JAMA* 1994;271:665–671.
34. Steiner P, Rao M, Mitchell M, Steiner M. Primary drug-resistant tuberculosis in children: emergence of primary drug-resistant strains of *M. tuberculosis* to rifampin. *Am Rev Respir Dis* 1986;134:446–448.

35. O'Toole RD, Thorton GF, Mukherjee MK, Nath RL. Dexamethasone in tuberculous meningitis. *Ann Intern Med* 1969;70:39–48.
36. Girgis NI, Farid Z, Kilpatrick ME, Sultan Y, Mikhail IA. Dexamethasone adjunctive treatment for tuberculous meningitis. *Pediatr Infect Dis J* 1991;10:179–183.
37. Shaw PP, Wang SM, Tung SG, et al. Clinical analysis of 445 adult cases of tuberculous meningitis. *Chin J Tuberc Respir Dis* 1984;3:131–132.
38. Nemir RL, Cardona J, Vaziri F, Toledo R. Prednisone as an adjunct in the chemotherapy of lymph node-bronchial tuberculosis in childhood: a double-blind study, II: further term observation. *Am Rev Respir Dis* 1967;95: 402–410.
39. Toppet M, Malfroot A, Derde MP, Toppet V, Spehl M, Dab I. Corticosteroids in primary tuberculosis with bronchial obstruction. *Arch Dis Child* 1990;65:1222–1226.
40. Smith MHD, Matsamotis N. Treatment of tuberculous pleural effusions with particular reference to adrenal corticosteroids. *Pediatrics* 1958;22:1074–1087.
41. Snider D, Caras G, Kaplan J. Preventive therapy with isoniazid: cost-effectiveness of different durations of therapy. *JAMA* 1986;255:1579–1583.
42. Moehle-Boetaini JC, Miller B, Halpern M, et al. School-based screening for tuberculous infection: a cost-benefit analysis. *JAMA* 1995;274:613–619.
43. Starke J. Universal screening for tuberculosis infection: school's out [editorial]! *JAMA* 1995;274:652–653.
44. Rapp RS, Campbell RW, Howell JC, Kendig EL Jr. Isoniazid hepatotoxicity in children. *Am Rev Respir Dis* 1978;118:794–796.
45. Beaudry PH, Brickman HF, Wise MB, MacDougall D. Liver enzyme disturbances during isoniazid chemoprophylaxis in children. *Am Rev Respir Dis* 1974;110: 581–584.
46. Litt IF, Cohen MI, McNamara H. Isoniazid hepatitis in adolescents. *J Pediatr* 1976;89:133–135.
47. Spyridis P, Sinaniotis C, Papadea I, Oreopoulos L, Hadjiyiannis S, Papadatos C. Isoniazid liver injury during chemoprophylaxis in children. *Arch Dis Child* 1979;54: 65–67.
48. Nakajo MM, Rao M, Steiner P. Incidence of hepatotoxicity in children receiving isoniazid chemoprophylaxis. *Pediatr Infect Dis J* 1989;8:649–650.
49. Moulding TS, Redeker AG, Kanel GC. Twenty isoniazid-associated deaths in one state. *Am Rev Respir Dis* 1989;140:700–705.
50. Snider DE Jr, Caras GJ. Isoniazid-associated hepatitis deaths: a review of available information. *Am Rev Respir Dis* 1992;145:494–497.
51. Centers for Disease Control and Prevention. Severe isoniazid-associated hepatitis: New York, 1991–1993. *MMWR* 1993;42:545–547.
52. Colditz GA, Brewer TF, Berkey CS, et al. Efficacy of BCG vaccine in the prevention of tuberculosis: meta-analysis of the published literature. *JAMA* 1994;271: 698–702.
53. Packe GE, Innes JA. Protective effect of BCG vaccination in infant Asians: a case control study. *Arch Dis Child* 1988;63:277–281.
54. Houston S, Fanning A, Soskolne C, Fraser N. The effectiveness of bacillus Calmette-Guérin (BCG) vaccination against tuberculosis: a case-controlled study in Treaty Indians, Alberta, Canada. *Am J Epidemiol* 1990; 131:340–348.

10

Tuberculosis Chemotherapy, Including Directly Observed Therapy

This chapter is dedicated to Wallace Fox, Dennis Mitchison, and their colleagues in India, East Africa, Hong Kong, Singapore, and England, who truly led the evolution of modern tuberculosis chemotherapy.

HISTORY

The most meaningful advance in the history of twentieth-century medicine arguably has been the development of curative chemotherapy for tuberculosis. Over the two centuries preceding this watershed, tuberculosis had taken roughly one billion human lives. In 1945, before the advent of effective medications, persons with advanced pulmonary tuberculosis had greater than a 50% probability of dying within 5 years; those with miliary, meningeal, or pericardial disease universally confronted death within a matter of weeks. War, by disrupting the social fabric, had always been associated with a surge in tuberculosis rates. Ironically, it was during World War II, in three centers unknown to the others, that heroic work was being performed that would lead to the goal that had eluded scientists for 2,000 years: a predictable cure for "consumption." Waksman and Schatz in New Jersey came upon streptomycin (SM) in 1943. Simultaneously, Lehman in Sweden pursued the synthesis of his conceptualization, the para-amino salt of salicylic acid. And Domagk, working in repeatedly bombed laboratories within Germany, laid the chemical groundwork that led to the synthesis, first, of thiacetazone (THA), then of isonicotinic acid hydrazide, or isoniazid (INH). See Chapter 1 for details.

Streptomycin was pressed into clinical use shortly after it was shown to be active against the tubercle bacillus in test tubes and animal models; its efficacy in human disease was initially reported in 1945 (1). Para-aminosalicylate (PAS) had actually been administered to a patient one month before SM, but publication of this event was delayed until 1946. In one of the first randomized clinical trials, the complementary activity of these drugs was reported from Britain in 1949 (2).

However, not until INH was added to this duo in 1952 were predictable, enduring cures a reality (3). Since that time, other effective drugs have been discovered, the duration of required treatment has been reduced, sanatoria have been closed, and immense numbers of lives have been spared. However, nonadherence to therapy, inadequate health care delivery systems, and financial constraints combined to diminish the potential impact of this potent tool. Immense challenges lie ahead to better implement the agents in hand and to develop new and better drugs and systems to deliver them.

OBJECTIVES OF TREATMENT

Broadly speaking, tuberculosis chemotherapy has three identifiable goals: to rapidly kill the massive numbers of bacilli that are multiplying in the tissues of the typically diseased host, to prevent the emergence of clinically significant strains of drug-resistant mutants, and to effectively sterilize the disease sites.

Rapid Reduction of the Number of Bacilli

Rapid reduction of the number of mycobacteria has as its immediate objective sparing of the hosts' tissues and, perhaps, their lives. Secondary benefits include shortening the total duration of treatment and rendering those persons noninfectious in order that they be allowed to return to their homes and productive lives.

Preventing Acquired Drug Resistance

Preventing the resistance of drug-resistant mutants is of critical importance. Inadequate treatment allows naturally occurring drug-resistant mutations to emerge, resulting in increased treatment failures and relapses. Drug resistance has dire implications, not only for the individual patients, but also for those to whom they pass on their infections.

Sterilization to Prevent Relapses

Sterilizing the tissues or reducing the number and viability of the tubercle bacilli to such a minimal level that the host is able to prevail over the microbe is the final goal of treatment. In this manner, the patients do not experience recrudescence after the medication is terminated, further transmission of infection is averted, and society is spared the burden of additional medical care.

As will be seen, the various individual medications have special contributions toward these goals.

THEORETICAL CONSIDERATIONS IN TREATMENT

Three-Populations Model

Based on an amalgam of clinical observations, animal model research, and in vitro studies, contemporary scientists postulated a treatment model wherein there originally were four populations of tubercle bacilli within a patient with pulmonary tuberculosis. These populations are referred to by their locations within lesions and by their metabolic status (4). In this model, these populations play varying roles in relationship to specific drug actions, the evolution of drug resistance, and persistence or recrudescence of disease. It is important to note that the actual existence of these discrete populations remains largely unproven or inferential. As originally conceived, the bacillary populations of this model included a large population of extracellular bacilli that were anatomically located in the liquefied caseum of pulmonary cavities and characterized metabolically by rapid proliferation; these were referred to as Population A. This constituted the great preponderance of the bacillary population. The immense numbers of dividing bacteria increased the likelihood of resistant mutations occurring. Population B was thought to consist of bacilli held in a state of retarded proliferation by local acidic conditions. Initially, it was thought that this acidic milieu was within the macrophage, but subsequent analyses have suggested that this is in the necrotic debris lining the cavity (see "Bacteriostatic versus Bactericidal Activity"). Population C has not been well characterized in terms of anatomical locations or other factors that influence its biology but—nonetheless–has been posited to represent bacilli that undergo only brief, sporadic episodes of metabolism or replication. Mitchison also postulated there to be a population D consisting of dormant, nonreplicating organisms that were not vulnerable to antimicrobial action (5). These bacilli were held responsible for relapses, the assumption being that the microbes were reconstituted as pathogenic after medications were withdrawn. However, in the updated model, this population has been deleted, leaving a three-population model (Fig. 10.1).

Specific Drug Activities in the Revised Model

Based on discrepancies between the observed responses to various drugs in the treatment of pulmonary tuberculosis in humans, the three-populations model has been revised into a more dynamic system with shifts between Populations A, B, and C based on changes in local environments (5). One of the major variables posited was a shift from Population A to Population C as the liquefied caseum (a very supportive environ-

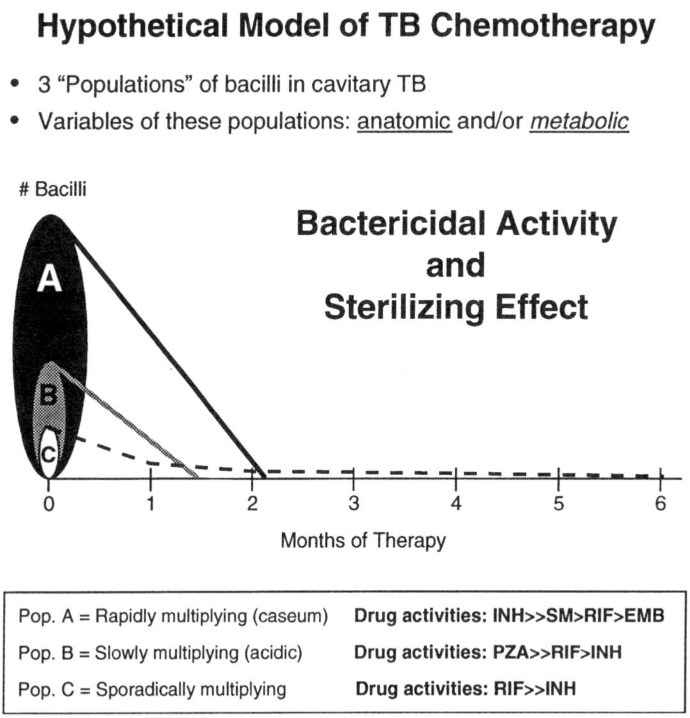

FIG. 10.1. In the three-population model, *population A* represents the immense number of rapidly multiplying bacteria found in the caseous debris in pulmonary cavities. In vitro studies, as well as human chemotherapy experience, indicate that isoniazid (INH) plays a dominant role in killing this population. By contrast, *population B* is believed to comprise bacilli that are multiplying less rapidly because of local acidic conditions; the unique action of pyrazinamide (PZA) against these organisms is thought to be the means by which this drug has allowed shortened duration of treatment. The "elimination" of populations A and B results in negative sputum cultures, typically after 2 months of chemotherapy. However, there ostensibly remains behind a *population C,* comprised of bacilli in the host's tissues which are capable of sporadic bursts of metabolism/replication. These organisms represent the source of potential relapses. Clinical studies, as well as in vitro observations, suggest that rifamycin agents play a major role in the elimination of these sporadically active bacilli.

ment for bacillary proliferation) is expelled, leaving more of the surviving bacilli in the intact cavity walls where they are subject to being engulfed by macrophages. In addition, Mitchison has speculated that, as inflammation subsided because of the effects of treatment, the shrinking acidic environment lessened the role of pyrazinamide (PZA) (see below).

Specific Drug Activities in the Revised Model

Based on the observed impact of the various antituberculosis medications in human therapy trials, as well as in vitro and animal studies, various students of this field have assigned to the individual agents particular roles in treatment in relationship to their activity against these described populations (Fig. 10.1).

Bactericidal Activity

In general terms, those medications most active against Population A are deemed to have **bactericidal activity (BA).** Note, this is not the same as "early BA," which is currently regarded as drug action in the first 48 hours. BA is recognized by the rapidity with which sputum smears and cultures become negative during treatment of cases of pulmonary disease.

Preventing Emergence of Resistance

Agents that are most capable of killing large numbers of Population A bacilli in the early phase of treatment are thus able to block the emergence of mutant strains. Such drugs are said to **prevent drug resistance.** Obviously, there is considerable overlap in these first two categories; I construe the distinction between these two functions to be alacrity in the former and broader ranges of activity in the latter. Analysis of large numbers of patients treated with various regimens allows these subtle distinctions to be made.

Sterilization to Prevent Relapses

Drugs that are capable of killing the mycobacteria in Populations B and C are regarded as **sterilizing agents.** The potency of the different drugs or regimens in this regard is reflected in relapse rates.

Chemotherapy and "Dormant" Bacilli

Since the bacilli in this putative population are ostensibly dormant, they are not accessible to any of the standard medications. Theoretically, the major reason that drug regimens must be continued for months after sputum cultures have become negative is to ensure that drugs are present when or if these bacilli become active and thus susceptible to killing. In the updated model (Fig. 10.1), the "dormant" group has been subsumed under the heading of "sporadically multiplying," or Population C. Mitchison's categorization of the contributions of the five standard drugs is displayed in Table 10.1.

Bacteriostatic Versus Bactericidal Activity

One of the major sources of confusion about antituberculosis medications has been the labels "bactericidal" and "bacteriostatic." Because of the conceptions engendered by such titles, it is worth reviewing these concepts. Classically, *bactericidal* action has been regarded as the ability of an antimicrobial agent to kill 99% to 99.9% of a target population upon exposure; *bacteriostatic* activity, by contrast, indicates the capacity of an agent to limit the proliferation of the target population such that there are 99% fewer microbes in the exposed than in the control population after a defined period of growth. Historically, there have been efforts to describe various antituberculosis agents by those functional terms. However, the many discrepancies

TABLE 10.1. *Activities of standard anti-tuberculosis drugs in theoretical model of treatment*

	Activity		
Agent	Early bactericidal effect	Resistance prevention	Sterilization
Isoniazid	Highest	High	Intermediate
Rifampin	Intermediate	High	Highest
Pyrazinamide	Low	Low	High
Streptomycin	Intermediate	Intermediate	Intermediate
Ethambutol	Intermediate–high	Intermediate	Low

In the model presented, drugs have been assigned a hierarchical utility in activity categories. Clearly, in "early bactericidal activity" (EBA) studies, isoniazid (INH) has the most potent profile. Rifampin (RIF) (or other rifamycins) has made the greatest impact on reducing the duration of therapy required to keep relapse rates at an acceptably low level; thus it is deemed the major contributor to sterilization. Pyrazinamide (PZA) is a very limited agent in terms of its in vitro activity, but the addition of PZA permitted a reduction in duration from 9 months (with INH, RIF, ± other oral agents) to 6 months (INH, RIF, PZA, ± other agents). Streptomycin (or other injectable agents) contributes only modestly to regimen potency. Ethambutol (EMB), although it had considerable EBA activity in high-range dosing, contributes rather little to regimen potency, but has demonstrated utility in BMRC trials at preventing acquired resistance to other agents, most notably, INH and/or RIF.

Based on observations from in vitro studies, animal models, and human tuberculosis treatment trials, Mitchison has created this hierarchy of drug activities. Critical components of short-course regimens include the activities of rifamycins and PZA in "sterilizing" lesions.

between in vitro studies, animal models, and human treatment experience suggest that attempting to categorize drugs by these simple terms is often misleading and should, in my estimation, be abandoned. The 1980 report of a study of the effects of single and combined drugs on the sputum bacillary counts in the first 14 days of therapy belied many of the older labels of drug activity (6). Among the surprising results of this project were that ethambutol (EMB), historically regarded as bacteriostatic, had substantially more early bactericidal activity (BA) than rifampin (RIF), SM, or PZA. Also instructive was the observation that the activities of RIF and EMB were clearly dose dependent, ranging from weakly inhibitory to substantially bactericidal. This analysis also demonstrated the considerable superiority of INH over any other agent in terms of early reduction of bacillary counts.

In fact, the results of this study led to reconsideration of the notion that PZA acted only upon a small population of mycobacteria held in the "allegedly acidic" environment of macrophages, while SM attacked a larger, extracellular population. Indeed, PZA—while having a very modest effect in the first 2 days—was observed to have a singular effect in the East African early bacterial activity (EBA) study (6): unlike other drugs that had maximal effect during the first 2 days, followed by reduced impact, PZA resulted in a gradual but steady decline in the bacillary burden over the entire 2 weeks. Subsequent studies by Heifets and Lindholm-Levy (7) confirmed that PZA was only active at acidic pH values of 5.5 to 6.0 or less; Crowle et al. (8) demonstrated that the pH within the tubercle bacilli–containing macro-phage was not acidic save for the lysosomal packet. Thus, it is currently reasoned that the acidic milieu in which PZA is initially active is the necrotic, caseous debris lining the pulmonary cavity. It appears likely that this particular contribution may explain PZA's special facility for shortening the duration of treatment (see below).

Additive, Synergistic, and Antagonistic Effects

Another concept that should be considered is that of **additive, synergistic,** or **antagonistic** interactions among the antituberculosis medications. In the study cited above (6), INH and RIF were generally additive in combination with each other or other drugs. Nonetheless, this study and other investigations (9) suggest that, under certain conditions, modest antagonism can be seen between these agents and others. Although of modest effect and not proven to be related to drug antagonism, the paradoxical effect of slightly more relapses when PZA was given for longer periods in certain British Medical Research Council (BMRC) trials (see below) should alert us to this potential result.

INDIVIDUAL DRUGS

There currently are five medications that are considered *first-line medications* for the treatment of tuberculosis in the industrialized nations: INH, RIF, PZA, EMB, and SM. Thiacetazone is widely employed in the developing nations because of its remarkably low costs; because of its limited efficacy and substantial toxicity, it has not been approved for use in the United States. Nonetheless, for purposes of a more comprehensive discussion of treatment regimens and the utility of those who practice in regions where this drug is available, it is reviewed in this section. While there are numerous other drugs with some activity in the treatment of tuberculosis, they are generally deemed *second-line agents* because of less efficacy and more toxicity than the agents listed above. These medications are generally reserved for the treatment of multidrug-resistant cases and are reviewed in detail in Chapter 11.

Major Agents: Isoniazid and Rifampin

While there is a tendency to regard the five first-line drugs as co-equals, **INH** and **RIF** are clearly the two most significant medications in the treatment of tuberculosis in this era. They are the keys to highly effective, short-duration treatment. If both drugs can be employed, 6-month, all-oral, curative therapy is readily achievable. Given one *or* the other, highly successful regimens of short duration are still feasible (10). If only INH is lost—through resistance or toxicity—6-month curative treatment can still be achieved. If only RIF is lost, slightly longer—9-month—short-course treatment is possible. However, if both of these critical drugs are lost, the prospects for cure are substantially compromised (see Chapter 11).

Adjunctive First-Line Agents: Pyrazinamide, Streptomycin, and Ethambutol

The other medications, **PZA, SM,** and **EMB,** offer complementary effects, such as reducing the risk of acquired drug resistance and modestly accelerating the response to treatment. The particular contributions of these major drugs and the vital importance in preventing increased levels of resistance to them are presented below. Pharmacological data and in vitro activities of the first-line medications are displayed in Table 10.2. Dosage of these drugs in patients with hepatic or renal impairment is discussed below.

Developing-World Adjunctive Agent: Thiacetazone

Thiacetazone has been used extensively in developing nations because of its remarkable affordability. In the period from 1965 to 1990, standard treatment in many countries entailed 12 months of daily INH and THA, self-administered, with an initial 1-month course of SM. Such regimens cost in the range of $12 to $15, total! However, recent trends favor the use of RIF-containing regimens for a variety of reasons.

Standard Medications in Contemporary Chemotherapy

Below are described the six drugs which are the core agents of regimens employed in the current era.

TABLE 10.2. *First-line tuberculosis medications: pharmacology and in vitro activities*

Drug	Adult dose/route	Serum level at 2 h	Usual MIC (μg/mL)	Altered absorption	Major toxicity	Drug interactions
Isoniazid	Daily: 300 mg p.o. t.i.w.: 600 mg p.o. b.i.w.: 900 mg p.o.	3–5 μg/mL	0.025–0.05	Food, Antacids	Hepatitis Neuropathy Mood Cognition SLE syndrome	Phenytoin Carbamazepine Disulfiram
Rifampin	Daily: 600 mg p.o. t.i.w.: 600 mg p.o. b.i.w.: 600 mg p.o.	Early: 10–20 μg/mL Late[a]: 6–8 μg/mL	0.06–0.25	Food, Antacids	Hepatitis Flu syndrome Thrombopenia Nephritis GI Distress	See Table 10.4 for more complete listing. Others: see PDR
Pyrazinamide	Daily: 30 mg/kg p.o. t.i.w.: 30–40 mg/kg p.o. b.i.w.: 30–40 mg/kg p.o.	30–40 μg/mL	62–50 μg/mL at pH 5.5	Unknown	Hepatitis Arthralgias Rash GI tract distress	Unknown
Ethambutol	Daily: 25 mg/kg initial 2 mo; then 15 mg/kg p.o. t.i.w.: 30 mg/kg p.o. b.i.w.: 50 mg/kg p.o.	3–5 μg/mL 5–7 μg/mL 8–12 μg/mL	0.95–3.8 μg/mL	Unknown	Optic neuritis Hyperuricemia GI tract distress	Unknown
Streptomycin	Daily: 1000 mg i.m. (750 mg if >55 y) t.i.w.++: 1000 mg i.m. b.i.w.++: 1000 mg i.m.	35–45 μg/mL	0.25–2.0 μg/mL	NA	Vestibular Auditory Renal Electrolyte and cation disturbances Rash and fever	NSAIDs increase risk of renal impairment

The dosing recommendations include daily, thrice-weekly (t.i.w.), and twice-weekly (b.i.w.) schedules for isoniazid and ethambutol; intermittent doses are increased to deliver approximately the same amount weekly as the daily schedule. This is not necessary with rifampin and, in fact, higher intermittent doses produce excess toxicity.

[a] Rifampin induces its own catabolism.

MIC, minimum inhibitory concentration; p.o., by mouth; SLE, systemic lupus erythematosis; PDR, *Physicians' Desk Reference*; GI, gastrointestinal; i.m, intramuscular; NSAIDs, nonsteroidal anti-inflamation drugs; ++, see text for dosage options; other doses may be used as noted in text.

Isoniazid

Isoniazid remains by far the most potent single drug against the tubercle bacillus, more than 40 years after its introduction. Minimal inhibitory concentrations (MICs) and minimal bactericidal concentrations (MBCs) are extremely low, the former typically in the range of 0.025 to 0.050 μg/mL (11). INH is generally well absorbed, reaching serum levels of 3 to 5 μg/mL, concentrations far in excess of MICs or MBCs. The site(s) of action of INH has not been definitely established. INH is a prodrug that apparently is activated by a catalase-peroxidase enzyme, *katG,* which is produced by the tubercle bacillus. In this active form, the hydrazide moiety exerts a lethal effect via inhibition of various intracellular targets. Most evidence suggests that the final pathway for this effect lies in the mycolic acid synthetic pathways (12).

Isoniazid is generally well absorbed, although individuals with extensive gastric surgery or those with resected or dysfunctional terminal ileum may fail to have normal absorbtion. Heavy meals, including both carbohydrate and fatty foodstuffs, result in delayed absorption and reduced maximal concentrations ranging from -9% to -50% in various reports (13–15).

Isoniazid is metabolized in the liver, with the rate of elimination determined by the individual's genetically determined acetylation phenotype: in slow acetylators, the half-life ranges from 120 to 270 minutes; for rapid acetylators, the range is 45 to 110 minutes (16). Distribution of acetylation genotypes varies by race with approximately 50% of whites, blacks, and South Indians being rapid acetylators and 80% to 90% of Chinese, Japanese, and Eskimos having this trait (17–19).

A recent analysis demonstrated that there actually are three groupings for INH-acetylation status: fast, intermediate, and slow (20). Excretion of INH was compared with genotyping of the *NATZ* allele. The *NATZ* IZA allele codes for fast acetylation. Rapid acetylators are homozygous, intermediate acetylators are heterozygous, and slow acetylators do not possess this allele. Significant differences in various pharmacokinetic parameters were seen with these phenotypes. Most notable was the area under the curve, with mean values following a 10-mg/kg dose of INH being 7.73, 16.52, and 31.12 mg/h/L for fast, intermediate, and slow eliminators, respectively.

Despite wide variations in the serum concentrations and kinetics of INH, acetylation status has not been shown to influence the outcome of treatment in which INH is given *daily.* In some of the early *twice-weekly* treatment trials in which INH was accompanied by relatively weak drugs, such as EMB or para-aminosalicylic acid, rapid acetylators fared slightly less well. But, in contemporary twice- or thrice-weekly regimens in which INH is accompanied by other potent drugs, acetylation status has not been shown to influence the outcome (19). By contrast, rapid acetylators have consistently less favorable outcomes in once-weekly regimens. The authors of the report on the trimodal pattern of acetylation suggested that this factor may influence the outcome of therapy in extensive disease with poor tissue penetration of drugs, malabsorption, and/or impaired immunity.

Isoniazid has been shown to interfere with the biological functions of the vitamin B6 or pyridoxine compounds resulting in various toxicities including peripheral neuropathy and anemia (21). The likelihood of toxicity is related to the nutritional status of the patient and is dosage related, rarely occurring with the standard adult 300-mg daily dose. There is a slightly increased risk for neuropathy among slow acetylators of INH. Small supplemental doses of pyridoxine (6 mg/day) have been shown to prevent the neuropathy. Individuals for whom vitamin supplementation has been deemed appropriate include chronically undernourished persons, persons with chronic alcoholism, pregnant women, adolescent girls, and persons with advanced age, uremia, and/or cancer (21). Although unproven in utility, pyridoxine supplementation has been advocated for persons with a seizure disorder for whom INH has been prescribed. Because of the potential for interference by high doses of pyridoxine with the antituberculosis activity of INH, no more than 10 mg per day should be used (21). Pyridoxine is very inexpensive, and its routine use with INH has been advocated. Probably the best argument *against* this practice is the potential confusion and nonadherence associated with prescribing "another pill." A combined formulation of INH with pyridoxine was available at one time in the United States but is no longer marketed. Given the high association between tuberculosis and poverty with the potential for malnutrition, consideration should be given to resumption of this practice. The peripheral neuropathy, when seen, is characteristically a "stocking- glove" process that commences with numbness and tingling, usually worse in the feet. Untreated, it may progress to disabling paresthesias, pain, and weakness.

The use of INH in patients with substantial liver injury or impairment is highly problematic. Although the rate of acetylation does not change in the presence of liver disease, clearance of the drug in patients with significantly impaired liver function is diminished, resulting in a prolonged half-life (22,23). Therefore, if INH must be used in a patient with advanced liver disease, the dosage probably should be reduced to 150–200 mg daily and serum levels monitored.

Since only a small portion of INH is excreted renally, the dose need be reduced only in patients with severe renal insufficiency (e.g., those with creatinine clearances less than 10% of normal or creatinine levels of 12 mg/dL). In patients undergoing periodic hemodialysis, giving INH in the usual dose just following dialysis is recommended for rapid acetylators; a reduced dose may be appropriate for slow acetylators, but pharmacokinetic assessment is advocated (24).

Although INH is generally benign and well tolerated, there are a few toxic reactions of which the clinician should be aware. **Hepatitis** is clearly the most problematic aspect of INH administration. The incidence of hepatitis attributable to INH appears to increase with the rising age of the population (25–27), the coadministration of other potentially hepatotoxic drugs, and increased doses of INH (28). In a large study of persons receiving INH preventive therapy, the mean values of transaminase levels were increased (29); in addition to mean increases of the values, some of the patients' serum glutamic-oxaloacetic transaminase (SGOT) and serum glutamic-pyruvic transaminase (SGPT) levels rose well above the range of normal. In this study, blood was drawn and frozen every 4 weeks during the year of INH therapy, but liver chemistry values were measured only after completion of treatment. Thus, some patients continued to receive INH despite abnormalities of liver function test results. Among those who took 24 weeks or more of INH, 13.3% had one or more SGOT values greater than 60 units versus 2.8% for persons not taking INH; the risk of transaminase elevation related to increasing age but not to INH acetylation status. Despite these elevations of the transaminase levels, none of the patients developed clinically significant hepatitis. This is consistent with the experience in Belgium where INH was continued despite asymptomatic elevations of the transaminases to values 5- to 10-fold above baseline (27); the drug was halted in only 5 of 30 patients with fivefold or higher transaminase elevations. Similarly, 10% of hospital employees receiving preventive therapy had asymptomatic elevation of serum transaminase levels attributable to INH (30); INH was stopped in two of the nine patients because of patient concerns in one and an abnormal finding on liver biopsy in the other. Another study of hospital employees revealed similar findings: 37 (8.7%) of 427 persons had elevated SGOT values in 4 to 8 months of treatment. Isoniazid was discontinued in 5 persons because of symptoms and in 8 others because of elevated bilirubin or alkaline phosphatase values, or both—a 2.9% incidence of "clinically significant" hepatitis (31).

Two large surveys of clinically significant hepatitis among persons receiving INH monotherapy were reported in the 1970s, both of which indicated an incidence less than 1%. Among 13,838 persons receiving INH preventive treatment at multiple centers across the United States, 82 (0.59%) had hepatitis (25). Similarly, among 20,838 residents of eastern Europe who were enrolled in an INH prevention study, 95 (0.46%) developed hepatitis (26). In both of these large series, the incidence of hepatitis increased gradually with age, reaching 2.5% to 3.5% about age 65 years. Notably, in the European trial the rising risk of INH-related hepatitis among older patients was related to an increasing prevalence of preexisting hepatobiliary disorders with greater age; data for underlying liver disease was not available in the U.S. study.

There is a variably increased risk of hepatitis among patients taking INH who also receive other hepatotoxic antituberculosis medications. In a meta-analysis of the reported incidence of "significant hepatitis" (many and varied definitions but always more than asymptomatic, minimal elevations of liver chemistry values), Steele et al. (32) compared the incidence of hepatic injury among thousands of *adult* patients from around the world over several decades taking antituberculosis medications. The categories and the frequency of hepatitis are displayed in Table 10.3. Statistical analysis of these data revealed the following: (a) The increased risk of hepatitis in those taking INH and RIF compared with those taking INH without RIF approached statistical significance ($p = .048$); the relative-risk ratio was 1.6 with 95% confidence intervals (CI) of 1.1 to 2.6. (b) The incidence of hepatitis in those taking INH and RIF was significantly higher than in those taking RIF without INH ($p = .008$). (c) There was no significant difference between the incidence of hepatitis between those taking INH without RIF (groups A and B) and those taking RIF without INH (group D).

In the studies cited above there was only a modest difference in the risk of hepatitis for those taking INH and RIF versus the other groups of patients. However the experience in one report from India with the INH-RIF combination was different and merits consideration. Among adult patients with vertebral or pulmonary tuberculosis receiving INH and RIF with other drugs, the incidence of hepatitis was significantly higher—10% and 2% to 8% (depending on the regimens), respectively—than contemporary patients and historical controls taking INH, PZA, and other drugs (28). Of particular interest in this complex report are the following observations: (a) The risk of hepatitis in patients taking INH-RIF was *greatly* increased by slow INH acetylation status (see below for details). (b) The immediate risk of hepatitis appeared very high in the postoperative period for patients with spinal disease who had undergone surgery with general anesthesia, raising the question of blood products or anesthetic agents as cofactors. (c) The risk of hepatitis among those receiving INH-RIF appeared markedly lower in this series if the treatment was *intermittent,* not daily. (d) PZA did not appear to contribute to the risk of hepatitis in these patients, which is consistent with observations in other trials (33,34).

Regarding the role of acetylation status and the risk of INH-RIF hepatitis, the group at the Research Center in Madras, India, speculated that RIF induces an INH degradation pathway whereby more of the INH is hydrolyzed to form increased amounts of hydrazine, a potentially hepatotoxic compound (35). While the evidence in support of this putative mechanism was only indirect and not wholly persuasive, the strong association between slow acetylation status and the risk for hepatitis among Indian patients re-

TABLE 10.3. *Incidence of hepatitis among persons receiving isoniazid or rifampin or both, with and without other drugs: results of a meta-analysis*

Groups	Number evaluated	Cases of hepatitis	Percentage
A. INH (alone)	38,257	210	0.55
B. INH (no RIF, plus other drugs)	2,053	33	1.61
C. INH (plus RIF, ± other drugs)	6,105	156	2.55
D. RIF (no INH; plus other drugs)	1,264	14	1.11

In the meta-analysis presented, it was shown that the risk of clinically significant hepatitis was modestly greater for persons taking INH and RIF than INH alone, although the differences did not achieve statistical significance. By contrast, the risk for patients receiving INH and RIF was statistically greater than RIF alone.

In the meta-analysis of isoniazid and rifampin–related hepatitis, it was noted that the combination of INH and RIF resulted in a modest but significant increase in hepatitis risk. Because RIF is not given alone (as is INH for preventive chemotherapy), the risks for the individual drugs cannot be directly compared; see text for details.

INH, isoniazid; RIF, rifampin.

From ref. 32, with permission.

ceiving daily doses of INH and RIF appears clinically relevant. This finding is similar to that of a report from Scotland which indicated that, while transaminase rises in patients taking INH and RIF were seen equally among rapid or slow acetylators, 13 of 14 cases with elevations of both transaminases and bilirubin occurred among slow acetylators (36).

Potential contributors or cofactors in the relatively high rates of hepatitis in these Indian trials included higher doses of INH per patient weight than are usually employed outside of India, general anesthesia and blood products administered to spinal tuberculosis patients who were going to have surgery (see above), and various endemic hepatic viruses. Regarding the latter element, viral serological studies performed in 40 Indian children who developed hepatitis while receiving INH and RIF demonstrated immunoglobulin M (IgM) antibodies to hepatitis A in 7.5% and to hepatitis B in 35% of the patients; and risk factors for non-A, non-B hepatitis were prevalent among the other children (37).

Outside India, the question of cofactors for INH-related hepatitis are relevant as well. Remarkable is the paucity of reported cases of hepatitis attributable to INH in the first 20 years of its use. There were sporadic reports of abnormal liver chemistry values, usually attributed to PAS and following a benign course (38). Among the approximately 36,000 persons given INH in the five U.S. Public Health Service (USPHS) preventive therapy trials in the late 1950s to the 1960s, there were only four cases of hepatitis with jaundice in association with the drug (39). Perhaps more cases were present but overlooked (see Chapter 12 for a comprehensive discussion). However, given the potentially lethal consequences of continued drug administration to those with drug-induced hepatitis, it is unlikely that there were substantial numbers of unnoticed cases of INH-related hepatitis. Therefore, it seems plausible that new chemical compounds, drugs, or not yet recognized viral agents were present in our increasingly complicated human milieu, augmenting the capacity for INH to cause liver injury. Of extraordinary interest in this regard, a group from Florida recently documented that tuberculosis patients co-infected with hepatitis C virus or human immunodeficiency virus (HIV) were fivefold or fourfold more likely, respectively, to experience drug-induced hepatitis when begun on antituberculosis therapy (40). Patients infected with both of these viruses were at 14.4-fold increased risk of drug-induced hepatitis in this series. In retrospect, I believe that a substantial amount of the INH-related hepatitis seen beginning in the 1970s was related to the introduction of hepatitis C ("non-A, non-B" hepatitis) into the population. Also, the widely used, commercially available analgesic acetaminophen is a potential candidate as a contemporary cofactor. Hepatotoxic itself in very high doses, acetaminophen usage was reported in association with one or two among fatal INH-related hepatitis in 20 patients in a 1989 report from California (41) and in 3 patients in a recent Centers for Disease Control and Prevention (CDC) report (42).

Rifampin and Other Rifamycins

Synthesized initially in Italy in 1957 from *Streptomyces mediterranei,* RIF has become a major component of modern antituberculosis therapy. The antimicrobial activity of RIF is attributed to the capacity of its macrocyclic ring to bind to the DNA-dependent RNA polymerase of the mycobacteria, thus blocking the initiation of RNA synthesis (43). RIF was introduced into clinical use in 1966, employed initially for the retreatment of drug-resistant treatment-failure cases (44). However, based on BMRC studies, which demonstrated the capacity of regimens containing INH and RIF to substantially shorten the duration of treatment, RIF became a standard element of therapy by the late 1970s (45).

The in vitro activity of RIF varies greatly with the media employed. In 7H-12 liquid medium in the BACTEC system (Becton-Dickenson, Baltimore, MD), the MICs of susceptible strains ranged from 0.06 to 0.25 μg/mL (46). Achievable serum levels of RIF following a 600-mg oral dose vary according to the period over which the drug has been administered. During the first few weeks of therapy, RIF induces accelerated rates at which it is desacetylated in the liver (47). Since desacetylrifampin is excreted in the bile much more rapidly than plain RIF, this is the probable explanation for the modest reductions in maximum concentrations, half-life, and area under the curve seen during the initial phase of RIF administration. (Note: This is independent of the effects of RIF on the cytochrome P450 pathway). Thus, while peak levels initially may reach 20 μg/mL or higher, the usual range seen later is from 8 to 12 μg/mL.

Rifampin is absorbed better in an acidic environment; hence, both food and antacids interfere with absorption and should be avoided in relation to the time of RIF administration. RIF is widely distributed in tissues, predictably reaching therapeutic levels in all sites save the central nervous system, wherein passage across the blood-brain barrier diminishes as meningeal inflammation abates (see Chapter 7).

Although INH demonstrated more early BA than RIF in human trials (6), RIF appears to have superior sterilizing capacity (5). Direct evidence in support of this activity includes in vitro experiments which indicated that RIF has considerably more bactericidal action than INH against tubercle bacilli, which are only briefly active metabolically (represented as Population C in the multi-compartment model) (48). Similarly, in a murine in vivo model of chronic tuberculosis, RIF has been shown to have much greater sterilizing activity than INH (49). The disparity of the in vitro and in vivo bactericidal activities of INH and RIF is a curious phenomenon. In the test tube, both are rapidly lethal for the tubercle bacillus, but in EBA studies in humans, INH greatly outdistances RIF (or any rifamycin). One possible explanation for this discrepancy is relative protein binding: INH is virtually unbound, while RIF is roughly 80% bound.

Rifampin results in red-orange discoloration of urine, feces, sputum, perspiration, and tears. It has been noted to permanently discolor soft contact lenses. As the peak levels diminish, this phenomenon becomes less noticeable. Toxicity from RIF includes hepatitis (see Table 10.3 for discussion of relative risks of hepatic injury from RIF, INH, and other drugs). Gastrointestinal tract disturbances including anorexia, vague discomfort, and generally mild diarrhea are not uncommon early in treatment. These complaints often subside with continued therapy. Pseudomembranous colitis (50,51) and one case resembling ulcerative colitis (52) have been reported in association with RIF use. Frank hypersensitivity reactions with fever, rash, and eo-sinophilia are rare. An effective desensitization protocol for minor hypersensitivity has been described (53). Thrombocytopenia including fulminant purpuric reactions have been noted to occur, particularly in association with interrupted, erratic treatment and increased doses during intermittent schedules (54–56). Three cases of RIF-induced thrombocytopenia associated with antiplatelet antibodies were recently reported (57). A "flu syndrome" marked by fever, chills, myalgias, and malaise has been observed, also most commonly in association with interrupted treatment, high-dose intermittent schedules, and once-weekly regular treatment. Renal damage with or without impaired function or failure has been reported sporadically in association with RIF; variable features of these reports include tubular necrosis, interstitial nephritis, glomerulitis, intravascular hemolysis, immune globulin deposition, and flu syndrome (58–60). Rare features of RIF-associated renal damage include light-chain cast nephropathy simulating myelo-ma (61). A lupus erythematosis syndrome with arthralgias, myalgias, malaise and positive antinuclear antibody (ANA) tests has recently been described in patients taking RIF (or rifabutin) along with other agents such as clarithromycin or ciprofloxacin, which inhibit the cytochrome P450 system (62).

RIF predictably induces hepatocellular smooth endoplasmic reticulum, resulting in increased cytochrome P450 enzyme activity; this causes accelerated degradation or elimination of a variety of exogenous and endogenous compounds. The magnitude of these changes may be clinically significant and should be considered whenever RIF is prescribed. The more common RIF-related drug interactions are listed in Table 10.4. The most common drug-drug interaction problems are due to reduced levels of the drugs/hormones in question; of vital interest at present is the interaction between RIF and antiretroviral agents (see Chapter 8). In addition, it is vital to note that rebound toxicity from other agents may occur when RIF is discontinued. In this situation, a dosage of medication that previously has

TABLE 10.4. *Some of the more clinically significant drug-drug interactions related to rifampin (other rifamycin) and the hepatic cytochrome P450 enzymatic pathway*

1. Rifampin induces the cytochrome P450 (Cy-P450) pathway, resulting in more rapid elimination of the following compounds:
   a. Protease inhibitors
   b. Azol antifungal agents
   c. Corticosteroids (exogenous *and* endogenous)
   d. Warfarin anticoagulants
   e. Opiates including methadone
   f. Oral hypoglycemic agents
   g. Macrolides
   h. Anticonvulsants
   i. Antiarrhythmics, β-blockers, and calcium channel blockers
   j. Benzodiazepines
   k. Cyclosporine
2. The following compounds inhibit the Cy-P450 pathway resulting in retarded elimination of the rifamycin:
   a. Protease inhibitors
   b. Azol antifungal agents
   c. Ciprofloxacin

Partial listing of agents with which rifampin has been noted to have potentially significant interactions. Rifampin in this most potent inducer of the cytochrome P450 pathway; rifapentine is about 50% as active and rifabutine about 10%. Please see *Physician's Desk Reference* or other updated resource for other potential interactions.

Listing of documented drug interactions involving rifampin is partial. Other medications or hormones might be anticipated to be influenced. The magnitude of these changes may well be of clinical significance. Maximum induction of the cytochrome pathway may require 7 to 10 days; conversely, these effects do not resolve for 7 to 14 days following discontinuation of rifampin. If major drug-drug interactions are feared, one may either substitute rifabutin (which has far less cytochrome-inducing activity than rifampin) or adjust upward the doses of the other medication(s).

resulted in therapeutic levels may cause dangerously high serum concentrations to accumulate after the enzyme induction effect subsides.

Other rifamycin agents recently have been introduced into human use. A spiropiperidyl rifamycin, originally designated LM 427 (Ansamycin) and currently referred to as rifabutine (RBU) (Rifabutin), was introduced in the United States in 1982 (63). Because of uncertainty regarding in vitro critical concentrations, RBU was originally thought to be active against many strains of *Mycobacterium tuberculosis* resistant to RIF (63). However, it was soon recognized that, when in vitro concentrations were adjusted according to bioavailability, the majority of strains resistant to RIF were also resistant to RBU, 64% (63), 73% (64), and 69% (65) being resistant at 0.5 μg/mL in three reports. In clinical use, RBU has generally been disappointing versus RIF-resistant tuberculosis (66,67). Most tubercle bacilli that acquire resistance to rifamycins do so by mutations of the RNA-polymerase chromosomes, which convey resistance to all of this category of drugs (68); only a modest proportion of strains (in the range of 10%) has mutations that confer resistance to RIF and rifapentine but not to RBU (68).

Rifabutin does have naturally lower MICs for *M. tuberculosis* than does RIF (65). Hence, it has been considered as a potentially superior agent for short-course treatment. However, these two rifamycins were found equivalent in direct comparison trials from South Africa (69) and Argentina (70). This equivalency may reflect the pharmacokinetics of RBU, which entail substantially lower maximum serum concentrations, 0.5 μg/mL ± 0.2 μg after a standard 300-mg dose of RBU versus 8 to 24 μg/mL after a standard 600-mg dose of RIF, but a longer serum half-life, 20 to 25 hours for RBU and 2 to 4 hours for RIF (71). A trial from Uganda reported comparable efficacy of RIF and RBU but superior early activity of RBU manifested by a higher percentage of culture negativity at 2 months (72). However, I am unsure of the meaning of this report, since the 2-month conversion rates for the RIF regimen were unexpectedly low (roughly 45%); the RBU did not perform well so much as the RIF arm performed poorly. Also, there were only 24 and 25 patients in the two arms, respectively.

Other potentially meaningful differences between RBU and RIF include the following. RBU is substantially less active in induction of the hepatic cytochrome P450 pathways than is RIF (71); this is more relevant in contemporary medicine in terms of treatment of tuberculosis in persons with acquired immunodeficiency syndrome (AIDS) (see Chapter 8 for full discussion). Also, my experience suggests that the side effects and toxicity profiles are somewhat different, with RBU more likely to result in cytopenias, whereas RIF seems more prone to hepatic injury; however, these differences are not statistically significant.

Rifapentine (RPT) (Priftin) was approved by the U.S. Food and Drug Administration (FDA) in 1998. It is a cyclopentyl rifamycin and has pharmacokinetic properties that distinguish it from RIF and RBU: substantially greater maximum serum concentration and extended half-life. Important pharmacokinetic parameters for these three currently available rifamycins include the following:

- *Serum maximum concentration* (C_{max}) (micrograms per milliliter): RIF, 8 to 24; RBU, 0.3 to 0.9; RPT, 10 to 30.
- *Serum half-life* (hours): RIF, 2 to 4; RBU, 20 to 25; RPT, 12 to 15.
- *Minimal inhibitory concentrations* at pH 6.0 versus wild-type strains, *M. tuberculosis* (micrograms per milliliter): RIF, 0.06 to 0.25; RBU, 0.03 to 0.06; RPT, 0.015 to 0.06 (46).

These attributes make RPT an excellent candidate for intermittent chemotherapy with the potential to widen the interval between doses (73,74).

Because of these features, Grosset et al. (49) have studied RPT in the chemotherapy of chronic tuberculosis in the mouse model. These studies indicated considerable activity even when RPT and INH, PZA, and SM were given once weekly, but weekly treatment was not comparable in efficacy to 6-day-per-week RIF-containing regimens.

Two large human trials using RPT-containing regimens against pulmonary tuberculosis have been completed (75,76); another study conducted by the CDC is still enrolling patients. The first trial was conducted in Hong Kong with RPT produced in Shanghai, China, not by the firm of origin, Hoechst-Marion-Roussel (77). The Hong Kong trial consisted of 6 months of therapy: 2 months of a standard RIF-containing, thrice-weekly regimen followed by randomization to 4 months of either RPT/INH *once weekly* or RIF/INH *thrice weekly* (78). The trial was complicated by the finding of substandard bioavailability of the Chinese RPT in the midst of the study; this led to increasing the RPT dose from 600 to 750 mg. Overall, however, the once-weekly RPT performed less well than the thrice-weekly RIF: there were 3% to 4% posttreatment relapses with RIF, 9% to 12% with RPT; these differences were statistically significant. It seems likely that diminished bioavailability of the Chinese-manufactured RPT, 66% to 74% of the Western product, may have been responsible for some of this effect (77). However, fundamental questions of the efficacy of once-weekly INH/RPT in the continuation phase were raised.

The second large trial was conducted in South Africa and the United States by Hoechst-Marian-Roussel. The results of the trial were presented to the FDA in May 1998 but have not yet been published. This study employed a control 6-month regimen consisting of 2 months of *daily* RIF/INH/PZA/EMB followed by 4 months of *twice-weekly* RIF/INH; this was compared with 2 months of RPT *twice weekly* with INH/PZA/EMB *daily* followed by 4 months of RPT/INH *once weekly*. In terms of relapses, the RPT arm was associated with a modest but statistically significant increased risk: 10% versus 5%. However, there were fewer treatment failures in the RPT arm (1% vs. 3%), giving the regimens overall statistical equivalency. As a consultant retained to help analyze and present the data to the FDA, I have the following impressions: (a) The study design was unfortunate; the use of *twice-weekly* RPT with other drugs *daily* resulted in reduced compliance with the non-RPT agents, a factor significantly associated with the risk of relapse; (b) the dose of RPT, 600 mg, may be suboptimal; pharmacokinetic data from the trial indicated maximal concentrations below those anticipated; future studies should include dose ranging; and (c) the side effects and toxicity profiles of RPT were very benign and similar to RIF.

The third trial is being conducted in the United States and Canada by the Tuberculosis Elimination Division of the CDC. The study design consists of a 6-month regimen consisting of 2 months of a standard RIF/INH/PZA/EMB *daily* regimen followed by randomization to 4 months of *twice-weekly* RIF/INH or *once-weekly* RPT/INH. Since the study is still enrolling patients, overall results are not available. However, the CDC group did report that among HIV-infected persons in this trial, five patients in the RPT arm failed or relapsed, 4 of these developing rifamycin resistance (79). Because of this, the researchers closed the RPT arm to further enrollment of HIV-infected persons. Whether this is of unique clinical significance is not yet clear: rifamycin resistance has been seen with RIF and RBU, as well as RPT (78,80). Also, the HIV-infected patients in the RPT arm who acquired rifamycin resistance were substantially more ill and their cases were medically complicated, including more extrapulmonary tuberculosis, lower CD4 cell counts, and more use of antifungal agents than the RIF-arm patients.

At the present time, the role(s) of RPT in tuberculosis chemotherapy is unclear. However, extrapolating from the available data in the three trials cited above and from the previously noted animal work of Grosset et al. (49), I would predict that 6-month regimens requiring fewer encounters will be feasible. To overcome the disparity in drug duration in once-weekly schedules, we may consider means to provide prolonged release INH (79,81,82) and/or use agents such as EMB or SM, which have longer "postantibiotic effects" than INH.

Pyrazinamide

Because of its ability to reduce the required duration of treatment, PZA is the third most important drug after INH and RIF in contemporary tuberculosis therapy. PZA is the amide derivative of pyrazine-2-carboxylic acid. PZA is a prodrug, requiring cleavage of this amide moiety to release the active compound, pyrazinoic acid. Although shown to have considerable activity during the 1950s, the propensity for PZA to produce serious, even lethal hepatitis when used in dosages ranging from 40 to 70 mg/kg resulted in its use being limited to drug-resistant, treatment-failure cases (83). But, based on PZA's potency in the murine model, British scientists reintroduced the drug in various short-course chemotherapy studies. Trials in which simultaneous regimens most clearly demonstrated the utility of PZA are displayed in Table 10.5; these include East Africa regimen 3 (regimens 10 vs. 13 and 20 vs. 23), as well as Hong Kong thrice-weekly regimen 1 (regimens 35–37 vs. regimen 39). Studies in which nonsimultaneous trials showed the impact of PZA include USPHS trials 20 and 21 (regimen 52 vs. regimen 51) and Poland trials 1 and 3 (regimen 47 vs. regimen 50).

While it has been suggested that PZA is essential to reduce the duration of chemotherapy for smear-positive pulmonary tuberculosis to 6 months, two regimens without PZA from the East African trials 1 and 2 yielded excellent results in only 6 months: regimens 16 and 18, which employed INH, RIF, and SM daily, were associated with no treatment failures and 3.4% and 2.3% relapse rates, respectively. These regimens are not regarded as readily applicable, though, because they were given entirely in the hospital to ensure that all doses were given, and they entailed 180 doses of SM, therapy not universally tolerable or acceptable.

A subtle but noteworthy aspect of PZA's impact on short-course regimens is the lack of additional utility when given beyond the first 2 months to patients with drug-susceptible tuberculosis. Comparison between Hong Kong thrice-weekly trials 1 and 2 clearly reveals that in the thrice-weekly format, PZA given for just 2 months (regimen 42), was equal to PZA given for 4 months (regimen 40) or 6 months (regimens 36 and 40). In fact, early trials with simultaneous regimens raised the question whether PZA might have a moderately adverse effect when given beyond the initial 2 months: East Africa trial 4 (regimen 72 vs. regimen 73) and Singapore trial 2 (regimen 77 vs. regimen 78). Although these differences were not statistically significant, they do clearly indicate that PZA need not be used beyond the first 2 months unless initial drug resistance is detected. Possible mechanisms to explain the slightly negative effect of PZA include a recent report from India demonstrating a very modest but statistically significant reduction in serum RIF levels when PZA was given simultaneously (84) and the observation that, in the human macrophage, PZA caused a slight reduction in the BA of RIF (9).

TABLE 10.5. *Summary of selected short-course regimens of varied duration*

Study (ref. no.)	Regimen number	Regimen (drugs given daily unless indicated by subscripts, days per week given)	Total relapse (%)	Comments	Percentage of patients with negative cultures at various times		Time of relapses posttreament[a]	
							Early	Late
1. Eight or 9 months' duration					2 mo	3 mo		
BTA No. 1 (1)	1	2 mo IRS or E plus 7 mo of IR	0.0	No relapses in 60 mo of designed follow-up; but 1 at 62 and 1 at 64 mo	—	—	—	—
BTA No. 2 (2)	2	2 mo IRE plus 7 mo of IR	1.5		—	—	—	—
Arkansas (3)	3	1 mo IR plus 8 mo of I_2R_2	1.7	2.9% failed to convert	67%	92%	—	—
							To 6 mo	7–24 mo
Hong Kong No. 1 (4)[b]	4	3 mo IPS plus 6 mo of $I_3P_3S_3$	4.6	*No rifampin used.* Only SC regimens without RIF. Outcome poor with 6 mo. See regimens 30–32. Initial failures seen with regimen 6.	77%	93%	2/65	1
	5	9 mo of $I_3P_3S_3$	6.1		70%	94%	3/65	1
	6	9 mo of $I_2P_2S_2$	6.1		72%	86%	2/49	1
							To 4 mo	5–24 mo
Hong Kong No. 2 (5)	7	2 mo of IRPS plus 6 mo $I_2P_2S_2$	3.4	No RIF in latter treatment to save money; some efficacy lost. Note efficacy of fully intermittent regimens, 5, 6, and 9.	95%	99%	2/87	1
	8	2 mo of IRPE plus 6 mo $I_2P_2E_2$	9.5		81%	97%	7/84	1
	9	4 mo of $I_3R_3P_3S_3$ plus 4 mo $I_3P_3S_3$	1.2		94%	100%	0/83	1
East Africa No. 3 (6)[a]	10	2 mo IRPS plus 6 mo 1 Th	0.0	Generally favorable outcome; lower cost by omitting rifampin in late treatment. Results substantially better than with 6–month therapy, regimens 20–23.	87%	93%	0/81	0
	11	1 mo IRPS plus 7 mo 1 Th	6.9		67%	88%	3/58	1
	12	1 mo IRPS plus 7 mo $I_2P_2S_2$	2.3		68%	92%	2/88	0
	13	2 mo IRS plus 6 mo 1 Th	6.5		75%	91%	3/77	2
					2 mo	3 mo	To 6 mo	7–19 mo
USPHS-21 (7)	14	9 mo IR	2.8	High attrition from study. EMB added initially improved conversion and relapsed rates (see text)	70%	85%	4/204	6/172
	15							
					2 mo	3 mo	To 6 mo	7–12 mo
San Francisco (8)		2 mo IRE plus 7 mo IR	2.3	1.5% failure rate	—	—	4/174	0/109
2. Six months' duration					2 mo	3 mo	To 12 mo	13–60 mo
East Africa No. 1 (9)[a]	16	6 mo IRS	3.4	All therapy in hospital	69%	94%	5/145	5
	17	6 mo IPS	10.7		67%	91%	—	—
East Africa No. 2 (10)[a]	18	6 mo IRS	2.3	All therapy in hospital	70%	95%	4/171	0
	19	6 mo IR	7.3		64%	96%	10/164	2
							To 6 mo	7–18 + mo
East Africa No. 3 (6)[a]	20	2 mo IRPS plus 4 mo of 1 Th	13.3	All in hospital × 6 mo. Contrast results when treatment extended to 8 mo (see regimens 10–13)	—	—	8/75	2
	21	1 mo IRPS plus 5 mo of 1 Th	17.7		—	—	11/79	3
	22	1 mo IRPS plus 7 mo of 1 Th	9.3		—	—	5/75	2
	23	2 mo IRS plus 4 mo of 1 Th	18.3		—	—	13/82	2

continues

TABLE 10.5. *Continued*

Study (ref. no.)	Regimen number	Regimen (drugs given daily unless indicated by subscripts, days per week given)	Total relapse (%)	Comments	Percentage of patients with negative cultures at various times		Time of relapses posttreament[a] Early	Late
							To 6 mo	7–24 mo
East Africa No. 5 (11)[a]	24	2 mo IRPS plus 4 mo of IR	2.4	+ Regimen *27* was 8 mo; extending INH reduced relapse rate significantly. PZA during last 4 mo added little to INH (regimen 25 *vs.* 26).	84%	—	2/166	2
	25	2 mo IRPS plus 4 mo of IP	7.9		84%	—	6/164	7
	26	2 mo IRPS plus 4 mo of I	9.6		84%	—	14/156	1
	27	2 mo IRPS plus 6 mo of I*	3.3		84%	—	2/123	2
					2 mo	3 mo	To 6 mo	7–17 mo
Hong Kong No. 1 (4)[a]	28	6 mo IPS	18.3	No RIF used. Outcome much better when Rx extended to 9 mo. 4.5% failed to convert with regimens 28–30.	77%	93/5	9/60	2
	29	6 mo $I_3P_3S_3$	23.5		70%	94%	13/68	3
	30	6 mo $I_2P_2S_2$	20.5		72%	86%	7/39	1
							To 6 mo	7–24 mo
Hong Kong No. 2 (5)[a]	31	6 mo IRS	5.6	Substantially worse outcome with EMB vs. SM (regimen 33 vs. 32)	88%	100%	6/143	2
	32	2 mo IRPS plus 4 mo of $I_2P_2S_2$	6.9		95%	99%	4/87	2
	33	2 mo IRPE plus 4 mo $I_2P_2E_2$	22.6		81%	97%	16/84	3
	34	4 mo $I_3R_3P_3S_2$ plus 2 mo of $I_2P_2S_2$	5.6		94%	100%	4/71	0
							To 6 mo	7–59 mo
Hong Kong-TIW No. 1 (12)[a]	35	6 mo $I_3R_3P_3S_3E_3$	3.9	Marked loss of efficacy without PZA in regimen 39. Note diminished 2 mo. conversion rate. EMB added little in cases with susceptible strains.	88%	—	0/152	6
	36	6 mo $I_3R_3P_3S_3$	1.3		90%	—	1/151	1
	37	6 mo $I_3R_3P_3E_3$	4.4		90%	—	4/160	3
	38	6 mo IRPE	3.7		94%	—	1/163	5
	39	6 mo $I_3R_3S_3E_3$	10.2		76%	—	11/166	6
							To 6 mo	7–24 mo
Hong Kong-TIW No. 2 (13)[b]	40	6 mo I_3R; 4 mo S_3; 6 mo P_3	3.4	No SM (regimen 43) resulted in 2% failure to convert and high relapse rate; not statistically significant but HK clinicians continue to use SM.	93%	—	3/208	2
	41	6 mo I_3R_3; 4 mo S_3; 4 mo P_3	4.4		87%	—	7/205	3
	42	6 mo I_3R_3; 4 mo S_3; 2 mo P_3	2.7		94%	—	4/220	2
	43	6 mo $I_3R_3P_3$	6.5		88%	—	5/199	7
					2 mo	3 mo	To 6 mo	7–30 mo
Poland No. 1 (14)	44	6 mo IRE	12.9	Inexplicably high relapse rates in this study.	63%	—	6/93	6
	45	2 mo IRE plus 4 mo $I_2R_2E_2$	17.8		69%	—	10/90	6
	46	2 mo IRE plus 4 mo $I_1R_1E_1$	21.3		66%	—	12/89	7
	47	2 mo IRE plus 4 mo I_2R_2	7.7		75%	—	4/90	3
							To 6 mo	7–18 mo
Poland No. 2 (15)	48	2 mo IRPS plus 4 mo I_2R_2	0.0	Omitting SM in regimen 50 resulted in 1.7% failure to convert; similar to HK regimen 43.	91%	—	0/85	0
Poland No. 3 (16)	49	2 mo IRPS plus 4 mo I_2R_2	1.8		74%	—	1/56	0
	50	2 mo IRP plus 4 mo I_2R_2	3.4		85%	—	1/116	3

USPHS-20 (17)	51	6 mo IR	9.2	Heavy losses from study population	—	—	—	—
					2 mo	3 mo	To 6 mo	7–19 mo
USPHS-21 (7)	52	2 mo IRP plus 4 mo IR	3.5	Heavy losses from study population	80%	91%	4/343	9/273
Denver (18)	53	0.5 mo IRPS; 1.5 mo $I_2R_2P_2S_2$; plus 4 mo I_2R_2	1.6	5.5 mo twice-weekly therapy; 62 total doses	75%	—	1/125	1
							To 6 mo	7–96 mo
Singapore No. 2 (19)[a]	54	2 mo IRPS plus 4 mo of IRP	0.0		98%	—	0/78	1
BTA No. 2 (2)	55	2 mo IRPS plus 4 mo of IR	2.5		98%	—	1/80	1
	56	2 mo IRPS plus 4 mo of IR	0.8		—	—	—	—
	57	2 mo IRPE plus 4 mo of IR	2.5		—	—	—	—
E. Germany (20)	58	6 mo $I_2R_2P_2S_2$	0.0	Note strongly adverse effect of no RIF during last 3 mos.	—	—	—	—
	59	3 mo $I_3R_3P_3S_3$ plus 3 mo of $I_3P_3S_3$	5.0		—	—	—	—
							To 6 mo	7–60 mo
Singapore No. 3 (21)[a]	60	2 mo IRPS plus 4 mo I_3R_3	2.1		99%	—	1/96	1
	61	1 mo IRPS plus 5 mo I_3R_3	2.1		85%	—	1/96	1
	62	2 mo IRP plus 4 mo I_3R_3	2.9		90%	—	1/109	2
Brazil (22)	63	2 IRP plus I_2R_2	4.1	4.6% failed to convert. Compliance comparable in daily & b.i.w. regimens.	—	—	—	—
		2 IRP plus 4 IR	6.5		—	—	—	—
3. Less than 6 months' duration								
					2 mo	3 mo	Y 1	Y 2–5
Madras No. 1 (23)	64	3 mo IRPS plus 2 mo $I_2P_2S_2$	5.2*	*"Relapses requiring retreatment." 5-year follow-up of adherent patients.	91%	96%	4/97	1
	65	3 mo IPS plus 2 mo $I_2P_2S_2$	20.0*		74%	93%	13/115	10
	66	3 mo IRPS	16.8*		91%	96%	16/113	3
Madras No. 2 (24)	67	2 mo IRPS plus 3 mo $I_2P_2S_2$	7.1	5-year follow-up	—	—	6/126	3
					2 mo	3 mo	Y 1	Y 2
Agra(25)	68	3 mo IRPS plus 1.5 mo IR	1.6	2-year follow-up. Contrast results at 3 mo with those of Madras 66. Controversial data.	—	—	1/64	0
	69	3 mo IRPS plus 1.5 mo $I_2R_2S_2$	8.6		—	—	6/81	1
	70	3 mo IRPS	5.7		—	—	3/53	0

continues

TABLE 10.5. *Continued*

Study (ref. no.)	Regimen number	Regimen (drugs given daily unless indicated by subscripts, days per week given)	Total relapse (%)	Comments	Percentage of patients with negative cultures at various times		Time of relapses posttreament[a]	
							Early	Late
					2 mo	3 mo	To 6 mo	7–24 mo
East Africa No. 4 (26)[a]	71	2 mo IRPS plus 2 mo IRP	16.3	Great impact of RIF in last 2 mo; no beneficial effect of PZA in last 2 mo.	85%	—	9/109	8
	72	2 mo IRPS plus 2 mo IR	10.6		85%	—	9/107	1
	73	2 mo IRPS plus 2 mo IP	31.6		85%	—	24/101	7
	74	2 mo IRPS plus 2 mo I	30.5		85%	—	26/107	6
	75	2 mo IRPS plu 2 mo I	40.0		85%	—	33/102	5
							To 6 mo	7–96 mos
Singapore No. 2 (19)[a]	76	2 mo IRPS plus 2 mo IRP	11.4	Adverse effect of PZA in last 2 mo	98%	—	8/79	2
	77	2 mo IRPS plus 2 mo IR	7.8		98%	—	5/77	5
France (27)	78	4.2 mo of IRPS	2.4		—	—	2/84	—
E. Germany (20)	79	3.0 mo of IRPS	20.0	Deemed "unsatisfactory" by authors.	—	—	—	—

[a] Relapses in the early phase are expressed in terms of numerator:denominator data. Due to losses from the observed group, the denominator numbers typically fall. Thus, the later relapses are expressed as simple numbers (the traditional model for reporting tuberculosis study data).

[b] Studies made in collaboration with the British Medical Research Council (BMRC).

I = INH = isoniazid; R = RIF = rifampin; P = PZA = pyrazinamide; S = SM = streptomycin; E = EMB = ethambutol; Th = Thiacetazone; SC = short course; BTA = British Thoracic Association; USPHS = United States Public Health Service; TW = thrice weekly; HK = Hong Kong; q.d. = daily; b.i.w. = twice weekly.

Summary of the results of short-course chemotherapy trials for pulmonary tuberculosis involving 9 months' duration or less; of treatment. In general, treatment "failure" (sputum cultures do not become negative during treatment) was so rare that no column was dedicated to this feature. In addition to relapse rates, the time at which the relapse was noted is included. Also, to help characterize the potency of these various regimens, the percentage of patients with negative cultures at various points of therapy (usually 2 or 3 mo) is included. To make it easier to identify the report from which these data were derived, the referenced articles are included as footnotes to Table. 10.5.

1. British Thoracic and Tuberculosis Association. Short-course chemotherapy in pulmonary tuberculosis: a controlled trial by the British Thoracic and Tuberculosis Association. *Lancet* 1976;2:1102–1104.
2. British Thoracic Association. A controlled trial of six months chemotherapy in pulmonary tuberculosis: second report—results during the 24 months after the end of chemotherapy. *Am Rev Respir Dis* 1982;126:460–462.
3. Dutt AK, Moers D, Stead WW. Undesirable side effects of isoniazid and rifampin in largely twice-weekly short-course chemotherapy for tuberculosis. *Am Rev Respir Dis* 1983;128:419–424.
4. Hong Kong Chest Service, British Medical Research Council. Controlled trial of 6-month and 9-month regimens of daily and intermittent streptomycin plus isoniazid plus pyrazinamide for pulmonary tuberculosis in Hong Kong. *Am Rev Respir Dis* 1977;115:727–735.
5. Hong Kong Chest Service/British Medical Research Council. Controlled trial of 6-month and 8-month regimens in the treatment of pulmonary tuberculosis: the results up to 30 months. *Tubercle* 1979;60:201–210.

6. East African/British Medical Research Council. Third East African/British Medical Research Council Study: controlled clinical trial of four short-course regimens of chemotherapy for two durations in the treatment of pulmonary tuberculosis—second report. *Tubercle* 1980;61:59–69.
7. Combs D, O'Brien R, Geiter L. USPHS tuberculosis short-course chemotherapy trial 21: effectiveness, toxicity, and acceptability—the report of final results. *Ann Intern Med* 1990;112:397–406.
8. Slutkin G, Schecter GF, Hopewell PC. The results of 9-month isoniazid-rifampin therapy for pulmonary tuberculosis under program condition in San Francisco. *Am Rev Respir Dis* 1988;138:1622–1624.
9. East African/British Medical Research Council. East African/British Medical Research Council Study: results at 5 years of a controlled comparison of a 6-month and a standard 18-month regimen of chemotherapy for pulmonary tuberculosis. *Am Rev Respir Dis* 1977;115:3–8.
10. East African/British Medical Research Council. Second East African/British Medical Research Council Study: second report—controlled clinical trial of four 6-month regimens of chemotherapy for pulmonary tuberculosis. *Am Rev Respir Dis* 1976;114:471–475.
11. East and Central Africa/British Medical Research Council. East and Central Africa/British Medical Research Council Fifth Collaborative Study: controlled clinical trial of 4 short-course regimens of chemotherapy (three 6-month and one 8-month) for pulmonary tuberculosis—final report. *Tubercle* 1986;67:5–15.
12. Hong Kong Chest Service/British Medical Research Council. Five-year follow-up of a controlled trial of five 6-month regimens of chemotherapy for pulmonary tuberculosis. *Am Rev Respir Dis* 1987;136:1339–1342.
13. Hong Kong Chest Service/British Medical Research Council. Controlled trial of 2, 4, and 6 months of pyrazinamide in 6-month, three-times weekly regimens for smear-positive pulmonary tuberculosis, including an assessment of a combined preparation of isoniazid, rifampin, and pyrazinamide: results at 30 months. *Am Rev Respir Dis* 1991;143:700–706.
14. Zierski M, Bek E, Long MW, Snider DE Jr. Short-course (6-month) cooperative tuberculosis study in Poland: results 30 months after completion of treatment. *Am Rev Respir Dis* 1981;124:249–251.
15. Snider DE Jr, Rogowski J, Zierski M, Bek E, Long MW. Successful intermittent treatment of smear-positive puolmonary tuberculosis in six months: a cooperative study in Poland. *Am Rev Respir Dis* 1982;125:265–267.
16. Snider DE Jr, Graczyk J, Bek E, Rogowski J. Supervised 6-month treatment of newly diagnosed pulmonary tuberculosis using isoniazid, rifampin, and pyrazinamide with and without streptomycin. *Am Rev Respir Dis* 1984;130:1091–1094.
17. Snider DE Jr, Long MW, Cross FS, Farer LS. Six-month isoniazid-rifampin therapy for pulmonary tuberculosis: report of a United States Public Health Service cooperative trial. *Am Rev Respir Dis* 1984;129:573–579.
18. Cohn DL, Catlin BJ, Peterson KL, Judson FN, Sbarbaro JA. A 62-dose, 6-month therapy for pulmonary and extrapulmonary tuberculosis: a twice-weekly, directly observed, and cost-effective regimen. *Ann Intern Med* 1990;112:407–415.
19. Singapore Tuberculosis Service/British Medical Research Council. Long-term follow-up of a clinical trial of 6-month and 4-month regimens of chemotherapy in the treatment of pulmonary tuberculosis. *Am Rev Respir Dis* 1986;133:779–783.
20. Eule H, Beck H, Evers H, et al. Daily and intermittent short-course chemotherapy using four drugs in recently detected bacillary pulmonary tuberculosis. *Bull Int Un Tuberc* 1982;57:63.
21. Singapore Tuberculosis Service/British Medical Research Council. Five-year follow-up of a clinical trial of three 6-month regimens of chemotherapy given intermittently in the continuation phase in the treatment of pulmonary tuberculosis. *Am Rev Respir Dis* 1988;137:1147–1150.
22. Castelo A, Goihman S, Dalboni MA, et al. Comparison of daily and twice-weekly regimens to treat pulmonary tuberculosis. *Lancet* 1989;2:1173–1176.
23. Balasubramanian R, Sivasubramaniar S, Vijayan VK, et al. Five-year results of a 3-month and two 5-month regimens for the treatment of sputum-positive pulmonary tuberculosis in South India. *Tubercle* 1990;71:253–258.
24. Santha T, Nazareth O, Krishnamurthy MS, et al. Treatment of pulmonary tuberculosis with short course chemotherapy in South India: 5-year follow-up. *Tubercle* 1989;70:229–234.
25. Mehrotra ML, Gautam KD, Chaube CK. Shortest possible acceptable effective chemotherapy in ambulatory patients with pulmonary tuberculosis, II: results during the 24 months after the end of chemotherapy. *Am Rev Respir Dis* 1984;129:1016–1017.
26. East African/British Medical Research Council. Controlled clinical trial of five short-course (4 month) chemotherapy regimens in pulmonary tuberculosis: second report of the 4th study. *Am Rev Respir Dis* 1981;123:165–170.
27. Perdrizet S, Liard R, Pretet S, Grosset J. Short-term chemotherapy in pulmonary tuberculosis: French Cooperative Trial. *Bull Int Union Tuberc* 1984;59:11–14.

The mechanism(s) of PZA's action and the means by which it contributes to short-course therapy are obscure and controversial. Among all of the current major drugs, PZA demonstrated the least potency in reducing the number of bacilli in the sputum of patients treated with single drugs for 14 days (6). Testing PZA's activity in vitro has been highly problematic because of pH-dependent variables of drug activity and mycobacterial growth. PZA has no activity at pH 7.0 to 7.4; its capacity to inhibit *M. tuberculosis* increases as the pH of the medium decreases. However, even at pH 5.6, the most acidic environment in which tubercle bacilli can consistently multiply, the MIC for three strains of *M. tuberculosis* was 31 μg/mL and a fourth MIC was 62 μg/mL (7). In this system, PZA concentrations as high as 500 to 1,000 μg/mL failed to produce a "bactericidal" effect, defined as 99% or 99.9% killing of the mycobacterial population. Thus, Heifets and Lindholm-Levy (7) reported that the MBC of PZA at pH 5.6 was in excess of 1,000 μg/mL, far beyond achievable serum levels.

Several studies have been conducted in an effort to explain the seeming paradox of significant clinical utility despite extremely limited in vitro activity. Since PZA has been shown to achieve levels within macrophages that are only ±50% of the concentration in the medium (85), one may conclude that PZA does *not* work through extreme concentration in macrophages. Crowle et al. (86) tested the activity of PZA against *M. tuberculosis* multiplying ex vivo in human monocyte-derived macrophages and, while more active intracellularly than in culture medium, only inhibitory effects were seen when PZA concentrations as high as 80 to 160 μg/mL were added to the milieu. Crowle et al. (87) subsequently showed that the addition of 1,25 $(OH)_2$-vitamin D_3 acted synergistically with low concentrations of PZA to result in modest intracellular killing. To achieve this effect, a supra-physiological concentration (4 μg/mL) of the vitamin D_3 compound was used. This may be biologically relevant, however, since activated macrophages do synthesize 1,25 $(OH)_2$-vitamin D_3, raising the possibility that sufficiently high concentrations of this compound to enhance PZA activity may exist within tuberculous lesions.

Extreme regional acidity within localized regions of the diseased host has been offered as another theory to explain PZA's activity. Originally, it was speculated that the intracellular milieu of the macrophage was acidic due to lysosomal enzymes. However, Crowle et al. (8) have shown that the pH within the vesicles of human macrophages, which contain tubercle bacilli, is neutral. This finding is consistent with the observation that virulent tubercle bacilli multiply prolifically in this setting, an improbability were the pH to be very low. Mitchison has suggested that, rather than within the macrophage, it is the local milieu within necrotic, caseating lesions that is acidic (5). He proposed that this environment results in inhibition or semidormancy for the tubercle bacilli (5), and posited that PZA may contribute uniquely to tuberculosis therapy by killing the bacilli in this state, wherein they are not vulnerable to the other agents which only act on proliferating bacilli (88). To test this hypothesis, Heifets and Lindholm-Levy (7) conducted an elegant study in which tubercle bacilli were induced into a viable but "semidormant" state by lowering the pH of the medium to 4.8. In this environment, PZA at a concentration of 50 μg/mL caused a 1,000-fold reduction in the bacillary population, representing 99.9% killing. However, given the unusual circumstances entailed, the authors elected to refer to this as a "sterilizing" rather than a classic "bactericidal" effect.

The major side effect of PZA is **arthralgia** associated with elevated levels of serum uric acid. The active drug form, pyrazinoic acid, blocks renal tubular excretion of uric acid resulting in a predictable increase in serum urate concentrations (89). In a 1979 report from Hong Kong (90), therapy was seen to result in arthralgias most commonly affecting the shoulders, knees, fingers, feet and ankles; 73% of the patients had simultaneous involvement of two or more joints. The patients, most of whom were receiving daily PZA, most frequently complained of joint pain, two-thirds noting stiffness or limited motion and only 40% citing swelling; effusions were noted in only 9 of 70 cases. Actual acute gout was seen in only one patient. The onset of symptoms occurred during the first 3 months in 51% of the cases. In USPHS trial 21, 6 of 617 patients (1%) assigned to daily INH, RIF, and PZA had arthralgias severe enough to interrupt therapy (34). Among 125 patients in Denver, Colorado, who received PZA daily for 2 weeks, then twice weekly for 6 more weeks, there were no complaints of arthralgias (91). In one trial in Hong Kong, the risk of arthralgia was highest among those receiving PZA daily (9.2%) and less among those receiving thrice-weekly (2.7%) and twice-weekly (1.2%) treatment; these differences were statistically significant (92). In another Hong Kong trial, 6.8% of those taking PZA daily reported arthralgias, while only 2.9% of those receiving thrice-weekly treatment did so (93). An overall analysis of arthralgias among Hong Kong patients receiving PZA found 7% of those on daily, 3% on thrice-weekly, and 1% on twice-weekly regimens (94). In subsequent Hong Kong thrice-weekly therapy trials, the frequency of arthralgias was so low that it was not even noted among adverse drug reactions. These clinical findings support the pharmacological studies of Ellard and Haslam (89), which demonstrated diminished uric acid retention with intermittent PZA therapy.

Cutaneous reactions have been noted in association with PZA (94). Typically, a faintly erythematous rash with mild pruritus, the reaction rarely requires discontinuation of the drug. Symptomatic relief may be possible through antihistamine and topical lotion therapy. **Gastrointestinal tract distress** is common during the initial phase of therapy, but these symptoms generally abate. **Hepatitis,** while infrequent with the doses employed, may be quite difficult to manage (94). Most often, there is isolated elevation of the transaminase values, although in severe cases jaundice may evolve. Notable about PZA hepatitis is the extended period required for liver chemistry values to return to normal. Unlike RIF- or INH-associated hepatitis, wherein values typically normalize in 10 to 14 days, PZA-induced hepatitis may persist for 4 to 6 weeks after the drug has been discontinued, (National Jewish Hospital, Denver, CO, unpublished data).

Streptomycin

Streptomycin is an injectable agent that has played a major role in tuberculosis chemotherapy ever since its discovery in the 1940s. Streptomycin is a prototype of the aminoglycoside antibiotics, which are defined by the presence of amino sugars bound by glycosidic linkage to a central hexose nucleus. Streptomycin, like the other aminoglycosides, binds irreversibly to the bacterial 30S ribosomes, thus inhibiting protein synthesis. Streptomycin (SM) is very poorly absorbed orally and must be given parenterally. The current FDA package insert indicates only intramuscular administration. However, because of poor tolerance of prolonged intramuscular injections in emaciated patients, we at National Jewish Hospital have given SM intravenously for many years under an investigational protocol. Streptomycin so given has been well tolerated with no undue risks of phlebitis, renal toxicity, or otovestibular damage. Because of their highly polar structures, SM and the other aminoglycosides cross biological membranes very poorly; their volumes of distribution approximate the extracellular fluid compartment. Streptomycin does not penetrate the central nervous system well, even in the presence of severe meningeal inflammation. In the early days of therapy, when there were no alternatives, SM was given intrathecally to treat tuberculous meningitis.

Given for tuberculosis, SM has traditionally been employed in a once-daily schedule at 15 mg/kg up to 1,000 mg daily for persons 55 years of age or younger with normal renal function. For older persons or those weighing less than 50 kg, the maximum daily dose has been limited to 750 mg. For use in patients with renal insufficiency an initial loading dose of 5.0 to 7.5 mg/kg was given followed by the usual daily dose reduced by the following formula: daily dose × creatinine clearance/100 (95). While these guidelines are practical for the initiation of therapy, I believe that dosage and scheduling of SM or other aminoglycosides in persons with renal impairment should be guided with pharmacokinetic monitoring to avoid toxicity and maximize efficacy. Since SM assays are not readily available in most communities, an agent such as amikacin may be preferable if an aminoglycoside is indicated.

Dosage practices when SM is used in intermittent regimens have varied considerably. In their early intermittent regimen, Hudson and Sbarbaro (96) used SM at a dose of 27 mg/kg given twice weekly. Thus, the typical 60-kg patient would receive 1,620 mg of SM (810 mg intramuscularly in each buttock) every Monday and Thursday for an average of 17 months; transient circumoral numbness was common, but only 9 of 85 patients reported ataxia, and no hearing loss or nephrotoxicity was reported. By contrast, the dosage of SM in the BMRC trials was typically 1,000 mg twice or thrice weekly. When used in highly potent regimens (such as INH, RIF, plus PZA or EMB), higher dosage may not be needed. However, when SM or other aminoglycosides are employed without the benefit of these other highly potent drugs (e.g., for cases of multidrug-resistant tuberculosis or mycobacterioses other than tuberculosis), higher dosage with intermittent scheduling may offer enhanced antimycobacterial activity without significantly increased toxicity (see Chapter 11). Three recent analyses of extended-interval (daily) dosing versus multiple daily dosing of aminoglycoside antibiotics concluded broadly that efficacy was comparable and toxicity the same or slightly less (97–99); two editorials accompanied these reviews, one endorsing daily therapy (100) and the other expressing skepticism (101). I would suggest that while the data for toxicity with *once-daily* versus 8- or 12-hour dosing intervals may be marginal, the published experience with *thrice- or twice-weekly* dosing clearly suggests reduced morbidity.

A single 1,000-mg dose given to an adult with normal renal function results in a peak serum concentration between 35 and 45 μg/mL (23). If given intravenously in a fluid volume of 100 mL over 30 minutes, the peak level occurs typically between 30 and 60 minutes and is 15% to 20% higher than the intramuscular route. Our experience suggests that both the renal and eighth-nerve toxicities of SM and other aminoglycosides are more closely related to trough levels and dosage intervals than to peak levels. Hence, I presently advocate intermittent scheduling of these drugs in typical cases of tuberculosis, even for *hospitalized* patients.

The range of MICs for 39 wild-type strains of *M. tuberculosis* for SM in broth or agar ranged from 0.25 to 2 μg/mL (102). MBCs for four strains ranged between 0.5 and 2.0 μg/mL, very close to the inhibitory concentrations (11).

The ranges of MICs and MBCs noted for amikacin, kanamycin, and capreomycin are very close to those of SM cited above. Examining these criteria alone, more or less comparable utility against tuberculosis would be predicted. Thus, the choice of a parenteral agent might be made on the basis of the following considerations:

- *Drug resistance:* proven or potential.
- *Availability:* SM was in limited supply in the United States from 1991 to 1993 because of manufacturing interruption. Currently, it is available at no charge from Pfizer (New York, N.Y.), but this entails special ordering and additional forms.
- *Toxicity:* Amikacin or kanamycin is relatively more ototoxic, while SM has more vestibular effects. While neither toxic effect is desirable, high-frequency hearing loss seems better tolerated than ataxia by most patients. Functionally, monitoring audiometry is more practical and quantitative than assessing vestibular function.
- *Expense.* The "average wholesale price"—a standard marker of drug cost—in 1998 for kanamycin was $5.60/g; for capreomycin, $25.34/g; and for amikacin, $65 to $127/g. However, if the drugs are to be given intravenously, the associated costs for equipment, dilutional solutions, preparation, and administration usually exceed the cost of the medication (103). Prices of amikacin are falling; check local costs.
- *Route of administration.* Amikacin and kanamycin are already FDA approved for intravenous use. Streptomycin use intravenously requires an investigational protocol. Kanamycin and, to a lesser extent, amikacin are extremely painful via the intramuscular route.

Toxicity from SM may entail vestibular dysfunction with ataxia and/or hearing loss, both of which are irreversible. However, used for 2 months on a twice-or thrice-weekly schedule in patients 50 years of age or younger with normal renal function, no prior treatment with aminoglycoside antibiotics, and normal baseline vestibuloauditory function, such toxicity is extremely uncommon. Thus, monitoring of hearing and vestibular function under these conditions is not required. However, if SM or other aminoglycosides are to be used for longer periods, in more intensive scheduling, in higher than usual doses, or among persons with impaired renal or vestibuloauditory function, pharmacokinetic surveillance of antibiotic concentrations, monthly audiograms, and bimonthly assessment of vestibular function should be performed (see Chapter 11 for more complete discussion).

Nephrotoxicity from SM is slightly less common than with the other aminoglycoside agents. Nonetheless, baseline and periodic surveillance of urinalysis, blood urea nitrogen values, and creatinine values is indicated. If detected early, most nephrotoxicity is reversible. The propensity for nonsteroidal antiinflammatory drugs to act synergistically with aminoglycoside antibiotics in causing renal dysfunction should be kept in mind when employing these drugs.

Overall, there appears to be a modest role for SM in contemporary short-course chemotherapy. The most instructive study of SM's utility was performed in the two Hong Kong thrice-weekly studies. In Hong Kong thrice-weekly trial 1, SM was given thrice weekly for 6 months accompanying INH, RIF, and PZA in regimen 36 and INH, RIF, PZA, plus EMB in regimen 35. By comparison, in Hong Kong thrice-weekly trial 2, SM was only given for 4 months in regimens 40 to 42, and no SM was used in regimen 43. Although there was not a statistically significant difference in the outcomes with or without SM, the only treatment failures during any of the INH-, RIF-, and PZA-containing regimens were in regimen 43 (those who did not receive any SM); in addition, all four of these patients developed drug resistance. Similarly, omitting SM in Poland trial 3 (regimen 50 vs. regimen 49) was associated with a 1.7% rate of failure to convert; also, in the Brazilian INH, RIF, and PZA 6-month protocols (regimens 63 and 64), there was a 4.6% rate of failure to convert. Even more impressive was the observation that the highest relapse rates of any of the INH-, RIF-, and PZA-containing regimens in the Hong Kong thrice-weekly trials was, again, regimen 43. Thus, while the differences were minor and did not achieve statistical significance, the trends indicate that adding SM to the three oral agents during the initial phase may modestly enhance the outcome. Because the differences are small, clinicians need to consider community and individual patient issues in choosing to use SM.

Ethambutol is commonly used as the fourth drug to accompany INH, RIF, and PZA in short-course regimens. However, in an aggregate analysis of the 6-month regimens presented in Table 10.5, relapse rates were modestly lower (5.6%) when SM rather than EMB (9%) was the fourth agent. Factors favoring the use of SM (or another aminoglycoside) include a high prevalence of initial drug resistance, very extensive disease, the potential utility of a drug injection as a justification for directly observed therapy (DOT) ("the leash effect"), potential malabsorption of the oral medications, and inability initially to deliver the oral drugs because of obtundation or gastrointestinal tract dysfunction.

Ethambutol

Ethambutol (EMB) is a singular compound, not related to any other family of antimicrobial agents. Synthesized in a directed search for antituberculosis drugs, d-ethylenediimino-di-l-butanol was reported first in 1961 (104).

Ethambutol showed considerable effect in the East African early-BA study, reducing the number of bacilli in sputum over 14 days at a rate second only to INH (6). In the BACTEC system, MICs for susceptible strains of *M. tuberculosis* generally ranged from 0.95 to 7.5 μg/mL (105); MBCs determined in this study ranged from 3.8 to 60 μg/mL. Ethambutol is well absorbed orally, reaching peak levels in 2 to 3 hours; food does not interfere with EMB uptake. Peak levels correlate with dosage, 15 mg/kg resulting in levels from 3 to 4 μg/mL; 25 mg/kg, from 4 to 6 μg/mL; and 50 mg/kg, from 8 to 12 μg/mL (106,107). Ethambutol is largely cleared by the kidneys, and dosage adjustment must be performed for patients with renal impairment (108).

Early experience employing high dosage ranging from 30 to 75 mg/kg daily was associated with significant optic neuritis and vision impairment (109). However, subsequent studies showed that by reducing the daily dose to 15–25 mg/kg, the ocular toxicity could be nearly eliminated while retaining antituberculosis activity comparable to PAS or PZA (110,111). Because it was much more readily tolerated than PAS and did not produce hepatitis, as did PZA, EMB eventually replaced these agents as an oral drug to accompany INH. Throughout the 1970s and early 1980s, standard treatment of tuberculosis in the United States consisted of 18 months of daily INH and EMB with an initial 2-month course of SM.

Sbarbaro switched from SM to EMB in the early 1970s in his supervised, intermittent program. In 1976, the Denver group reported a series of 81 patients who had received INH and EMB twice weekly for 18 months after an initial 2-month phase of daily treatment; EMB was used at 50 mg/kg and given as a single dose each Monday and Thursday (112). There were no treatment failures and no relapses, and no ocular toxicity was detected by symptom review and monthly testing of visual and color acuity.

Studies of EMB activity in various dynamic in vitro models have indicated that high concentrations of EMB (10 μg/mL) have considerable BA against *M. tuberculosis* (113). Since these high concentrations were achievable with the dosages employed in intermittent therapy, there appeared to be a role for EMB in short-course, twice- or thrice-weekly treatment. However, the available data largely indicate that, for patients with drug-susceptible tuberculosis, EMB contributes only modestly in regimens that employ INH, RIF, and PZA. The most favorable account of EMB's activity in short-course chemotherapy was seen in USPHS trial 21; in this study, EMB was added initially to regimens of INH/RIF/PZA or INH/RIF for persons at risk for drug resistance (34). EMB use was associated with more rapid sputum conversion rates, decreased relapse rates, and lower adverse reaction rates; but because of sociodemographic variables among the EMB-treated group, the implications of these findings are unclear. An 8-month regimen studied in the Philippines—1 month of daily INH/RIF/PZA/EMB followed by 7 months of twice-weekly high-dose INH/PZA/EMB—yielded disappointing results, indicating inferentially the lack of sterilizing effect of EMB even in a 50 mg/kg twice-weekly dosage (114).

The major utility of EMB as demonstrated in the BMRC trials is for cases with initial drug resistance to INH and/or SM (115). Indeed, the primary effect of EMB in this setting is to prevent treatment failure and further acquisition of drug resistance. Thus, in communities in which there is any real dimension of drug resistance or for an individual who is at identifiable risk for initial resistance, EMB should be added during the initial phase of treatment until drug susceptibility is established (116). As noted above (see "Streptomycin"), SM appears slightly more potent than EMB as a fourth drug to accompany INH, RIF, and PZA.

Thiacetazone

Known also as TB-1, thiacetazone (THA) was developed through the efforts of Gerhard Domagk, who heroically conducted studies in Germany throughout World War II seeking a cure for tuberculosis (117). Domagk, who had previously won a Nobel Prize for his role in the discovery of Prontosil, the predecessor of the sulfonamide antibiotics, recognized around 1940 that a component of the sulfa agents, the thiosemicarbazone moiety, had potential as a tuberculosis medication. Had it not been for the disruption of his research by continued Allied bombing, he may well have preceded Waksman as the father of tuberculosis chemotherapy. Nonetheless, by 1946 reports of THA's clinical efficacy were published (118).

Thiacetazone was shown subsequently to have modest activity against tuberculosis, roughly equivalent to that of PAS. Being very inexpensive (synthesized directly as a petrochemical product), it has enjoyed widespread use in the developing nations accompanying INH, typically given for one year with a brief initial course of SM (119). The drug was recently used in the continuation phase of a 6-month regimen employed in Tanzania (120); by adding THA to INH during the last 4 months, relapse rates were reduced from 11% to 2.9%.

Limited data are available on the in vitro activity and pharmacokinetics of THA. Heifets and Lindholm-Levy (121) determined that MICs for 15 wild-type strains of *M. tuberculosis* ranged from 0.08 to 1.2 μg/mL (121). The maximum concentration following the usual oral dose of 150 mg ranges between 1 and 4 μg/mL (122).

Thiacetazone has considerable side effects and substantial toxicity. This drug is similar in structure to a second-line tuberculosis drug, ethionamide, and has a similar profile of intolerance including nausea, vomiting, abdominal distress, and anorexia (123). In addition, when given with SM, THA appears to result in side effects or toxicity that is nominally associated with the aminoglycoside, namely, dizziness, giddiness, vertigo, ataxia, tinnitus, and deafness (123). Furthermore, THA was noted to delay the reversal of the usual anemia of tuberculosis seen with other treatment regimens (123). Most unfavorably, the drug was associated with severe dermatological reactions, including occasionally lethal erythema multiforme or toxic epidermal necrolysis (123). Overall, the side effects and toxicity of THA have been so extensive that only its affordability and ease of administration (it has been compounded with INH in a single formulation containing 300 mg of INH and 150 mg of THA) have kept it in use. Three recent considerations, however, have cast doubts on this drug's future utilization. First, an analysis by the World Bank and the World Health Organization has indicated that short-course multi-drug regimens are more cost-effective in the long term because of lower failure and relapse rates (124). Second, the risk from major cutaneous hypersensitivity reactions to THA among persons with HIV infection is extremely high, ranging from 20% (125) to 39% (126). While some authorities have argued that the incidence of major dermatological reactions is not great enough to exclude THA from primary drug regimens in Africa, others have indicated that further use of this agent—for reasons of both safety and efficacy—is no longer acceptable (see Chapter 8 for a more thorough discussion). Third, as the prevalence of drug resistance increases—most notably, to INH—the efficacy of the INH-THA regimen declines. Nonetheless, it seems probable that because of meager resources, many impoverished nations will continue to employ this agent until improved assets are made available to them.

CHOICE OF SHORT-COURSE CHEMOTHERAPY REGIMENS

Question: What does the periodicity of Earth's rotation on its axis as it revolves around the sun have to do with tuberculosis chemotherapy?

Answer: Nothing.

The reluctance of clinicians to change from daily to intermittent treatment of patients with tuberculosis seems in large measure to reflect a visceral reaction that to do so will "weaken" the therapeutic effect. There is, in fact, abundant evidence that, with the available medications, treatment given twice or thrice weekly is just as efficacious as daily, is very probably less toxic, significantly reduces the cost of medications, and greatly facilitates supervision of treatment to overcome nonadherence with medication. Table 10.6 displays selected 6-month regimens given for pulmonary tuberculosis, generally sputum smear positive. These regimens are stratified according to the schedules of treatment, including daily, daily-switching-to-intermittent, and all-intermittent. As readily appreciated, there is no loss of efficacy with intermittent therapy and the number of days of treatment (doses) is reduced substantially. The approximate costs for the drugs entailed in some of these regimens were calculated as follows in 1990 (91): Among the daily regimens, the cost for regimen 52 was $192; for regimen 55, $266; and for regimen 38, $757. For the daily-to-intermittent regimens, the cost for regimen 48 was $215 and for 53, $113. Among the all-intermittent regimens, the cost for regimen 36 was $250 and for regimen 37, $476. Indeed, the Denver regimen (regimen 53), which entails 5.5 months of twice-weekly treatment and a total of only 62 doses, costs less than any other proven regimen except the Arkansas regimen (regimen 53), which is acceptable only in populations with a very low prevalence of drug resistance and favorable adherence behaviors. A subsequent analysis indicated that, even allowing for the personnel costs of directly observed therapy (DOT), the cost of the 62-dose Denver regimen was less than a 6-month daily regimen, such as regimen 52 or

TABLE 10.6. *Relative efficacy of selected daily, daily to intermittent, and all-intermittent 6-month regimens employing isoniazid, rifampin, pyrazinamide, and/or other drugs*

Study (ref. no.)	Regimen number[a]	Regimen[b]	Days of treatment (no.)	Relapse (%)
Daily				
EA No. 5 (1)	24	2 IRPS/4 IR	182	2.4
USPHS-21 (2)	52	2 IRP/4 IR	182	3.5
Sing. No. 2 (3)	54	2 IRPS/4 IR	182	2.5
BTA No. 2 (4)	55	2 IRPS/4 IR	182	0.8
HK-TIW No.1 (5)	38	6 IRPE	182	3.8
Daily to intermittent				
Sing. No. 3(6)	60	2 IRPS/4 I_3R_3	113	2.1
	61	1 IRPS/5 I_3R_3	96	2.1
Poland No. 2 (7)	48	2 IRPS/4 I_2R_2	96	0.0
Poland No. 3 (8)	49	2 IRP/4 I_2R_2	96	1.8
Brazil (9)	63	2 IRP/4 I_2R_2	96	4.1
Denver (10)	53	0.5 IRPS/1.5 $I_2R_2P_2S_2$/4 I_2R_2	62	2.0
All intermittent				
HK-TIW No. 1 (5)	36	6 $I_3R_3P_3S_3$	78	1.3
	37	6 $I_3R_3P_3E_3$	78	4.4
HK-TIW No. 2 (11)	41	6 I_3R_3; 4 P_3S_3	78	4.4
	42	6 I_3R_3; 2 P_3; 4 S_3	78	2.7
East Germany (12)	58	6 $I_2R_2P_2S_2$	52	0.0

[a] See Table 10.5.
[b] Drugs given daily unless noted by subscript, which indicates day/week.

1. East and Central Africa/British Medical Research Council. East and Central Africa/British Medical Research Council Fifth Collaborative Study: controlled clinical trial of four short-course regimens of chemotherapy (three 6-month and one 8-month) for pulmonary tuberculosis—final report. *Tubercle* 1986;67:5–15.
2. Snider DE Jr, Long MW, Cross FS, Farer LS. Six-month isoniazid-rifampin therapy for pulmonary tuberculosis: report of a United States Public Health Service cooperative trial. *Am Rev Respir Dis* 1984;129:573–579.
3. Singapore Tuberculosis Service/British Medical Research Council. Long-term follow-up of a clinical trial of 6-month and 4-month regimens of chemotherapy in the treatment of pulmonary tuberculosis. *Am Rev Respir Dis* 1986;133:779–783.
4. British Thoracic Association. A controlled trial of six months chemotherapy in pulmonary tuberculosis: second report—results during the 24 months after the end of chemotherapy. *Am Rev Respir Dis* 1982;126:460–462.
5. Hong Kong Chest Service/British Medical Research Council. Five-year follow-up of a controlled trial of five 6-month regimens of chemotherapy for pulmonary tuberculosis. *Am Rev Respir Dis* 1987;136:1339–1342.
6. Singapore Tuberculosis Service/British Medical Research Council. Five-year follow-up of a clinical trial of three 6-month regimens of chemotherapy given intermittently in the continuation phase in the treatment of pulmonary tuberculosis. *Am Rev Respir Dis* 1988;137:1147–1150.
7. Snider DE Jr, Rogowski J, Zierski M, Bek E, Long MW. Successful intermittent treatment of smear-positive pulmonary tuberculosis in 6 months: a cooperative study in Poland. *Am Rev Respir Dis* 1982;125:265–267.
8. Snider DE Jr, Graczyk J, Bek E, Rogowski J. Supervised 6 month treatment of newly diagnosed pulmonary tuberculosis using isoniazid, rifampin, and pyrazinamide with and without streptomycin. *Am Rev Respir Dis* 1984;130:1091–1094.
9. Castelo A, Goihman S, Dalboni MA, et al. Comparison of daily and twice-weekly regimens to treat pulmonary tuberculosis. *Lancet* 1989;2:1173–1176.
10. Cohn DL, Catlin BJ, Peterson KL, Judson FN, Sbarbaro JA. A 62-dose, 6-month therapy for pulmonary and extrapulmonary tuberculosis: a twice-weekly, directly observed, and cost-effective regimen. *Ann Intern Med* 1990;112:407–415.
11. Hong Kong Chest Service/British Medical Research Council. Controlled trial of 2, 4, and 6 months of pyrazinamide in 6-month, three-times weekly regimens for smear-positive pulmonary tuberculosis, including an assessment of a combined preparation of isoniazid, rifampin, and pyrazinamide: results at 30 months. *Am Rev Respir Dis* 1991;143:700–706.
12. Eule H, Beck H, Evers H, et al. Daily and intermittent short-course chemotherapy using four drugs in recently detected bacillary pulmonary tuberculosis. *Bull Int Union Tuberc* 1982;57:63.

Abbreviations are expanded in Table 10.5 footnote.

57, because of fewer doses of expensive drugs and reduced need to monitor response to therapy, since all doses were supervised (127).

Functionally, it has been argued that daily self-administered therapy has a built-in "fudge factor," namely, if the patients forget some of their doses, there is enough overage in the daily schedule that the outcome will not be adversely impacted. While this is undoubtedly true, it seems unacceptable that we concede this uncertain, even chaotic principle as a fixed element in the therapy of this complex disease. The effectiveness and numerous advantages of intermittent DOT are vital elements in contemporary tuberculosis treatment.

Principles of Therapy

There is no single best tuberculosis chemotherapy regimen today. As can be seen from a survey of Table 10.5, there are many options that might serve an individual patient or community particularly well. The principles that must be kept in mind include the following:

- **Efficacy:** Will the regimen act promptly to bring the patient's disease under control?
- **Toxicity:** Is the drug combination the least likely to result in organ damage and still achieve the other goals of therapy?
- **Acceptability:** Aside from overt toxicity, are the subjective side effects of therapy minimal?
- **Deliverability:** For those patients among whom nonadherence is a likely issue, how practical is the regimen schedule in terms of allowing health care workers to oversee medication delivery?
- **Adequacy:** Given the possibility of initial drug resistance, does the regimen employ a sufficient number of potent agents to reasonably ensure the prevention of further acquisition of resistance?
- **Enduring effect:** Having produced an initial response, what is the likelihood of relapse once treatment is halted?

Illustrative Cases

Perhaps the best way to examine the various treatment options would be to consider various hypothetical patients and review the factors in choosing regimens.

Case 1

Mrs. B is a 79-year-old widow who has resided in a nursing home in Iowa since the death of her husband 3 years ago. After 4 months of continuous cough and a 10-pound weight loss, she is found to have a dense fibronodular infiltrate without cavity in the right upper lobe of her lungs. One of three sputum smears is positive for acid-fast bacillus (AFB); culture is pending. She lived on a farm most of her life; the only recollection of "TB" she has is her grandmother, who immigrated from Europe and died of "consumption" when Mrs. B was in primary school. Mrs. B was in good health except for chronic osteoarthritis involving her hands, shoulders, and knees, for which she took nonsteroidal antiinflammatory drugs.

On the reasonable assumption that she is suffering from tuberculosis, choose one of the *initial regimens* below:

A. INH, RIF, PZA, and SM daily?
B. INH, RIF, PZA, and SM thrice weekly?
C. INH, RIF, and EMB daily?
D. INH and RIF daily?

I would opt for choice C, with D a possibility as well. Although it is unlikely that Mrs. B harbors a drug-resistant strain, I would be comforted using a benign third drug until the laboratory assured me that the strain was drug-susceptible *M. tuberculosis.* Also in favor of the addition of EMB is the real possibility that this infection is *Mycobacterium kansasii* or *Mycobacterium avium* complex; in both of those cases, EMB is a very useful agent. I would not add PZA because there is a very good possibility that the drug would aggravate her arthritis and/or upset her stomach, and PZA is not active against mycobacteria other than tuberculosis. Further, in Mrs. B's case, a more rapid response to treatment is not important. Likewise, SM would be an uncomfortable and potentially toxic agent to employ empirically in a 79-year-old person.

When the laboratory confirmed (in several weeks) that the etiological agent was *M. tubercu-*

losis, drug-susceptible, I would stop the EMB and treat her with INH and RIF through a total of 9 months. Since she is in a nursing home where forgetfulness or nonadherence should not be a factor in treatment, she might receive daily therapy administered by the staff there (see regimen 1, 2, 14, or 15 in Table 10.5), or—if it is more tolerable for her—twice-weekly medication (see regimen 3).

Incidentally, even though her sputum smear was not strongly positive, a contact investigation for newly transmitted infection must be performed in the nursing home (see Chapter 3).

Case 2

Joe is a 38-year-old homeless single man who is admitted to the municipal hospital after experiencing gross hemoptysis in the men's shelter. His course in the hospital was complicated by delirium tremens as he withdrew from long-term alcohol abuse. A chest x-ray revealed a large cavity in the left apex, and sputa were found to be strongly positive on smear for AFB. Physical examination demonstrated hepatomegaly but no stigmata of cirrhosis; the liver panel was remarkable for fivefold to eightfold elevations of the transaminases above normal levels, alkaline phosphatase values twofold to fourfold above the normal range, and normal bilirubin, prothrombin, and cholesterol values; platelet counts ranged from 125,000 to 175,000 per cu. mm.

Which of the following regimens would you choose to initiate his antituberculosis therapy?

A. INH, RIF, PZA, and SM daily?
B. INH, RIF, and EMB daily?
C. INH, SM, and EMB daily?
D. RIF, PZA, SM, and EMB daily?

Certainly, this is a complex decision. One of the important issues is whether there has been drug-resistant tuberculosis noted in the men's shelter system recently; if so, regimen D would be attractive, since the most common resistance is to INH. If not, a vital issue is whether one can give three potentially hepatotoxic drugs—INH, RIF, and PZA—to an individual who presumably has alcoholic hepatitis. Multiple studies indicate that alcoholics do not have higher rates of drug-induced hepatitis from INH and RIF. There remains, however, another aspect of this issue: whether an individual with alcoholic or other liver disease has sufficient hepatic reserve to withstand the effects of drug-induced liver damage. If a person has marginal reserve (as indicated by poor synthetic function [i.e., low albumin and low cholesterol values and prolonged prothrombin time]), I would be reluctant to employ the combination of INH and RIF, which appears to place an individual at higher risk of hepatitis than the use of either drug alone (see above, Table 10.3). Drug-induced hepatitis in a person with impaired reserve may, even when detected early, provoke liver failure with potentially profound consequences. PZA does not contribute measurably beyond INH and RIF to the risk of hepatic damage (128). Therefore, among patients with adequate reserve liver function, I would opt for regimen A with this near-term objective: rapid impact on his sputum culture status in order that he be rendered noninfectious and safe for placement in a community residential facility as soon as his general health allows. A second element in this choice is the long-term concern about losing the patient from treatment: unattached male patients are at very high risk for nonadherence or loss from treatment. By employing the most active combination available, we can reduce to the minimum the duration of therapy required for enduring cure.

After starting the patient on the four drugs, INH/RIF/PEA/SM, the choice of continuation therapy will depend largely on his ongoing social circumstances and available tuberculosis treatment services. The cardinal issue is ensuring continuous treatment. Before he is discharged from the hospital, case workers must develop a clear plan for domicile and therapy. Treatment options following 2 weeks of inpatient therapy include the following:

A. INH, RIF, PZA, and SM *twice weekly* for the next 1.5 months, then INH and RIF *twice weekly* for 4 months (regimen 53, Table 10.5).
B. INH, RIF, PZA, and SM *daily* for the next 1.5 months, then INH and RIF *daily* for 4 months (regimens 24 and 54, Table 10.5).
C. INH, RIF, PZA, and SM *daily* for the next 1.5 months, then INH and RIF *twice weekly* for 4 months (regimens 48 and 49, Table 10.5).

D. INH, RIF, PZA, and SM *daily* for the next 1.5 months, then INH and RIF *thrice weekly* for 4 months (regimen 60, Table 10.5).

All of these options are proven, efficacious regimens; any one of them is potentially appropriate. However, given concerns about the deliverability and acceptability of the treatment, my choice would be option A. Each dose of medication should be directly observed by a health care worker, and since my clinic and outreach assets are limited, I want to minimize the number of encounters without jeopardizing results. Regimen 53 would require only 48 additional encounters, easing the burden on the health care staff and the patient. Option B would involve 168 additional encounters or—if self-administered—rely on the patient's compliance, a dubious proposition at best. Option C would involve 48 consecutive daily visits followed by 36 twice-weekly encounters, a total of 84 contacts. While some authorities might argue that extending the initial daily regimen strengthens the antituberculosis activity of the treatment and improves the patient's chances to cure if he absconds from treatment (see regimens 64–79, Table 10.5), the available data indicate no or only marginal improvement in bacteriological response or relapse rates with daily versus thrice- or twice-weekly administration of these potent drugs. Regarding options C or D, review of the data indicates that twice-weekly continuation regimens are comparably potent and obviously require fewer encounters than thrice-weekly regimens.

Case 3

Roberta is a 32-year-old Filipina who came to the United States in 1987. After the recent birth of a child, she began to experience fatigue, then malaise and cough. Her chest x-ray revealed fibronodular shadows in both apices; computed tomography demonstrated a thick-walled cavity in the extreme apex of the right lobe of the lung. Sputum smears were 2+ to 3+ positive for AFB; cultures are pending. Select an initial regimen for her:

A. INH, RIF, PZA, and SM *daily?*
B. INH, RIF, PZA, and EMB *daily?*
C. INH, RIF, and EMB daily?
D. INH and RIF daily?

Because Roberta comes from the Philippines, there is a substantial risk of drug resistance (127). Therefore, initial therapy should consist of at least four drugs. INH and SM have been used most extensively in the Philippines; hence, resistance to one or both of these agents is the most common pattern seen (114). Consequently I would choose regimen B: INH, RIF, PZA, and EMB. Ethambutol, while not shown to have substantial sterilizing activity, did show real utility in preventing treatment failure and progressive drug resistance in BMRC trials (see above). Regimen C, by omitting PZA in the initial phase of therapy, would commit us to a 9-month rather than 6-month course of treatment. Regimen D could be totally unacceptable for use in a patient like Roberta, for—if there were initial resistance to INH—the two-drug regimen would pose a very high risk for acquired resistance to RIF before therapy could be amended.

At 4 weeks, the laboratory reported the organism as *M. tuberculosis* with direct susceptibility testing demonstrating high-level resistance to INH and SM. The patient has improved dramatically with defervescence, cessation of cough, and an 8-pound weight gain. She no longer can spontaneously produce sputum, but her most recent specimens, taken at 3 and 4 weeks of treatment, showed only scanty numbers of bacilli on smear. Which of the following treatment options would you select at this time:

A. INH, RIF, PZA, and EMB *daily* through 12 months?
B. INH, RIF, PZA, and EMB *daily* through 6 months?
C. INH, RIF, PZA, and EMB *thrice weekly* through 6 months?
D. RIF, PZA, and EMB *thrice weekly* through 6 months?

One report called for 12 months of therapy with RIF, EMB, ±PZA for patients with INH-resistant tuberculosis (129). However, the BMRC data have demonstrated that, despite initial resistance to INH and/or SM, 6-month regimens which incorporate RIF, PZA, and EMB or SM throughout the bulk or whole of the period result in very low failure and relapse rates (115). In the first Hong Kong thrice-weekly study there was only one failure of 104 and 3 relapses of 103 (2.9%) among patients with INH and/or SM resistance during a 5-year follow-up (Hong Kong thrice-weekly trial 1, regimens 35–39). By contrast, in the second Hong Kong thrice-weekly trial (wherein SM therapy was reduced to only 4 months and PZA therapy shortened to 2 or 4 months among many patients [regimens 41–43]), there was a 4.4% rate of treatment failure and an 8.1% relapse rate among 137 patients. Thus, I believe regimen A would be excessive. Regimens B, C, and D all would be appropriate for Roberta's treatment in terms of drugs and duration. However, there is generally no utility to administering INH in the presence of high-level resistance, only the potential hazard of drug toxicity—particularly hepatitis. Thus, my choice would be regimen D, which deletes INH and employs the three active oral agents on an easily supervised thrice-weekly schedule. If the patient were very ill or had very extensive disease, one might add one of the other aminoglycoside or fluoroquinolone antibiotics to strengthen the regimen.

Fixed-Dose Combinations

Compounding multiple medications in a single preparation has been proposed as a means to reduce nonadherence with prescribed therapy (116,130,131). By incorporating two or three of the major drugs into single pills or capsules, it has been argued that patients are more likely to take their medications regularly, since the process will entail fewer pills and a simpler routine—both factors proven to impact favorably on drug-taking behavior (132). More importantly, the fixed-dose combinations (FDCs) would prevent "selective discontinuation" of one or more of the drugs, which, in addition to causing treatment failures, promotes the selection of drug-resistant mutants. Currently, in North America and Europe two popular combinations are produced, INH and RIF (Rifamate), and INH, RIF, and PZA (Rifater). Rifamate and Rifater are both currently available in the United States.

Careful studies have documented comparable pharmacokinetic profiles for INH, RIF, and PZA when they were given singly, simultaneously as individual formulations, or as a fixed combination (133,134). A second study (134) confirmed the bioavailability of two different INH + RIF + PZA formulations, one designed for daily use (Rifater 2), the other for thrice-weekly use (Rifater 3). In the former, the ratios for INH, RIF, and PZA were 50, 120, and 300 mg per tablet, respectively, and in the latter, 125, 100, and 375 mg, respectively.

Subsequently, a study in Hong Kong compared patient acceptance, compliance, and adverse drug reactions when receiving the FDC thrice-weekly formulation (INH, RIF, and PZA: 125, 100, and 375 mg, respectively) with comparable doses separately (135). Notable findings included better acceptability of the combined formulation with fewer complaints that the pills stuck in the throat or required special fluids to assist with swallowing. Toxicity was similar. Compliance was obscured by the fact that the patients took all medications under observation. However, surrogate markers suggested similar adherence behavior. Subsequently, three trials have compared the performance of the combined formulation of INH + RIF + PZA with the individual drugs. In Singapore, the daily combination (Rifater 2, given during the first 1 or 2 months) performed similarly to single drugs in terms of acceptability, toxicity, and sputum conversion rates (136). However, for unclear reasons, relapse rates among those receiving Rifater 2 were significantly higher than among those receiving separate drugs: 8 of 128 (6.3%) versus 2 of 137 (1.5%) ($p = .04$). In Hong Kong, the thrice-weekly formulation (Rifater 3) was studied (137). The acceptance, compliance, and adverse reactions in this study were noted above. In terms of efficacy, sputum conversion rates were similar at 1 month (69% vs. 61%) and 2 months (93% vs. 91%), slightly but not significantly in favor of the combined formulation. However, relapse rates were slightly higher among those receiving the combined formulation (14 of 273 [5.1%] vs. 20 of 559 [3.6%]), a difference that was not statistically significant. In the United States, a daily combined formulation with slightly different drug ratios (Rifater V: INH, RIF, and PZA, 75, 150, and 400 mg, respectively) was compared with separate drugs in the first 2 months of a 6-month regimen in USPHS trial 21 (34,138). Unlike the Singapore and Hong Kong trials, the USPHS study entailed self-administration of drugs, thus giving a more realistic view of treatment adherence. This study demonstrated no advantage in terms of compliance, slightly more rapid sputum conversion rates (86.6% vs. 77.7% at 2 months), modestly more adverse drug reactions requiring change of therapy (13.2% vs.6.5%), and minimally higher relapse rates (3.4% vs. 2.6%) with the FDC; neither the adverse drug reactions nor the relapse rates were statistically significant. Of note, the currently available formulation of Rifater employs a different ratio of component drugs. Each tablet contains 50 mg of INH, 120 mg of RIF, and 300 mg of PZA. Thus, the average adult patient weighing 55 kg or more, on a daily therapy regimen would receive six tablets for a dose of 300 mg of INH, 720 mg of RIF, and 1,500 mg of PZA. The relatively higher dose of RIF reflects pharmacokinetic data indicating lesser absorption of RIF in the FDC than in single-drug preparations (information from Hoechst-Marian-Roussel). Patients weighing 45 to 54 kg should take five tablets of Rifater daily, and those weighing 44 kg or less are to take four tablets daily.

Overall, the utility of FDC treatment remains more theoretical than proven. Certainly, the concept is sound: it is arguably better for patients to take *none* of their medications than *some* of them and thus to breed drug resistant strains. However, the actual demonstration of this function will be difficult to prove and therefore will have to be taken as an article of faith in the near term. While it is logical to infer that an FDC like Rifater will lessen the likelihood of acquired drug resistance, this *has* been documented to occur (139). The FDCs may be modestly more expensive than single drugs, and authorities will need to consider whether the dollars are more productively spent on these preparations than on DOT. In addition, drug intolerance or toxicity has proven problematic, since patients are unable to sort out for themselves which of their medications is causing the untoward effects. Therefore, most clinicians employ single agents when assessing this issue and resuming therapy. Based on the equivocal or slightly adverse differences in outcome using combined formulations versus single drugs in DOT programs (above), it would be difficult to justify greatly increased medication expenses when drugs are given in a supervised treatment program. Thus, as the United States moves toward more DOT and confronts rising prevalences of drug resistance that require initial four-drug, not three-drug, therapy, the role for such compounds as Rifater has not yet been clearly defined. FDCs with INH/RIF/PZA *and* EMB are in use elsewhere but are not available at present in the United States. Certainly, FDCs are wholly appropriate for patients who are being entrusted to self-administered therapy. Indeed, Sbarbaro (140) has recently proposed that in countries or communities without DOT programs, FDCs be the only readily accessible form of antituberculosis medication. (In this model, patients requiring single drugs or unusual regimens would be referred to specialized centers.) It is vital, however, among persons taking FDCs, that care be taken to ensure that patients do not systematically take fewer tablets than appropriate for their weights. Such suboptimal therapy exposes patients to treatment failure and acquired resistance.

There is another potentially important role for FDCs, namely, in helping to reduce the likelihood of *provider* prescribing errors. The various regimens noted above use various schedules of daily, thrice-weekly, and twice-weekly therapy. In these situations, the relative dosing of the component drugs changes (see above). Rather than having providers recalculate the dosing for different medications when the schedule changes from daily to intermittent, it would be much easier to have an array of combined formulations suitable for the diverse rhythms (141). At this time, the Rifater formulations for thrice- or twice-weekly dosing are not available in the United States.

Special Circumstances and Chemotherapy

The great majority of patients in the treatment trials cited above had sputum smear–positive pulmonary tuberculosis without particular coexisting diseases or complicating conditions. Therefore, it is appropriate to consider the extent to which special circumstances influence the applicability of these data to various patients, including extrapulmonary tuberculosis (XPTB), sputum smear–negative pulmonary tuberculosis, pulmonary tuberculosis associated with silicosis, tuberculosis in immunocompromised hosts (other than HIV-infected/AIDS patients, discussed in Chapter 8), and tuberculosis occurring in pregnancy.

Extrapulmonary Tuberculosis

In the majority of cases, XPTB involves populations of tubercle bacilli far smaller than those present in cavitary pulmonary tuberculosis. This makes the probability of drug-resistant mutants presumably lower. Nonetheless, early experience with monotherapy of XPTB—particularly with SM—tells us that inadequate regimens can result in the selection of clinically significant drug resistance.

The most problematic issues, though, in the therapy of XPTB are penetration of drugs into particular tissues and the possibility that some patients with certain forms of XPTB are cryptically impaired hosts. For example, is miliary tuberculosis a de facto indication of abnormal tuberculoimmunity? Regarding tissue penetration, the only site in which there is clear evidence of poor drug penetration is the central nervous system, which is discussed at length in Chapter 7. Regarding immune competency, based on the degree of anergy present, as well as direct studies of cellular function in those with miliary tuberculosis, it is clear that many such patients do have impaired immune function. However, except in cases where patients present in extremis, virtually all respond well to modern drug therapy. While the studies of XPTB are less clearly defined because of the lack of clear end points (such as sputum cultures in pulmonary disease), the available data strongly indicate that regimens which are curative for cavitary pulmonary disease are sufficient for virtually all cases of XPTB (142). Hence, authorities consistently endorse the standard short-course regimens for XPTB with the caveat that special attention be paid to meningeal or miliary disease (142,143). The 1994 American Thoracic Society (ATS) guidelines recommend 12 months of therapy for pediatric patients with bone/joint or central nervous system disease; however, this is based on fear of the consequence of relapse rather than objective evidence of need. Does this mean that it is unacceptable to extend the duration of treatment from 6 to 9 months for the miliary tuberculosis patient who came to medical attention extremely ill? The answer is obviously no; clinicians can and should be able to individualize treatment based on special concerns. These recommendations should be seen as indicating that, for the vast majority of cases, usual regimens will provide a lifetime cure.

Sputum Smear–Negative Pulmonary Disease

Patients with pulmonary tuberculosis with multiple **negative sputum smears** before treatment usually have substantially less extensive disease than the patients in the studies cited in Table 10.5. Hence, it has been suggested that they might be treated with shorter than usual regimens (144,145). Once again, the BMRC and their international colleagues have performed the studies which enlighten us on this issue. Relevant are two large studies to which I will refer as Hong Kong Sputum Smear Negative Study 1 (HK-SSN 1) (146) and Hong Kong Sputum Smear Negative Study 2 (HK-SSN 2) (147). These trials, among the most complex and subtle of all tuberculosis therapy studies, contain important information on the natural history and treatment of this condition. In HK-SSN 1, 1,019 patients were identified as having chest x-rays strongly suggestive of "active" tuberculosis but had five negative sputum smears for AFB; in 655 patients all cultures were subsequently negative as well, while in 364 persons, one or more cultures were positive. Among those with negative cultures, 173 persons were assigned to "selective chemotherapy" or treatment with the standard 12-month regimen *only* if they subsequently became sputum culture positive or deteriorated clinically and/or radiographically. In essence, this group served as a control to delineate the natural history of smear- and culture-negative patients with highly suspect chest x-rays. Of this control group in the ensuing 5 years, 71 of 173 (41%) had positive sputum cultures, while another 28 (16.2%) were deemed to have active disease on clinical and/or radiographic bases—a total rate of 57%. The 2- and 3-month regimens substantially reduced the risk of activation from the control level, with only 6.2% and 3.1% developing culture-positive disease, respectively. By contrast, among the 364 patients whose smears were negative but who had one or more positive cultures, neither the 2- nor the 3-month regimen yielded acceptable results, with 22.5% and 10.3%, respectively, of those treated developing reactivations with positive sputum cultures.

In the next trial, HK-SSN 2, 1,710 smear-negative patients were studied, including 1,118 of those with negative cultures and 592 with one or more positive initial cultures (Fig. 10.2). No control group was included because of the high risk of subsequent disease seen in trial 1. Recognizing the marginal adequacy of the 2- and 3-month regimens in the second study, the 1,118 patients with negative cultures were randomly assigned to a 3-month daily, 3-month thrice-weekly, or 4-month thrice-weekly regimen. All regimens performed well with a bacteriological relapse rate less than 3% through 5 years. Among those 592 with negative smears but positive culture(s), there was randomization to 4- or 6-month regimens similar to those described above. Notably, the 4-month regimen performed very well in this setting. Thus, treating smear-negative patients for 3 to 4 months, depending on their culture results, appears appropriate as long as potent therapy, like the INH/RIF/PZA ± SM regimens in the Hong Kong trial, is used.

By comparison, smear-negative, *culture-positive* cases of pulmonary tuberculosis in Arkansas were treated using a *6-month* regimen consisting of 1 month of daily INH + RIF followed by 5 months of twice-weekly INH + RIF; this longer, less potent regimen yielded similar results with a 2.4% relapse rate (144). For smear-negative, *culture-negative* patients in Arkansas, a 4-month regimen (INH/RIF for 1 month daily, then for 3 months twice-weekly) yielded a comparably favorable outcome; among those deemed to have had active pulmonary tuberculosis, only 3 of 126 (2.4%) had reactivation during approximately 3.5 years of follow-up (145). Although the two-drug regimen noted above was comparably effective to the shorter Hong Kong regimens, such a treatment strategy would not be appropriate outside the state of Arkansas or in another area where there is a demonstrated low prevalence of drug resistance.

Silicotuberculosis

Silicotuberculosis has long been regarded as a particularly vexing therapeutic challenge. For unclear reasons, patients with silicosis and tuberculosis have been noted to respond less well to therapy than others (148). Small series of patients with silicotuberculosis who were treated successfully with RIF-containing regimens of longer than 12 months' duration were reported from Belgium in 1977 (149) and Pennsylvania in 1982 (150). The first report of short-course therapy was in 1987, from Taiwan, where 59 patients with anthracosilicosis or silicosis received the following 9-month regimen: 2 months of daily INH/RIF/PZA/SM followed by 7 months of daily INH/RIF (151). In this trial, 3 of 59 (5.1%) failed to convert while receiving therapy and 3 of 56 (5.4%) relapsed, all within 7 months of stopping treatment. No drug susceptibility data were reported to exclude primary drug resistance, and there was a possibility of nonadherence with therapy, since the last 7 months were self-administered. However, the results do suggest a negative impact of the pneumoconioses on treatment. Better results were seen in a report of tuberculosis therapy in South African gold miners among whom the prevalence of overt silicosis was not quantified (152). In this trial, a 4.5-month regimen of INH/RIF/PZA/SM was given Monday through Friday at the workplace, resulting in a relapse rate of 3.8%. It should be stressed that, while all miners had significant dust exposure, the prevalence of silicosis among this study arm is unclear. The most definitive study of the treatment of silicotuberculosis came from Hong Kong in 1991 (153). Among patients without

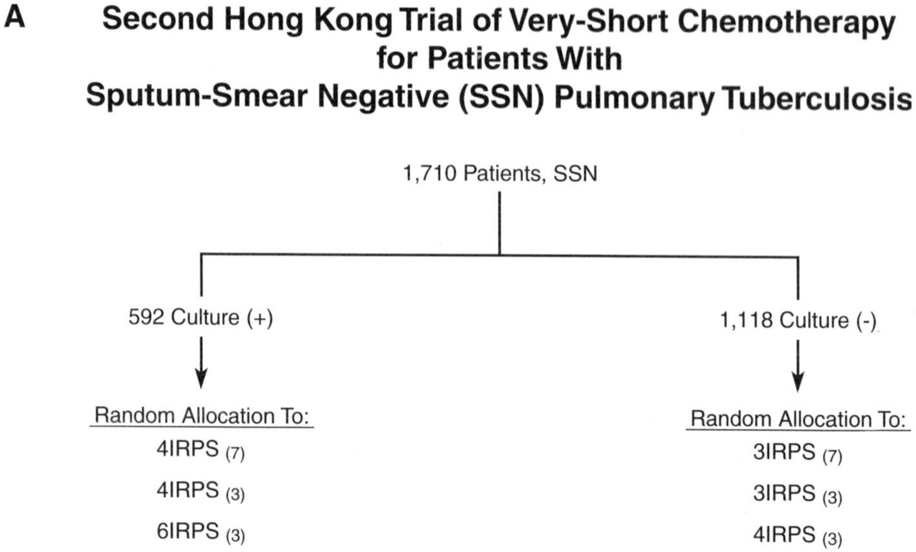

B **Results of the Second Hong Kong Trial**

Regimens and Relapse Rates

Group	4 mos. IRPS (7)	4 mos. IRPS (3)	6 mos. IRPS (3)
Smear Negative/Culture Positive			
Drug Susceptible	3% (3%)	2% (1%)	5% (2%)
Resistance to I+/or S	7% (4%)	10% (6%)	8% (4%)

Group	3 mos. IRPS (7)	3 mos. IRPS (3)	4 mos. IRPS (3)
Smear Negative/Culture Negative			
No Susceptibility Available	6% (3%)	8% (3%)	4% (1%)

(The number in parenthesis=culture positive relapses;
the other number=relapse based on radiographic and clinical features).

FIG. 10.2. **A.** Based on the first study of sputum smear–negative (SSN) cases, it was known that 2- or 3-month therapy was inadequate for patients who were either culture positive (+) or culture negative (−). Therefore, in the trial, those who were culture negative were assigned to either 3- or 4-month therapy, while those who were culture positive were assigned to 4- or 6-month therapy. **B.** Results of the treatment arms. In the first Hong Kong SSN study, 57% of control (untreated) patients had developed active tuberculosis within 5 years. Thus, the 3- or 4-month regimens in this trial have conferred considerable benefit. Hence, for patients with suspect chest x-rays, with or without symptoms, and negative initial sputum smears, one might commence therapy with a four-drug regimen and—if all of the cultures returned negative, terminate treatment at 3 months. If, on the other hand, positive cultures were reported, terminate therapy at 4 to 6 months. Note that these data do not apply to human immunodeficiency virus (HIV)–infected persons, nor would I apply this approach to patients with other immunosuppressive states. I, INH; R, RIF; P, PEA; S, SM.

prior therapy, there was initial randomization to 6 or 8 months of thrice-weekly INH/RIF/ PZA/ SM. The results were so poor with the shorter regimen that all later patients were assigned to the 8-month regimen. The initial results, including the 8-month regimen, were quite unfavorable when compared with 6-month thrice-weekly regimens among normal hosts in Hong Kong Thrice-Weekly (HK-T/W) trials 1 and 2 (Table 10.5). At 3 years' follow-up, the relapse rate in the 6-month group was 22%, and in the 8-month group, 6% to 7%. Hence, the reasonable inference to make is that therapy of silicotuberculosis should be extended beyond the usual duration. How long, though, is uncertain. As an arbitrary rule, I would propose that, for any of the successful regimens studied in patients without pneumoconiosis, the duration of chemotherapy be extended by 50%.

Tuberculosis in the Immunocompromised Host

The risk of tuberculosis is substantially increased among persons with impaired cellular immunity. Thus treatment of tuberculosis in the **immunocompromised host** is an ongoing issue. HIV infection and AIDS, because of the extraordinary relationship with tuberculosis, is covered separately in Chapter 8. Among the other more common conditions seen in association with tuberculosis are gastrointestinal tract resectional surgery associated with weight loss, solid tumors, lymphohematological neoplasias, organ transplantation, and renal failure (see Chapter 5). Because there are such diverse features among these patients, it is very difficult to perform well-controlled studies and to make valid generalizations about the management of tuberculosis in such cases. However, special considerations are appropriate. For patients with prior gastrointestinal tract resectional surgery, it is vital to ensure that there is adequate absorption of the oral medications. Many of the immunocompromised patients are taking other drugs for their underlying conditions; the potential for drug interactions, particularly in relation to RIF, should be kept in mind (see above). Most evidence suggests that persons with these immunocompromising conditions respond well to initial intensive tuberculosis chemotherapy; however, there is concern that they are at higher risk of relapse. Therefore, I believe it is appropriate to extend the duration of the continuation phase of treatment by some modest period, perhaps 2 to 3 months, in immunocompromised hosts with tuberculosis. In patients with profound immunological deficits that may be expected to persist, the question of administering indefinite "suppressive treatment" following formal chemo-therapy may arise. This is predicated on the notion that chemotherapy may not sterilize the body of tubercle bacilli but leave behind some bacilli which are profoundly inhibited but capable of resuming growth in the absence of competent immunity. No systematic data exist on the utility of this practice, but, for high-risk patients who are readily tolerant of INH, this may be an appropriate option.

Pregnancy and Lactation

The treatment of active tuberculosis during **pregnancy** entails the same principles as noted above: efficacy, toxicity, acceptability, deliverability, adequacy, and enduring effect. Of these variables, the only particular consideration relevant to pregnancy is toxicity. In an excellent review of the literature published in 1980, Snider et al. (154) concluded that previous experience demonstrated INH, RIF, EMB, and SM "to have a reasonable margin of safety when utilized during pregnancy." These authors pointed out that the evidence was most clear in support of INH and EMB and that the findings with RIF, while generally favorable, left some ambiguity regarding its safety. Also, while most cases when SM was given during pregnancy did not result in complications, there was a statistically significant risk—in the range of 15% to 30%—for auditory dysfunction in the infant because of transplacental passage of SM. They concluded that INH and EMB should be used in all cases of tuberculosis during pregnancy, that RIF should be used in cases with more extensive or dangerous disease, and that SM should *not* be used.

Subsequently, however, consideration of the potentially serious complications of *inadequate treatment of tuberculosis* led to recommendation by an ATS/CDC committee that all pregnant women be treated with INH and RIF; EMB should be used in cases at risk for initial drug resistance (116). The use of SM was strongly discouraged, and—because of inadequate data on its safety, not actual evidence of hazard—PZA usage was, similarly, not recommended.

Related to pregnancy, the issue of tuberculosis chemotherapy in the **postpartum** period was addressed in the ATS/CDC guidelines. Breastfeeding while receiving antituberculosis medications was deemed safe in view of the very modest amounts of medication that appear in the milk; Snider and Powell (155) calculated that breast-fed infants would receive no more than 20% of the usual therapeutic doses of the standard medications.

DIRECTLY OBSERVED THERAPY

Arguably the most important elements of control programs are systems to ensure reliable delivery of chemotherapy to patients with communicable pulmonary tuberculosis. For an infectious disease to persist or increase in a population, it must propagate itself among new vulnerable subjects at a rate equal to or greater than simultaneously occurring deaths or cures. In the situation of tuberculosis, early detection and treatment of persons whose respiratory secretions contain infectious particles will substantially curtail the dynamic balance of the disease in the community. Or, in the words of one astute observer, "one man's cure is several men's prevention" (156).

To provide predictable, effective therapy, society—in its own self-interest—may have to provide active outreach programs for drug delivery. This is a virtually unique model for disease management in the entire pantheon of medicine. The history of the concept, the philosophical and legal ramifications, and the field experience with DOT in tuberculosis are described below.

History

As noted in Chapter 1, the early twentieth century witnessed the development of extensive systems of institutional care—sanatoria—for patients with tuberculosis. With the advent of chemotherapy in the 1950s, sanatoria and drug treatment were first amalgamated into a program wherein medications were administered to patients housed in these facilities. However, this model was soon abandoned when it was recognized that, because of the rapid reduction in sputum bacillary counts, isolation of these persons receiving chemotherapy was not necessary to protect their contacts in the community (157,158); that such programs involved immense, unnecessary disruptions of these patients' lives; and that the expenses of maintaining these facilities were not feasible for less wealthy nations or suitable for the industrialized countries.

However, clinicians and program directors clearly saw that many patients, left to their own devices, would not take their medications with sufficient reliability to effect cures. Thus, programs of home or "domiciliary" treatment were studied. It was the desire for domiciliary care that led the BMRC consortium to examine the feasibility of intermittent regimens. However, these programs did not enjoy widespread use for a variety of reasons. Poorer nations or communities deemed them financially unachievable. Wealthier nations with more extensive levels of education believed that patients, informed of the hazards and benefits of the situation, could be persuaded to complete treatment. Other authorities argued that such measures should be reserved only for persons in whom noncompliance had been demonstrated or could be readily predicted, that such an approach was too paternalistic or an affront, that the presumption of treatment malfeasance was inconsistent with modern jurisprudence.

Sbarbaro in Denver was the earliest and most persistent advocate in North America of DOT as a standard component of a community control program (159). Recognizing that it would be impossible to oversee daily therapy, he embarked upon a model of employing 2 months of initial daily therapy given in the hospital followed by 16 to 17 months of twice-weekly treatment. Initially, the continuation phase of therapy consisted of INH and SM (96); subsequently, EMB supplanted SM (112). By 1974, he had persuaded the ATS and the CDC to endorse the option of supervised, intermittent chemotherapy (160).

Nevertheless, this approach was not generally embraced in North America or Europe, despite accumulating evidence of widespread abandonment of treatment. However, with the resurgence of tuberculosis in the United States and the rising prevalence of drug resistance, interest in this model was reawakened. Indeed, based on widening reports of the effectiveness, achievability, and—very likely—the cost-effectiveness of DOT, this approach has been endorsed as a national model of care (116) and a global standard of practice (161).

Philosophical and Legal Premises

One might readily ask why the treatment of tuberculosis has been and should be accorded such unique considerations. Obviously, concerns regarding transmission of other infectious diseases have led to legal constraints including quarantine, variably obligatory vaccinations, and exclusion from immigration. However, society has never gone so far in enforcing therapy.

In truth, treatment has not actually been mandated. In the U.S. legal system, forcing individuals to take drugs against their wishes has not been deemed acceptable. Rather, the model indicates that, if persons with potentially transmissible tuberculosis refuse to take treatment, they can and should be quarantined (isolated) to protect the public. Tuberculosis should be distinguished from sexually transmitted diseases in this vital respect: as an airborne infection, unknowing or casual sharing of air is sufficient to cause spread of this potentially lethal disease!

It is vital in this instance to contemplate some of the implications of this model. If society is to compel individuals with tuberculosis to take therapy, it becomes the responsibility of society to provide the medications and other elements (diagnostic tests and monitoring measures) of such a treatment program. Once, however, such services are made available to persons with tuberculosis, society may then reasonably expect of these individuals that they take their medications.

Sbarbaro has described this process as "chemical" quarantine: so long as patients take their medications they are presumed not to pose a public health risk. However, if they fail to appear for therapy, they are breaching their quarantine. Therefore, these individuals are in violation of their quarantine order and are subject to detention and isolation. This process has been a component of the Denver control model for over 25 years and has proven to be an important aspect of the DOT program.

Although rarely used, detention has been the "teeth" that provide the public health authorities with credibility in the community (162).

However, in order that this process meet contemporary legal standards for "due process," patients must receive initial information regarding their expected cooperation with this program. There must be explicit warnings about the consequences of their actions, including detention for nonadherence. To meet these objectives, patients with proven or suspected tuberculosis should be served with a formal quarantine notification that is read and explained to them; receipt of this quarantine notification is documented by the patients' signatures.

Clearly, tuberculosis control should not rely exclusively on this coercive threat to promote compliance. Rather, the fundamental elements should consist of patient education, facilitation, and inducement. Education helps the patients and their families to understand the nature of the disease and the importance of successful therapy, but an equally valuable aspect of the education is that the process helps the patients see their caregivers as friends and allies (163). Facilitation should include making clinical services geographically and temporally convenient. When needed, outreach workers may visit residences, schools, or places of employment (164). Treatment may be delivered in drug/alcohol rehabilitation facilities or homeless shelters (165). Inducements might include provision of transportation, social services, housing or food assistance, or—conceivably—cash payments to compensate patients for the inconvenience of making themselves regularly available for therapy (166). Sbarbaro (132) described and employed such a system with great success.

However, in order to sustain discipline it is critical that public health officers be willing and able to follow through on their mandate to protect the public from tuberculosis transmission. Virtually all states and communities have laws or regulations that empower authorities to quarantine persons deemed at risk for transmitting a communicable disease. In some instances, these laws or regulations are out of date and would not stand up to a court challenge (167). But, what is lacking, more often, is the will to pursue these remedies or the facilities to conduct a locked quarantine. Yet, if we are to succeed in the struggle against tuberculosis, communities in which the disease remains prominent must be willing to provide adequate resources to conduct these programs. Nardell et al. (165) and others have argued against the principle of standard DOT, saying that it is "herd medicine," "too coercive," or "unnecessary." It is argued that DOT programs are not feasible in [our] community. No doubt, each of these issues has some kernel of truth in various settings. However, what I ardently believe is that DOT is the most reliable way to cure patients with tuberculosis; that patients managed in DOT programs are more likely to be cured and less likely to experience relapses or acquired drug resistance; that communities that employ good DOT programs will enjoy significantly diminished rates of morbidity; and that well-run DOT programs will prove highly cost-effective. I will make the case for considering DOT "the standard of care" below (see "Directly Observed Therapy and the Future of Tuberculosis Control in the United States").

Field Experience

Probably the first large-scale, systematic program to deliver supervised outpatient treatment was organized in Hong Kong in the 1950s by Moodie and colleagues. However, their methods and results were not formally published until years later (168). The early Hong Kong system involved 6 months of 6-days-per-week supervised therapy conducted in 25 dispersed treatment centers followed by 16.5 months of self-administered therapy.

Fox and colleagues at the Tuberculosis Center in Madras reported in the early 1960s on their experience with a central clinic-based program. Particularly notable in this program was the initiation of intermittent therapy in an effort to facilitate supervision (169).

These programs were obviously based in poorer nations in which financial constraints sorely limited treatment options. Focus on the problems of noncompliance in industrialized nations emerged, recognizing, in particular, difficulties with adherence to PAS, the side effects of which were particularly formidable (170). However, Fox (171), as well as Stradling and Poole (170), recognized that, for a variety of reasons, patients with tuberculosis were at substantial risk for erratic drug therapy with predictable, adverse results including treatment failure and acquired drug resistance.

Attention to this problem in the United States evolved in the early 1960s as the extensive sanatorium treatment program was being dismantled (there had been nearly 100,000 dedicated beds at the middle of the century). Moulding (172) reported a small series of recalcitrant patients in Denver who were treated successfully with a twice-weekly regimen. However, then—as at present—Moulding contended that supervised therapy need be reserved only for a minority of patients who, by various markers such as pill counts, medication monitors, or treatment failure, were proven to be noncompliant.

Sbarbaro, who collaborated with Moulding in Denver, gradually evolved to the obverse position based on his analysis of the literature on noncompliance and his experience with tuberculosis patients at Denver's city-run hospital. From 1965 to 1967, 25 patients deemed "unreliable" because of alcoholism, sociopathic/criminal behavior, and/or demonstrated noncompliance with outpatient therapy were successfully treated with regimens of twice-weekly INH and SM directly administered for an average of 51 weeks (159). Subsequently, Hudson and Sbarbaro (96) reported on a larger cohort of "unreliable" patients, with 100 of 101 (99%) completing therapy with a bacteriological response. However, around this period Sbarbaro made a major change in his regimen, substituting an oral agent, EMB, for the injectable SM (173). This was a sentinel event, since the requirement for a nurse to administer the injection had been a readily understandable justification (to the patient) for supervised treatment. In this EMB series, 81 "unreliable" patients completed the treatment protocol from 1969 to 1975; there were no failures or relapses among these patients through 1976 (112).

Around this time, Sbarbaro chaired a committee of the ATS which produced officially endorsed guidelines for supervised "intermittent chemotherapy for adults with tuberculosis" (160). Because of limited resources, this approach was expressly "reserved for patients who cannot be relied upon to take drugs daily on their own." The guidelines basically endorsed the INH and SM regimen, while noting that INH and EMB "has also been reported to be a successful regimen."

In 1980 a summary analysis of the Denver experience with 18-month, twice-weekly, non-RIF regimens was published (173). In the selected population of 165 "unreliable patients," there were only 4 treatment failures or relapses (2.4%). Notable aspects of this series were that missed appointments were twice as frequent among persons who received EMB (9.6%) than among those who received SM (4.5%), that as many as 15% to 20% of continuation-phase doses could be missed without adversely affecting outcome, and—remarkably—that long-term tolerance of twice-weekly high-dose SM (27 mg/kg) and EMB (50 mg/kg) was excellent. Indeed, only 9 of 101 patients on a regimen of SM therpay had ataxia, which was managed by dosage reduction, not discontinuation, and there were no instances of significant renal dysfunction (96). Also, among the EMB recipients there were no cases of visual disturbances (112).

By the mid-1970s, attention was shifted away from these supervised 18-month, intermittent regimens to "short-course chemotherapy." Following the first reports of successful 6-month treatment with regimens including RIF, focus was directed to these shorter regimens, hoping implicitly that reducing the duration of treatment would combat noncompliance. By 1980, the ATS and CDC had endorsed a 9-month regimen (174).

These shorter regimens clearly offered a greater likelihood that patients would complete prescribed treatment. However, a casual perusal of the published literature on noncompliance would have indicated that the 6- to 9-month regimens would not have a major impact on this phenomenon in tuberculosis (175).

Results in the United States

Denver, Colorado

As described above, the programs of supervised, intermittent chemotherapy conducted in Denver were the first and only systematic uses of this tactic in the United States, employing, initially, 18-month regimens (1968–1981), then a 6-month regimen (1981 to the present). In large measure, the Denver program functioned as a clinic-based program in which patients came to a single central tuberculosis facility; only in special cases did the clinic nurses or their surrogates go out into the community to deliver the medications. More often, for patients who were reluctant or unable to come to clinic, a community worker met or tracked down the patients and delivered them to the facility. Denver has consistently achieved approximately 95% rates of treatment completion within the time frame stipulated in the CDC program measures.

Notably, not all patients in Denver were put on a regimen of DOT; rather, the decision to apply DOT was based on the judgment of community physicians, clinic physicians, and nurses. As seen in Fig. 10.3, the proportion of patients on a regimen of DOT varied considerably over the period 1976–1993 (176). In the most recent era, a rising percentage of cases was managed under direct supervision. This was based in part on the perception of an increasing prevalence of high-risk markers for noncompliance such as a history of sociopathy, mental incompetence, substance abuse, and language or cultural barriers. Also, however, it reflects the broadening perception that DOT should be the standard of practice.

Baltimore, Maryland

Glasser in Baltimore began a community-based program of DOT in 1981 (164). In this program, teams of workers from the city's tuber-

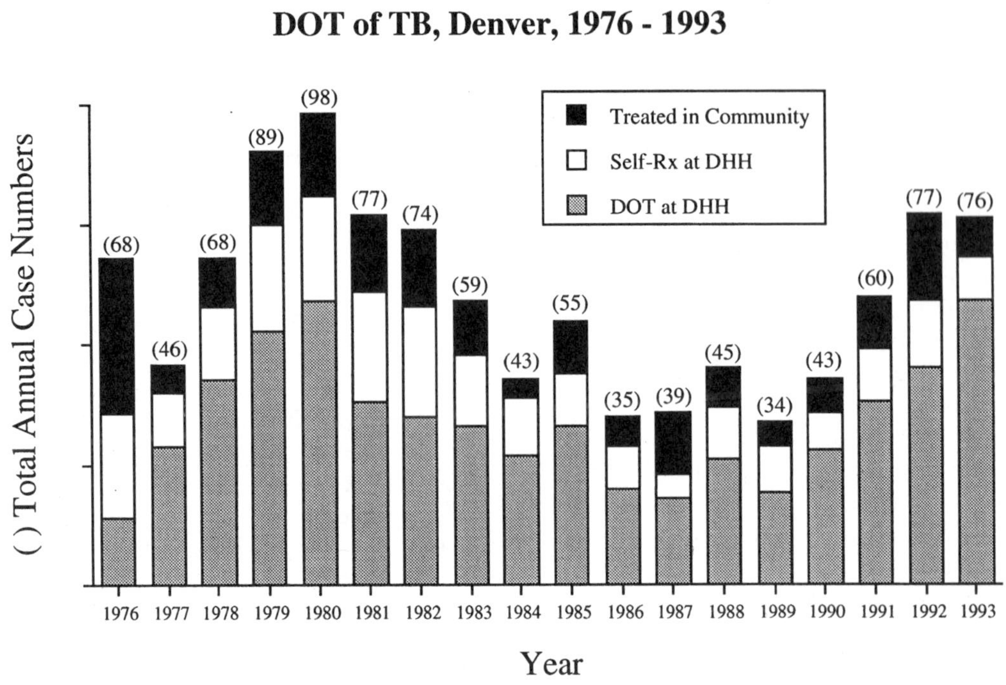

FIG. 10.3. Proportion of tuberculosis patients in Denver, Colorado, receiving directly observed therapy (DOT) in 1976–1993. During this period, a variable percentage of patients with tuberculosis received DOT at Denver Health and Hospitals (DHH). During this period, as the number of patients deemed to be at particularly high risk for nonadherence rose, the proportion treated at DHH and receiving DOT increased.

culosis clinic tracked and delivered chemotherapy to nearly all patients in the city. Approximately 90% of all DOT was delivered to patients at sites including home, workplace, school, nursing home, jail, or drug rehabilitation facility. The results of this approach were recently reported (164). More than any other evidence, this analysis clearly documents the immense benefits that flow from DOT. The authors compared case rates for Baltimore and five other cities that were closely matched as the six cities with the highest case rates in 1981. As seen in Fig. 10.4, both Baltimore's absolute case rates and its relative national ranking fell very substantially from 1981 to 1992. When compared with 20 U.S. cities with populations greater than 250,000 and high rates of tuberculosis, Baltimore experienced the greatest decline in case rates (from 35.6 to 17.2 cases/100,000) and city ranking (from 6th to 28th). More dramatic were the recent patterns

FIG. 10.4. A. Eleven-year trends in tuberculosis incidence for the six cities with the highest rates in 1981, compared with United States average. Over this 11-year period, the incidence of tuberculosis in Baltimore, Maryland, fell by approximately 50% from 35.6 to 17.2 cases per 100,000 population. By contrast, the national urban average for this period had risen and other cities with similar profiles, such as Newark, New Jersey, Atlanta, Georgia, and New York, New York, had seen dramatic upturns in case rates. **B.** National rankings for tuberculosis incidence: the six leading cities in 1981, and their trends from 1981 to 1992. Baltimore had consistently been among the top five cities in the United States throughout much of the twentieth century. With the introduction of a DOT program in 1981, this city enjoyed a steady decline in case rates **(A)** and in national urban rankings. Multivariant analysis for tuberculosis risk factors including HIV infection, immigration, minority populations, substance abuse, unemployment, and homelessness did not incriminate these elements in the differential rates and trends for Baltimore and these other cities.

A **Tuberculosis Cases Rates, Comparison of Baltimore Versus Five Other Leading United States Cities, 1981-1991.**

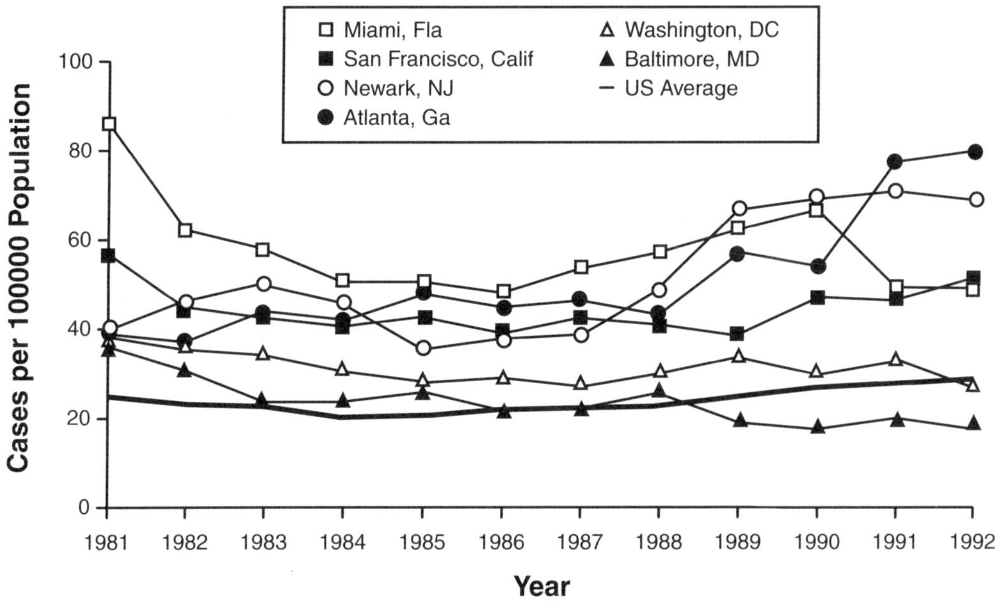

B **National Ranking of Baltimore Versus Other Leading Cities, Tuberculosis Incidence Rates, 1981-1992.**

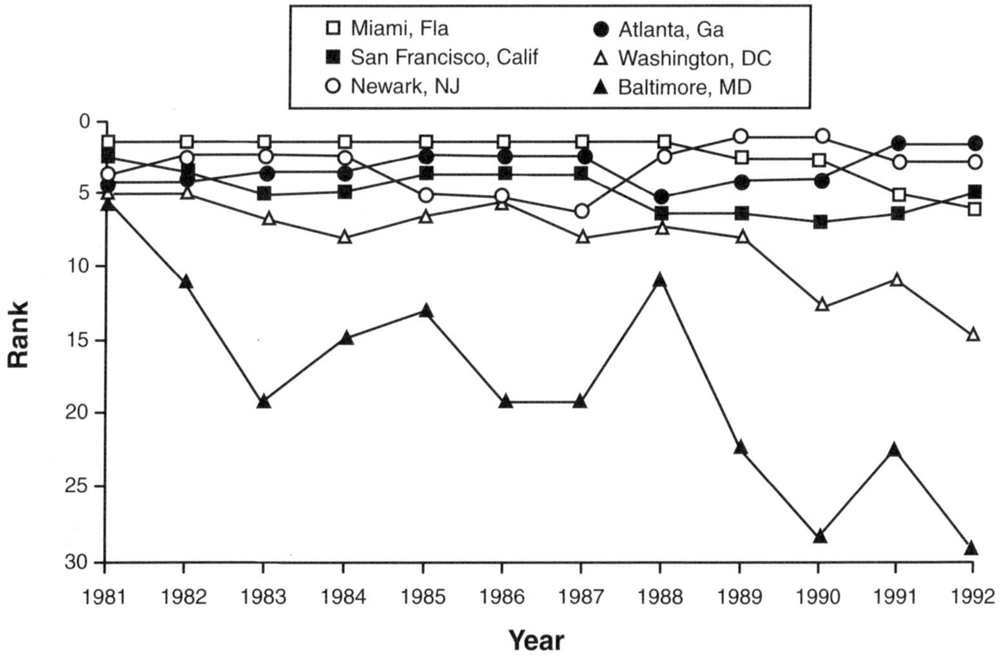

during 1985–1992 when national case rates were soaring: cases *declined* 29.5% in Baltimore while they *rose* 35.3% in the leading five cities and 28.5% in the other top 19 cities!

Multivariate analysis demonstrated that, while there were natural differences among Baltimore and these cities in terms of factors associated with tuberculosis risk, the differences in case rates could not be ascribed to the prevalence of AIDS, immigrants, poverty, or unemployment.

The authors also compared the impacts of *selective* DOT for persons at "risk" of noncompliance that was performed from 1978 to 1981 with the *city-wide* program of 1981–1992. They noted that both phases of DOT resulted in substantial reductions in case rates: 89.5% with the former, 52% with the latter.

Fort Worth, Texas

Weis et al. (177) recently reported the results of a DOT program employed in Tarrant County, Texas, from 1986 to 1992. This program was an amalgam of clinic and community-based treatment, some patients coming to or being delivered to clinic for therapy, and others being treated at home or in other sites by outreach workers. The results of this DOT program were compared historically with the previous 6 years in which treatment was self-administered. Admittedly an imperfect control, the differences were, nonetheless, striking and are displayed in Fig. 10.5. Notably, the DOT program was implemented at a time of rising numbers of cases and increasing prevalences of intravenous drug use, homelessness, and HIV infection among the population served. In terms of financial requirements, the authors observed that the DOT program was conducted with the same staff and support services that existed in the previous era.

New York City

New York City was the most heavily impacted community in the United States during the resurgence of tuberculosis in the 1980s. In fact, case rates had begun to rise in New York City in the late 1970s, impelled by deteriorating public health programs, immigration, and the early effects of HIV. As documented so vividly by Brudney and Dobkin (178), a laissez-faire "non program" resulted in partial or abandoned therapy among 89% of a cohort of patients from one city hospital in 1988–1989 (178). These and other poorly treated cases were obviously the sources of multiple new infections in the community and the breeding grounds for drug-resistant strains. Frieden et al. (179) reported that the incidence of primary drug resistance (in vitro resistance in strains from patients not previously treated) rose from 10% in 1982–1984 to 23% by 1991 (179). During this period, a very small minority of patients in New York City were on regimens of DOT, consistently less than 5% (180).

Aided by an infusion of federal support, New York City rapidly implemented programs of DOT using a variety of mechanisms including both clinic and community-based treatment. As seen in Fig. 10.6, the proportion of patients on regimens of DOT rose steeply from 1992 to 1994. This was associated temporarily with a 21% decline in overall cases—from 3,811 in 1992 to 2,995 in 1994—and a 44% reduction in the incidence of primary multidrug resistant cases (from 775 cases in 1991–1992 to 435 cases in 1993–1994). Certainly, there were multiple factors associated with the favorable trends, including improved infection-control practices in hospitals and other congregate facilities to reduce nosocomial transmission, as well as improved chemotherapeutic management of multidrug-resistant cases to help control spread in institutions and the community. Nonetheless, the authors of the recent analysis of tuberculosis in New York City ascribed a substantial portion of the improvement to the impact of ensured treatment (DOT), under which treatment completion rates rose from less than 50% in 1989 to approximately 90% in 1994.

Directly Observed Therapy and the Future of Tuberculosis Control in the United States

The flood of tuberculosis apparently crested in the United States in 1993 with more than 27,000 cases and is receding, with 19,875 cases in 1997. It is important that, of the declining

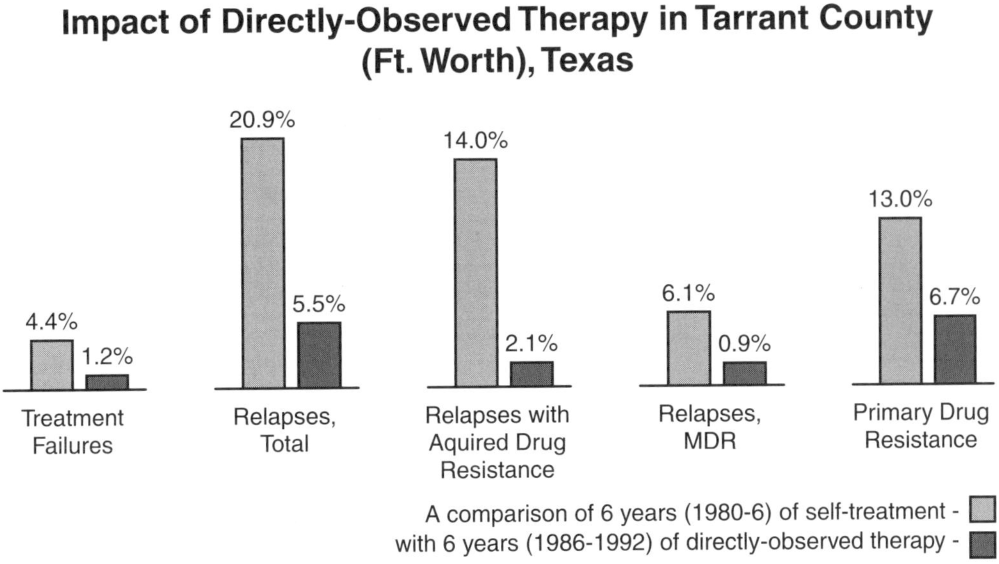

FIG. 10.5. From 1980 to 1986, 407 cases occurred among 379 patients; from 1986 to 1992, 581 cases occurred among 578 patients. The introduction of DOT resulted in significant reductions in treatment failures and relapses. Perhaps most important, acquired resistance—including multidrug resistance—diminished. This resulted in diminished transmission of resistant strains and a 50% reduction in the prevalence of primary resistance.

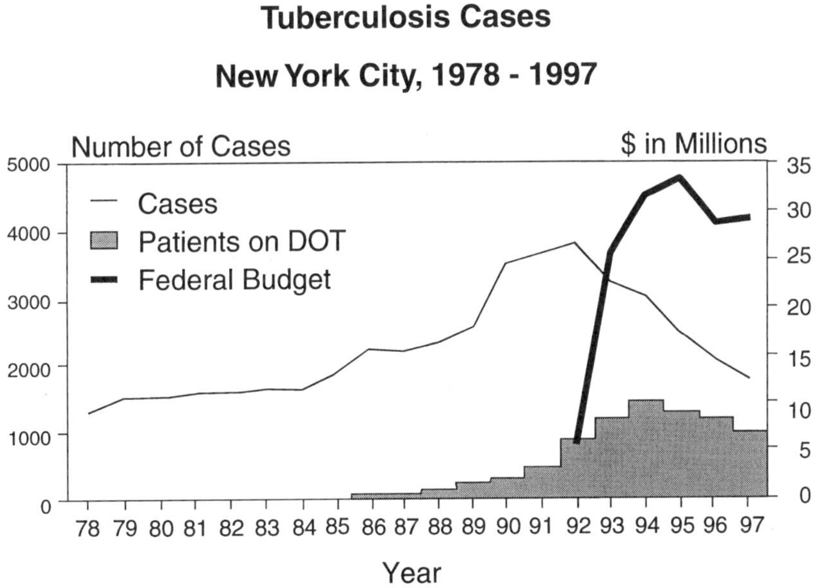

FIG. 10.6. The impact (and costs) of DOT in New York, New York, 1978–1997. Tuberculosis cases began to rise in New York City in the late 1970s, but with the wholesale introduction of HIV infection, cases soared in the period from 1989 to 1992. DOT performed in municipal clinics, shelters, and various nongovernmental facilities was a major factor in controlling this epidemic; other significant elements included improved case detection, curtailed transmission within hospitals and correctional facilities, and expanded programs of contact investigation/preventive therapy. In addition to curtailing overall case rates, the number of cases of multidrug-resistant tuberculosis cases fell dramatically in this period. To accomplish this control effort, substantial federal dollars were required. (Data compiled from New York City Department of Health.)

number of cases in the early 1990s, nearly half of that total reflected diminished cases in New York. Some authorities may see that as a signal to resume business as usual, but I would maintain that the decade-long deluge was a warning that more aggressive and structured programs of treatment delivery must be applied if we are to avoid reprises of this scenario.

Chaulk, Kazandjian (181) and a panel of practitioners of public health, behavioral sciences, and clinical care analyzed the scientific literature from 1966 to 1996 on DOT of tuberculosis. Their analysis indicated that variations on DOT are significantly more likely to result in completion of therapy than self-administered treatment (SAT); in their aggregate assessment, DOT—enhanced with incentives and enablers—had resulted in a median completion rate of 91%, while the mean SAT completion rate was 61% (Fig. 10.7).

The authors also suggested that "DOT appears to be cost effective compared with self-administered therapy, although data on cost-effectiveness are limited." Previously, the group from Baltimore had indicated in a decision analysis that both DOT and the use of FDC medications would be more cost-effective than SAT, with DOT yielding the best clinical and epidemiological outcomes (182). Using substantially different assumptions, Burman et al. (183) from Denver concluded that, despite higher initial costs, DOT is more cost-effective than SAT.

In a 1993 opinion piece, Sbarbaro, Cohn, and I argued that "substantially greater numbers [of patients]—perhaps all patients in some communities—should be receiving such [DOT] therapy" (166). While conceding that universal DOT is neither feasible nor appropriate for all patients in the United States, I would argue that the following paradigm be adopted:

- **Directly observed therapy (DOT) be considered a standard of practice for all tuberculosis patients in the United States** (that it be considered normative, not punitive).
- **All patients with proven/suspected tuberculosis be considered for DOT; when clinicians choose to exempt patients from DOT, they (the clinicians) assume the onus and responsibility for the consequences of the patients' noncompliance.** (Don't blame the patient after the fact.)
- **Therefore, by implication, DOT programs must be made available in all states and communities in the United States.**

This model has obvious imperfections and ambiguities, but it is a jumping-off point from which various programs can/will evolve to meet the diverse needs of communities and institutions. Colorado recently incorporated the following policy into its tuberculosis control program:

> The Board of Health determines that to prevent the emergence of multiple drug-resistant tuberculosis, it is necessary and appropriate and good medical practice that persons with active tuberculosis disease receive directly observed treatment for their disease. All medical providers and health care organizations are required to provide directly observed therapy for patients with active tuberculosis disease for the full course of therapy, unless a variance for a particular patient from this requirement is ap-

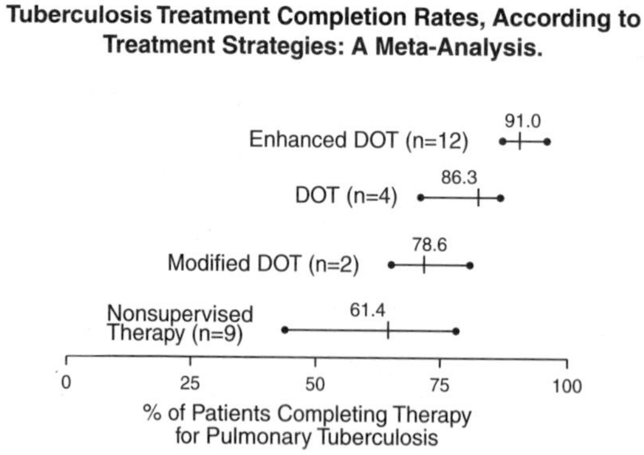

FIG. 10.7. Impact of various modalities of DOT on completion rates of tuberculosis chemotherapy. Convened by the Annis E. Casey Foundation, a public health tuberculosis panel analyzed the published literature regarding the influence of DOT on treatment completion. "Enhanced" DOT refers to comprehensive, patient-centered strategies with elements of incentives and enablers. Simple "DOT" programs did not systematically use incentives and enablers. "Modified" DOT typically entailed initial DOT, then self-administration.

> proved by the tuberculosis control program of the State Department of Public Health and Environment or Denver Public Health. Directly observed therapy is not required for patients with extrapulmonary tuberculosis disease provided that the presence of pulmonary tuberculosis has been investigated and excluded. In applicable situations, a variance shall be granted in accordance with C.R.S. 25-4-506(3).
>
> Medical providers and health care organizations shall report to the state or local health department within seven days the name of any patient on directly observed therapy who has missed one dose. When requested by medical providers and health care organizations, the state or local health department shall provide directly observed treatment to outpatients with active tuberculosis disease and this shall fulfill the requirement for the medical providers and health care organizations (State of Colorado Rules and Regulations Pertaining to Epidemic and Communicable Disease Control, 1995).

It is clearly unacceptable that public health officers or other practitioners involved with tuberculosis begin their arguments for resources from the null position. These premises should provide a reasonable basis for the acquisition of adequate resources to conduct effective treatment and control programs. Encouraging is the survey indicating that from 1992 to 1996, the use of short-course intermittent regimens in major metropolitan health departments rose from 4.3% to 46% (184). Not coincidentally, the clinic budgets had risen by an average of 84% in this period. Good tuberculosis control does not come cheaply.

Global Tuberculosis and Directly Observed Therapy

In 1993, the World Health Organization (WHO) declared tuberculosis "a global emergency," the only disease ever so designated (185). In 1994, WHO described a program of "directly-observed therapy, short-course (DOTS)" as the central component of its framework for tuberculosis control (186). Elements of DOTS included DOT, but stipulated the following additional features: (a) passive case-finding by sputum microscopy with detection of at least 70% of smear-positive cases; (b) ensured drug supplies; (c) monitoring the outcome of treatment of the entire cohort of cases with the target of treatment success equal to or greater than 85%; and (d) perhaps most important, a serious commitment on the part of the government toward the creation of an effective control program.

The focus on directly observed therapy, "putting the DOT in DOTS," is consistent with the policy advocated by the International Union Against Tuberculosis and Lung Disease stating that, to prevent acquired drug resistance to RIF, this drug should only be given under direct supervision to prevent acquired resistance (187). However, in practice, direct observation of all treatment is not deemed feasible. This is due to various considerations including lack of access to patients living in remote or sparsely populated areas or inability to provide an adequate cadre of health care providers. In response to these problems, some programs have featured an initial intensive 2-month phase of hospital-based treatment with a four-drug regimen, followed by 6 months or more of a self-administered non-RIF regimen, either INH-EMB or INH-THA. This has proven effective in some settings, but where HIV infection is prevalent, use of THA appears highly dubious.

Clearly, each country, perhaps even region or community, must identify what it needs, what it can afford, and what is currently feasible. However, protestations that DOTS "just can't be done here" are belied by success stories from increasingly diverse and problematic areas including China (188), Bangladesh (189), Somalia (190), and Peru (191).

The World Health Organization is tracking efforts to ascertain the use of DOTS and has reported that countries implementing a DOTS strategy have increased from fewer than 10 in 1990 to nearly 100 in 1996 (191). However, as of 1997, less than one-third of the world's tuberculosis cases fall under DOTS care.

My personal perspective is that the first decade of the next millenium, 2001–2010, will prove to be a critical period in the global struggle against tuberculosis. Unless case-finding is improved and treatment delivery systems are greatly expanded and refined, the burden of morbidity and mortality will soar. As discussed in Chapter 11, multidrug-resistant tuberculosis—once implanted in marginalized populations—may not be controllable. Although some resist the use of martial metaphors, this is a threat against which we must launch a war or, at least, a crusade.

SUMMARY

Salient points about contemporary management for adult tuberculosis include the following:

1. Regimens of 6 months' duration comprising an initial 2-month intensive phase of INH, RIF, PZA, with or without SM or EMB, followed by INH and RIF can be expected to yield long-term success rates of 95% or greater for patients with drug-susceptible pulmonary disease.
2. Much or all of this therapy can be given intermittently, twice or thrice weekly, to facilitate direct observation and to reduce drug costs.
3. PZA, EMB, and/or SM contribute very little to treatment after the initial 2 months if there is susceptibility to INH and RIF and these two drugs are employed throughout therapy.
4. The great majority of patients who experience relapse of their tuberculosis following such therapy do so with fully susceptible strains; this presumably reflects the phenomenon of "persistence."
5. Although the data are limited, most experience to date indicates that regimens that are successful against extensive cavitary pulmonary disease are adequate against extrapulmonary tuberculosis. The most problematic form of extrapulmonary disease is meningitis wherein the ability of the medications to cross the blood-brain barrier is involved.
6. Despite initial in vitro resistance to INH and/or SM, a 6-month chemotherapy regimen employing RIF, PZA, and EMB, with or without an aminoglycoside or fluoroquinolone, is still feasible.
7. In cases of isolated resistance to or intolerance of RIF, curative regimens of 8 to 9 months' duration employing INH, PZA, SM, and EMB are achievable.
8. If there is in vitro resistance to or intolerance of both INH and RIF, short-course (9 months or less) therapy is not achievable (see Chapter 11).
9. Among persons with HIV infection or AIDS, optimal combinations and durations of therapy have not been clearly determined, but experience to date indicates good initial response rates with only modestly higher relapse rates (see Chapter 8).
10. For patients with silicotuberculosis, extending the duration of treatment is required to obtain low relapse rates.
11. For patients with pulmonary tuberculosis with multiple negative sputum smears before treatment, intensive treatment regimens of 4 months' duration (for those with positive cultures) and 3 months'duration (for those with negative cultures) are sufficient.

REFERENCES

1. Hinshaw HC, Feldman WH. Streptomycin in treatment of clinical tuberculosis: a preliminary report. *Mayo Clin Proc* 1945;1945:313–318.
2. British Medical Research Council. Treatment of pulmonary tuberculosis with para-aminosalicylic acid and streptomycin. *Br Med J* 1949;2:1521–1525.
3. Robitzek EH, Selikoff IJ. Hydrazine derivations of isonicotinic acid (Rimafon, Marsilid). *Am Rev Tuberc* 1952;65:402–428.
4. Fox W, Mitchison DA. Short-course chemotherapy for pulmonary tuberculosis. *Am Rev Respir Dis* 1975;111: 325–353.
5. Mitchison D. Mechanisms of the action of drugs in the short-course chemotherapy. *Bull Int Union Tuberc* 1985;60:36–40.
6. Jindani A, Aber VR, Edwards EA, Mitchison DA. The early bactericidal activity of drugs in patients with pulmonary tuberculosis. *Am Rev Respir Dis* 1980;121: 939–949.
7. Heifets LB, Lindholm-Levy PJ. Is pyrazinamide bactericidal against Mycobacterium tuberculosis? *Am Rev Respir Dis* 1990;141:250–252.
8. Crowle AJ, Dahl R, Ross E, May MH. Evidence that vesicles containing living, virulent Mycobacterium tuberculosis or *Mycobacterium avium* in cultured human macrophages are not acidic. *Infect Immun* 1991;59: 1823–1831.
9. Sbarbaro J, Iseman M, Crowle A. The combined effect of rifampin and pyrazinamide within the human macrophage. *Am Rev Respir Dis* 1992;146:1448–1451.
10. Iseman MD. Treatment of multidrug-resistant tuberculosis. *N Engl J Med* 1993;329:784–791.
11. Heifets L, Lindholm-Levy P. Comparison of bactericidal activities of streptomycin, amikacin, kanamycin, and capreomycin against *M. avium* and *M. tuberculosis*. *Antimicrob Agents Chemother* 1989;33:1298–1301.

12. Wang L, Takayama K. Relationship between the uptake of isoniazid and its action on in vivo mycolic acid synthesis in *Mycobacterium tuberculosis*. *Antimicrob Agents Chemother* 1972;2:438–441.
13. Mannisto P, Mantyla R, Klinge E, Nykanen S, Koponen A, Lamminsivu U. Influence of various diets on the bioavailability of isoniazid. *J Antimicrob Chemother* 1982;10:427–434.
14. Zent C, Smith P. Study of the effect of concomitant food on the bioavailability of rifampicin, isoniazid and pyrazinamide. *Tuberc Lung Dis* 1995;76:109–113.
15. Peloquin CA, Namdar R, Dodge AA, Nix DE. Pharmacokinetics of isoniazid under fasting conditions, with food, and with antacids. *Chest* 1999;15:12–18.
16. Tiitinen H. Isoniazid and ethionamide serum levels and inactivation in Finnish subjects. *Scand J Respir Dis* 1969;50:110–124.
17. Weber W, Hein D. Clinical pharmacokinetics of isoniazid. *Clin Pharmacokinet* 1979;4:401–422.
18. Evans DA. Genetic variations in the acetylation of isoniazid and other drugs. *Ann N Y Acad Sci* 1968;151: 723–733.
19. Ellard G. The potential clinical significance of the isoniazid acetylator phenotype in the treatment of pulmonary tuberculosis. *Tuberc Lung Dis* 1984;65:211–227.
20. Parkin DP, Vandenplas S, Botha FJH, et al. Trimodality of isoniazid elimination: phenotype and genotype in patients with tuberculosis. *Am J Respir Crit Care Med* 1997;155:1717–1722.
21. Snider DE Jr. Pyridoxine supplementation during isoniazid therapy. *Tubercle* 1980;61:191–196.
22. Acocella G, Bonollo L, Garimoldi M, Mainardi M, Tenconi LT, Nicolis FB. Kinetics of rifampicin and isoniazid administered alone and in combination to normal subjects and patients with liver disease. *Gut* 1972;13:47–53.
23. Peloquin CA. Antituberculosis drugs: pharmacokinetics. In: Heifets LB, ed. *Drug susceptibility in the chemotherapy of mycobacterial infections.* Boca Raton, FL: CRC Press, 1991:59–88.
24. Bowersox DW, Winterbauer RH, Stewart GL, Orme B, Barron E. Isoniazid dosage in patients with renal failure. *N Engl J Med* 1973;289:84–87.
25. Kopanoff DE, Snider DE Jr, Caras GJ. Isoniazid-related hepatitis: a U.S. Public Health Service Cooperative Surveillance Study. *Am Rev Respir Dis* 1978;117: 991–1001.
26. Riska N. Hepatitis cases in isoniazid treated groups and in a control group. *Bull Int Union Tuberc* 1976;51: 203–208.
27. van den Brande P, van Steenbergen W, Vervoort G, Demedts M. Aging and hepatotoxicity of isoniazid and rifampin in pulmonary tuberculosis. *Am J Respir Crit Care Med* 1995;152:1705–1708.
28. Parthasarathy R, Sarma GR, Janardhanam B, et al. Hepatic toxicity in South Indian patients during treatment of tuberculosis with short-course regimens containing isoniazid, rifampicin, and pyrazinamide. *Tubercle* 1986;67:99–108.
29. Mitchell JR, Long MW, Thorgeirsson UP, Jollow DJ. Acetylation rates and monthly liver function tests during one year of isoniazid preventive therapy. *Chest* 1975;68:181–190.
30. Scharer L, Smith JP. Serum transaminase elevations and other hepatic abnormalities in patients receiving isoniazid. *Ann Intern Med* 1969;71:1113–1120.
31. Bailey WC, Sbarbaro JA. All patients should receive directly observed therapy in tuberculosis: pro and con. *Am Rev Respir Dis* 1988;138:1075–1076.
32. Steele M, Burk R, Des Prez R. Toxic hepatitis with isoniazid and rifampin: a meta-analysis. *Chest* 1991;99: 465–471.
33. Citron KM, Somner AR, Angel JM. Short duration chemotherapy in pulmonary tuberculosis: the occurrence of hepatitis in 6 months regimens containing pyrazinamide as well as rifampin. *Am Rev Respir Dis* 1980;121[Suppl]:452(abst).
34. Combs D, O'Brien R, Geiter L. USPHS tuberculosis short-course chemotherapy trial 21: effectiveness, toxicity, and acceptability—the report of final results. *Ann Intern Med* 1990;112:397–406.
35. Sarma GR, Immanual C, Kailasam S, Narayana AS, Venkatesan P. Rifampin-induced release of hydrazine from isoniazid: a possible cause of hepatitis during treatment of tuberculosis with regimens containing isoniazid and rifampin. *Am Rev Respir Dis* 1986;133: 1072–1075.
36. Smith J, Tyrrell WF, Gow A, Allan GW, Lees AW. Hepatotoxicity in rifampin-isoniazid treated patients related to their rate of isoniazid inactivation. *Chest* 1972;61:587–588.
37. Kumar A, Misra PK, Mehotra R, Govil YC, Rana GS. Hepatotoxicity of rifampin and isoniazid: is it all drug-induced hepatitis? *Am Rev Respir Dis* 1991;143: 1350–1352.
38. Kalinowski S, Lloyd T, Moyes E. Complications in the chemotherapy of tuberculosis: a review with analysis of the experience of 3,148 patients. *Am Rev Tuberc* 1961;83:359–371.
39. Ferebee SH. Controlled chemoprophylaxis trials in tuberculosis: a general review. *Adv Tuberc Res* 1970; 17:28–106.
40. Ungo JR, Jones D, Ashkin D, et al. Antituberculosis drug-induced hepatotoxicity: the role of hepatitis C virus and the human immunodeficiency virus. *Am J Respir Crit Care Med* 1998;157:1871–1876.
41. Moulding TS, Redeker AG, Kanel GC. Twenty isoniazid-associated deaths in one state. *Am Rev Respir Dis* 1989;140:700–705.
42. Centers for Disease Control and Prevention. Severe isoniazid-associated hepatitis: New York, 1991–1993. *MMWR* 1993;42:545–547.
43. Hobby GL. Summation of experimental studies on the action of rifampin. *Chest* 1972;61:550–554.
44. Vall-Spinosa A, Lester TW. Rifampin: characteristics and role in the chemotherapy of tuberculosis. *Ann Intern Med* 1971;74:758–760.
45. Fox W. The current status of short-course chemotherapy. *Tubercle* 1979;60:177–190.
46. Heifets LB, Lindholm-Levy PJ, Flory MA. Bactericidal activity in vitro of various rifamycins against *Mycobacterium avium* and *Mycobacterium tuberculosis*. *Am Rev Respir Dis* 1990;141:626–630.
47. Acocella G. Clinical pharmacokinetics of rifampicin. *Clin Pharmacokinet* 1978;3:108–128.
48. Dickinson JM, Mitchison DA. Experimental models to explain the high sterilizing activity of rifampin in the chemotherapy of tuberculosis. *Am Rev Respir Dis* 1981;123:367–371.
49. Grosset J, Lounis N, Truffot-Pernot C, O'Brien RJ, Raviglione MC, Ji B. Once-weekly rifapentine-con-

taining regimens for treatment of tuberculosis in mice. *Am J Respir Crit Care Med* 1998;157:1436–1440.
50. Melange M, Vanheuverzwyn R. Pseudomembranous colitis and rifampicin [Letter]. *Lancet* 1980;2:1192.
51. Prigogine T, Burette A, Schmerber J. Pseudomembranous colitis and rifampicin. *Chest* 1981;80:766–767.
52. Tajima A, Mine T, Ogata E. Rifampicin-associated ulcerative colitis [Letter]. *Ann Intern Med* 1992;116:778.
53. Matz J, Borish LC, Routes JM, Rosenwasser LJ. Oral desensitization to rifampin and ethambutol in mycobacterial disease. *Am J Respir Crit Care Med* 1994; 149:815–817.
54. Zierski M. Side effects under intermittent rifampicin: a general review. *Bull Int Union Tuberc* 1973;48:119–127.
55. Singapore Tuberculosis Service/British Medical Research Council. Controlled trial of intermittent regimens of rifampicin plus isoniazid for pulmonary tuberculosis in Singagore: the results up to 30 months. *Am Rev Respir Dis* 1977;116:807–820.
56. Lee C-H, Lee C-J. Thrombocytopenia: a rare but potentially serious side effect of initial daily and interrupted use of rifampicin. *Chest* 1989;96:202–203.
57. Mehta YS, Jijina FF, Badakere SS, Pathare AV, Mohanty D. Rifampicin-induced immune thrombocytopenia. *Tuberc Lung Dis* 1996;77:558–562.
58. Nessi R, Bonaldi GL, Redaelli B, di Filippo G. Acute renal failure after rifampicin: a case report and survey of the literature. *Nephrology* 1976;16:148–159.
59. Gabow PA, Lacher JW, Neff TA. Tubulointerstitial and glomerular nephritis associated with rifampin. *JAMA* 1976;235:2517–2518.
60. Cohn JR, Fye DL, Sills JM, Francos GC. Rifampicin-induced renal failure. *Tubercle* 1985;66:289–293.
61. Soffer O, Nassar V, Campbell W, et al. Light chain cast nephropathy and acute renal failure associated with rifampin therapy: renal disease akin to myeloma kidney. *Am J Med* 1987;82:1052–1056.
62. Berning SE, Iseman MD. Rifamycin-induced lupus syndrome. *Lancet* 1997;349:1521–1522.
63. Woodley C, Kilburn J. In vitro susceptibility of *Mycobacterium avium* complex and *Mycobacterium tuberculosis* strains to a spiro-piperidyl rifamycin. *Am Rev Respir Dis* 1982;126:586–587.
64. Heifets LB, Iseman MD, Cook JL, Lindholm-Levy PJ, Drupa I. Determination of in vitro susceptibility of *Mycobacterium tuberculosis* to cephalosporins by radiometric and conventional methods. *Antimicrob Agents Chemother* 1985;27:11–15.
65. Dickinson JM, Mitchison DA. In vitro activity of new rifamycins against rifampicin-resistant *M. tuberculosis* and MAIS-complex mycobacteria. *Tubercle* 1987; 68: 177–182.
66. Hong Kong Chest Service/British Medical Research Council. A controlled study of rifabutin and an uncontrolled study of ofloxacin in the retreatment of patients with pulmonary tuberculosis resistant to isoniazid, streptomycin and rifampicin. *Tuberc Lung Dis* 1992; 73:59–67.
67. Iseman MD. Unpublished data.
68. Telenti A. Genetics of drug resistance in tuberculosis. In: Iseman MD, Huitt GA, eds. *Clinics in chest medicine.* Philadelphia: WB Saunders, 1997:55–64.
69. McGregor MM, Olliaro P, Wolmarans L, et al. Efficacy and safety of Rifabutin in the treatment of patients with newly diagnosed pulmonary tuberculosis. *Am J Respir Crit Care Med* 1996;154:1462–1467.
70. Gonzalez-Montaner LJ, Natal S, Yongchaiyud P, Olliaro P. Rifabutin for the treatment of newly-diagnosed pulmonary tuberculosis: a multinational, randomized, comparative study versus Rifampicin. *Tuberc Lung Dis* 1994;75:341–347.
71. Peloquin CA. Using therapeutic drug monitoring to dose the antimycobacterial drugs. In Iseman MD, Huitt GA, ed. *Clinics in chest medicine.* Philadelphia: WB Saunders, 1997:79–87.
72. Schwander S, Rüsch-Gerdes S, Mateega A, et al. A pilot study of antituberculosis combinations comparing rifabutin with rifampicin in the treatment of HIV-1 associated tuberculosis: a single-blind randomized evaluation in Ugandan patients with HIV-1 infection and pulmonary tuberculosis. *Tuberc Lung Dis* 1995;76: 210–218.
73. Dickinson JM, Mitchison DA. In vitro properties of rifapentine (MDL473) relevant to its use in intermittent chemotherapy of tuberculosis. *Tubercle* 1987;68: 113–118.
74. Dickinson JM, Mitchison DA. In vitro observations on the suitability of new rifamycins for the intermittent chemotherapy of tuberculosis. *Tubercle* 1987;68: 183–193.
75. Tam CM, Chan SL, Lam CW, et al. Rifapentine and isoniazid in the continuation phase of treating pulmonary tuberculosis: initial report. *Am J Respir Crit Care Med* 1998;157:1726–1733.
76. Hoechst-Marion-Roussel. Presentation to U.S. Food and Drug Administration, Rockville, MD. May 1998.
77. Tam CM, Chan SL, Lam CW, Dickinson JM, Mitchison DA. Bioavailability of Chinese rifapentine during a clinical trial in Hong Kong. *Int J Tuberc Lung Dis* 1997;1:411–416.
78. Munsiff S, Joseph S, Ebrahimzadeh A, Frieden T. Rifampin-monoresistant tuberculosis in New York City: 1993–1994. *Clin Infect Dis* 1997;25:1465–1467.
79. Kailasam S, Daneluzzi D, Gangadharam PRJ. Maintenance of therapeutically active levels of isoniazid for prolonged periods in rabbits after a single implant of biodegradable polymer. *Tuberc Lung Dis* 1994;75: 361–365.
80. Ridzon R, Whitney CG, McKenna MT, et al. Risk factors for rifampin mono-resistant tuberculosis. *Am J Respir Crit Care Med* 1998;157:1881–1884.
81. Santha T, Fox W, Nazareth O, et al. Study of adverse reactions to a once-weekly regimen of streptomycin plus a slow-release preparation of isoniazid in high dosage for six months. *Tubercle* 1976;57: 123–130.
82. Parthasarathy R, Devadatta S, Fox W, et al. Studies of immediate adverse reactions to different doses of a slow-release preparation of isoniazid. *Tubercle* 1976; 57:115–121.
83. Steele M, Des Prez R. The role of pyrazinamide in tuberculosis chemotherapy. *Chest* 1988;94:845–850.
84. Jain A, Mehta VL, Kulshrestha S. Effect of pyrazinamide on rifampicin kinetics in patients with tuberculosis. *Tuberc Lung Dis* 1993;74:87–90.
85. Acocella G, Carlone N, Cuffini A, Cavallo G. The penetration of rifampicin, pyrazinamide, and pyrazinoic acid into mouse macrophages. *Am Rev Respir Dis* 1985;132:1268–1273.

86. Crowle AJ, Sbarbaro JA, May MH. Inhibition by pyrazinamide of tubercle bacilli with cultured human macrophages. *Am Rev Respir Dis* 1986;134:1052–1055.
87. Crowle AJ, Salfinger M, May MH. 1,25 (OH)2-vitamin D3 synergizes with pyrazinamide to kill tubercle bacilli in cultured human macrophages. *Am Rev Respir Dis* 1989;129:542–552.
88. Hobby G, Lenert T. The in vitro action of antituberculous agents against multiplying and non-multiplying microbial cells. *Am Rev Tuberc Pulm Dis* 1957; 76:1031–1048.
89. Ellard G, Haslam R. Observations on the reduction of the renal elimination of urate in man caused by the administration of pyrazinamide. *Tubercle* 1976;57:97–103.
90. Horsfall PAL, Plummer J, Allan WGL, Girling DJ, Nunn AJ, Fox W. Double blind controlled comparison of aspirin, allopurinol, and placebo in the management of arthralgia during pyrazinamide administration. *Tubercle* 1979;60:13–24.
91. Cohn DL, Catlin BJ, Peterson KL, Judson FN, Sbarbaro JA. A 62-dose, 6-month therapy for pulmonary and extrapulmonary tuberculosis: a twice-weekly, directly observed, and cost-effective regimen. *Ann Intern Med* 1990;112:407–415.
92. Hong Kong Chest Service, British Medical Research Council. Controlled trial of 6-month and 9-month regimens of daily and intermittent streptomycin plus isoniazid plus pyrazinamide for pulmonary tuberculosis in Hong Kong. *Am Rev Respir Dis* 1977;115:727–735.
93. Hong Kong Chest Service, British Medical Research Council. Controlled trial of 6-month and 8-month regimens in the treatment of pulmonary tuberculosis. *Am Rev Respir Dis* 1978;118:219–227.
94. Hong Kong Tuberculosis Treatment Services/British Medical Research Council. Adverse reactions to short-course regimens containing streptomycin, isoniazid, pyrazinamide, and rifampicin in Hong Kong. *Tubercle* 1976;57:81–95.
95. Van Scoy R, Wilson W. Antimicrobial agents in adult patients with renal insufficiency: initial dosage and general recommendations. *Mayo Clin Proc* 1987;62: 1142–1145.
96. Hudson LD, Sbarbaro JA. Twice weekly tuberculosis chemotherapy. *JAMA* 1973;223:139–143.
97. Bailey TC, Little JR, Littenberg B, Reichley RM, Dunagan WC. A meta-analysis of extended-interval dosing versus multiple daily dosing of aminoglycosides. *Clin Infect Dis* 1997;24:786–795.
98. Ali MZ, Goetz MB. A meta-analysis of the relative efficacy and toxicity of single daily dosing versus multiple daily dosing of aminoglycosides. *Clin Infect Dis* 1997;24:796–809.
99. Hatala R, Dinh TT, Cook DJ. Single daily dosing of aminoglycosides in immunocompromised adults: a systematic review. *Clin Infect Dis* 1997;24:810–815.
100. Gilbert DN. Editorial response: meta-analyses are no longer required for determining the efficacy of single daily dosing of aminoglycosides. *Clin Infect Dis* 1997;24:816–819.
101. Bertino JS Jr, Rotschafer JC. Editorial response: single daily dosing of aminoglycosides—a concept whose time has not yet come. *Clin Infect Dis* 1997;24:820–823.
102. Suo J, Chang C-E, Lin T, Heifets LB. Minimal inhibitory concentrations of isoniazid, rifampin, ethambutol, and streptomycin against *Mycobacterium tuberculosis* strains isolated before treatment of patients in Taiwan. *Am Rev Respir Dis* 1988;138:999–1001.
103. Gilbert DN, Dworkin RJ, Raber SR, Leggett JE. Outpatient parenteral antimicrobial-drug therapy. *N Engl J Med* 1997;337:829–838.
104. Thomas JP, Baughn CD, Wilkinson RG, Shepherd RG. A new synthetic compound with antituberculous activity in mice: ethambutol (dextro-2, 2′-(ethylenediimino)-di-l-butanol). *Am Rev Respir Dis* 1961;83:891–893.
105. Heifets L, Iseman M, Lindholm-Levy P. Ethambutol MIC's and MBC's for *Mycobacterium avium* complex and *Mycobacterium tuberculosis. Antimicrob Agents Chemother* 1986;30:927–932.
106. Place VA, Thomas JP. Clinical pharmacology of ethambutol. *Am Rev Respir Dis* 1963;87:901–904.
107. Sbarbaro JA. Unpublished data.
108. Varughese A, Brater DC, Benet LZ, Lee CS. Ethambutol kinetics in patients with impaired renal function. *Am Rev Respir Dis* 1986;134:34–38.
109. Leibold J. The ocular toxicity of ethambutol and its relation to dose. *Ann N Y Acad Sci* 1966;135:904–909.
110. Bobrowitz I, Robias D. Ethambutol-isoniazid versus PAS-isoniazid in original treatment of pulmonary tuberculosis. *Am Rev Respir Dis* 1967;96:428–438.
111. Doster B, Murray FJ, Newman R, Woolpert SF. Ethambutol in the initial treatment of pulmonary tuberculosis: U.S. Public Health Service Tuberculosis Therapy Trials. *Am Rev Respir Dis* 1973;107:177–190.
112. Albert R, Sbarbaro J, Hudson L, Iseman M. High-dose ethambutol: its role in intermittent chemotherapy—a six-year study. *Am Rev Respir Dis* 1976;114:699–704.
113. Gangadharam PR, Pratt PF, Perumal VK, Iseman MD. The effects of exposure time, drug concentration, and temperature on the activity of ethambutol versus *Mycobacterium tuberculosis. Am Rev Respir Dis* 1990; 141:1478–1482.
114. Manalo F, Tan F, Sbarbaro JA, Iseman MD. Community based short-course treatment of pulmonary tuberculosis in a developing nation: initial report of an eight-month, largely intermittent regimen in a population with high prevalence of drug resistance. *Am Rev Respir Dis* 1990;142:1301–1305.
115. Mitchison DA, Nunn AJ. Influence of initial drug resistance on the response to short-course chemotherapy of pulmonary tuberculosis. *Am Rev Respir Dis* 1986; 133:423–430.
116. American Thoracic Society. Treatment of tuberculosis and tuberculosis infection in adults and children. *Am J Respir Crit Care Med* 1994;149:1359–1374.
117. Ryan F. *The forgotten plague.* Boston: Little, Brown and Company, 1992.
118. Domagk G, Behnisch R, Mietzsch F, et al. Uber eine neue gegen tuberkelbacillin in vitro wirksames verbindungsclasse. *Naturwissenschafter* 1946;33:315.
119. Singapore Tuberculosis Services/Brompton Hospital/British Medical Research Council. A controlled clinical trial of the role of thiacetazone-containing regimens in the treatment of pulmonary tuberculosis in Singapore: second report. *Tubercle* 1974;55:251–260.
120. Tanzania/British Medical Research Council Study. Controlled clinical trial of two 6-month regimens of

chemotherapy in the treatment of pulmonary tuberculosis. *Am Rev Respir Dis* 1985;131:727–731.
121. Heifets LB, Lindholm-Levy PJ, Flory M. Thiacetazone: in vitro activity against *Mycobacterium avium* and *M. tuberculosis*. *Tubercle* 1990;71:287–291.
122. Sen PK, Chatterjee R, Saha JR, Roy HS. Thiacetazone concentration in blood related to grouping of tubercular patients: its treatment, results, and toxicity. *Indian J Med Res* 1974;62:557–564.
123. Miller AB, Fox W, Tall R. An international cooperative investigation into thiacetazone (thioacetzaone) side effects. *Tubercle* 1966;47:33–74.
124. Murray CJL, Styblo K, Rouillon A. Tuberculosis in developing countries: burden, intervention and cost. *Bull Int Union Tuberc Lung Dis* 1990;65:1–20.
125. Nunn P, Kubuga D, Gathnua S, et al. Cutaneous hypersensitivity reactions due to thiacetazone in HIV-1 seropositive patients treated for tuberculosis. *Lancet* 1991;337:627–630.
126. Eriki PP, Okwera A, Aisu T, Morrissey AB, Ellner JJ, Daniel TM. The influence of human immunodeficiency virus infection on tuberculosis in Kampala, Uganda. *Am Rev Respir Dis* 1991;143:185–187.
127. Iseman MD, Sbarbaro JA. The increasing prevalence of resistance to antituberculosis chemotherapeutic agents: implications for global tuberculosis control. *Curr Clin Top Infect Dis* 1992;12:188–207.
128. Pilheu J, DeSalvo M, Koch O. Liver alterations in antituberculosis regimens containing pyrazinamide. *Chest* 1981;80:720–722.
129. Weinberger S. Recent advances in pulmonary medicine (2). *N Engl J Med* 1993;328:1462–1470.
130. Davies D, Glowinski JJ. Jaundice due to isoniazid. *Tubercle* 1961;42:504–506.
131. Moulding T, Dutt AK, Reichman LB. Fixed-dose combinations of antituberculous medications to prevent drug resistance. *Ann Intern Med* 1995;122:951–954.
132. Sbarbaro JA. Compliance: inducements and enforcements. *Chest* 1979;76S:750S–756S.
133. Acocella G, Conti R, Luisetti M, Pozzi E, Grassi C. Pharmacokinetic studies on antituberculosis regimens in humans, I: absorption and metabolism of the compounds used in the initial intensive phase of the short-course regimens—single administration study. *Am Rev Respir Dis* 1985;132:510–515.
134. Ellard GA, Ellard DR, Allen BW, et al. The bioavailability of isoniazid, rifampin, and pyrazinamide in two commercially available combined formulations designed for use in the short-course treatment of tuberculosis. *Am Rev Respir Dis* 1986;133:1076–1080.
135. Hong Kong Chest Service/British Medical Research Council. Acceptability, compliance, and adverse reactions when isoniazid, rifampin, and pyrazinamide are given as a combined formulation or separately during three-times weekly antituberculosis chemotherapy. *Am Rev Respir Dis* 1989;140:1618–1622.
136. Singapore Tuberculosis Service/British Medical Research Council. Assessment of a daily combined preparation of isoniazid, rifampin, and pyrazinamide in a controlled trial of three 6-month regimens for smear-positive pulmonary tuberculosis. *Am Rev Respir Dis* 1991;143:707–712.
137. Hong Kong Chest Service/British Medical Research Council. Controlled trial of 2, 4, and 6 months of pyrazinamide in 6-month, three-times weekly regimens for smear-positive pulmonary tuberculosis, including an assessment of a combined preparation of isoniazid, rifampin, and pyrazinamide: results at 30 months. *Am Rev Respir Dis* 1991;143:700–706.
138. Geiter LJ, O'Brien RJ, Combs DL, Snider DE Jr. United States Public Health Service Tuberculosis Therapy Trial 21: preliminary results of an evaluation of a combination tablet of isoniazid, rifampin, and pyrazinamide. *Tubercle* 1987;68[Suppl]:41–46.
139. Mitchison D. How drug resistance emerges as a result of poor compliance during short-course chemotherapy for tuberculosis. *Int J Tuberc Lung Dis* 1998;2: 10–15.
140. Sbarbaro JA. A challenge: to our practices and to our principles. *Tuberc Lung Dis* 1996;77:2–3.
141. Iseman MD. Directly-observed therapy, patient education and combined drug formulations: complementary, not alternative, strategies in tuberculosis control (editorial). *Tuberc Lung Dis* 1996;77:101.
142. Dutt A, Moers D, Stead W. Short-course chemotherapy for extrapulmonary tuberculosis. *Ann Intern Med* 1986;104:7–12.
143. Snider DE Jr, Cohn DL, Davidson PT, Hershfield ES, Smith MH, Sutton FD Jr. Standard therapy for tuberculosis: 1985. *Chest* 1985;87[Suppl]:117S–124S.
144. Dutt AK, Moers D, Stead WW. Smear-negative, culture-positive pulmonary tuberculosis: six-month chemotherapy with isoniazid and rifampin. *Am Rev Respir Dis* 1990;141:1232–1235.
145. Dutt AK, Moers D, Stead WW. Smear- and culture-negative pulmonary tuberculosis: four-month short-course chemotherapy. *Am Rev Respir Dis* 1989;139: 867–870.
146. Hong Kong Chest Service/Tuberculosis Research Centre/Madras/British Medical Research Council. A controlled trial of 2-month, 3-month, and 12-month regimens of chemotherapy for sputum-smear negative pulmonary tuberculosis: results at 60 months. *Am Rev Respir Dis* 1984;130:23–28.
147. Hong Kong Chest Service/Tuberculosis Research Centre/Madras/British Medical Research Council. A controlled trial of 3-month, 4-month, and 6-month regimens of chemotherapy for sputum-smear negative pulmonary tuberculosis: results at 5 years. *Am Rev Respir Dis* 1989;139:871–876.
148. Snider DE, Jr. The relationship between tuberculosis and silicosis. *Am Rev Respir Dis* 1978;118:455–460.
149. Dubois P, Gyselen A, Prignot J. Rifampin-combined chemotherapy in coal-worker's pneumoconio-tuberculosis. *Am Rev Respir Dis* 1977;115:221–228.
150. Jones FJ Jr. Rifampin-containing chemotherapy for pulmonary tuberculosis associated with coal-worker's pneumoconiosis. *Am Rev Respir Dis* 1982;125:681–683.
151. Lin T-P, Suo J, Lee C-N, Lee JJ, Yang SP. Short-course chemotherapy of pulmonary tuberculosis in pneumoconiotic patients. *Am Rev Respir Dis* 1987; 136:808–810.
152. Cowie RL, Langton ME, Becklake MR. Pulmonary tuberculosis in South African gold miners. *Am Rev Respir Dis* 1989;139:1086–1089.
153. Hong Kong Chest Service/Tuberculosis Research Centre/British Medical Research Council. A controlled clinical comparison of 6 and 8 months of antituberculosis chemotherapy in the treatment of patients with silicotuberculosis in Hong Kong. *Am Rev Respir Dis* 1991;143:262–267.

154. Snider DE Jr, Layde PM, Johnson MW, Lyle MA. Treatment of tuberculosis during pregnancy. *Am Rev Respir Dis* 1980;122:65–79.
155. Snider DE Jr, Powell KE. Should women taking antituberculosis drugs breast-feed? *Arch Intern Med* 1984;144:589–590.
156. Sutherland I, Lindgren I. The protective effect of BCG vaccination as indicated by autopsy studies. *Tubercle* 1979;60:225–231.
157. Kamat SR, Daawson JJY, Devadatta S, et al. A controlled study of the influence of segregation of tuberculous patients for one year on the attack rate of tuberculosis in a 5-year period in close family contacts in South India. *Bull WHO* 1966;34:517–532.
158. Gunnells JJ, Bates JH, Swindoll H. Infectivity of sputum-positive tuberculous patients on chemotherapy. *Am Rev Respir Dis* 1974;109:323–330.
159. Sbarbaro JA, Johnson S. Tuberculous chemotherapy for recalcitrant outpatients administered directly twice weekly. *Am Rev Respir Dis* 1968;97:895–903.
160. American Thoracic Society. Intermittent chemotherapy for adults with tuberculosis. *Am Rev Respir Dis* 1974;110:374–376.
161. World Health Organization. *TB. A crossroads.* WHO Report on the Tuberculosis Epidemic, 1998. Geneva, Switzerland, 1998.
162. Burman WJ, Cohn DL, Rietmeijer CA, Judson FN, Sbarbaro JA, Reves RR. Short-term incarceration for the management of noncompliance with tuberculosis treatment. *Chest* 1997;112:57–62.
163. Sumartojo E. When tuberculosis treatment fails: a social behavioral account of patient adherence. *Am Rev Respir Dis* 1993;147:1311–1320.
164. Chaulk CP, Moore-Rice K, Rizzo R, Chaisson RE. Eleven years of community-based directly observed therapy for tuberculosis. *JAMA* 1995;274:945–951.
165. Nardell E, McInnis B, Thomas B, Weishaas S. Exogenous reinfection with tuberculosis in a shelter for the homeless. *N Engl J Med* 1986;315:1570–1575.
166. Iseman MD, Cohn DL, Sbarbaro JA. Directly observed treatment of tuberculosis: we can't afford not to try it. *N Engl J Med* 1993;328:576–578.
167. Centers for Disease Control and Prevention. Tuberculosis control laws: United States, 1993. *MMWR* 1993; 42:1–28.
168. Moodie AS. Mass ambulatory chemotherapy in the treatment of tuberculosis in a predominantly urban community. *Am Rev Respir Dis* 1967;95:384–397.
169. Tuberculosis Chemotherapy Centre/Madras. A concurrent comparison of intermittent (twice-weekly) isoniazid plus streptomycin and isoniazid plus PAS in the domiciliary treatment of pulmonary tuberculosis. *Bull WHO* 1964;31:247–271.
170. Stradling P, Poole G. Towards foolproof chemotherapy for tuberculosis. *Tubercle* 1963;44:71–75.
171. Fox W. The problem of self-administration of drugs, with particular reference to pulmonary tuberculosis. *Tubercle* 1958;39:269–274.
172. Moulding T. New responsibilities for health departments and public health nurses in tuberculosis: keeping the outpatient on therapy. *Am J Public Health* 1966;56: 416–427.
173. Sbarbaro JA, Hudson L. High dose ethambutol: an oral alternate for intermittent chemotherapy. *Am Rev Respir Dis* 1974;110:91–94.
174. Iseman MD, Albert R, Locks M, Raleigh J, Sutton F, Farer LS. Guidelines for short-course tuberculosis chemotherapy. *Am Rev Respir Dis* 1980;121:611–613.
175. Iseman MD, Huitt GA. *Tuberculosis.* Philadelphia: WB Saunders, 1997.
176. Catlin BJ. Unpublished data.
177. Weis SE, Slocum PC, Blais FX, et al. The effect of directly observed therapy on the rates of drug resistance and relapse in tuberculosis. *N Engl J Med* 1994;330: 1179–1184.
178. Brudney K, Dobkin J. Resurgent tuberculosis in New York City: human immunodeficiency virus, homelessness, and the decline of tuberculosis control programs. *Am Rev Respir Dis* 1991;144:745–749.
179. Frieden TR, Sterling T, Pablos-Mendez A, Kilburn JO, Cauthen GM, Dooley SW. The emergence of drug-resistant tuberculosis in New York City. *N Engl J Med* 1993;328:521–526.
180. Frieden TR, Fujiwara PI, Washko RM, Hamburg MA. Tuberculosis in New York City: turning the tide. *N Engl J Med* 1995;333:229–233.
181. Chaulk CP, Kazandjian VA. Directly observed therapy for treatment completion of pulmonary tuberculosis. *JAMA* 1998;279:943–948.
182. Moore RD, Chaulk CP, Griffiths R, Cavalcante S, Chaisson RE. Cost-effectiveness of directly observed versus self-administered therapy for tuberculosis. *Am J Respir Crit Care Med* 1996;154:1013–1019.
183. Burman WJ, Dalton CB, Cohn DL, Butler JRG, Reves RR. A cost-effectiveness analysis of directly observed therapy vs. self-administered therapy for treatment of tuberculosis. *Chest* 1997;112:63–70.
184. Lee DR, Leff AR. Tuberculosis control policies in major metropolitan health departments in the United States, VI: standard of practice in 1996. *Am J Respir Crit Care Med* 1997;156:1487–1494.
185. Raviglione MC, Snider DE Jr., Kochi A. Global epidemiology of tuberculosis: morbidity and mortality of a worldwide epidemic. *JAMA* 1995;273:220–226.
186. World Health Organization. WHO Tuberculosis Programme: framework for effective tuberculosis control. *WHO/TB* 1994;94:179.
187. Enarson DA, Rieder HL, Arnadottir T. Tuberculosis guide for low income countries. In IUATLD, ed. *Tuberculosis guide for low income countries,* 3rd ed. Frankfurt am Main: pmi Verl.-Gruppe, 1994:74.
188. China Tuberculosis Control Collaboration. Results of directly observed short-course chemotherapy in 112,842 Chinese patients with smear-positive tuberculosis. *Lancet* 1996;347:358–362.
189. Chowdhury AMR, Chowdhury S, Islam N, Islam A, Vaughan JP. Control of tuberculosis by community health workers in Bangladesh. *Lancet* 1997;350:169–172.
190. Crowe S. DOTS is effective even in nomadic populations. *Lancet* 1997;350:343.
191. World Health Organization. Global tuberculosis control. *WHO/TB* 1998;98:237.

11

Drug-Resistant Tuberculosis

DEFINITIONS

Diverse patterns of drug resistance are described in relation to *Mycobacterium tuberculosis*. Traditional nomenclature has referred to two "types" of resistance, **primary** and **acquired.** "Primary" refers to resistance on a strain isolated from a patient who has not received previous treatment. "Acquired" designates resistance in strains from patients with prior drug therapy. The fundamental truth is that all strains of *M. tuberculosis* that manifest *significant* levels of drug resistance reflect the impact of previous chemotherapy on the phenotype of that strain. Wild-type strains studied at the "dawn" of the chemotherapy era revealed infrequent mutants which could not constitute a significant percentage of the populations *without the selective* advantage conferred by drugs (1). Thus, the term "primary resistance" may underrepresent the role of therapeutic misadventures in the phenomenon. My recommended terminology relating to resistance is represented in Table 11.1; unique in this system is the explicit designation of "transmitted" drug resistance (2).

The most commonly seen pattern involves resistance to single drugs, most notably isoniazid (INH) or streptomycin (SM), drugs in use for many decades and widely employed because of their relatively low prices (3,4). Until the advent of rifampin (RIF), this type of resistance had serious implications for prognosis (5). However, the availability of this new potent drug diminished the importance of such loss of susceptibility. Regimens employing RIF in cases of INH and/or SM resistance have resulted in success rates of approximately 95% (6,7). Thus, in contemporary practice the most meaningful pattern is resistance to the two keystone drugs, INH and RIF. In recent practice, "multidrug-resistant tuberculosis (MDR-TB)" has been reserved to designate cases involving resistance *at least* to INH and RIF. This offers potential confusion for cases in which there is resistance to several agents but not both of these agents; in such instances, I would suggest the following nomenclature: "compound-drug resistance, involving drug x, y, and z" and so forth. In terms of the potential to concoct effective regimens, cases with more extensive patterns of compound resistance are generally less responsive to treatment. Indisputably, though, the greatest impact on response rates and duration of required treatment lies with the acquisition of resistance to INH and RIF.

MOLECULAR MECHANISMS OF DRUG RESISTANCE

Recent advances in molecular biology have allowed identification of the genetic loci and biological mechanisms of resistance to various drugs. These observations are displayed in Table 11.2 (8–13).

To date, these mutations have been found to confer resistance only to a single drug or closely related members of a class. Recent analyses of patterns indicated that similar loci and mechanisms were involved whether there was resistance to single or several drugs in the individual strains (14,15). These findings support the theory that resistance evolves by unlinked processes, resistance being acquired independently

TABLE 11.1. *Definitions of drug resistance*

Acquired resistance:	Cases in which the strain of tubercle bacilli shifts from a susceptible to resistant phenotype during or following a course of chemotherapy; in these instances, "inadequate" treatment selects for emergence of drug-resistant mutants. Among patients with histories of 1 month or more of prior treatment, it is inferred that this treatment has caused acquired resistance (however, unless the initial susceptibility pattern at the onset of therapy is known, initial or transmitted resistance cannot be excluded).
Primary resistance:	In some cases, patients are found on initial medical encounters to harbor a strain of tuberculosis involving significant resistance to a single drug or resistance to several agents. These patterns are not known to occur spontaneously, but the patients have never been treated before, nor have they knowingly been in contact with a case of active tuberculosis. We infer that the patients have been infected by previously treated persons but cannot prove this; hence, the less restrictive term, "primary."
Combined resistance:	The World Health Organization sums primary and acquired to determine the overall or combined prevalence of resistance.
Transmitted resistance:	Tuberculosis involving strains with high-level, clinically significant drug resistance that have been spread recently from known contacts with similar patterns of resistance. Strain identity is proven by resistance pattern or restriction fragment length polymorphism (RFLP) "fingerprinting."
Monoresistance:	Strains that are resistant to only one of the five first-line drugs.
Compound resistance:	Strains that are resistant to two or more drugs but *not* to both isoniazid and rifampin.
Multidrug resistance:	Strains that are resistant to *both* isoniazid and rifampin; there may be additional resistance, but this is not required.

to one drug at a time; this was true whether the cases represented primary or acquired resistance, including persons infected with human immunodeficiency virus (HIV).

Although clinically significant resistance appears to evolve initially through the selective pressure of chemotherapy, there is no evidence that when drug treatment is withdrawn there is substantial back-mutation toward the susceptible phenotype. We and others have seen some drift in in vitro resistance patterns toward susceptibility after the specific agents are withdrawn from therapy. However, in our experience, resumption of the drug(s) in question was generally associated with less than anticipated antimycobacterial activity and accelerated reappearance of in vitro resistance (16).

MUTATION AND THE PROCESS OF SELECTION

Tubercle bacilli have been shown in vitro to undergo spontaneous mutations giving rise to organisms resistant to various drugs. This phenomenon is believed to occur without the requirement of or acceleration by the presence of drugs. As noted above, the loci and mechanisms are independent and specific for individual drugs or closely similar agents within a group (e.g., an organism might develop simultaneous resistance to the structurally analogous drugs amikacin and kanamycin but not to SM).

David and Newman (1) reported in 1971 on the frequency of mutation yielding INH resistance for a standard laboratory strain of *M. tuberculosis*, H37Rv, a relatively rapid-growing and quite virulent organism. In their report, the authors considered various scenarios that might be associated with the evolution of drug-resistant strains. They calculated the time required for a strain to shift *spontaneously* (random genetic drift) from an INH-susceptible phenotype to a population with 1% resistance and compared this to the time observed to cause this drift by *indirect selection* (a complex system of enrichment with resistant mutants) and *direct selective pressure* (growth in the presence of INH). They found, according to this analysis, that the shifts spontaneously would take 5,000 to 10,000 years; by contrast, 1% resistance evolved in only 200 days by indirect enrichment methods and as few as 5 to 6 days via the direct selection system. The average *mutation rate* per bacterium per generation was 2.56×10^{-8}, giving rise to the calculated 5,000 to 10,000 years for spontaneous drift to 1% prevalence of INH-resistant mutants. In the direct selection method, cultures were exposed to either 0.2 or 1.0 mg/mL concentrations of INH, and mutations confirming resistance were noted to occur at 1.8×10^{-8} and 0.86×10^{-8} replications, respectively. Overall, the data from this report and a prior analysis (17) indicated that the average mutation rate was 1.9×10^{-8} per bacterium per generation. Based on these observations, the authors concluded that the initial appearance of substantial populations of INH-resistant bacilli (more than 1.2×10^{-5} of the population) in a patient cannot be ascribed to spontaneous mutation but must reflect either prior exposure to INH or infection of that patient with a strain that has been preselected by treatment in another person. *In other words, clinically significant levels of INH resistance are virtually always a human-made phenomenon.*

TABLE 11.2. *Loci, prevalence and effects of known mechanisms of resistance to major anti-tuberculosis medications*

Drug	Mutation locus	Prevalence among resistant strains	Comments
Isoniazid (INH)	*katG* (catalase-peroxidase)	~50%	Results in loss of catalase-peroxidase activity by bacilli; this prevents conversion of INH to its active metabolite. Confers high-level resistance (e.g., 5.0 μg/ml.
	InhA (enoyl-acp reductase)	~25%	This enzyme encodes for synthesis of a cell-wall constituent mycolic acid; mutations at this locus cause upregulation of the enzyme that is a target of INH. This confers low-level resistance (1.0 μg/mL); such organisms may still be inhibited by INH.
	ahpC (alkyl hydroperoxide reductase)	~10–15%	This gene is thought to break down the active metabolite of INH; it normally does not function in *Mycobacterium tuberculosis* because of natural lack of a controlling gene, *oxyR*. Mutations may confer spontaneous activity, thereby engendering resistance to the drug.
Rifampin (RIF)	*rpoB* (RNA polymerase, subunit B)	~97%	Prevents formation of messenger RNA by inhibiting the polymerase. Most mutations confer resistance to all rifamycins; <15% do not involve rifabutin.
Streptomycin (SM)	*rpsL* (ribosomal protein subunit 12)	~50%–60%	Mutation of targets of SM confer clinically significant resistance. These defects do not confer resistance to other aminoglycoside agents like amikacin or kanamycin, nor to the other injectable antituberculosis drug, capreomycin, which is a polypeptide agent.
	rrs (16s ribosomal RNA)	~20%	
Ethambutol (EMB)	*embAB* (arabinosyl transferase)	~50%	EMB acts by inhibiting cell-wall building blocks, arabinogalactan and lipoarabinomannan. Mutation in this region results in overexpression of the enzyme or other mechanisms to blunt EMB effect.
Pyrazinamide (PZA)	*pcrA*	Unknown	The precise mechanism of PZA activity is unknown; therefore, actions of mutation(s) are undetermined. PZA is "thought" to be a prodrug that requires activation by cleavage via a mycobacterial amidase; loss of the enzyme activity is associated with resistance to PZA.

David (17) earlier reported on the *mutation rates* (per bacterium, per generation) and *average mutant frequencies* (in an unselected population of bacteria, the proportions of resistant bacilli) for several other standard antituberculosis drugs. The mutation rates and prevalence of mutants, respectively, included the following:

- INH (0.2 μg/mL) = 1.84×10^{-8} and 3.5×10^{-6}.
- RIF (1.0 μg/mL) = 2.2×10^{-10} and 1.2×10^{-8}.
- SM (2.0 μg/mL) = 2.9×10^{-8} and 3.8×10^{-6}
- Ethambutol (EMB) (5.0 μg/mL) = 1.0×10^{-7} and 3.1×10^{-5}.

Using a somewhat different methodology, Tsukamura (18) showed that there was a similar frequency of spontaneously occurring mutants to RIF. These mutations were of an obligatory "single-step" pattern and occurred at a rate of 10^{-7} to 10^{-8}, conferring spontaneous high-level resistance.

FREQUENCY OF MUTATION IN RELATION TO TYPE(S) OF DISEASE AND ACQUIRED DRUG RESISTANCE

As noted in Chapter 8, modern tuberculosis chemotherapy is based on this resistance-probability model. Canetti (19) showed that in the usual case of far-advanced tuberculosis the cavitary lesions contained roughly 10^8 rapidly dividing, robust mycobacteria. In this setting, given the probabilities delineated above, small numbers of bacilli resistant to INH, RIF, or other drugs might be expected to evolve spontaneously each day, assuming a mycobacterial doubling time of approximately 18 to 24 hours. But, because these mutations are so infrequent, the spontaneous occurrence of a mutant resistant to *both* INH and RIF would be singularly uncommon: 1 in roughly 10^{18}, the product of $10^8 \times 10^{10}$ (17). The bacillary burden required to spontaneously spawn this biresistant mutant is so great as to be inconsistent with the survival of the diseased host.

From this model, one would predict that (a) even patients with extensive disease caused by wild-type strain, susceptible tubercle bacilli could be treated successfully with an INH-RIF regimen, (b) patients with paucibacillary disease or subclinical infection could be cured with monotherapy, and (c) monotherapy or erratic administration of a multidrug regimen for patients with heavy mycobacterial burdens would probably result in acquired drug resistance. All of these predictions have been borne out by clinical observations (20–22).

As discussed in Chapter 8, pyrazinamide (PZA) has been added to modern regimens because of the unique effect this drug has in accelerating each bactericidal activity and thus shortening the required duration of therapy. Currently, the American Thoracic Society (ATC) and the Centers for Disease Control and Prevention (CDC) recommend that EMB be added to initial therapy in most cases based on the rising likelihood of INH resistance; this tactic is directed primarily to the prevention of acquired resistance to RIF (23).

CURRENT EPIDEMIOLOGY OF DRUG RESISTANCE IN TUBERCULOSIS

Forty years into the era of tuberculosis chemo-therapy, regional prevalences of resistant strains are strikingly diverse. In communities that have stable local populations and effective treatment programs, the frequency of clinically significant resistance remains very low, slightly more than that of the natural levels at the inception of the chemotherapy era. In other locales, there are varying combinations of "indigenous" (locally created) and "imported" resistance (reflecting immigration of persons with active disease or latent infection attributable to resistant bacilli). Furthermore, within any given community there may be wide ranges in the prevalence of resistance among populations disparate by race, age, national origins, or other risk factors (24).

There have been very heterogeneous efforts at surveillance of the prevalences and trends in resistance. Sadly, in the communities, regions, and/or nations that are most in need of such data, resistance data have been least available. Simply stated, poor populations that are most likely to suffer from increased rates of tuberculosis, inadequate treatment programs, and high rates of noncompliance—conditions associated with high rates of drug resistance—are most likely to have deficient or absent laboratory services. In an effort to remedy this deficiency, the International Union Against Tuberculosis and Lung Disease (IUATLD) and the World Health Organization (WHO) recently initiated an international surveillance program to monitor patterns of drug resistance (25). Results of the initial survey are available in a monograph (25); a concise analysis recently has been published (3).

Consideration of regional variations of resistance are essential to guide local treatment and prevention programs. Hence, available data on the geographical and population-based epidemiology of resistance are presented below.

Global Drug Resistance

As noted in Chapter 5, recent analyses have estimated there to be 1.7 billion persons infected with the tubercle bacillus and 8 to 10 million new cases of active tuberculosis annually. Among new cases, many individuals are cured, but others either die of their disease (estimated 2.5 million deaths annually) or have spontaneous remissions. Prechemotherapy era data indicate that roughly 20% to 40% remitted without treatment, a rate that varied widely in relation to age and race; today, patients who are partially treated may improve and enter a state of sustained, stable but active disease (26). As described by Grzybowski and Enarson, these inadequately treated persons are among the most problematic elements in contemporary tuberculosis, for—unlike untreated patients who die quickly with drug-susceptible disease—they develop drug resistance and live on in their communities, transmitting these strains which are no longer amenable to therapy with the standard, affordable drugs (27).

Some generalizations can be made about the distribution of drug resistance in various countries/populations. In countries with a low prevalence of tuberculosis, relative prosperity, demographic stability, and a well-organized system for treatment, the prevalence of resistance tends to be low, consistently 5% or less. Immigration patterns in these countries can have a strong influence on the prevalence of resistance. Among countries that are extremely poor, with such limited heath resources that antituberculosis medications are generally unavailable, the prevalence of drug resistance is also low, despite high rates of tuberculosis. The most troublesome pattern appears in "intermediate" countries in which the rates of tuberculosis remain high and there is widely available but poorly organized access to health care and medications. Features of such nations include the absence of controlled prescription policies and partially funded government drug programs. In such settings the historical prevalence of drug resistance ranged as high as 30% to 50% with numerous multidrug-resistant cases (28).

When Sbarbaro and I attempted to review national drug resistance rates in 1992, the data presented were often suspect for various reasons (28). In some cases, the information was quite old. In other cases, the methodology and/or representational validity was questioned. And, perversely, the quality of the reported data generally was inversely related to the prevalence of disease and the probable frequency of drug resistance (i.e., countries with poor treatment programs that begat high rates of resistance were very likely to have deficient laboratory services).

Cohn et al. (29) from WHO reviewed 63 surveys of resistance performed between 1985 and 1994; included in their review was work cited in other prior reports. In the aggregate, these data revealed the following patterns:

- **Primary resistance** (range; median)
  - INH = 0% to 16.9%; 4.1%.
  - SM = 0.1% to 23.5%; 3.5%.
  - RIF = 0% to 3.0%; 0.2%.
  - EMB = 0% to 4.2%; 0.1%.
- **Acquired resistance** (range; median)
  - INH = 4.0% to 53.7%; 10.6%.
  - SM = 0% to 19.4%; 4.9%.
  - RIF= 0% to 14.5%; 2.4%.
  - EMB = 0% to 13.7%; 1.8%.

Striking information from the reports the authors cited included MDR-TB rates in Nepal of 48.0%; in Gujarat, India, of 33.8%; in Bolivia of

15.3%; and in Korea of 14.5%. Data from surveys in Africa and South America are shown in tabular form in their survey.

Since that report, other surveys have been published. Acknowledging a variety of flaws in these reports, the data, arranged by continent/region, include the following:

- **Middle East**
  - *Turkey:* Overall resistance, 35.5%; initial resistance, 26.6%; acquired resistance, 53.4%; and MDR-TB, 3.2% (30).
  - *Ethiopia:* Overall primary resistance, 15.6%; primary resistance to INH, 8.4%; to SM, 10.2%; and to RIF, 1.8% (of note, this survey included only newly diagnosed, previously untreated subjects) (31).
- **Sub-Saharan Africa**
  - *Malawi:* Among previously untreated patients, initial resistance, 11.8%; INH, 3.5%; SM, 3.5%; INH + SM, 4.0%; and RIF, 0.8% (32).
  - *Cameroon*: Of 516 culture-positive, previously untreated cases, 90% were *M. tuberculosis* and 10% were *Mycobacterium africanum;* overall primary resistance, 31.8%; INH, 12.4%; SM, 20.5%; RIF, 0.8%; and EMB, 0.4% (33).
  - *Rwanda:* Overall initial drug resistance, 9.75%; overall acquired drug resistance (ADR) among previously treated patients, 37.1%; combined resistance, 15.4%; and combined MDR-TB, 1.34% (34).
  - *Madagascar:* Overall primary resistance, 20%, including INH (4%) and SM (15%); among previously treated patients, 40% had ADR, including single resistance to INH (11%), SM (14%), and RIF (1.5%); MDR-TB was seen in 5% of previously treated cases (35).
  - *Burkina-Faso:* Among culture-positive cases, 75% were *M. tuberculosis* and 18% were *M. africanum;* overall primary resistance, 16%; INH, 7.6%; SM, 12.4%; RIF, 2.5%; and EMB, 1.0%; MDR-TB was seen in 1.8% of untreated and 53.3% of previously treated cases (36).
- **Asia**
  - *Japan:* Overall primary resistance, 5.6%; INH, 1.5%; SM, 3.8%; RIF, 0.7%; and EMB, 0.1%; ADR among previously treated cases, 27.8% with 10.1% MDR-TB; combined resistance, 10.6% with 2.4% MDR-TB (37).
  - *Philippines:* Among a selected population referred to the University of the Philipines–Philippine General Hospital, 83.3% had drug resistance; 29.8% of cases were resistant to a single drug; 53.5% of cases were resistant to two or more drugs; 31.8% of the cases were MDR-TB (38).
- **Central America/Mexico**
  - *Honduras:* Combined drug resistance was found in 13 of 85 (15.3%) culture-positive cases; 7 smear-positive MDR-TB cases were found (39).
  - *Guatamala:* Among 335 culture-positive patients at a referral hospital, 172 had drug susceptibility testing; of these, 30% were resistant to one or more drugs and 15% were resistant to two or more drugs (40).
  - *Mexico:* A 1997 survey of three states from northern, central, and southern Mexico yielded the following results (41): overall primary resistance was 12%; with INH, 11%; SM, 11%; RIF, 2%; EMB, 3%; PZA, 1%; and MDR-TB, 2%; among previously treated patients; overall resistance, 50% with MDR-TB, 20%.

WHO and IUATLD, in an effort to overcome the deficiencies of prior studies, combined resources to conduct surveys of drug resistance in various nations on all the continents (25). Although many important and large populations (such as Pakistan, the Philippines, and mainland China) were not included and some sampling bias could not be avoided, the results are generally the best-quality data for many regions.

Incorporating all of these data, I have attempted to develop a descriptive, semiquantitative hierarchy for the larger nations of the world with regard to the likelihood of drug resistance for citizens of those nations with tuberculosis; this information is found in Table 11.3. Obviously, data derived from a survey at a given time or location may give a skewed view of national patterns. For instance, the survey in the United States in 1991–1992 indicated that 3.5% of the patients with tuberculosis harbored MDR-TB (24). How-

TABLE 11.3. *Estimated national patterns of combined drug resistance*[a]

National patterns	My estimation of the combined resistance	Countries
Group A Wealthy, demographically stable, with well-organized public health programs	<10%	Japan, England and Wales, Northern Ireland, Scotland, Germany, France, Scandinavia, Belgium, Canada, Australia, New Zealand
Group B Wealthy; demographically more heterogenous (may have large component of immigrants who "imported" resistance with themselves); public health programs of variable quality	10%–15%	United States, Cuba, Spain, Hong Kong, Taiwan, Argentina, Singapore, Israel, Switzerland, Netherlands, Malaysia, Poland, Hungary, Romania, Brazil, and Korea
Group C Intermediate economic development; drugs widely available but poorly controlled; limited public health programs	>15%	Mexico, Dominican Republic, Philippines, South Africa, Venezuela, Bolivia, Peru, Central America, India, mainland China, Pakistan, Tibet, Indonesia, Latvia, Lithuania, Estonia, Russia, Portugal, Thailand, Vietnam, Haiti, Madagascar, Sierra Leone
Group D Very limited economies; drugs scarce and underused; extremely limited diagnostic and treatment programs	<10%	Bangladesh, Cambodia, Laos, Zimbabwe, Botswana, Lesotho

[a] Combined is the sum of primary and acquired resistance in a population; see Table 11.5 for WHO/IUATLD data.

ever, New York City alone had provided 70 of the 114 (61%) reported MDR-TB cases. Similarly, in the WHO/IUATLD survey, Argentina had high rates (roughly 10%) of MDR-TB disease attributable in large measure to a huge epidemic of nosocomially-transmitted disease in Buenos Aires (42). These observations are intended to point out the limitations of such surveys in predicting the likelihood of drug resistance for any given person originating in that *nation.*

In general, the intent of this estimated/measured system is to provide guidelines for clinicians who must initiate drug therapy in cases of active or presumed tuberculosis before susceptibility data are available and to help select an agent (or agents) for preventive chemotherapy. My practice and recommendations are to be aggressive when commencing empirical treatment. Although there are demonstrable risks from the toxicity of extra agents, I believe that the patient's and society's welfare are best served by the principle of using "one drug too many" rather than "one too few," a practice which can increase the risk of treatment failure and further acquired drug resistance.

The most common pattern of resistance is to INH and, to a lesser extent, SM, two inexpensive and widely used agents. As a rule, for countries/populations in which resistance to these drugs is more common, multidrug resistance will also be more prevalent. The influence of these considerations in selecting empirical disease treatment or preventive chemotherapy is discussed below (see "Implications of Potential Resistances for Choice of Initial Therapy").

Patterns of Resistance in the United States

The CDC and U.S. Public Health Service began systematically tracking drug resistance in the early 1960s. Results of the periodic surveys, which were generally selective, not comprehensive, are displayed in Table 11.4. As seen, the survey conducted in the first quarter of 1991 represented the culmination of a deteriorating pattern (24).

Based on the dramatic upturn in drug resistance seen in 1991, the CDC in 1993 initiated a national surveillance program for drug resistance. Results

TABLE 11.4. *Historical levels of antituberculosis drug resistance: United States*

	Primary						Acquired (prior treatment)					
	INH	SM	RIF	EMB	PZA	MDR	INH	SM	RIF	EMB	PZA	MDR
1961–1968 (127)	1.8%	2.3%	—	—	—	—	36.8%	19.2%	—	—	—	—
1975–1977 (128)	4.4	5.1	0.3	0.7	—	NR	—	—	—	—	—	—
1982–1986 (129)	5.3	4.9	0.6	0.6	0.5		19.5	10.4	3.3	2.2	1.6	NR
1991[a]	8.2	5.0	3.5	3.5	5.0	3.5	21.5	7.7	9.0	3.8	17.6	7.2
1993–1996[b]	7.9	6.1	2.7	2.7	2.9	1.9	17.0	8.7	8.6	4.5	54.6	6.9

[a] Ref. 24.
[b] Ref. 3.
INH, isoniazid; SM, streptomycin; RIF, rifampin; EMB, ethambutol; PZA, pyrazinamide MDR, multidrug resistance; NR, not reported.

of the 1993–1996 program were reported in 1997 (3); data from these surveys are displayed in Tables 11.5–11.8. The most salient observations from these surveys include the following:

- Resistance to all five first-line drugs except SM gradually diminished during this period.
- The incidence of INH and RIF resistance—"MDR-TB"—fell from 2.8% to 1.4%.
- A history of prior treatment was strongly associated with the risk of drug resistance.
- Foreign-born patients were substantially more likely to harbor resistant strains, particularly to INH and SM; high-risk countries of origin included Vietnam, Mexico, the Philippines, South Korea, China, Haiti, and India.
- HIV-infected persons, both U.S. and foreign born, were more likely to have drug-resistant strains.
- Younger persons were more likely to have drug-resistant disease than the elderly.
- Residency in New York City was still a powerful risk factor for drug resistance; although MDR-TB had been reported from 42 states between 1993 and 1996, 30% of the total number of MDR-TB cases in 1996 came from New York City.

These data are quite useful for clinicians in selecting empirical chemotherapy. Also, they may be helpful in deciding whether an alternative agent such as RIF should be used in preventive

TABLE 11.5. *Number and percentage of tuberculosis patients with drug-resistant isolates by year of report: United States (1993–1996)*

	No. (%) resistant by year			
Drug[a]	1993	1994	1995	1996
Isoniazid[b]	1572 (8.9)	1520 (8.7)	1324 (7.9)	1217 (8.0)
Rifampin[b]	637 (3.6)	592 (9.4)	432 (2.6)	347 (2.3)
Pyrazinamide[b]	318 (4.3)	287 (3.4)	216 (2.4)	210 (2.3)
Streptomycin	944 (6.1)	969 (6.2)	986 (6.4)	855 (6.2)
Ethambutol hydrochloride[b]	448 (2.6)	309 (1.8)	326 (2.0)	339 (2.2)
Isoniazid and rifampin[b]	488 (2.8)	419 (2.4)	313 (1.9)	237 (1.6)
One first-line drug	2369 (13.4)	2297 (13.1)	2129 (12.5)	2012 (13.2)
Any drug[b]	2475 (14.0)	2373 (13.5)	2181 (12.9)	2049 (13.4)

[a] The patient isolate has resistance to at least the specified drug but may have resistance to other drugs.
[b] $< .05$ for the χ^2 test for linear trend of resistance by year.

Overall, the patterns of resistance were stable with slight reductions for isoniazid, rifampin, and pyrazinamide and INH-RF. Most common was resistance to isoniazid and/or streptomycin, the agents in longest and most extensive use historically.

TABLE 11.6. *Number and percentage of tuberculosis patients with drug-resistant isolates, 1993–1996, United States*

Drug[a]	No. (%) of foreign-born patients[a] No Prior TB[c]	Prior TB[c]	Total	No. (%) of US-born patients[b] No Prior TB[c]	Prior TB[c]	Total
Isoniazid	2386 (11.6)	333 (25.8)	2741 (12.4)	2501 (6.0)	296 (12.2)	2822 (6.4)
Rifampin	509 (2.5)	165 (12.8)	677 (3.1)	1138 (2.7)	150 (6.2)	1296 (2.9)
Pyrazinamide	375 (3.2)	64 (8.1)	440 (3.4)	527 (2.7)	45 (3.8)	577 (2.8)
Streptomycin	1829 (9.7)	192 (15.6)	2040 (10.0)	1553 (4.3)	109 (4.9)	1677 (4.3)
Ethambutol hydrochloride	484 (2.4)	91 (7.1)	577 (2.6)	745 (1.8)	74 (3.1)	824 (1.9)
Isoniazid and rifampin	392 (1.9)	146 (11.4)	540 (2.4)	780 (1.9)	108 (4.4)	893 (2.0)
One first-line drug	3624 (17.6)	407 (31.5)	4069 (18.4)	4185 (10.1)	408 (16.8)	4631 (10.4)
Any drug	3720 (18.0)	410 (31.7)	4169 (18.8)	4340 (10.4)	420 (17.2)	4799 (10.8)

[a] The patient isolate has resistance to at least the specified drug but may have resistance to other drugs. Patients with an unknown prior history of tuberculosis (TB) are included under the category of total patients.

[b] For all drugs, the percentage of resistance is higher for the comparison: foreign-born versus US-born patients (with the exception of rifampin for patients without prior TB and total patients and both isoniazid and rifampin for patients without prior TB); < .05 for the χ^2 test statistic.

[c] For all drugs, the percentage of resistance is higher for the comparison: prior versus no prior TB (with the exception of streptomycin for U.S.-born patients; χ <.05 for the χ^2 test statistic.

TABLE 11.6. Foreign-born persons were nearly twice as likely to harbor drug-resistant strains. For both groups, the history of prior tuberculosis increased the risk nearly twofold.

therapy. However, clinicians must realize that in a globally mobile society, each patient or situation must be considered in detail with respect to work, travel, and contacts, in order to assess the probability of harboring drug-resistant strains.

Human Immunodeficiency Virus Infection and Drug-Resistant Tuberculosis

Because of the potentially great impact on morbidity and mortality, the relationship between HIV infection/acquired immunodeficiency syndrome (AIDS) and drug-resistant tuberculosis should be emphasized. The only clear-cut relationship in the 1994 CDC report was the association between MDR-TB and AIDS in New York City. This association was confirmed in multiple reports from New York (43–46). The trend toward increased risk for drug-resistant tuberculosis among persons with HIV infection/AIDS was sustained during the period 1993–1996. As seen in Table 11.8, the as-

TABLE 11.7. *Number and percentage of tuberculosis patients with drug-resistant isolates, by country of birth: United States (1993–1996)*

Birth country	No. (%) of patients with resistant isolates by drug[a] Isoniazid	Rifampin	Isoniazid and rifampin	Streptomycin
Mexico	487 (9.8)	150 (3.0)	105 (2.1)	386 (9.3)
Phillippines	421 (14.7)	78 (2.7)	61 (2.1)	203 (7.5)
Vietnam	494 (18.3)	52 (1.9)	50 (1.9)	556 (22.0)
China	146 (11.7)	36 (2.9)	33 (2.7)	100 (8.3)
Haiti	150 (15.0)	34 (3.4)	24 (2.4)	46 (4.7)
India	112 (10.9)	19 (1.8)	16 (1.6)	72 (7.4)
South Korea	135 (15.6)	36 (4.2)	32 (3.7)	57 (7.0)

[a] The patient isolate has resistance to at least the specified drug but may have resistance to other drugs.
From ref. 3, with permission.

TABLE 11.7. The countries listed yielded the greatest numbers and highest likelihood of drug-resistant strains for this period. Because of selection bias, these data may not correspond consistently with the 1998 World Health Organization survey (3).

TABLE 11.8. *Number and percentage of tuberculosis patients (aged 25–44 years) with drug-resistant isolates by HIV status: United States (1993–1996)*

	No. (%)					
	US-born patients[b]			Foreign-born Patients[b]		
Drug[a]	HIV positive	HIV negative	Unknown	HIV positive	HIV negative	Unknown
Isoniazid	622 (11.5)	227 (5.7)	520 (6.9)	124 (13.0)	248 (13.4)	877 (13.5)
Rifampin	501 (9.3)	66 (1.7)	209 (2.8)	67 (7.0)	60 (3.3)	187 (2.9)
Pyrazinamide	149 (5.1)	38 (2.1)	75 (2.2)	21 (3.2)	34 (2.8)	150 (4.1)
Streptomycin	322 (6.8)	146 (4.1)	324 (5.0)	70 (7.9)	182 (10.3)	696 (11.8)
Ethambutol hydrochloride	215 (4.0)	61 (1.6)	146 (2.0)	43 (4.6)	58 (3.2)	164 (2.6)
Isoniazid and rifampin	344 (6.4)	55 (1.4)	129 (1.7)	45 (4.7)	56 (3.0)	148 (2.3)
Rifampin only[c]	138 (2.6)	10 (0.3)	62 (0.8)	21 (2.2)	3 (0.2)	31 (0.5)

[a] The patient isolate has resistance to at least the specified drug but may have resistance to other drugs. HIV indicates human immunodeficiency virus.

[b] For all drugs, $P < .05$ for χ^2 comparison of HIV-positive versus HIV-negative patients and HIV-positive versus patients with unknown status, with the exception of foreign-born patients with isolates tested for isoniazid and pyrazinamide and HIV-positive versus HIV-negative patients with isolates tested for ethambutol.

[c] These figures were calculated only for patients with isolates tested for at least isoniazid, rifampin, and ethambutol with or without streptomycin. Monoresistant isolates were resistant to rifampin but susceptible to the other first-line drugs tested.

For U.S.-born patients, human immunodeficiency virus (HIV) infection was associated with a substantially greater risk of resistance including MDR-TB. This relationship generally did not obtain for foreign-born subjects, the same as for rifampin monoresistance.

sociation applied to both domestic and foreign-born patients (3). The relative risk of HIV was most powerfully seen, however, among U.S.-born seropositive versus seronegative subjects in relationship to both RIF monoresistance and MDR-TB: 2.6% versus 0.3% and 6.4% versus 1.4%, respectively.

The apparent propensity of HIV/AIDS patients for drug-resistant tuberculosis is quite probably a combination of biological factors (extreme vulnerability to tuberculosis) and opportunity (as AIDS patients experience progressive immunosuppression, they tend to spend more time in hospitals or other congregate settings, increasing their risk for nosocomial infection). Shafer et al. (47) studied temporal trends and transmission patterns in New York City using restriction fragment length polymorphism (RFLP) and found clustering of MDR-TB cases, particularly among HIV-infected persons who suffered disproportionately from drug-resistant disease, findings consistent with the above scenario. A subsequent survey of 167 consecutive cases of tuberculosis seen at five New York hospitals during 1992 and 1993 demonstrated that HIV-infected persons were significantly more likely to have been recently infected with MDR-TB; indeed, 79% of the drug-resistant cases were shown by RFLP to be clustered with the clear implication of recent transmission (48).

Other possible mechanisms exist that might cause an association between AIDS and drug-resistant tuberculosis. Monoresistance to RIF (or rifamycins) was a very rare phenomenon in prior surveys. However, during the 1990s, it has been seen with increasing frequency in areas of the United States, particularly in association with HIV/AIDS (49,50). A recent CDC study found 77 cases of RIF monoresistance (51); 13 of the cases were attributed to transmitted resistance. Among the other 64 cases, 59% of the individuals had HIV infection and 38% were foreign born. In a case-control comparison, prior rifabutine use (presumably for prophylaxis against *Mycobacterium avium*), antifungal therapy, and diarrhea were associated with RIF monoresistance. The authors concluded that prior rifabutine use *was* a risk factor for this phenomenon, but could not otherwise explain its origins. Because these cases all had RIF monoresistance at presentation, the authors could not invoke diarrhea with malabsorption of tuberculosis medications as an immediate causative factor. However, malabsorption of antituberculosis drugs has been shown to occur with high frequency among persons with AIDS, presumably because of various HIV-caused, parasitic or other enteropathies (52,53). Potentially, this could lead to grossly disparate drug levels, resulting in acquired resistance despite adherence to the prescribed regimen.

At a different level, promonocytic cells that are chronically infected with HIV have been shown, when superinfected with *M. tuberculosis,* to express increased plasma membrane P-glycoprotein (P-gp); this functions as a metabolically active drug reflux pump (54). The monocytic cells so infected with mycobacteria took up only 10% as much INH as cells not infected. The authors speculated that this phenomenon *could* be associated with acquired resistance, but there is no evidence of this occurring clinically.

Perhaps the best overview of this association in the United States between HIV-infection and drug-resistant tuberculosis may be seen in the Community Program for Clinical Research on AIDS (CPCRA) survey of 1992–1994 (55). There was a significantly greater likelihood for HIV-positive persons to have both single-drug resistance and MDR-TB. The differences were most pronounced in New York City (single resistance, 37% vs. 19%; MDR-TB, 19% vs. 6%). For those outside New York City, HIV infection was only associated with slightly higher rates of MDR-TB (2.8% vs. 1.4% for HIV-negative persons).

CLINICAL SCENARIOS THAT RESULT IN ACQUIRED DRUG RESISTANCE

Preventing additional ADR is vital for the future of tuberculosis treatment, prevention, and control. Therefore, it is well worth reviewing the actual clinical situations in which ADR evolves. Basically, ADR usually develops when an inadequate regimen is given to a patient with active disease. Mechanisms of "inadequacy" include noncompliance or nonadherence with therapy (4,22,56), adding a single drug to a failing regimen (16,22), and failure to initiate therapy with a sufficient number of drugs when drug resistance may be expected (22,44).

In terms of the actual dynamics by which resistant mutations are spawned and for which inadequate therapy selects, Lipsitch and Levin (57) recently published an elegant mathematical model. This model focuses on the concept of compartments or subpopulations of mycobacteria (see Fig. 10.1). In their model, the potential roles of irregular drug ingestion, taking some but not all of one's pills, and suboptimal drug concentrations can be explored. Mitchison (58) also speculated that subpopulations may help us conceptualize the processes by which resistance is created by inadequate therapy. Creating a novel paradigm for ADR, these two studies have suggested that some of these compartments or subpopulations are, in effect, being treated with monotherapy. Therefore, if such populations were inordinately large or rapid in proliferation, nominally correct therapy might beget failure and ADR.

While critics may claim that the proposed remedial practices—which hinge largely upon directly observed therapy (see Chapter 10)—are too expensive, impractical, unnecessary, or unduly infringe upon civil liberties (59), I believe that the ultimate morbidity, public health problems, and economic consequences of failing to act will be far less acceptable than the short-term costs entailed.

VIRULENCE AND DRUG-RESISTANT STRAINS

The traditional received wisdom about drug-resistant strains of tuberculosis has been that they are less "virulent" (e.g., less likely to produce progressive disease in persons infected with such strains). This was based substantially on the observation by Cohn et al. (60) that virulent strains of *M. tuberculosis*, when selectively bred in the laboratory for high-level resistance to INH, became significantly less capable of producing progressive infection in animal models. This was associated with loss of catalase activity by the bacilli, the catalase being either a direct or surrogate indicator of attenuated virulence. Nonetheless, there have been sporadic reports of cases in which persons, ostensibly normal hosts, infected with strains resistant to INH went on to develop serious, even lethal disease. Among patients admitted to National Jewish (NJC) over the years have been a modest number of normal-host contacts to MDR-TB cases, either health care workers or family members, who developed active disease with the MDR source-case strains (16). (At this point, it is important to distinguish between a normal host who develops disease attributable originally to a virulent susceptible strain, but over years of poor therapy acquires multidrug resistance and, by contrast, an individual who is initially infected with an MDR-TB strain and proceeds to develop active disease—"acquired" versus "transmitted" drug resistance) (Table 11.1).

Snider et al. from the CDC performed a retrospective, case-control analysis of the likelihood of infecting contacts by patients with susceptible strains (61). They observed that *infection* rates were comparable overall for young, high-risk contacts to susceptible or resistant cases (33.6% and 39.8%, respectively). And, among contacts to drug-resistant cases, with a history of prior treatment, the risk of infection was even higher—49%—presumably reflecting extended periods of exposure. The authors concluded that their data indicated no lesser risk of infection when contacts were exposed to tubercle bacilli resistant to high concentrations of INH or to INH and SM.

However, this does not fully address the issue of virulence, for it is possible that strains could cause local pulmonary infections sufficient to cause tuberculin conversion but have a lesser capacity to produce active pulmonary or extrapulmonary disease. In the CDC study, there were positive cultures recorded for 4 of 239 (1.67%) persons deemed infected with resistant strains and 6 of 252 (2.38%) infected with susceptible strains, a difference that was not statistically significant.

Overall, it appears as though there may be wide differences in transmissibility and/or virulence among strains of *M. tuberculosis* both susceptible and resistant. The CDC study cited above noted that index cases tended to infect most (or all) or few (or none) of their contacts. While this may reflect other elements including the physical environment of the shared air, relative vulnerability of the exposed groups, or the nature of the index case's cough, a hypothetical case can be made for strain "transmissibility" or "virulence" as significant variables.

Because transmission occurs from a *diseased* human, all strains so spread must be considered pathogenic. However, previous investigations (see Chapter 2) indicate considerable variations among susceptible strains in in vitro growth rates and ability to produce disease in animals. Recently, Ordway et al. (62) have observed some MDR-TB strains that exhibit in vitro growth rates and animal virulence characteristics comparable to the most virulent, wild-type drug-susceptible strains. Certainly, the rapid community spread of MDR-TB in New York noted above constitutes powerful circumstantial evidence of the transmittability and virulence of these microbes.

The 1996 report of the multiinstitutional spread of the notorious "strain W" in New York City may offer some insight into the question of INH resistance and virulence (63). Despite mutations in the *katG* locus, this strain is catalase positive and grows rapidly in culture media and animals (Barry Kreiswirth, personal communication, 1998). Also, multivariant analysis of factors favoring survival included the administration of INH (63). From this, I infer that INH resistance derived by this unique *katG* mutation may be associated with more retained virulence; this *may* be mediated by catalase-peroxidase protection against the host macrophages' oxidative burst.

Overall, the preponderance of evidence indicates that, while some strains with laboratory-bred resistance exhibit slowed in vitro replication and attenuated in vivo virulence in animal models, current drug-resistant strains have demonstrated the capacity to produce progressive disease in both normal and immunosuppressed contacts.

IMPACT OF DRUG RESISTANCE ON THE OUTCOME OF CHEMOTHERAPY

Early in the era of drug treatment, it was recognized that in vitro resistance to drugs such as

INH and SM was associated with increased risk of treatment failure (5). This phenomenon was most prominent in the early era of therapy when INH was the dominant bactericidal agent. In the current situation, the loss of a single drug to resistance is potentially less significant, because of the availability and use of other potent agents such as RIF, PZA, and EMB.

The most reliable data on the impact of drug resistance on treatment outcome were derived from British Medical Research Council (BMRC) Short-Course Chemotherapy trials performed in East Africa, Hong Kong, and Singapore (64). In these studies, previously untreated patients with pulmonary tuberculosis were enrolled and assigned to study regimens that were administered regardless of initial susceptibility results. Drug testing and surveillance bacteriological studies were conducted in the BMRC laboratories in London and were of superior quality. The outcome of these studies may be summarized as follows: pretreatment resistance was associated with an 88-fold higher risk of failure (to convert sputum cultures to negative), and, among those whose cultures did become negative, there was a twofold higher risk of relapse after drug therapy was completed. What merits emphasis in these data, however, is the strongly favorable effect associated with assignment to a regimen initially containing INH, RIF, PZA, and SM. Among such cases, the failure rate was less than 5%, in contrast to an approximately 20% rate among cases assigned to less potent regimens. It should be stressed, however, that the bulk of resistance in these trials constituted loss of susceptibility to a single drug, usually INH or SM.

Among the BMRC short-course trials, two studies provide particular insights into the management of cases involving resistance to INH and/or SM. During the 1980s, consecutive studies of 6-month thrice-weekly (TIW) regimens were conducted in Hong Kong, trials I refer to as HK-TIW 1 (65) and HK-TIW 2 (66). In HK-TIW 1, all regimens consisted of at least four drugs for the entire 6 months. In HK-TIW 2, only the INH and RIF were consistently given for the entire period. The duration of PZA included 2-, 4-, and 6-month arms; SM was given for 4 months except for one arm in which it was omitted (see Table 10.5 for full description of regimens). For patients with *drug-susceptible* disease, comparison of HK-TIW 1 and HK-TIW 2 showed that PZA need only be given for 2 months and that SM contributed little to the success of this type of regimen. However, in both trials there were approximately 100 patients enrolled whose strains of *M. tuberculosis* had initial resistance to INH and/or SM. For such cases, HK-TIW 1 still yielded excellent results with only 1 of 104 failing to convert and only 3 of 103 (2.9%) relapsing. However, in HK-TIW 2, which employed shortened PZA duration and reduced duration or deletion of SM, the failure rate was 3% and the relapse rate 6%. I infer from these observations that, if patients are begun on a four-drug regimen (INH, RIF, PZA, and SM or EMB) and the initial susceptibility test indicates resistance to INH (and/or SM), it is still possible to obtain excellent results with a 6-month, all-intermittent regimen. In the Hong Kong trials, no changes were made in the regimen, despite reported resistance. However, in cases with INH resistance, I would advocate stopping the INH (it contributes little in this setting and poses a small but real risk for hepatitis or other toxicities). Rather, if the patient were receiving INH, RIF, PZA, and SM when INH resistance was noted, I would drop INH and add EMB. If both INH and SM resistance were reported, I would add EMB and levofloxacin. Note that the Hong Kong experience indicates that 6-month therapy is feasible despite resistance, assuming normal early bacteriological response to therapy!

Isolated resistance to RIF is relatively uncommon, and there is little clinical experience managing such cases. However, the 1993–1996 CDC survey noted above (3) found that 2.6% of U.S.-born HIV-infected patients with tuberculosis harbored strains with resistance to RIF only. Also, a small number of cases have been reported wherein HIV-infected persons with drug-susceptible tuberculosis developed isolated resistance to RIF while receiving therapy (67). Also problematic is the scenario wherein toxicity precludes the use of rifamycins. In these instances, it is still possible to employ short-course therapy, but a 6-month regimen is not feasible. A study from Hong Kong omitted RIF from regimens because of concerns of cost (68); the regimens consisted of INH, PZA, and SM given daily, thrice weekly, or twice weekly for 6 or 9 months (see regimens 4 to 6, Table 10.5, for details). The results of this study indicate that a 9-month intermittent regimen can yield effective results without RIF so long as one is able or willing to administer SM (or comparably effective amikacin) for this period.

As noted earlier, the major hurdle in modern therapy is resistance to both INH and RIF, referred to in this chapter as multidrug resistance (MDR-TB). In actuality, there are relatively few cases in which resistance only to these drugs is present. More often, there is resistance to several additional agents by the time patients arrive at specialized medical attention.

Among the BMRC studies, only 11 of the approximately 2,900 patients enrolled were found to have INH and RIF resistance (64), and only 3 (27%) of them were cured. Among 171 patients recently reported from the National Jewish Hospital with INH and RIF resistance, only 4 had resistance merely to these two drugs (16). By the time of referral to this specialty center, the patients had been treated for an average of 6 years elsewhere and were shedding organisms resistant to a mean number of 5.8 drugs. Among the 134 patients eligible for long-term analysis, only 56% were cured despite the use of aggressive medical retreatment. Factors associated with adverse outcome in univariate analysis included previous use of a greater number of drugs, in vitro resistance to more drugs, regimens containing fewer previously unused drugs, and male gender. Similarly, among patients receiving a standard 8-month regimen in a short-course study in the Philippines, progressively higher rates of treatment failure were seen with initial resistance to more drugs (69).

Four separate reports from New York City appeared in 1995–1996 on the response to therapy for patients with MDR-TB (70-73). The group from Beth Israel Hospital in Manhattan demonstrated better outcome with early recognition of resistance and administration of two or more drugs to which there was in vitro susceptibility (70). Similarly, the group from the Bronx-Lebanon Hospital reported improved survival rates if the patients were given 2 or more effective agents within 4 weeks of diagnosis (71). In both of these series, a high percentage of patients with MDR-TB (89% and 94%, respectively) had HIV infection or AIDS. Similarly, a report from Bellevue Hospital in Manhattan demonstrated improved survival with MDR-TB if patients were given appropriate treatment (73); however, neither of the death rates—in the HIV-negative group (20%) or the HIV-positive group—(72%) were acceptable.

By contrast, another report focused on 26 HIV-negative patients with MDR-TB who "responded well" to appropriate chemotherapy (72). Noting that these patients had been put on revised treatment within 44 days (range, 0 to 181 days) of diagnosis, the authors noted that—despite MDR-TB—they had converted to sputum culture negativity within 69 days (range, 2 to 705 days). Important distinctions should be made between this series of HIV-negative patients and those reported by Goble et al. (16). The New York City patients' strains were resistant to a median of 3.5 drugs versus 6 drugs in the Denver series; 35% of the New York City strains were resistant only to INH and RIF, but only 4% of the Denver patients had this limited resistance pattern. Also, 3 of the 19 patients with pulmonary disease in New York City underwent early resectional surgery, and 7 of the 26 patients in New York City had extrapulmonary tuberculosis only, disease that typically is paucibacillary in nature (74).

Based on these observations, recommendations regarding the choice of drug regimens for patients with proven or suspected drug resistance are displayed in Table 11.9; drug dosage, minimum inhibitory concentration (MIC) data, and relevant pharmacokinetic data are shown in Table 11.10.

IMPLICATIONS OF POTENTIAL RESISTANCE FOR CHOICE OF INITIAL THERAPY

The early reports of extremely high death rates among persons with nosocomially transmitted MDR-TB led to reconsideration of initial

TABLE 11.9. *Suggested regimens for patients with tuberculosis with various patterns of drug resistance*

Resistance	Suggested regimen	Duration of therapy	Comments
Isoniazid, streptomycin	RIF, PZA, EMB, AK[a]	6 to 9 mo	Anticipate 100% response rate and less than 5% relapse rate
Isoniazid and ethambutol (± streptomycin)	RIF, PZA, FQN, AK[a]	6 to 12 mo	Efficacy should be similar to above regimen
Isoniazid and rifampin (± streptomycin)	PZA, EMB, FQN, AK[b]	18 to 24 mo	Consider surgery
Isoniazid, rifampin and ethambutol (± streptomycin)	PZA, FQN, AK,[a] Plus 2[b]	24 mo after conversion	Consider surgery
Isoniazid, rifampin, and pyrazinamide (± streptomycin)	EMB, FQN, AK,[a] Plus 2[b]	24 mo after conversion	Consider surgery
Isoniazid, rifampin, pyrazinamide, and ethambutol (± streptomycin)	FQN, AK,[a] Plus 3[b]	24 mo after conversion	Surgery, if possible

[a] If there is resistance to amikacin, kanamycin, and streptomycin, capreomycin is a good alternative. Injectable agents are usually continued for 4 to 6 months if toxicity does not intervene. All the injectable drugs may be given daily or twice or thrice weekly and may be administered intravenously or intramuscularly.

[b] Potential agents from which to choose include ethionamide, cycloserine, or aminosalicylic acid. Others that are potentially useful but of unproved utility include clofazimine and amoxicillin-clavulanate. Clarithromycin and azithromycin are unlikely to be active (see text). Rifabutin may be active versus some strains resistant to rifampin (see Table 11.2).

RIF, rifampin; PZA, pyrazinamide; EMB, ethambutol; AK, amikacin; FQN, fluoroquinolone.

TABLE 11.10. *Dosages and pharmacokinetics of antituberculosis medications*

Drug	Usual adult daily dosage[a]	Peak serum concentration μg/mL	Usual MIC[b] (range, μg/mL)
First-line oral drugs			
Isoniazid	300 mg	3–5	0.01–0.25
Rifampin	600 mg	8–20	0.06–0.25
Pyrazinamide	30 mg/kg	20–60	6.2–50
Ethambutol	15–25 mg/kg	3–5	0.5–2.0
Injectable drugs[b]			
Streptomycin	15 mg/kg	35–45	0.25–2.0
Amikacin	15 mg/kg	35–45	0.5–1.0
Kanamycin	15 mg/kg	35–45	1.5–3.0
Capreomycin	15 mg/kg	35–45	1.25–2.5
Second-line oral drugs			
Rifabutin	300–450 mg		0.125–1.0
Ofloxacin	400 mg b.i.d.	8–10	0.25–2.0
Ciprofloxacin	750 mg b.i.d.	3–5	0.25–2.0
Levofloxacin	500–750 mg b.i.d.		
Sparfloxacin	200 mg b.i.d.		
Ethionamide	250 mg b.i.d. or t.i.d.	1–5	0.3–1.2
Aminosalicylic acid (Paser[d])	4 g b.i.d. or t.i.d.	20–40	Not known
Cycloserine	250 mg b.i.d. or t.i.d.	20–35	Not known

[a] b.i.d., twice a day, t.i.d., three times a day, q.i.d., four times a day.

[b] Data are from Heifets (79). MIC denotes minimal inhibitory concentration.

[c] These injectable agents may be given with comparable efficacy on a thrice-weekly basis.

[d] Paser® Granules, Jacobus Pharmaceuticals, Princeton, NJ.

treatment of patients in the community (75). This led to the practice of commencing treatment with six- to seven-drug regimens consisting of the standard agents, INH/RIF/PZA/EMB, plus agents to which the infamous strain W was susceptible, typically ciprofloxacin, cycloserine, and capreomycin—"the three C's." Such empirical treatment appeared to substantially improve survival/response rates in this population (63).

However, in most communities or populations it is difficult to accept this as a standard practice. Yet, there is appropriate concern that use of a conventional four-drug regimen might lead not only to treatment failure and death but also to further acquired resistance (76); Paul Farmer has dubbed this the "amplification effect."

What then is to be done? In technologically advanced settings, a case can be made for waiting for susceptibility data, which may return in 2 to 3 weeks (see Chapter 2 for details). Conceivably, we soon will have molecular probes that can identify RIF or INH resistance in 24 to 48 hours (again, see Chapter 2). One of the reports from New York City suggested that patients who did not have defervescence within 14 days of commencing standard treatment should be considered probable MDR-TB cases (70); while only 67% of the patients with active tuberculosis had fever in that report, this might be an effective strategy in some communities. Other authorities have suggested that the presence of MDR-TB can be anticipated by a history of prior treatment (76). However, in many of the cases of MDR-TB cited above, there was clear evidence of recently transmitted MDR-TB, greatly lessening the negative predictive value of the history of no prior treatment.

The history of HIV-infection/AIDS may be a useful marker of the risk of MDR-TB, although multivariant analysis did not confirm the validity of this relationship in two of the New York City series above (70,71). However, for individuals known to have AIDS, the presumption of initial drug resistance may be prudent and appropriate for the following reasons: (a) They may spend time in institutions such as hospitals, clinics, residencies, or prisons where transmission of tuberculosis is more probable, (b) they may come from nations or subcultures such as users of injection drugs wherein resistance may be more common (56), and (c) failure to promptly give adequate therapy is more likely to result in death.

For developing nations where good laboratory support is not available, the practice has been to select therapy based solely on prior treatment patterns. Among a series of patients in Brazil, MDR-TB rates varied widely according to the nature of prior therapy: 54% of those who *failed to respond to administered first-line therapy*, 36% of those who *failed to respond to second-line therapy*, and only 6% of those who *absconded from initial treatment or relapsed after initial treatment* had MDR-TB (76). Nonetheless, at the current time, WHO (77) and IUATLD (78) guidelines advocate empirical regimens stratified by prior treatment history. Given financial limitations, this appears to be the best option at present, but in view of the predictable morbidity and mortality, as well as the potential for amplification of resistance, we must move promptly to refine and remedy this process.

In summary, my practice—when confronted with an individual who may reasonably be deemed at high risk for MDR-TB—would be to initiate treatment with an extended regimen. This regimen might contain an uncommon injectable agent like capreomycin, a fluoroquinolone like levofloxacin, and an exotic oral agent like cycloserine or para-aminosalicylate (PAS), drugs to which resistance is uncommon. Rather than using rapid laboratory reporting times to add additional drugs to an inadequate regimen, I would use them to delete unnecessary medications from a surfeit regimen.

TREATMENT OF PATIENTS WITH DRUG-RESISTANT TUBERCULOSIS

Management of cases with *single* drug resistance is generally only moderately more complicated than management of drug-susceptible cases. Even cases in which there is two- or three-drug resistance may be addressed in a fairly straightforward manner *so long as either INH or RIF is available for use*. **However, cases in which there is resistance to both INH and RIF should be regarded as high-priority medi-**

cal/public health problems. Patients with such MDR-TB should be immediately referred to specialized centers for highly structured, aggressive therapy. In the industrialized, relatively affluent nations, effective treatment may potentially be provided for such persons. However, in less wealthy nations, cases of tuberculosis with resistance to both INH and RIF have been deemed generally untreatable (78). This stark reality cannot be overemphasized.

This chapter is particularly intended for clinicians in industrialized nations with in vitro susceptibility testing and predictable availability of second-line or retreatment medications. However, in less affluent nations, clinicians typically define cases as "retreatment" or "chronic" as a surrogate indicator of drug resistance. In this setting, therapeutic decisions are usually made by algorithm or inferences from previous treatment. WHO recently published a helpful monograph to aid this process (77).

In Vitro Testing, Susceptibility or Resistance, and the National Jewish Center Classification System

Early efforts to characterize strains of tubercle bacilli as "susceptible" or "resistant" recognized that there was a wide disparity between the concentrations of INH or SM required to kill the organisms in vitro from wild-type, newly recovered isolates and those from patients who had received the drugs and failed to be cured. Subsequently, investigators observed that the presence of "resistance" predicted less favorable responses to treatment (5). This led to the adoption of "critical concentrations" of drugs, levels at which resistance in vitro was predictive of lack of therapeutic efficacy (19). The validity of these designations was directly proven in prospective clinical studies of human disease *only* for INH and SM (5). For such agents as RIF, EMB, and PZA, these designations have been inferred, based on limited data and in vitro observations. For less frequently used second-line drugs (ethionamide, cycloserine, kanamycin, capreomycin) or newer agents (such as the fluoroquinolones), there is very little systematic information from human trials available.

As a result, we have employed a system at our institution that represents an amalgam of clinically proven results, in vitro and animal model studies, and extrapolation from fundamental pharmacological principles applied to other antimycobacterial or antiinfective agents. This system was described by Heifets (79) and has proven clinically helpful, albeit statistically unproven in program use. This classification is represented in Table 11.11.

Drugs Used in the Treatment of Drug-Resistant Tuberculosis

All of the agents listed in Table 11.11 may be characterized by their ability to kill *tubercle* bacilli in vitro at concentrations readily achievable in serum or tissue *except* for the drug PZA. PZA has several peculiarities that are worth briefly noting. It is a prodrug, requiring cleavage by an amidase to release the active compound, pyrazinoic acid; it is significantly active only at acidic pH in the range of 5.5 to 6.0 or lower; even at these concentrations it has extremely little activity in vitro at achievable serum concentrations (80). See Chapter 10 for a more thorough review of PZA's activity.

Conversely, β-lactam antibiotics, including penicillins and cephalosporins, have reasonable activity in vitro against *M. tuberculosis* but seem to have limited utility in therapy (81–86). Although there have been anecdotal reports of efficacy (87), we found disappointing activity in patients given ceforanide, the most active β-lactam agent found in our earlier screening study (86). Despite in vitro MICs of 4 to 8 μg/mL and our ability to achieve maximum serum levels up to 25-fold higher than the MICs, no bacteriological or clinical responses were seen in three patients to whom the drug was given for many weeks (unpublished data, 1982–1985). Subsequently, we studied the activity of ceforanide in the ex vivo human macrophage model (88). This study indicated that this cefamycin agent had considerably less activity within the macrophage than in simple culture medium, a feature common to β-lactam drugs. Thus, the question of drug penetration and activity within the macrophage remains a significant issue for characterizing the potential for new

TABLE 11.11. *Susceptibility criteria and side effects of antituberculosis medications*[a]

Drug	Susceptible	Moderately susceptible	Moderately resistant	Resistant	Side effects[b]
	[minimal inhibitory concentration (μg/mL)]				
Isoniazid	≤0.1	0.2–1.0	2.0	≥4	Hepatitis, neuritis, lupus erythematosus syndrome, drowsiness, mood changes
Rifampin	≤0.5	1.0–4.0	8.0	≥16	Drug interactions, hepatitis, thrombopenia, abdominal distress, diarrhea
Rifabutin	—	—	—	—	Neutropenia, thrombopenia, hepatitis, uveitis, lupus syndrome
Pyrazinamide	≤100	300	900	>900	Hepatitis, rash, arthralgia or arthritis, hyperuricemia, abdominal distress
Ethambutol	≤2.0	4.0	8.0	≥16	Optic neuritis, abdominal distress
Streptomycin	≤2.0	4.0	8.0	≥16	Hearing loss, ataxia, nystagmus, azotemia, proteinuria, eosinophilia, serum electrolyte abnormalities
Amikacin	≤2.0	4.0	8.0	≥16	
Kanamycin	≤2.0	4.0	8.0	≥16	
Capreomycin	≤2.0	4.0	8.0	≥16	
Ofloxacin	≤2.0	4.0	8.0	≥16	Abdominal distress, headache, anxiety, tremulousness, thrush
Levofloxacin	—	—	—	—	Similar to ofloxacin
Ciprofloxacin	≤2.0	4.0	8.0	≥16	Abdominal distress, headache, anxiety, tremulousness, thrush, drug interactions
Sparfloxacin	—	—	—	—	Similar to other FQNs plus photosensitization and QT interval prolongation
Ethionamide	≤1.25	2.5	5.0	≤10	Abdominal distress, dysgeusia, diarrhea, hepatitis, arthralgia
Aminosalicylic acid	—	—	—	—	Abdominal distress, nausea, bloating, diarrhea, rash, edema
Cycloserine	—	—	—	—	Mood and cognitive deterioration, psychosis, seizures

[a] The susceptibility categories are from Heifets (79).
[b] A partial listing; for more information see the *Physicians' Desk Reference* or the package insert provided with each medication.
FQN, fluoroquinolone.

antituberculosis agents. However, given their ability to inhibit tubercle bacilli in vitro, ongoing research with the β-lactam agents is warranted.

Initiating Drug Therapy

In most cases of tuberculosis, the clinician does not know the drug-resistance pattern for the patient when drug therapy is begun. Regional patterns of drug resistance, the patient's HIV status, history of exposure or prior therapy, and demographic features including profession, national origin, age, race, and ethnicity all influence the initial choice of medical regimens (see "Implications of Potential Resistance for Choice of initial Therapy" above).

Suggested regimens for various patterns of resistance are noted in Table 11.9. However, successful treatment often requires that the medications be introduced with staggered schedules and escalating doses. If patients are begun on a regimen with full doses of several poorly tolerated drugs such as ethionamide, PAS, or even fluoroquinolones, severe gastrointestinal tract disturbances (nausea, vomiting, diarrhea, or abdominal pain) may ensue, resulting in powerfully aversive conditioning. Such experiences may create anticipatory distress that makes subsequent use of these drugs problematic.

Although it may appear expensive in the short run, our experience indicates that for most patients, introducing these drugs in the hospital with careful symptomatic monitoring and support offers the best chance for an enduring accommodation to them. Our practice has been to commence with low doses spaced over the day and build up to the usual therapeutic levels over 2 to 4 days (16). After several days, serum drug concentrations and kinetics are measured to ensure that dosing is in the acceptable range. Although we are concerned that extended use of suboptimal doses or insufficient numbers of agents might result in further acquired resistance, this has not been observed.

While in the hospital, most patients tolerate agents with gastrointestinal tract side effects best when these are given in split doses. This poses a potential problem on discharge, since compliance with drug regimens diminishes with the frequency of dosing. Thus, as patients are nearing discharge, we often attempt to consolidate dosing to more easily followed schedules. For instance, ethionamide 250 mg twice daily may be switched to 500 mg once daily, ofloxacin 400 mg twice daily to 800 mg daily, and—occasionally—PAS 4 g twice daily to 8 g once daily. Often, these drugs may be given with metoclopramide to enhance tolerance. Caution should be taken with the use of antacids, histamine type 2 (H_2) blockers, or coating agents such as Carafate, which may bind or otherwise alter absorption of some of these drugs. Ethionamide and PAS may be tolerated better when given at the hour of bedtime. However, the fluoroquinolones given at that time commonly result in insomnia or unpleasant dreaming and generally should be given in the morning.

Pharmacokinetic Guidance of Therapy

For patients with drug-susceptible tuberculosis, monitoring serum for therapeutic drug levels is rarely indicated. Agents such as INH and RIF are so potent that, even with modest reductions below "ideal" levels, most such patients are readily cured (53). By contrast, for patients with MDR-TB who are receiving so-called second-line agents, which are less effective and generally more toxic, pharmacokinetic studies to place dosing in the range where therapeutic effect may be reasonably expected and toxicity risks are minimized should be performed for all cases when feasible. Again, while this may appear extravagant, the consequences of inadequate drug levels, toxicity that requires discontinuation of a drug(s), and further acquired resistance with treatment failure are so profound that these aggressive measures are justifiable, in my estimation.

Monitoring for Drug Toxicity

Periodic assessment is essential for persons receiving the agents typically employed for MDR-TB. Drugs that require particularly close attention include the aminoglycosides, which pose significant risks of otovestibular or renal toxicity, and cycloserine, which can produce confusion, thought disorders, suicidal ideation, psychosis, and seizures. Other drugs as well as these pose risks for other classic adverse drug effects including hematological, hepatic, or hypersensitivity reactions. For a listing of the most clinically relevant side effects and toxicity of the antimycobacterial drugs, see Table 11.9.

What needs careful emphasis is that monitoring to ensure appropriate drug levels generally reduces the likelihood of all of these toxicities and that early detection of adverse reactions usually minimizes their morbidity.

In short, treatment of MDR-TB is a labor- and laboratory-intensive process. It cannot be performed well without clinical assets and should not be performed in a cavalier manner.

Ensuring Adherence to Treatment

Many patients with MDR-TB developed some or all of the resistance because of erratic drug administration. Although one might believe that being confronted with a potentially untreatable, lethal variety of tuberculosis should enhance patients' compliance, many patients remain consistent in their behavior. Even persons *without* a history of noncompliance may be tempted to deviate from prescribed regimens because of the typically unpleasant effects of the drugs.

Thus, we follow very rigorous nursing procedures in the hospital. All doses of every medicine are directly observed; pills are not left at the bedside to be taken later. As patients near discharge, they are generally begun on a routine where they must come to the nurses' station at the appropriate times to ask for their drugs by name and dose. In this way they are educated and, it is hoped, conditioned to their postdischarge routine.

Following discharge, most patients are returned to some type of structured, monitored treatment depending on local facilities and means. Ideally, directly observed treatment (DOT) should be given for those with prior records of nonadherence. However, DOT is quite difficult, since the second-line oral agents are not amenable to intermittent (less than daily) schedules and may, in fact, require multiple doses per day. In general, the programs that enjoy the most success involve one or two caregivers regularly assigned to a patient, a situation that promotes closer human relationships and more clearly delineates responsibilities.

Monitoring Response to Therapy

The vast majority of HIV-negative patients with MDR-TB have pulmonary disease that can be monitored readily by sputum studies and chest radiography. At National Jewish we obtain weekly sputa samples for smear and culture to assess the response to treatment. In addition, surrogate markers such as fever, cough, sputum production, weight gain, and erythrocyte sedimentation rate are monitored.

Although the bacteriological and clinical markers do not usually improve as rapidly with MDR-TB as with susceptible disease, most patients who are going to respond begin to show favorable markers within 3 to 6 weeks following initiation of therapy. Indeed, in the series of patients of Goble et al. (16) with MDR-TB treated at NJC between 1973 and 1983, those who eventually became culture negative converted their sputum tests at a median of 2 months following initiation of therapy. Failure to show positive trends may be seen as an indication for intensified drug therapy, consideration for surgical resection, and—potentially—immunomodulation treatment (see below).

ADJUVANT THERAPIES FOR MULTIDRUG-RESISTANT TUBERCULOSIS

In addition to the administration of antimicrobial drug therapy, various other treatment modalities may play a significant role in patient management. Our recent experience has indicated that resectional surgery contributes significantly to cure rates (see below). However, the feasibility and success of surgery appears to be substantially enhanced by nutritional support. Intriguingly, the potential for immunity-enhancing therapy may be nearing clinical reality. "Collapse therapy" such as pneumoperitoneum does not appear to be of general utility, although it may be helpful in highly selected cases (89); artificial pneumothorax was recently reviewed, wistfully (90).

Resectional Surgery

Efforts at removing diseased portions of tuberculous lung tissue in the prechemotherapeutic era were largely abandoned because of failure of bronchial closure and wound dehiscence secondary to uncontrolled infection. Rather than resection, surgical approaches in that era focused on "collapse" procedures (see below). With the advent of modern chemotherapy, surgery enjoyed a brief revival, being employed to remove cavitary lesions that persisted after medical treatment. However, continued observations eventually showed that such resections were unnecessary and the practice was abandoned.

Resectional surgery for MDR-TB was applied infrequently at NJC during the 1970s and 1980s;

only 9 of 171 (5.3%) of the 1973–1982 series of patients with pulmonary MDR-TB underwent surgery (16). However, we have employed resectional surgery with escalating aggressiveness over the last decade. This is based on the following factors: (a) review of our experience with heroic medical management indicated unacceptably high rates of treatment failure—44% overall—with consequences that included respiratory failure, death, or—at best—drastic social isolation and (b) accumulating evidence of the safety and efficacy of the surgical approach.

Beginning with relatively simple lobar resections in patients with abundant respiratory reserve in 1983, we have progressed to pneumonectomies or bilateral resections in persons with very marginal cardiorespiratory capacity. In this process we have violated traditional physiological barriers to surgery used for a disease such as bronchogenic carcinoma. Our logic in this aggressive approach to surgery relates to the following features of MDR-TB that do not apply to lung cancer: (a) patients with pulmonary MDR-TB that remains culture positive have sorely constrained options in living: they cannot reside at home with family, cannot work or attend school, nor can they enjoy normal social intercourse or partake in community recreational activities, and (b) unlike the most lethal consequence of cancers, metastatic disease, the critical issue in chronic pulmonary tuberculosis has to do with progressive lung damage culminating in respiratory failure, and we have noted that cavitary lesions are the nidus for intrapulmonary spread and that their removal stops or substantially slows subsequent lung injury (91,92).

By contrast with the earlier series of 134 evaluable MDR-TB patients who were treated between 1973 and 1982 (16), only 5.2% of whom went to surgery, 62 of 109 (57%) similar patients treated between 1983 and 1993 underwent pulmonary resectional procedures (93). These groups were similar in terms of extent of drug resistance: all patients shed strains resistant to INH and RIF plus various other drugs, the mean number to which there was resistance being six to seven drugs in both series. In terms of radiographic markers, cavitation and bilateral involvement were comparable. Also, sputum smear and culture profiles on admission to NJC were comparable between these two groups. The only systematic differences in the management of the 1973–1982 and 1983–1993 groups were, in the latter phase, the use of fluoroquinolone antibiotics, the application of pharmacokinetic drug monitoring, and the increased frequency of surgery.

Indications for surgery included the following: (a) persistence of culture-positive MDR-TB, despite extended drug retreatment, and/or (b) extensive patterns of drug resistance that, based on our previous experience, were likely to be associated with the risk of treatment failure or relapse with additional resistance, and/or, (c) the existence of local cavitary, necrotic/destructive disease in a lobe or region of the lung that was amenable to resection without producing respiratory insufficiency and/or severe pulmonary hypertension.

Notably, among patients undergoing resection, a modest proportion had negative sputum cultures when they went to surgery. In these persons, we were concerned that, because of cavitary or devitalized tissue and extensive patterns of resistance, there was a high risk of recrudescence and, based on our earlier series of cases, that further acquired resistance was likely.

Among patients who went to surgery while still culture positive, we used our historical experience with time-to-conversion data as an indicator of the probability of chemotherapy failure to elect surgery. The analysis of the 1973–1982 group by Goble et al. (16) revealed that the median time for cultures to become negative at NJC was 2 months with the great majority becoming negative by 4 months. Thus, if a patient in the later group remained culture positive into the third or fourth month and had high levels of resistance, we concluded that the patient was unlikely to be cured with medication alone and proceeded with surgery.

Contraindications to surgery include such extensive bilateral diseases that resection of cavitary disease is not feasible. Also, attempting resection without establishing some antimycobacterial control is fraught with risk of bronchial or chest wall wound dehiscence.

Results in patients managed with drug therapy alone and with combined medication and surgery are displayed in Fig. 11.1. The patients in the later era (1983–1993), who received medical treatment alone, were a mix of disparate groups: (a) those with less extensive disease and/or resistance who could be readily cured with medication alone and (b) those with such extensive drug resistance that we could not achieve sufficient bacteriological suppression to facilitate surgery, or (c) those with such extensive bilateral disease that resection(s) would have resulted in cardiorespiratory failure or (d) those who refused the recommended surgery (93).

As may be seen, the overall "cure" rate during the surgical era was substantially higher than in the prior decade (81% vs. 56%). Although historical controls are an admittedly imperfect mechanism of comparison, we believe that the difference is valid and clinically meaningful because of the close similarities between the two groups and their medical management.

Obviously, surgery is not without the risk of serious complications and death. As noted in Fig. 11.1, four operative deaths (within 30 days of surgery) have occurred. The most common element associated with operative deaths in both our MDR-TB and nontuberculous mycobacterial infections has been postpneumonectomy, noncardiogenic pulmonary edema; noted to occur with other lung disorders, this unpredictable condition is quite hazardous (94). Other major complications include late bronchial dehiscense with bronchopleural fistula (less than 2%); rarely, this has entailed prolonged open draining with an Eloesser flap procedure. Because of extensive pleural scarring, extrapleural sharp dissection may be required; in some of these cases, multiple blood transfusions have been required. Because of marginal ventilatory reserve, a few patients (<2%) have required prolonged postoperative assisted ventilation or, rarely, reintubation. Occasionally, inability of the remaining lung to inflate adequately and/or failure of the mediastinum to shift or diaphragm to elevate has resulted in a chronic space problem; thus, tailor-

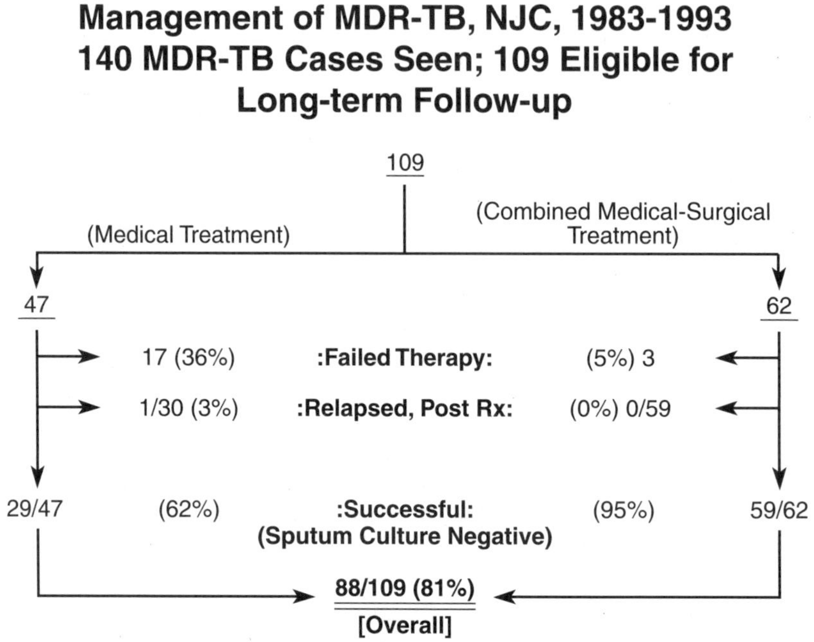

FIG. 11.1. As noted in text, patients were allocated to "medical treatment" or "combined medical-surgical treatment" for diverse reasons. Surgical morbidity included one postoperative bronchopleural fistula, which responded to reoperation, and one death from postoperative noncardiogenic pulmonary edema (included under "failed therapy"). There were three late nonsurgical deaths in the resectional series. In addition to improving sputum conversion rates, surgery substantially shortened duration of hospital stay, partially offsetting the operative expenses.

ing thoracoplasties has been required in 3 patients. Remote from surgery, 4 patients have developed severe pulmonary hypertension with cor pulmonale. From our pre-operative evaluations, it seems improbable that this is due simply to extirpation of the vascular bed, but we have no alternative explanations.

While these deaths and complications are obvious drawbacks to surgery, we believe that overall mortality is lessened compared with simple medical management and that the opportunity to rejoin society makes the risk readily defensible.

The medical factor that had the greatest potential for altering the outcomes in these different eras was use of the fluoroquinolone antibiotics, ofloxacin and ciprofloxacin. Virtually all strains of *M. tuberculosis,* wild-type or multidrug resistant, are susceptible to these agents in vitro unless they have been previously exposed (95). Our experience with these fluoroquinolones in our MDR-TB patients indicates that they are quite helpful in reducing the mycobacterial burden but are not consistently capable of producing sputum conversion. A 1993 report of the early bactericidal activity (EBA) of ciprofloxacin (750 μg) suggested that it was almost equal to INH (96), but a later study from another center indicated that, although there was a dose-dependent EBA of ciprofloxacin, even at 1,500-mg dosing, ciprofloxacin's activity was roughly one-third that of INH (97).

The great majority of patients in our series went to operation still culture positive despite 3 to 4 months of drug therapy including aggressive dosing of ofloxacin or ciprofloxacin. Based on our prior experience with "time-to-conversion" for medically "cured" patients, I believe that a clear preponderance of patients undergoing surgery would have experienced treatment failures or relapses without the resectional procedure, despite the use of the fluoroquinolone drugs. Whether use of the newer fluoroquinolones such as levofloxacin or sparfloxacin will provide substantially better results has not yet been proven; a recent review highlights previous experience with fluoroquinolones, emphasizing the risk of ADR if used in inadequate regimens (98).

Nutritional Enhancement

"Consumption" has been applied historically to tuberculosis, reflecting the inexorable, debilitating inanition from the progressive infection. During the modern era in industrialized societies where patients generally have ready access to health care, relatively few patients reach the advanced stages of cachexia seen historically or presently in developing countries. However, many patients with MDR-TB for whom effective chemotherapy has not been achieved do experience advanced stages of wasting.

Nutritional support is an important element of care for all persons with inanition including tuberculosis (99–101). Especially, however, reversal of malnutrition and wasting is vital for the success of surgical procedures. The stress of general anesthesia, thoracotomy, blood loss, tissue resection, and interrupted oral alimentation predictably worsens nutritional parameters. For patients undergoing pneumonectomy, there is substantial protein loss as the evacuated hemithorax fills with albumin-laden serum. Protein deficiencies threaten healing of the bronchial and/or chest wall closures. Disruptions of the bronchial stump or thoracotomy incision constitute major, life-threatening, extremely morbid complications.

Hence systematic, aggressive efforts to enrich nutrition are clearly indicated. Nutritional assessment and ongoing monitoring by a dietitian are standard components of care for all of our MDR-TB patients.

Anorexia is quite common because of the "toxic" effects of the ongoing tuberculous infection; this probably is due in part to the effects of the cytokine, tumor necrosis factor-α (TNF-α), known historically as "cachexin." To worsen matters, many of the medications administered to patients with MDR-TB are associated with gastrointestinal tract side effects such as nausea, anorexia, vomiting, and diarrhea (ethionamide, PAS, high-dose fluoroquinolones, and clofazimine are particularly notable in this regard). To combat these effects, the following strategies may be employed: (a) flexible menus to allow patients to select meals that are most palatable; (b) multiple small feedings or day-long "grazing" rather than large, fixed meals; (c) metoclopramide to prevent regurgitation and to accelerate passage of drugs out of the stomach; (d) appetite-enhancing substances such as the progesterone-like agent, megestrol acetate (Megace); and (e) fever control by judicious use of antipyretics, usually acetaminophen or aspirin. Although weight gain and subjective improvement may result with the use of megestrol acetate (102–104), other authors have reported, and we concur, that—for some patients—these effects seem very much like cortisone activity with fat deposition, loss of muscle mass, euphoria, and suppression of endogenous adrenal function (104,105). Also, the observation that progesterone causes a shift from type 1 T-helper (Th1)–to type 2 T-helper (Th2)–dominated immunity, presumably to prevent placental-fetal rejection, is a cause for further concern (see Chapter 5 for discussion). Therefore, we use this agent cautiously and are seeking alternative anabolic agents.

When the above measures fail to achieve sufficient oral intake to provide weight gain and an anabolic state, direct nutritional supplementation may be indicated. When feasible, we attempt to use a small-bore nasogastric device such as a pediatric (Dobhoff) feeding tube. If the patient has reasonable dietary practices, we may simply use nasogastric feeding at night to supplement intake. For patients with more profound deficits and long-term needs, feeding jejunostomy tubes may be placed.

In general, enteral feedings are favored over parenteral because of the ostensible immunological advantages, as well as convenience, safety, and financial considerations. However, for some patients, perioperative parenteral supplementation may be appropriate. Central lines may be useful in this regard to administer hyperalimentation as well as intravenous antibiotics. Double-lumen subclavian catheters provide such access, but for patients in whom phlebotomy access is problematic, triple-lumen devices may be more advantageous. Peripherally inserted central catheters are used in some centers for these functions.

Although there is a relative paucity of carefully controlled data on the impact of protein malnutrition on the outcome of pulmonary resectional surgery, our clinical experience indicates that persons with severe wasting are at higher risk of complications (91). Therefore, nutritional enhancement will remain a major component of our preoperative preparation.

Immunomodulation

As noted in Chapter 13, therapeutic modulation of the immune system to enhance the host's control of tuberculosis has enjoyed renewed interest recently. Efforts have been directed toward using immunoenhancement with *Mycobacterium vaccae* vaccination to shorten the duration of chemotherapy required to "cure" patients with drug-susceptible disease (106). However, this group also described transiently favorable results when administering this vaccine to patients in Iran with drug-resistant tuberculosis who had failed chemotherapy (107). According to the authors, *M. vaccae* works by redirecting the host's cellular response from a Th2-dominant to a Th1-dominant pathway, resulting in less tissue destruction and more effective inhibition of mycobacterial replication (see Chapter 13 for details). However, recent reports from controlled, randomized trials have failed to confirm the utility of this therapy (108).

Investigators from the National Institutes of Health have recently reported on the beneficial effects of administering interferon-γ (IFN-γ) parenterally to persons with disseminated disease attributable to mycobacteria other than tuberculosis that was refractory to chemotherapy (109). Although these mycobacteria are naturally more resistant to chemotherapy than the usual strain of *M. tuberculosis,* the failure to control these infections with chemotherapy almost surely reflected abnormalities of cellular immunity, which were presumably redressed by the IFN-γ. Therefore, it may not be appropriate to extrapolate from these results to persons with MDR-TB whose immunity, while possibly somewhat impaired by inanition and extensive infection, may not truly be abnormal or anomalous. Sharing the IFN-γ protocol of Holland, we have treated five patients with MDR-TB at National Jewish since 1995. In an open-labeled, nonrandomized observational study, the results for these patients have not been substantially favorable (James Cook, personal communication, 1998). A single case report in which inhaled IFN-γ appeared to be beneficial in a case of refractory pulmonary disease attributable to *Mycobacterium avium* complex was provocative (110). A group from Bellevue Hospital in New York City reported transient but clinically encouraging improvement in five patients with MDR-TB following one month of *inhaled* IFN-γ, 500 μg thrice weekly (111). Responses included unsustained conversion of sputum smears to negative, delayed growth of cultures, and shrinkage of cavities.

Cytokine therapy has been shown to have clinical utility in modifying the inflammatory manifestations of the lepromatous type of disease (112). In this model, interleukin-2 (IL-2) was used to restore antigen responsiveness, presumably via enhancing IFN-γ production. To combat excessive effects from TNF-α, thalidomide was employed. Thalidomide has also been employed in the treatment of Behçet syndrome (113) and the wasting syndrome of AIDS (114). One report has indicated that thalidomide may work by inhibiting the proinflammatory cytokine interleukin-12 (IL-12) (115), thus raising the possibility of an adverse effect on cellular immunity. However, the possibility that thalidomide or agents with similar effects may ameliorate tissue injury in tuberculosis should be studied.

The potential roles of such diverse agents as transfer factor, indomethacin, and levamisole were reviewed in 1986 (116). At that time, insufficient benefits could be discerned to justify clinical use.

Historical efforts at immunomodulation for tuberculosis included heliotherapy (exposure to sunshine or ultraviolet irradiation) and dietary supplementation including milk and cod-liver oil. It is very likely that these interventions resulted in increased levels of 1,25 dihydroxy-vitamin D_3, a compound now recognized to have salutary effects on T-cell and macrophage function. Perhaps this dimension of immune enhancement deserves to be revisited.

Collapse Therapy

Before effective drugs were available, clinicians commonly employed various techniques to "collapse" a cavity-containing lung (see Chapter 1). The concept was that compression of the cavity changed the local environment in a manner which inhibited the mycobacteria. Controlled studies were not performed during this era. Hence, it is not possible to be certain that such strategies were beneficial or, if so, how much benefit was derived. Nonetheless, generations of sophisticated clinicians believed strongly in such techniques as pneumothorax, pneumoperitoneum, plombage, and/or phreniclasis. Consequently, for patients with MDR-TB unmanageable by chemotherapy, we remain alert to the potential of this approach.

PREVENTIVE CHEMOTHERAPY FOR CONTACTS TO MULTIDRUG-RESISTANT TUBERCULOSIS CASES

Administering INH to persons who are exposed to and infected by *drug-susceptible* strains of tuberculosis has proven highly effective, conferring roughly 75% protection against subsequent active disease. A comprehensive overview of INH preventive chemotherapy is provided in Chapter 12.

However, INH is the only drug that has been studied systematically in "preventive therapy." Rifampin, based on its impact in patients with active tuberculosis, as well as its activity in in vitro or in vivo (animal) studies, may be of equal or potentially greater efficacy in prevention (117). Because RIF costs far more than INH, it will never replace INH for general use. But, for contacts exposed to a case with resistance to INH but with susceptibility to rifamycins, RIF preventive therapy has appeared protective in two anecdotal series (118,119) and has been endorsed by a committee of the American College of Chest Physicians (120).

MDR-TB, though, involves strains with resistance to both INH and RIF. Because these two drugs are much more active than other agents, a single drug to replace them is not readily apparent. Thus, a Delphi survey of experienced practitioners in North America (sequentially polling experts, providing them with the results of previous questionnaires) indicated a preference for administering two drugs to high-risk contacts deemed likely to have been infected with MDR-

TB strains (121). Similarly, the Tuberculosis Division of the CDC and its Advisory Council for the Elimination of Tuberculosis (consisting of several of the "experts" who participated in the Delphi survey) advocated two drugs in this setting (122). The CDC recommendations provide an excellent matrix for both the assessment/classification of contacts and their management. Components of the process include the following: (a) estimating the likelihood of new infection and therapeutic decision making (a schematic representation of this process is shown in Figure 2 of the CDC report); (b) estimating the likelihood of infection with MDR-TB among newly infected contacts, which includes estimating the infectiousness of the MDR-TB source case, the closeness and intensity of the MDR-TB exposure, and the potential that the contact had been exposed to/infected by a drug-susceptible case (see Table 10 of the CDC recommendations for schema to classify risk to contacts from high to low); and (c) estimating the likelihood that infected persons will develop active tuberculosis: by considering the potential for an individual to progress from latent infection to overt disease, the requirements and priorities for offering preventive medications can be stratified.

The CDC recommendations advocate managing newly infected contacts who are deemed to be at low to low-intermediate risk of infection with MDR-TB according to the guidelines for contacts to conventional drug-susceptible cases (see Figure 3 in CDC recommendations). For those considered to be at intermediate to high likelihood of MDR-TB infection, stratification by risk for developing active disease is advised. Special risk factors cited include AIDS, HIV infection, other immunosuppressive conditions (such as insulin-dependent diabetes mellitus, renal failure, carcinoma of the head and neck, and iatrogenic immunosuppressives), tuberculosis infection within the prior 2 years, and extremes of age ($\leq$5 years, $\geq$60 years). Relative risks estimated for these conditions when compared with normal hosts include the following: AIDS, 170-fold; HIV, 113-fold; other immunosuppressive conditions, 3.6- to 16-fold; recent infection, 15-fold; and extremes of age, 2.2- to 5-fold.

Two-drug therapy is recommended for persons who are likely to have been infected with MDR-TB and who are at higher risk for developing active disease. For MDR-TB contacts who are not infected with HIV or have other conditions that place them at extraordinary risk for developing tuberculosis, the CDC recommends one of two options: (a) give no medication and follow closely for early signs of tuberculosis or (b) give two-drug therapy. However, I disagree with one aspect of this recommendation. It states that, if there is less than 100% resistance to INH or RIF, that drug should be used for preventive therapy. While it is true that, theoretically, some of the mycobacterial population should be killed by the drug if there is incomplete resistance, clinical experience in patients with active disease and such partial resistance indicates that these agents are of very limited efficacy unless the percentage of resistance is quite low.

Specific agents recommended include PZA and EMB, presuming the source case strain is susceptible to these agents. As an alternative, PZA and a fluoroquinolone such as ofloxacin or ciprofloxacin are proposed. Parenteral agents such as SM, amikacin, kanamycin, or capreomycin are also mentioned, but the immense problems with using an injectable drug for prevention makes this impractical for all but the highest-risk contacts such as persons with AIDS, organ transplant recipients, or heavily immunosuppressed oncology patients. The CDC dismisses the other second-line oral agents because of their unproven efficacy and potential toxicity; however, under extreme circumstances, when no alternatives have been available, we have employed PAS and cycloserine for children in the household of persons with MDR-TB.

No data currently exist, nor will methodologically sound, statistically significant results ever be achieved, regarding the efficacy of "alternative" preventive therapy regimens; there are simply too few subjects and too many variables to conduct such a trial. Rather, we will be dealing with small series and anecdotal observations about the apparent power of this approach to prevent disease in MDR-TB contacts. A decision-analysis study recently concluded that preventive therapy with ciprofloxacin and PZA would be modestly beneficial for health care workers infected with MDR-TB (123). However, this approach must be reconsidered in light of new information regarding the side effects, tolerance, and toxicity of such regimens. The first report of problems with PZA-ofloxacin regimen came from a hospital in New York where an epidemic of MDR-TB resulted in high rates of skin test conversions among health care workers (124). A regimen of PZA 1,500 mg and ofloxacin 800 mg daily was initiated for 16 health care workers; remarkably, 13 (80%) of them reported intolerable side effects resulting in discontinuation of the drugs at a mean duration of 3 months. Similarly, following an outbreak of MDR-TB in a California high school, a directly observed daily regimen of PZA at 20 to 30 mg/kg body weight and ofloxacin 600 mg was given to 20 students and faculty members; among these patients, 12 (60%) reported intolerable side effects leading to discontinuation (125). Among these 12 patients there were 9 (75%) cases of symptomatic hepatitis associated with substantial derangements of liver function test values. These two reports raise serious questions about the advisability of the PZA-ofloxacin combination. The mechanism(s) for the unexpectedly high prevalence of adverse drug reactions is unclear. Clearly, further pharmacological investigations into possible drug-drug interactions need to be conducted, since the frequencies of intolerance/toxicity are higher than seen with either agent given alone and higher than seen in our experience with coadministration of the drugs (126).

Overall, I believe that the assessment algorithms described in the CDC report above remain useful and appropriate systems for contact-investigations of MDR-TB cases (122). However, the choice of preventive therapy agents remains problematic. If forced to choose a *single* drug from the list of agents excluding INH and RIF, levofloxacin, based on its in vitro activity (95) and relative freedom from toxicity in extended use (National Jewish Center, unpublished data, 1997–1999), would appear the best option to me. There is reluctance, however, to use a fluoroquinolone in preventive monotherapy because of the fear of acquired resistance to this category of drugs if the treatment were to fail. Acquired resistance during failed INH preventive therapy has been seen rarely among large trials (see Chapter 12 for full discussion). In most cases, it is thought that failure is more likely to occur because of noncompliance with the preventive treatment or simple "persistence" of the susceptible organisms. Because of the relatively small mycobacterial burden present in a person with latent, subclinical infection, the probability of selecting for drug-resistant mutants is believed to be very low. Hence, in cases in which there was high risk for subsequent tuberculosis, intolerance to ofloxacin-PZA, or resistance to PZA and EMB in the source-case strains, I think that 6 months of levofloxacin 500 to 750 mg daily is a justifiable approach to preventive therapy. Critical to this tactic is a rigorous exclusion of cryptically active disease in which a high bacillary burden would increase the risk of ADR.

PARTICULAR HAZARDS FOR NOSOCOMIAL TRANSMISSION OF MULTIDRUG-RESISTANT TUBERCULOSIS

Two factors have played major roles in recent institutional tuberculosis outbreaks: (a) the extraordinary propensity for persons with HIV/AIDS to acquire tuberculosis infection and rapidly progress to disease and (b) multidrug-resistant strains that, when transmitted, pose severe challenges in treatment and preventive therapy.

Factors involved with the transmission of tuberculosis are reviewed in detail in Chapters 3 and 14, but it is worth reiterating the particular challenges posed by MDR-TB.

The rapid effects of modern bactericidal regimens against drug-susceptible tuberculosis have played a large, underappreciated role in preventing nosocomial spread in the recent era. While it is true that it takes 1 to 2 months to achieve negative culture status in most cases of pulmonary tuberculosis, there is an exponential decline in the number of cultivable bacilli during the first few days of therapy. This must dramatically reduce the likelihood of transmission. Patients with new cavitary disease may shed up to 10,000,000 bacilli per milliliter of sputum before therapy, but this number typically falls to 100,000 bacilli per milliliter in less than a week (see Fig. 14.1). Also, as noted, the frequency of coughing diminishes as well. Thus, part of the recent lore of nosocomial tuberculosis transmission to health care workers has been that, "it's the case you don't know about [and commence treatment] that gets you." In large measure, that has been true—many of the documented institutional outbreaks (see Chapter 3) have involved delayed or failed diagnosis.

With MDR-TB, however, initiation of treatment with inadequate regimens is associated with protracted shedding of large numbers of viable bacilli and unrelieved coughing. This phenomenon has highlighted the deficiencies of our current institutional control policies and systems, leading to an urgent search for means to protect other patients and health care workers in institutions where MDR-TB cases receive care. These elements are discussed more thoroughly in Chapter 14.

REFERENCES

1. David HL, Newman CM. Some observations on the genetics of isoniazid resistance in the tubercle bacilli. *Am Rev Respir Dis* 1971;104:508–515.
2. Kritski AL, Marques MJO, Rabahi MF, et al. Transmission of tuberculosis to close contacts of patients with multidrug-resistant tuberculosis. *Am J Respir Crit Care Med* 1996;153:331–335.
3. Moore M, Onorato IM, McCray E, Castro KG. Trends in drug-resistant tuberculosis in the United States, 1993–1996. *JAMA* 1997;278:833–837.
4. Pablos-Méndez A, Raviglione MC, Laszlo A, et al. Global surveillance for antituberculosis-drug resistance, 1994–1997. *N Engl J Med* 1998;338:1641–1649.
5. Stewart SM, Crofton JW. The clinical significance of low degrees of drug resistance in pulmonary tuberculosis. *Am Rev Respir Dis* 1964;89:811–829.
6. Vall-Spinosa A, Lester TW. Rifampin: characteristics and role in the chemotherapy of tuberculosis. *Ann Intern Med* 1971;74:758–760.
7. A Cooperative Tuberculosis Chemotherapy Study in Poland from the National Research Institute for Tuberculosis. A comparative study of daily followed by twice- or once-weekly regimens of ethambutol and rifampicin in the retreatment of patients with pulmonary tuberculosis: second report. *Tubercle* 1976;57:105– 113.
8. Telenti A. Genetics of drug resistance in tuberculosis. In: Iseman MD, Huitt GA, eds. *Clinics in chest medicine.* Philadelphia: WB Saunders, 1997:55–64.
9. Musser JM. Antimicrobial agent resistance in mycobacteria: molecular genetic insights. *Clin Microbiol Rev* 1995;8:496–514.
10. Blanchard JS. Molecular mechanisms of drug resistance in *Mycobacterium tuberculosis. Annu Rev Biochem* 1996;65:215–239.
11. Sreevatsan S, Pan X, Zhang Y, Kreiswirth BN, Musser JM. Mutations associated with pyrazinamide resistance in *pncA* of *Mycobacterium tuberculosis* complex organisms. *Antimicrob Agents Chemother* 1997;41: 636–640.
12. Banerjee A, Dubnau E, Quemard A, et al. *inhA,* a gene encoding a target for isoniazid and ethionamide in *Mycobacterium tuberculosis. Science* 1994;263:227–230.
13. Musser JM, Kapur V, Williams DL, Dreiswirth BN, van Soolingen D, van Embden JDA. Characterization of the catalase-peroxidase gene *(katG)* and *inhA* locus in isoniazid-resistant and -susceptible strains of *Mycobacterium tuberculosis* by automated DNA sequencing: restricted array of mutations associated with drug resistance. *J Infect Dis* 1996;173:196–202.
14. Heym B, Honore N, Truffot-Pernot C, et al. Implications of multidrug resistance for the future of short-course chemotherapy of tuberculosis. *Lancet* 1994; 344:293–298.
15. Morris S, Bai GH, Suffys P, Portillo-Gomez L, Fairchok M, Rouse D. Molecular mechanisms of multiple drug resistance in clinical isolates of *Mycobacterium tuberculosis. J Infect Dis* 1995;171:954–960.
16. Goble M, Iseman MD, Madsen LA, Waite D, Ackerson L, Horsburgh CR Jr. Treatment of 171 patients with pulmonary tuberculosis resistant to isoniazid and rifampin. *N Engl J Med* 1993;328:527–532.
17. David HL. Probability distribution of drug-resistant mutants in unselected populations of *Mycobacterium tuberculosis. Appl Microbiol* 1970;20:810–814.
18. Tsukamura M. The pattern of resistance development to rifampicin in *Mycobacterium tuberculosis. Tubercle* 1972;53:111–117.
19. Canetti G. The J. Burns Amberson Lecture: present aspects of bacterial resistance in tuberculosis. *Am Rev Respir Dis* 1965;92:687–703.
20. Dutt AK, Moers D, Stead WW. Short-course chemotherapy for tuberculosis with mainly twice-weekly isoniazid and rifampin: community physicians' seven-year experience with mainly outpatients. *Am J Med* 1984;77:233–242.
21. Ferebee SH. Controlled chemoprophylaxis trials in tuberculosis: a general review. *Adv Tuberc Res* 1970; 17:28–106.
22. Mahmoudi A, Iseman MD. Pitfalls in the care of patients with tuberculosis: common errors and their association with the acquisition of drug resistance. *JAMA* 1993;270:65–68.
23. American Thoracic Society. Treatment of tuberculosis and tuberculosis infection in adults and children. *Am J Respir Crit Care Med* 1994;149:1359–1374.
24. Bloch AB, Cauthen GM, Onorato IM, et al. Nationwide survey of drug-resistant tuberculosis in the United States. *JAMA* 1994;271:665–671.
25. World Health Organization. Anti-tuberculosis drug resistance in the world. In: *The WHO/IUATLD global project on drug resistance surveillance, 1994–1997.* Geneva, Switzerland, 1997,1–227.
26. Grzybowski S, Burnett G, Styblo K. Contacts of cases of active pulmonary tuberculosis: report 3 of TSRU. *Bull Int Union Tuberc* 1975;60:90–106.

27. Iseman MD. Tailoring a time bomb: inadvertent genetic engineering. *Am Rev Respir Dis* 1985;132: 735–736.
28. Iseman MD, Sbarbaro JA. The increasing prevalence of resistance to antituberculosis chemotherapeutic agents: implications for global tuberculosis control. *Curr Clin Top Infect Dis* 1992;12:188–207.
29. Cohn DL, Bustreo F, Raviglione MC. Drug-resistant tuberculosis: review of the worldwide situation and the WHO/IUATLD global surveillance project. *Clin Infect Dis* 1997;24:S121–S130.
30. Tahaoglu K, Kizkin Ö, Karagöz T, Tor M, Partal M, Sadoglu T. High initial and acquired drug resistance in pulmonary tuberculosis in Turkey. *Tuberc Lung Dis* 1994;75:324–328.
31. Demissie M, Gebeyehu M, Berhane Y. Primary resistance to anti-tuberculosis drugs in Addis Ababa, Ethiopia. *Int J Tuberc Lung Dis* 1997;1:64–67.
32. Glynn JR, Jenkins PA, Fine PEM, et al. Patterns of initial and acquired antituberculosis drug resistance in Karonga District, Malawi. *Lancet* 1995;345:907–910.
33. Bercion R, Kuaban C. Initial resistance to antituberculosis drugs in Yaounde, Cameroon in 1995. *Int J Tuberc Lung Dis* 1997;1:110–114.
34. Carpels G, Fissette K, Limbana V, Van Deun A, Vandenbulcke W, Portaels F. Drug resistant tuberculosis in sub-Saharan Africa: an estimation of incidence and cost for the year 2000. *Tuberc Lung Dis* 1995;76:480–486.
35. Chanteau S, Rasolofo V, Ramarokoto H, et al. Anti-tuberculosis drug resistance in Madagascar in 1994–1995. *Int J Tuberc Lung Dis* 1997;1:405–410.
36. Ledru S, Cauchoix B, Yaméogo M, et al. Impact of short-course therapy on tuberculosis drug resistance in South-West Burkina Faso. *Tuberc Lung Dis* 1996;77: 429–436.
37. Hirano K, Kazumi Y, Abe C, Mori T, Aoki M, Aoyagi T. Resistance to antituberculosis drugs in Japan. *Tuberc Lung Dis* 1996;77:130–135.
38. Mendoza MT, Gonzaga AJ, Roa C, et al. Nature of drug resistance and predictors of multidrug-resistant tuberculosis among patients seen at the Philippine General Hospital, Manila, Philippines. *Int J Tuberc Lung Dis* 1997;1:59–63.
39. Pineda-Garcia L, Ferrera A, Galvez CA, Hoffner SE. Drug-resistant *Mycobacterium tuberculosis* and atypical mycobacteria isolated from patients with suspected pulmonary tuberculosis in Honduras. *Chest* 1997;111: 148–153.
40. Harrow EM, Rangel JM, Arriega JM, et al. Epidemiology and clinical consequences of drug-resistant tuberculosis in a Guatemalan hospital. *Chest* 1998;113: 1452–1458.
41. Centers for Disease Control and Prevention. Population-based survey for drug resistance of tuberculosis: Mexico, 1997. *MMWR* 1998;47:371–475.
42. Ritacco V, Di Lonardo M, Reniero A, et al. Nosocomial spread of human immunodeficiency virus-related multidrug-resistant tuberculosis in Buenos Aires. *J Infect Dis* 1997;176:637–642.
43. Edlin BR, Tokars JI, Grieco MH, et al. An outbreak of multidrug-resistant tuberculosis among hospitalized patients with the acquired immunodeficiency syndrome. *N Engl J Med* 1992;326:1514–1521.
44. Frieden TR, Sterling T, Pablos-Mendez A, Kilburn JO, Cauthen GM, Dooley SW. The emergence of drug-resistant tuberculosis in New York City. *N Engl J Med* 1993;328:521–526.
45. Coronado VG, Beck-Sague CM, Hutton MD, et al. Transmission of multidrug-resistant *Mycobacterium tuberculosis* among persons with human immunodeficiency virus infection in an urban hospital: epidemiologic and restriction fragment length polymorphism analysis. *J Infect Dis* 1993;168:1052–1055.
46. Busillo C, Lessnau K-D, Sanjana V, et al. Multidrug resistant *Mycobacterium tuberculosis* in patients with human immunodeficiency virus infection. *Chest* 1992; 102:797–801.
47. Shafer RW, Small PM, Larkin C, et al. Temporal trends and transmission patterns during the emergence of multidrug-resistant tuberculosis in New York City: a molecular epidemiologic assessment. *J Infect Dis* 1995;171:170–176.
48. Friedman CR, Stoeckle MY, Kreiswirth BN, et al. Transmission of multidrug-resistant tuberculosis in a large urban setting. *Am J Respir Crit Care Med* 1995; 152:355–359.
49. Bradford WZ, Martin JN, Reingold AL, Schecter GF, Hopewell PC, Small PM. The changing epidemiology of acquired drug-resistant tuberculosis in San Francisco, USA. *Lancet* 1996;348:928–931.
50. Burwen DR, Jones JL, Group THS. Epidemiology and diagnosis of tuberculosis. *Am J Respir Crit Care Med* 1995;151:A144(abst).
51. Ridzon R, Whitney CG, McKenna MT, et al. Risk factors for rifampin mono-resistant tuberculosis. *Am J Respir Crit Care Med* 1998;157:1881–1884.
52. Berning SE, Huitt G, Iseman MD, Peloquin CA. Malabsorption of antituberculosis medications by a patient with AIDS [Letter]. *N Engl J Med* 1992;327:1817–1818.
53. Peloquin CA, Nitta AT, Burman WJ, et al. Low antituberculosis drug concentrations in patients with AIDS. *Ann Pharmacother* 1996;30:919–925.
54. Gollapudi S, Reddy M, Gangadharam PRJ, Tsuruo T, Gupta S. *Mycobacterium tuberculosis* induces expression of P-glycoprotein in promonocytic Ul cells chronically infected with HIV type 1. *Biochem Biophys Res Comm* 1994;199:1181–1187.
55. Gordin FM, Nelson ET, Matts JP, et al. The impact of human immunodeficiency virus infection on drug-resistant tuberculosis. *Am J Respir Crit Care Med* 1996; 154:1478–1483.
56. Pablos-Méndoz A, Knirsch CA, Barr RG, Lerner BH, Frieden TR. Nonadherence in tuberculosis treatment: predictors and consequences in New York City. *Am J Med* 1997;102:164–170.
57. Lipsitch M, Levin BR. Population dynamics of tuberculosis treatment: mathematical models of the roles of non-compliance and bacterial heterogeneity in the evolution of drug resistance. *Int J Tuberc Lung Dis* 1998; 2:187–199.
58. Mitchison D. How drug resistance emerges as a result of poor compliance during short-course chemotherapy for tuberculosis. *Int J Tuberc Lung Dis* 1998;2:10–15.
59. Annas GJ. Control of tuberculosis: the law and the public's health. *N Engl J Med* 1993;328:585–588.
60. Cohn ML, Kovitz C, Oda U, Middlebrook G. Studies on isoniazid and tubercle bacilli, II: the growth requirements, catalase activities, and pathogenic properties of isoniazid-resistant mutants. *Am Rev Tuberc* 1954;54:641–664.

61. Snider DE, Kelly GD, Cauthen GM, Thompson NJ, Kilburn JO. Infection and disease among contacts of tuberculosis cases with drug-resistant and drug-susceptible bacilli. *Am Rev Respir Dis* 1985;132:125–132.
62. Ordway DJ, Sonnenberg MG, Donahue SA, Belisle JT, Orme IM. Drug-resistant strains of *Mycobacterium tuberculosis* exhibit a range of virulence for mice. *Infect Immun* 1995;63:741–743.
63. Frieden TR, Sherman LF, Maw KL, et al. A multi-institutional outbreak of highly drug-resistant tuberculosis: epidemiology and clinical outcomes. *JAMA* 1996; 276:1229–1235.
64. Mitchison DA, Nunn AJ. Influence of initial drug resistance on the response to short-course chemotherapy of pulmonary tuberculosis. *Am Rev Respir Dis* 1986; 133:423–430.
65. Hong Kong Chest Service/British Medical Research Council. Five-year follow-up of a controlled trial of five 6-month regimens of chemotherapy for pulmonary tuberculosis. *Am Rev Respir Dis* 1987;136:1339–1342.
66. Hong Kong Chest Service/British Medical Research Council. Controlled trial of 2, 4, and 6 months of pyrazinamide in 6-month, three-times weekly regimens for smear-positive pulmonary tuberculosis, including an assessment of a combined preparation of isoniazid, rifampin, and pyrazinamide: results at 30 months. *Am Rev Respir Dis* 1991;143:700–706.
67. Nolan CM, Williams DL, Cave MD, et al. Evolution of rifampin resistance in human immunodeficiency virus-associated tuberculosis. *Am J Respir Crit Care Med* 1995;152:1067–1071.
68. Hong Kong Chest Service, British Medical Research Council. Controlled trial of 6-month and 9-month regimens of daily and intermittent streptomycin plus isoniazid plus pyrazinamide for pulmonary tuberculosis in Hong Kong. *Am Rev Respir Dis* 1977;115:727–735.
69. Manalo F, Tan F, Sbarbaro JA, Iseman MD. Community based short-course treatment of pulmonary tuberculosis in a developing nation: initial report of an eight-month, largely intermittent regimen in a population with high prevalence of drug resistance. *Am Rev Respir Dis* 1990;142:1301–1305.
70. Salomon N, Perlman DC, Friedmann P, Buchstein S, Kreiswirth BN, Mildvan D. Predictors and outcome of multidrug-resistant tuberculosis. *Clin Infect Dis* 1995; 21:1245–1252.
71. Turett GS, Telzak EE, Torian LV. Improved outcomes for patients with multidrug-resistant tuberculosis. *Clin Infect Dis* 1995;21:1238–1244.
72. Telzak EE, Sepkowitz K, Alpert P, et al. Multidrug-resistant tuberculosis in patients without HIV infection. *N Engl J Med* 1995;333:907–911.
73. Park MM, Davis AL, Schluger NW, Cohen H, Rom WN. Outcome of MDR-TB patients, 1983–1993: prolonged survival with appropriate therapy. *Am J Respir Crit Care Med* 1996;153:317–324.
74. Iseman MD, Goble M. Multidrug-resistant tuberculosis [Letter]. *N Engl J Med* 1995;334:267.
75. Weltman AC, Rose DN. Tuberculosis susceptibility patterns, predictors of multidrug resistance, and implications for initial therapeutic regimens at a New York City hospital. *Arch Intern Med* 1994;154:2161–2167.
76. Kritski AL, de Jesus LSR, Andrade MK, et al. Retreatment tuberculosis cases: factors associated with drug resistance and adverse outcomes. *Chest* 1997;111: 1162–1167.
77. Crofton J, Chaulet P, Maher D, et al. Guidelines for the management of drug-resistant tuberculosis. *WHO/TB* 1997.
78. Enarson DA, Rieder HL, Arnadottir T. Tuberculosis guide for low income countries. In: IUATLD, ed. *Tuberculosis guide for low income countries,* 3rd ed. Frankfurt am Main: pmi Verl. Gruppe, 1994.
79. Heifets L. Qualitative and quantitative drug-susceptibility tests in mycobacteriology. *Am Rev Respir Dis* 1988;137:1217–1222.
80. Heifets L, Lindholm-Levy P. Pyrazinamide sterilizing activity in vitro against semidormant *Mycobacterium tuberculosis* bacterial populations. *Am Rev Respir Dis* 1992;145:1223–1225.
81. Kasik JE, Weber M, Freehill PJ. The effect of the penicillinase-resistant penicillins and other chemotherapeutic substances on the penicillinase of the R_1R_v strain of *Mycobacterium tuberculosis. Am Rev Respir Dis* 1967;95:12–19.
82. Cynamon MH, Palmer GS. *In vitro* activity of amoxicillin in combination with clavulanic acid against *Mycobacterium tuberculosis. Antimicrob Agents Chemother* 1983;24:429–431.
83. Casal M, Rodriguez F, Benavente M. In vitro susceptibility of *Mycobacterium tuberculosis, Mycobacterium fortuitum* and *Mycobacterium chelonei* to augmentin. *Eur J Clin Microbiol* 1986;5:453–454.
84. Casal MJ, Rodriguez FC, Luna MD, Benavente MC. In vitro susceptibility of *Mycobacterium tuberculosis, Mycobacterium africanum, Mycobacterium bovis, Mycobacterium avium, Mycobacterium fortuitum,* and *Mycobacterium chelonae* to ticarcillin in combination with clavulanic acid. *Antimicrob Agents Chemother* 1987;31:132–133.
85. Zhang Y, Steingrube VA, Wallace RJ Jr. Beta-lactamase inhibitors and the inducibility of the beta-lactamase of *Mycobacterium tuberculosis. Am Rev Respir Dis* 1992;145:657–660.
86. Heifets LB, Iseman MD, Cook JL, Lindholm-Levy PJ, Drupa I. Determination of *in vitro* susceptibility of *Mycobacterium tuberculosis* to cephalosporins by radiometric and conventional methods. *Antimicrob Agents Chemother* 1985;27:11–15.
87. Nadler JP, Berger J, Nord JA, Cofsky R, Saxena M. Amoxicillin-clavulanic acid for treating drug-resistant *Mycobacterium tuberculosis. Chest* 1991;99:1025–1026.
88. Crowle AJ, Sbarbaro JA, May MH. Effects of isoniazid and of ceforanide against virulent tubercle bacilli in cultured human macrophages. *Tubercle* 1988;69:15–25.
89. Nitta AT, Iseman MD, Newell JD, Madsen LA, Goble M. Ten-year experience with artificial pneumoperitoneum for end-stage, drug-resistant pulmonary tuberculosis. *Clin Infect Dis* 1993;16:219–222.
90. Grant GR, Lederman JA, Brandstetter RD. TG Heaton, tuberculosis and artificial pneumothorax: once again, back to the future? *Chest* 1997;112:7–8.
91. Pomerantz M, Madsen L, Goble M, Iseman M. Surgical management of resistant mycobacterial tuberculosis and other mycobacterial pulmonary infections. *Ann Thorac Surg* 1991;52:1108–1112.
92. Pomerantz M. Surgery for tuberculosis. In: Pomerantz M, ed. *Challengng pulmonary infections.* Philadelphia: WB Saunders, 1993:723–727.

93. Iseman MD, Madsen L, Iseman MC, Ackerson L. Impact of surgery on the management of MDR-TB (abstract). *Am J Respir Crit Care Med* 1995;151:A336.
94. van der Werff YD, van der Houwen HK, Heijmans PJM, et al. Postpneumonectomy pulmonary edema: a retrospective analysis of incidence and possible risk factors. *Chest* 1997;111:1278–1284.
95. Heifets LB, Lindholm-Levy PJ. Bacteriostatic and bactericidal activity of ciprofloxacin and ofloxacin against *Mycobacterium tuberculosis* and *Mycobacterium avium* complex. *Tubercle* 1987;68:267–276.
96. Kennedy N, Fox R, Kisyombe GM, et al. Early bactericidal and sterilizing activities of ciprofloxacin in pulmonary tuberculosis. *Am Rev Respir Dis* 1993;148:1547–1551.
97. Sirgel FA, Botha FJ, Parkin DP. The early bactericidal activity of ciprofloxacin in patients with pulmonary tuberculosis. *Am J Respir Crit Care Med* 1997;156:901–905.
98. Alangaden GJ, Lerner SA. The clinical use of fluoroquinolones for the treatment of mycobacterial diseases. *Clin Infect Dis* 1997;25:1213–1221.
99. Souba WW. Nutritional support. *N Engl J Med* 1997;336:41–48.
100. Morgan G. What, if any, is the effect of malnutrition on immunological competence? *Lancet* 1997;349:1693–1695.
101. Schwartz MW, Seeley RJ. Neuroendocrine responses to starvation and weight loss. *N Engl J Med* 1997;336:1802–1810.
102. Von Roenn JH, Armstrong D, Kotler DP, et al. Megestrol acetate in patients with AIDS-related cachexia. *Ann Intern Med* 1994;121:393–399.
103. Oster MH, Enders SR, Samuels SJ, et al. Megestrol acetate in patients with AIDS and cachexia. *Ann Intern Med* 1994;121:400–408.
104. Leinung MC, Liporace R, Miller CH. Induction of adrenal suppression by megestrol acetate in patients with AIDS. *Ann Intern Med* 1995;122:843–845.
105. Padmanabhan S, Rosenberg AS. Cushing's syndrome induced by megestrol acetate in a patients with AIDS. *Clin Infect Dis* 1998;27:217–218.
106. Stanford JL, Grange JM, Pozniak A. Is Africa lost? *Lancet* 1991;338:557–558.
107. Etemadi A, Farid R, Stanford JL. Immunotherapy for drug-resistant tuberculosis [Letter]. *Lancet* 1992;340:1360–1361.
108. Stanford JL. Frontiers in mycobacteriology. Symposium sponsored by National Jewish Center for Immunology and Respiratory Medicine, Vail, Colorado, October, 1997.
109. Holland SN, Eisenstein EM, Kuhns DB, et al. Treatment of refractory disseminated nontuberculous mycobacterial infection with interferon gamma. *N Engl J Med* 1994;330:1348–1355.
110. Chatte G, Panteix G, Perrin-Fayolle M, Pacheco Y. Aerosolized interferon gamma for *Mycobacterium avium*-complex lung disease. *Am J Respir Crit Care Med* 1995;152:1094–1096.
111. Condos R, Rom WM, Schluger NW. Treatment of multidrug-resistant pulmonary tuberculosis with interferon-γ via aerosol. *Lancet* 1997;349:1513–1515.
112. Kaplan G. Recent advances in cytokine therapy in leprosy. *J Infect Dis* 1993;167:S18–S22.
113. Hamuryudan V, Mat C, Saip S. Thalidomide in the treatment of mucocutaneous lesions of the Behçet syndrome: a randomized, double-blind, placebo-controlled trial. *Ann Intern Med* 1998;128:443–450.
114. Reyes-Teran G, Sierra-Madero JG, Martinez del Cerro V. Effects of thalidomide on HIV-associated wasting syndrome: a randomized, double-blind, placebo-controlled clinical trial. *AIDS* 1996;10:1501–1507.
115. Moller DR, Wysocka M, Greenlee BM. Inhibition of IL-12 production by thalidomide. *J Immunol* 1997;159:5157–5161.
116. Edwards D, Kirkpatrick CH. The immunology of mycobacterial diseases. *Am Rev Respir Dis* 1986;134:1062–1071.
117. Ji B, Truffot-Pernot C, Lacroix C. Effectiveness of rifampin, rifabutin, and rifapentine for preventive therapy of tuberculosis in mice. *Am Rev Respir Dis* 1993;148:1541–1546.
118. Villarino ME, Ridzon R, Weismuller PC. Rifampin preventive therapy for tuberculosis infection: experience with 157 adolescents. *Am J Respir Crit Care Med* 1997;155:1735–1738.
119. Polesky A, Farber HW, Gottlieb DJ, et al. Rifampin preventive therapy for tuberculosis in Boston's homeless. *Am J Respir Crit Care Med* 1996;154:1473–1477.
120. Iseman MD, Sbarbaro JE. American College of Chest Physicians Consensus Conference on Tuberculosis. *Chest* 1985;115S–159S.
121. Passannante MR, Gallagher CT, Reichman LB. Preventive therapy for contacts of multidrug-resistant tuberculosis: a Delphi survey. *Chest* 1994;106:431–434.
122. Centers for Disease Control and Prevention. Management of persons exposed to multidrug-resistant tuberculosis. *MMWR* 1992;41:61–71.
123. Stevens JP, Daniel TM. Chemoprophylaxis of multidrug-resistant tuberculous infection in HIV-uninfected individuals using ciprofloxacin and pyrazinamide. A decision analysis. *Chest* 1995;108:712–717.
124. Horn DL, Hewlett D Jr, Alfalla C, Peterson S, Opal SM. Limited tolerance of ofloxacin and pyrazinamide prophylaxis against tuberculosis [Letter]. *N Engl J Med* 1994;330:1241.
125. Meador J. Summary of tolerance of PZA/ofloxacin in a cohort of high school students and staff exposed to tuberculosis resistant to INH, rifampin, ethambutol, ethionamide and streptomycin. *Orange County MTB* 1995.
126. Berning SE, Madsen L, Iseman MD, Peloquin C. Long-term safety of ofloxacin and ciprofloxacin in the treatment of mycobacterial infections. *Am J Respir Crit Care Med* 1995;151:2006–2009.
127. Doster B, Caras GJ, Snider DE Jr. A continuing survey of primary drug resistance in tuberculosis, 1961 to 1968. A U.S. Public Health Service Cooperative Study. *Am Rev Respir Dis* 1976;113:419–422.
128. Kopanoff DE, Kilburn JO, Glassroth JL, Snider DE Jr., Farer LS, Good RC. A continuing survey of tuberculosis primary drug resistance in the United States: March 1975 to November 1977. A U.S. Public Health Service Cooperative Study. *Am Rev Respir Dis* 1978;118:835–842.
129. Snider DE Jr., Cauthen GM, Farer LS, Kelly GD, Kilburn JO, Good RC, Dooley SW. Drug-resistant tuberculosis (letter). *Am Rev Respir Dis* 1991;144:732.

12

Preventive Chemotherapy of Tuberculosis

Although an ounce of prevention may often be worth a pound of cure, there is an inherent and unfortunate tendency for prevention to be discouraging.

George Comstock, 1986 (1)

Perhaps the most contentious aspect of contemporary tuberculosis control relates to the role of preventive chemotherapy. The effectiveness of this strategy was demonstrated in a series of double-blind, placebo-controlled clinical trials conducted in the 1950s and 1960s. These studies showed considerable efficacy of isoniazid (INH) administered to persons with latent or minimal tuberculosis in preventing the subsequent evolution of active pulmonary or extrapulmonary disease (see below). Thus, the United States has relied for the past 30 years on isoniazid preventive therapy (INH PT) as the primary element in its national tuberculosis control program, essentially rejecting vaccination with BCG on the bases of epidemiological considerations and the questionable efficacy of vaccines. After its broad initial acceptance, professional resistance to INH PT has begun to emerge in the United States, based mainly on concern over the relative risk of INH-related hepatotoxicity versus the capacity to prevent tuberculosis. Other confounding variables that have arisen include the deteriorating performance of the tuberculin skin test in identifying tuberculosis-infected persons as the prevalence of tuberculosis infection has diminished, nonadherence to prescribed medication by persons/groups at highest risk for active tuberculosis, and the rising prevalence of tuberculosis strains resistant to INH.

Because of the intense, often acrimonious disputation on this issue, a careful review of the clinical studies that underpin the preventive therapy strategy is in order. Rather than simply asserting that the United States Public Health Service (USPHS) trials showed 60% overall protection against subsequent tuberculosis, this chapter provides a careful review of these trials and other studies of INH PT to determine to what extent they hold information relevant to current debates.

The United States in 1989 embarked on a program to substantially curtail ("eliminate") tuberculosis by the year 2010 (2). Isoniazid PT constitutes one of the major tactical elements of this campaign. Because progress toward this goal has been interrupted by the impact of HIV infection, immigration, and disruption of inner-city life (see Chapter 5), it is ever more critical that optimal usage of INH PT be determined and, to the extent that it is inadequate, alternative prevention modalities be developed.

THE EPIDEMIOLOGICAL BASIS OF ISONIAZID PREVENTIVE THERAPY: INH-PT VERSUS BCG VACCINATION

From a programmatic perspective, understanding the patterns of transmission and pathogenesis of tuberculosis is essential to developing a prevention strategy. In the 1960s, the

USPHS Tuberculosis Program developed a model for tuberculosis in the United States that compared the potential impact of a BCG vaccination program with that of a preventive chemotherapy program. Because of the potential relevance of this model to contemporary tuberculosis in America, it is worth consideration in some detail. Using 1963 data, a year in which there were roughly 50,000 new cases of tuberculosis, an epidemiological model (Fig. 12.1) was created based on the following assumptions: (a) in a total population of 190,000,000, there were roughly 25,000,000 persons who were believed to harbor latent tuberculosis infections based on skin-test surveys; (b) each year, one of every 625 of these persons experienced reactivation-type tuberculosis, step 1; (c) on average, each new active case infected three of the previously uninfected population, step 2; and (d) of those newly infected, one in 12 went on to develop active tuberculosis during the year of infection, step 3 (3).

Because the average age of the infected persons, 55 years, was greater than that of the uninfected population, 25 years, it was reasoned that with no programmatic intervention the annual incidence of tuberculosis would gradually ebb through attrition of the older group. But, based on these calculations, without intervention the number of cases would fall only from roughly 50,000 in 1964 to 38,000 in 1979, when the pool of infected would number 19,000,000. The USPHS staff then projected the potential impact of a BCG campaign on this trend (Fig. 12.2A).

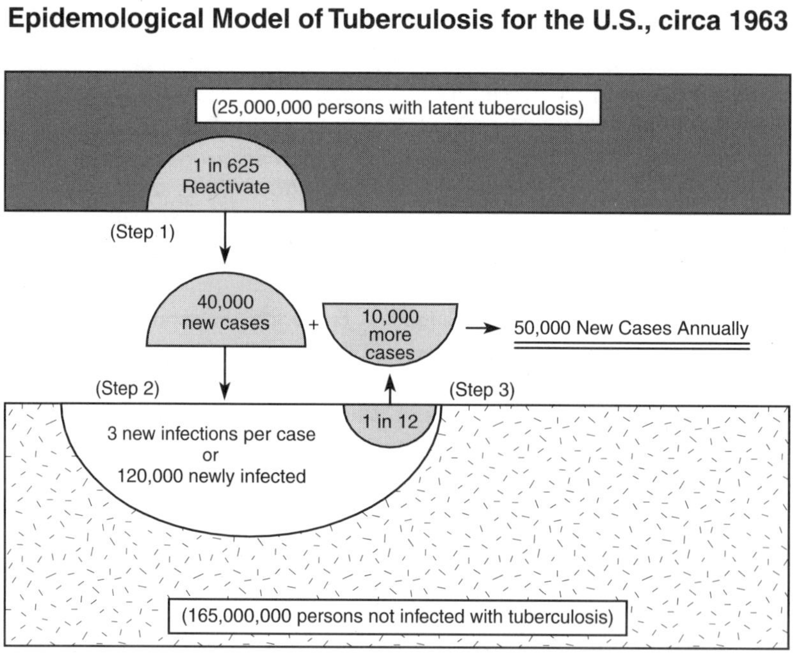

FIG. 12.1. In this model, it was assumed that four of five new cases of tuberculosis in the United States evolved from latent, remotely acquired (≥1 year) tuberculosis infection. Step 1 represents reactivation, which was estimated to occur in one of 625 persons with latent infection annually. Based on contact investigation data, authorities calculated that each new pulmonary case infected three contacts before diagnosis (the model did not factor in the relatively small portion of extrapulmonary, noninfectious cases). Among the 120,000 newly infected individuals, the data suggested that as many as 10,000 would develop disease within the year of infection, giving a total of 50,000 cases per year. Many, if not most, of these 10,000 cases among newly infected would be in the pediatric age group, which has a much greater risk of rapid transition from infection to disease than adults. Understanding this model is critical to understanding why the United States chose INH PT over BCG as the public health prevention strategy (Fig. 12.2).

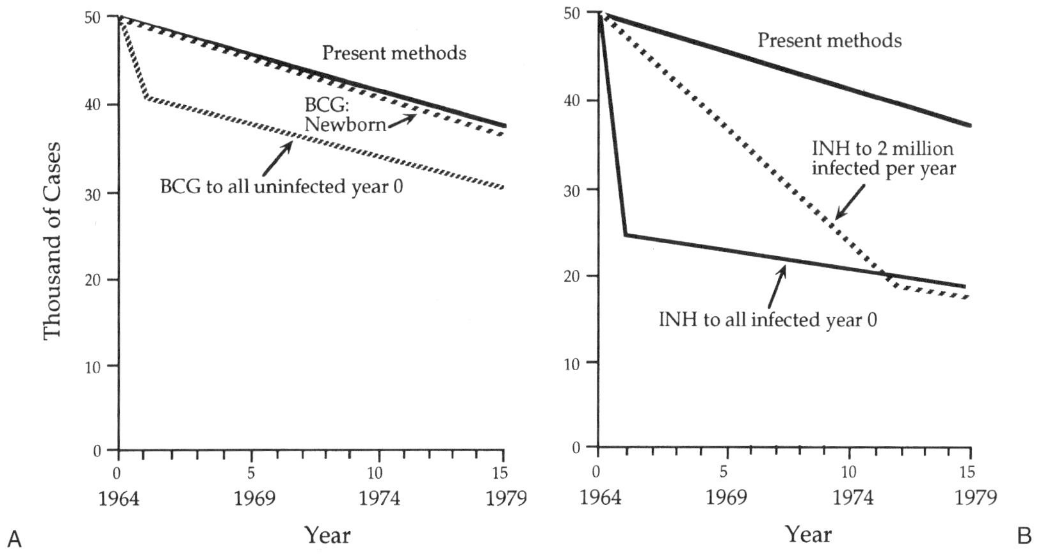

FIG. 12.2. A: Ferebee and colleagues in the U.S. Public Health Service estimated that with no intervention (beyond the existing disease treatment program), there would be a gradual decline in cases *(present methods).* This was deemed to be related to the age factor: at that time, the majority of persons with latent tuberculosis were in the older groups; through natural attrition in the age range, the pool would gradually shrink. Because a relatively small percentage of cases occurred among infants, they calculated that a BCG vaccination plan that targeted only newborns would have minimal impact on the aggregate morbidity *(BCG:Newborn).* Even if BCG were given to all uninfected, as identified by tuberculin nonreactivity, and BCG were 80% effective, it would have a rather trivial impact on national morbidity in return for the commitment to vaccinate 165 million persons *(BCG to all uninfected year 0).* **B:** By comparison, if INH PT were only 50% protective, the USPHS staff calculated that this intervention would have a substantially greater impact than BCG. If INH PT were given to all tuberculin reactors in one mass campaign, it would have a dramatic impact *(INH to all infected year 0)* (see text and Fig. 12.3 for more details). As an alternative, they estimated the impact if INH PT were given only to the relatively higher-risk persons with latent infection *(INH to 2 million infected per year).* This latter model was the underlying logic to the efforts to target high-risk groups in preventive chemotherapy guidelines (see text).

Because BCG is given to those uninfected, the vaccination program would be directed toward all or some of the 165,000,000 tuberculin-negative group. Assuming optimal performance of the vaccine—80% protection—this model predicted that if all 165,000,000 were vaccinated in the year 1964, the incidence of tuberculosis would fall by merely 8,000 cases in 1965 because the BCG could act to protect only the 120,000 newly infected persons from progressing to active disease, reducing the cases in step 3 of Fig. 12.1 from 10,000 to 2,000. If the BCG protection extends for at least 15 years, the model predicted that vaccination of the entire uninfected population in 1963–1964 would have a very modest impact on national tuberculosis morbidity: 42,000 cases in 1965 falling to approximately 32,000 in 1979.

On the basis of the observed efficacy of isoniazid preventive therapy in several USPHS Trials (see below), the Tuberculosis Branch staff then projected the potential impact of preventive chemotherapy on tuberculosis morbidity. In the most aggressive scenario, the results of giving IPT to all 25,000,000 infected persons were calculated (Fig. 12.2B). Assuming 50% efficacy of the INH PT, they projected that this strategy would cut in half the annual reactivation incidence, thus dropping the number of new cases in 1964 to 25,000 (Fig. 12.3). Assuming enduring benefit from the course of INH PT, they calculated that by 1979 there would be only 19,000

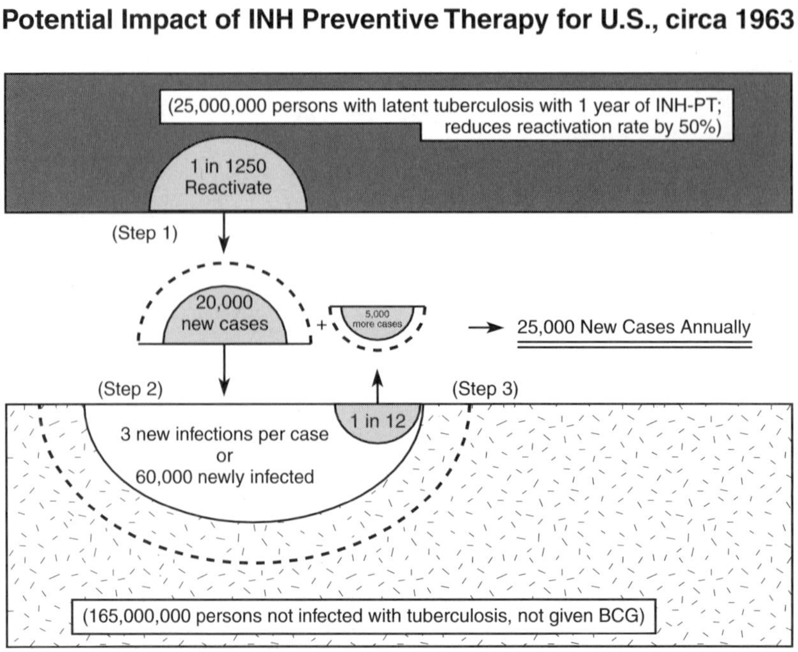

FIG. 12.3. Before the results of the USPHS INH PT trial had been fully reported, the staff projected that one year of INH monotherapy might reduce the likelihood of reactivation by at least 50%. Thus, in contrast to Fig. 12.1, only one in 1,250 with latent infection would develop active disease annually *(Step 1)*. This would halve the yearly reactivation cases, and without any intervention in the uninfected population, the number of newly infected would fall from 120,000 to 60,000 *(Step 2)*. Also, it would follow that the number of cases evolving rapidly from new infection would be decreased to 5,000 *(Step 3)*. Note, that if contact investigation of households of new cases were done, and the newly infected were identified and given INH PT, the annual morbidity would be reduced further.

cases annually. Conceding the impracticality of giving INH to all those infected in one year, the head of the research branch, Shirley Ferebee, instead proposed to give such therapy to 2,000,000 per year for the next 12 years (3). The long-term theoretical effects of no intervention, universal BCG, newborn BCG only, universal INH PT, and INH PT for 2,000,000 persons annually are displayed in Fig. 12.2.

Examining these projections, we can readily understand why the United States chose INH PT for its primary tuberculosis prevention strategy. Rather than a mass population approach as outlined above, the USPHS and the American Thoracic Society eventually chose instead to advocate INH for high-risk groups in the previously infected pool plus newly infected persons who were to be identified through the mechanism of contact investigation. The first official American Thoracic Society statement, "Preventive Treatment in Tuberculosis," was published in 1965 (4).

The epidemiological pattern of tuberculosis in the United States and most industrialized nations has been assumed to remain broadly similar to that projected for 1964. Currently, the Centers for Disease Control estimate there to be approximately 10,000,000 persons in the United States with latent tuberculosis. Although the dynamics of the transmission and disease incidence have surely been modified by the influence of HIV infection, the overall national pattern probably resembles that represented in Fig. 12.4. However, recent studies from San Francisco (5) and New York City (6,7) that employed molecular epidemiology to track specific strains of *M. tuber-*

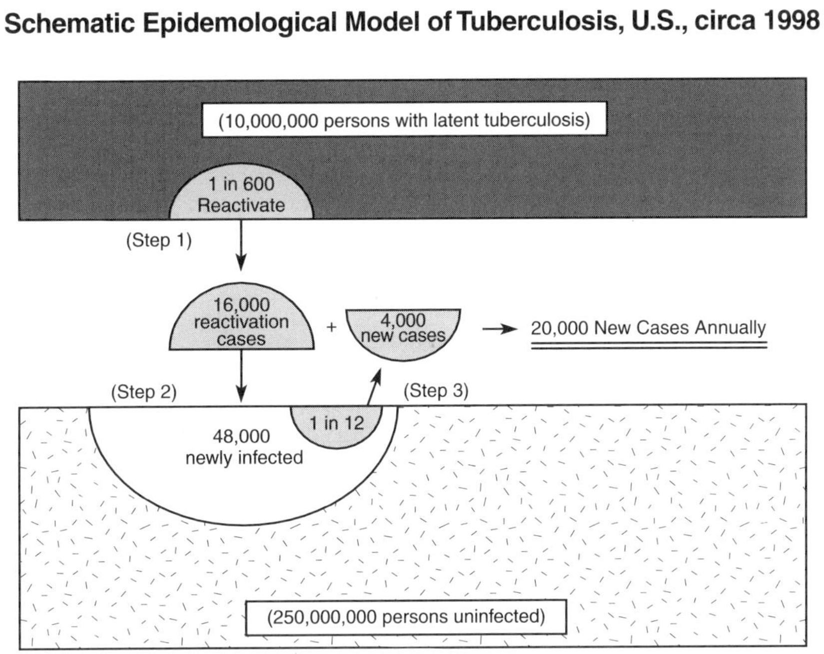

FIG. 12.4. I have attempted to update the 1963 Ferebee model to the United States, circa 1998. Because tuberculin skin testing is not done systematically in this era, it is difficult to establish the number of Americans with latent tuberculosis infection. However, if 10 million are remotely infected with roughly one in 600 still reactivated annually, that would yield about 16,000 new cases *(Step 1),* and assuming three new infections per case, that would entail 48,000 new infections *(Step 2).* Moreover, if one in 12 of these persons developed active disease in the year of their new infection, that would yield a net morbidity of approximately 20,000 cases. The potential impacts of HIV infection on *Step 1* and *Step 3* in this model are considerable (see Chapter 8).

culosis within these communities (see Chapter 5 for details) indicated that substantially greater proportions of new tuberculosis disease in these urban areas represented recent transmission of infection. The significance of these findings for prevention strategies cannot be fully calculated now, but if more evidence of recent transmission is accumulated, we must reconsider the roles of preventive chemotherapy, BCG vaccine, and environmental techniques in tuberculosis control strategies.

A REVIEW OF SELECTED INH PT TRIALS

Isoniazid was introduced into tuberculosis treatment in 1952. The singular capacity of this new drug to cure even in the most advanced cases soon became apparent, its activity far surpassing those of its predecessors, streptomycin and paraamino-salicylate (PAS). Furthermore, the drug was very inexpensive (entirely incidental to tuberculosis, the compound had been synthesized in Czechoslovakia in 1912, thus precluding any patent rights) and remarkably benign. Hence, it is not surprising that several clinicians or groups began pondering the potential of this new drug to prevent tuberculosis in the mid-1950s. A. Omodei Zorini, Professor of Pneumophthisiology at the University of Rome, reported in 1956 on the use of INH PT in 500 children of tuberculous families (8). Edith Lincoln, head of the pediatric tuberculosis program at Bellevue Hospital in New York, was impressed with the capacity of INH to prevent miliary or meningeal disease in youngsters (9), so she organized a multicenter prevention trial from 1955 to 1957 that was to become the first USPHS study (10). From this era to the present, there have been nine reasonably large, adequately conducted studies that examined the efficacy of INH in the prevention of tuberculosis among persons without HIV infection.

Ferebee, who helped to develop, oversaw, and reported most of the USPHS INH PT trials, authored a superb review in 1970 of the above-cited chemoprophylaxis trials, excluding the subsequent Veterans Administration and IUAT studies (11). Some of the material in the 1970 review had not been published in prior reports of these studies and included extended periods of observation and aggregate analyses of drug toxicity. Employing Ferebee's data as well as the primary reports themselves, I attempt to describe in detail these large-scale USPHS studies noted in Table 12.1.

United States Public Health Service Trials

The Tuberculosis Branch of the USPHS organized and conducted these large, randomized, placebo-controlled studies of INH PT. These trials are reported below in a standard format of admission criteria, study design, enrollee characteristics, and results.

Children with Asymptomatic Primary Tuberculosis

In this era, clinicians recognized that, although most children who had been recently infected by a parent did not develop overt illness

TABLE 12.1. *USPHS isoniazid preventive therapy trials*

Trial	Groups studied	Total subjects	Efficacy	Comments
Primary TB in children (12)	Asymptomatic infants and children with positive PPD and abnl CXR; assigned by household	2,750	88% reduction in total "complications" (41 vs. 5 events)	Protection demonstrated most clearly against XPTB; greatest effect in first year of therapy
Household contacts of prior cases (14)	Adolescents and adults in homes of previous cases	2,814	During year of INH PT, 3 cases with INH, 9 with placebo; not s.s.	Applied retroactively to homes in which the "primary TB in children" study had been done
Household contacts of new cases (15)	Persons "who took meals with source case"; assignment by household; did not require PPD reactivity	25,033	In first 2 years, 70% reduction in pulmonary, 72% in XPTB (97 vs. 29 events)	Results showed ↑ risk of TB with increasing PPD size; protection varied with adherence
Mental institutions (16)	Long-term residents of asylums; assignment by wards	25,210	In first 2 years, 63% reduction; in long-term follow-up, >60% protection (89 vs. 35 events)	Long-term protection diminished by a cluster on one of the wards assigned INH (see text)
Alaskan communities (17)	Villages near Bethel, AK; assignment by village; did not require tuberculin reactivity	6,054	Over 6 years, 59% reduction in morbidity (141 vs. 58 events)	Nearly half of subjects ≤14 years of age; protection shown to persist for 19 years; epidemic was arrested by case finding, treatment, and PT (see text)
"Inactive" lesions (11)	Persons with abnl CXRs; some old, some newly found, some previously treated	4,575	No Hx active disease: 63% reduction Known active, arrested without Rx: 46% reduction. Known active, treated: 17% reduction	Overall protection for 5 years was about 60%.

abnl, abnormal; CXR, chest x-ray; Hx, history; INH, isoniazid; PPD, purified protein derivative; PT, preventive therapy; Rx, treatment; SS, statistically significant; XPTB, extrapulmonary tuberculosis.

These USPHS studies were all randomized, double-blind, and placebo-controlled. Assignment to INH or placebo was done either by units such as village, wards, or families or by individual; approximately 50% in each study received INH. The actual numbers of morbid events are listed: placebo group, then INH recipients.

(12), a considerable number would experience highly morbid, potentially lethal forms of tuberculosis including miliary, meningeal, vertebral, and other forms of extrapulmonary disease (13). Lincoln and colleagues reasoned that INH might be able to avert these events if given promptly to newly infected children.

Criteria for Admission/Exclusion

Symptomatic children were excluded and given multidrug therapy. Children 2 years of age or younger required only a 5-mm or greater reaction to the 5-TU tuberculin skin test. Children 3 years of age or older required a 5-mm tuberculin reaction plus an abnormal chest x-ray.

Study Design

- Randomized, double-blind, placebo-controlled.
- INH 4 to 6 mg/kg daily for 12 months.
- Baseline physical exam, chest x-ray, and tuberculin skin test.
- Seen monthly for medical refill and interrogation regarding illness.
- Chest x-rays at 1, 3, 6, and 12 months.
- Physical exam and tuberculin skin test at 12 months.
- Seen periodically in years 2 and 3 with chest x-rays and tuberculin skin tests done yearly.
- Planned clinical follow-up to age 20 with chest x-rays at ages 12, 14, and 16.

Characteristics of Groups Enrolled

- 1,394 assigned INH, 1,356 on placebo.
- Ages 1 to 3, 50.5%; 4 to 6, 22.3%; <1 year, 8.5%; and 7 years or older, 18.7%.
- Race/ethnicity of children: white, 21.8%; nonwhite (presumably black), 36.1%; Puerto Rican, 15.3%; Mexican, 24.9%; Native American, 1.9%.
- Most had large tuberculin reactions, averaging 13.3 to 13.5 mm induration.
- Although chest x-ray abnormalities were not required for enrollments for those 2 years or younger, roughly one-third were noted to have hilar adenopathy or parenchymal lesions. Of those older children, approximately two-thirds had radiographic abnormalities. (Note: Although the original protocol had required radiographic abnormalities for children 3 years or older to be admitted to the study, clinicians later enrolled these youngsters if they were known to be recent converters.)

Results of Study

- Compliance: If all of the pills picked up were ingested, then 93% of children took at least 6 months, and 75% took all 12 months; however, we must assume that the actual number of pills taken was significantly less.
- Attrition: Losses from study were minimal, with 96% retained through 1 year of therapy and 89.7% retained through 2 years of follow-up.
- Pulmonary Disease: During the year of therapy, parenchymal shadows worsened in 29 of the INH recipients and 43 of the placebo recipients; this was not associated with clinical illness, and such a lack of clinicoradiographic concordance is now commonly recognized in pediatric tuberculosis (see Chapter 9).
- Extrapulmonary Disease: During the year of treatment, definite extrapulmonary complications were seen in 31 placebo and two INH recipients. Of the 31 placebo cases, eight were CNS, six skeletal, and one miliary; among the INH recipients only one skeletal case and one pleural effusion case were noted.
- Long-Term Follow-up: During the 10-year follow-up reported in 1970, there had occurred 41 complications in the placebo group, a rate of 30.2 per 1,000 children; in the INH group, the rate of complications was 3.6, an 8.4-fold reduction in morbidity. Notably, 76% of the complications in the placebo group and 80% in the INH group occurred during the year of treatment or the first year of observation.
- Level of Protection: The greatest degrees of protection were seen among the children aged 0 to 3 years and among those of all ages with parenchymal abnormalities on their chest x-rays; this apparent protection actually was the product of the relatively higher morbidity among these groups receiving placebo. Note: Among placebo-treated children, the

risk of complications was 3.6-fold higher with pulmonary parenchymal shadowing than in those with only hilar/paratracheal lymphadenopathy, 9.13% versus 2.56%, over the 10 years.

Household Contacts of Previously Known Active Cases

While the children's trial was being conducted, the USPHS organized a pilot study expanding the preventive therapy to contacts of all ages. This study also enrolled tuberculin-negative contacts to determine whether INH could prevent infection from occurring while there was an active case in the house, true prophylaxis if you will. In this study, families of patients who had been under treatment (14), often for an extended period, were enrolled; thus, some of the initial morbid complications among contacts very likely had already passed. Because of the limited and unusual nature of this study, it is not reviewed in detail. In the trial, 2,814 were enrolled; INH and placebo were randomly assigned by household, not individual, assuming that pills would be interchanged among family members. Salient findings of the study included the following: (a) the group receiving INH had three cases during the year of therapy versus nine cases in the placebo group, although because of the small numbers the findings were not statistically significant; (b) during the 3 years following the treatment year, three new cases occurred in both groups; (c) eight of the nine cases occurring in the placebo group occurred in those with original tuberculin reactions of 5 mm induration; and (d) INH did not appear to prevent infection in this setting. However, because all of the source cases were already on therapy, this was not a true test.

Household Contacts of Newly Diagnosed Cases

Based on the experience with the pilot study cited above, this trial (15) was expanded to include 37 communities; between 1957 and 1959, 25,033 contacts to 5,677 index cases were enrolled.

Criteria for Admission/Exclusion

Inclusion criteria included: (a) all household members ("persons who ate their meals with the index case") of newly discovered cases of pulmonary tuberculosis, regardless of tuberculin status; (b) no evidence of active disease; and (c) excluded children less than 2 months of age, those with epilepsy, and persons with prior tuberculosis.

Study Design

- Randomized, double-blinded, placebo controlled.
- Randomization by household, not individual.
- Isoniazid, 5 to 6 mg/kg daily for 12 months.
- Baseline chest x-ray and 5-TU tuberculin skin test.
- Subjects seen regularly to dispense medication and/or nurse home visit.
- Chest x-ray and tuberculin skin test after year of treatment.
- Plan for long-term annual follow-up.

Characteristics of Groups Enrolled

- 12,594 in placebo group, 12,439 receiving INH.
- Approximately 17% white, 17% black, 47% Puerto Rican, and 18% Hispanic (other than Puerto Rican) in both groups.
- Slight female preponderance in both groups.
- 65% of both groups less than 20 years of age.
- Roughly 60% in both groups reacted to 5-TU tuberculin skin test with 5 mm or more induration; prevalence of reactivity increased with age.
- Prevalence of skin-test reactivity of white male contacts less than 20 years of age was significantly higher than for white men of similar ages from those same communities who had undergone tuberculin skin testing in the U.S. Navy Recruit Study.

Results of Study

- Compliance: Compliance was good with 77% of participants claiming to have taken 75% to 100% of their INH during the year; another

10% claimed to have taken at least half of their INH doses.

- Attrition: Roughly 25% of participants were lost from both groups by the end of the treatment year.
- Primary Tuberculosis: Among tuberculin-negative contacts, radiographic primary tuberculosis developed in 16 persons receiving placebo and only five taking INH. By contrast, among tuberculin-positive contacts, 13 on placebo and 17 on INH developed radiographic primary complex tuberculosis during the treatment year. This suggested a true prophylactic effect of INH and demonstrated that, among young patients who are recently infected, radiographic abnormalities may evolve despite chemotherapy.
- Pulmonary Tuberculosis: During the year of therapy, pulmonary disease evolved among 62 placebo and 14 INH recipients; in the year following treatment, there were 17 cases among placebo and 10 cases in INH recipients.
- Extrapulmonary Tuberculosis: During the year of therapy, extrapulmonary disease was detected in 16 placebo and four INH patients; in the following year, there were two and one cases, respectively.
- Risk Factors: Among the 12,594 persons receiving placebo, it was possible to assess the factors predictive of developing tuberculosis during the treatment year. The overall rate for the entire cohort was 0.85% for the year; by comparison, these particular elements were significant:
  - Age: children aged 5 to 9 (0.23%) and 10 to 14 (0.45%) were relatively less vulnerable; the other age groups, 0 to 5 and 15 to 44, all averaged 1.2%.
  - Tuberculin Skin Test: Among 6,496 persons with ≤4 mm induration, the annual risk was 0.49%; by contrast, for those with 5 to 9 mm induration the risk was 0.83%; 10 to 14 mm, 1.03%; 15 to 19 mm, 1.25%; and 20 mm, or more 2.0%.
  - Weight: Among those contacts whose baseline weight was below the norm for that height in the study group, both male and female, there was significantly higher risk for active tuberculosis in both the treatment and posttreatment year. Other epidemiological evidence suggests that this association was not secondary to either cryptic tuberculosis or malnutrition but a true, natural propensity for thin persons to develop tuberculosis (see Chapter 6 for further discussion of this phenomenon).
- Drug Toxicity: Medication was discontinued because of side effects in 2% of the INH and 1.6% of the placebo groups.

Inmates of Mental Institutions

To date, most of the USPHS IPT trials had been directed at persons who, in large measure, had been recently infected. Looking for a population with more long-standing, quiescent infections, the investigators selected mental institutions (33 hospitals and 4 specialized schools) wherein previous tuberculosis mortality was 12-fold higher than for the general public (16).

Criteria for Admission

- Long-term residents in stable wards.
- Deemed likely to cooperate.
- Stipulations regarding tuberculin status.

Study Design

- Randomized, double-blinded, placebo-controlled trial.
- Randomization by ward.
- INH 4.2 to 5.0 mg/kg daily for 12 months.
- Baseline chest x-ray and 5-TU tuberculin skin test.
- Follow-up chest x-ray and tuberculin skin test at end of treatment year and annually thereafter.

Characteristics of Groups

- 12,326 received placebo, 12,884 INH.
- Both groups consisted of approximately 88% whites, 11% blacks.
- About half of the patients carried a diagnosis of mental illness (presumably, mostly schizophrenia); other common diagnoses were brain damage, mental deficiency, and epilepsy.

- 90% of the enrollees had been in institutions 2 years or more; over 50% had been institutionalized more than 10 years.
- One-half of each group was tuberculin-positive, with 5 mm or more induration; reactor rates were slightly higher among men than women; reactor rates rose with age, peaking about age 50 with about 80% of men and 70% of women reacting.
- About 9% of enrollees had abnormal initial chest x-rays.

Results of Trial

- Compliance: 19% reportedly took INH less than 20 weeks; 10%, 21 to 38 weeks; 70%, 39 to 52 weeks. However, actual pill counts indicated unreliable pill administration for about 30% of the wards.
- Side Effects: Slightly more refused INH (19%) than placebo (14%); 1.1% refused INH because they were sick from the pills versus 0.5% of those on placebo. No reports of jaundice were noted.
- Tuberculosis Morbidity: In the treatment year, 21 persons on placebo (0.17%) and four on INH (0.03%) developed active tuberculosis. During the subsequent year, 30 cases developed in the placebo group and 15 in the INH group.
- Risk Factors: Among the pretreatment variables that were significantly associated with the development of tuberculosis in the placebo group were tuberculin reactivity (24 cases among 6,484 reactors ≥5 mm, only four among 3,954 nonreactors), low weight (a fivefold higher risk among both men and women who were in low-weight groups), and abnormal baseline chest x-ray (37% of the morbidity came from the 9% with radiographic findings). In the discussion of this article, the authors for the first time began to consider IPT for identifiable high-risk groups rather than whole populations.
- Extended Follow-up: During the following 10 years of observation (11), INH continued to effect protection: the placebo group had 89 cases among 9,227 observed (0.96%), and the INH group 35 cases among 9,510 (0.37%), a 61.5% reduction in morbidity. The difference would have been more substantial except for a late undetected case on an INH ward who infected many contacts, 14 of whom went on to develop active disease. These late cases comprised 40% of the total tuberculosis morbidity among those who received INH.
- Tuberculin Skin Test Boosting: Recently converted skin tests in this mental institution population carried a relatively low risk for subsequent tuberculosis (11); this finding, contrasted with the high risk for disease following conversion in the household contact trials generated some of the first data indicating the phenomenon of boosting or increasing reactivity through serial testing in remotely infected populations.

Alaskan Community Trials

In the early 1950s, an extraordinary epidemic of tuberculosis was raging in the Bethel, Alaska area, largely among the Inuit (Eskimo) population (17). Each year, 25% of the tuberculin nonreactors became infected, the highest level of community transmission ever recorded. An intensive disease treatment program was initiated, resulting in one tuberculosis hospital bed for every 30 natives by 1956. Although the situation was improving, the USPHS embarked on this prevention trial intending to measure both the short- and long-term benefits from INH.

Criteria for Admission

Residency in one of 28 villages in the deltas of the Kuskokwim or lower Yukon rivers.

Study Design

- Randomized, double-blind, placebo-controlled.
- Randomization by households, not individuals.
- Stratified so that four of every eight households with eight or fewer members and two of every four households with nine or more members received each product.
- INH, 300 mg daily for those 16 or older, re-

sulted in dose ranges of 4 to 8 mg/kg. Children took age-adjusted dosage that averaged 5 mg/kg daily.

- Baseline chest x-rays and 5-TU tuberculin skin tests.
- Exclusions included those on treatment for active tuberculosis, persons with epilepsy, and infants less than 2 months old (they were started on the protocol when they reached this age).
- Quarterly visits by field nurses for medication refills, pill counts, interrogation regarding individual adherence, and health assessment.
- Continued quarterly surveillance posttreatment, including review of local records for tuberculosis morbidity.
- Chest x-ray and repeat tuberculin skin test after treatment year.

Characteristics of Group

- 7,333 residents were included in the villages or schools; 3,256 of them had known tuberculosis, 1,017 having been previously treated, 746 currently on treatment, and 1,493 without recommended treatment. Because of the presumed risk of reinfection, even those with prior therapy were randomized to the trial.
- 3,017 were assigned to placebo, and 3,047 to INH.
- 95% of both groups were Inuit or Native American.
- There was a slight male preponderance in both groups.
- Age groups included 0 to 14 (48%), 15 to 34 (29%), 35 to 54 (15%), and 55 or older (5%).
- Although approximately 90% of Inuit aged 10 and above reacted with 5 mm or more induration to PPDs in 1957, roughly one-third in both groups were nonreactors because many younger contacts were included in the trial.

Results of Trial

Data from this Alaskan study offered the most detail of any of the USPHS Trials regarding the various factors predictive of morbidity; thus, this section includes more data than other trial reviews.

- Compliance: By pill counts and questioning, it was estimated that 9.5% took 0 to 19% of their INH, 8.6% took 20% to 39%, 16.9% took 40% to 59%, 29.1% took 60% to 79%, and 35.9% took at least 80%; comparable percentages of placebo were taken.
- Attrition: Because of the closed populations involved, negligible numbers of patients were lost to follow-up.
- Tuberculosis Morbidity: As represented in Fig. 12.5, INH clearly reduced the incidence of tuberculosis during the year of therapy; notably, the protection extended throughout the entire 6-year observation period as well. For the 6 years, 141 of the 3,017 (4.67%) assigned placebo developed tuberculosis, while only 58 of the 3,047 (1.90%) on INH did so; this represents an overall 59% protective effect or a 2.5-fold reduction in morbidity.
- The authors of this report went on to break down their data to identify risk factors. Factors among the placebo-assigned patients that were significantly associated with the probability of developing tuberculosis included: tuberculin reactivity (5.6% vs. 2.2%); previously untreated versus treated tuberculosis (10.5% vs. 2.2%); and baseline abnormal chest x-ray, inactive lesions versus negative (7.8% vs. 3.4%).
- Regarding the impact of the percentage of the INH taken on the apparent protection, Fig. 12.6 reveals that patients who took 40% to 59% of the prescribed INH over the treatment year enjoyed protection roughly equal to those who took 60% to 79% or at least 80% of their drug. The numbers in the lower groups were too small to draw meaningful conclusions, but these data serve as an interesting prologue to the extended follow-up data and results of the IUAT Trial discussed below.
- Extended Follow-up: Continued observation of the patients treated in this trial indicated that significant benefits extended through 19 years (17). However, the data were complicated by a community-wide program of INH preventive therapy subsequently conducted in this original population in 1964. Based on the observed benefits of the 1957–1959 Trial, INH was given to everyone in those villages

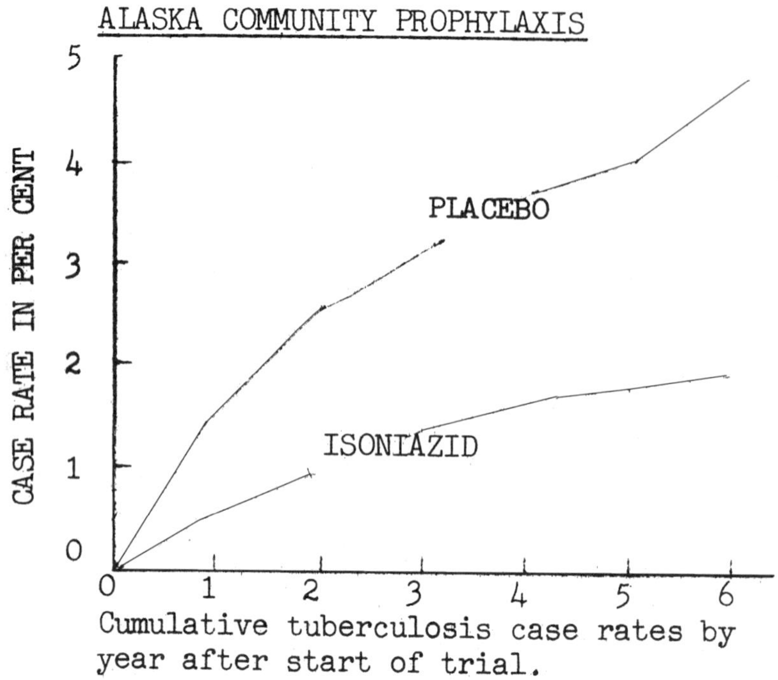

FIG. 12.5. In the Alaskan village INH PT trials, the group receiving placebo had an approximate morbidity of 5% by the end of the study. It should be noted that this included many who were tuberculin-negative at the outset of the study. By contrast, those receiving INH had an aggregate morbidity slightly less than 2%, a protective effect of approximately 60%. Notable also is the fact that this included a modest number of persons who, by pill counts, took less than 40% of their prescribed doses (see Fig. 12.6).

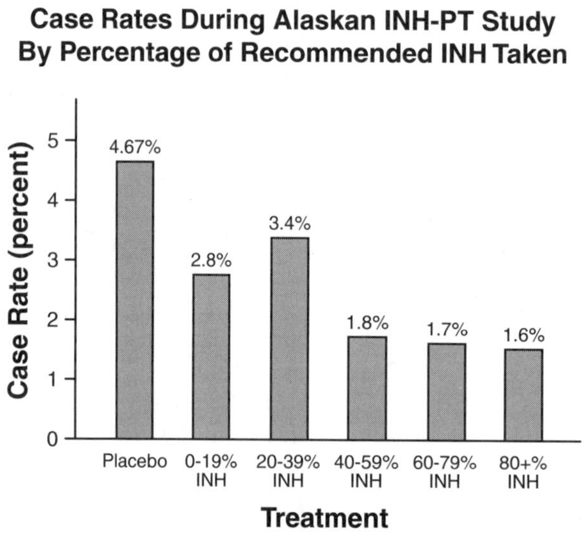

FIG. 12.6. Case rates during Alaskan isoniazid preventive therapy (INH PT) study by percentage of recommended INH taken. Each person for whom INH PT was prescribed was to have his or her compliance assessed by pill counts. Of note, the degree of protection was virtually identical among the groups that were estimated to have taken 40–59%, 60–79%, or ≥80% of the INH. Modest benefit was seen even in those who took even less INH. This benefit presumably resulted from treatment of latent infection in the individual. However, it is possible that some of the benefit occurred because others in the village were receiving INH PT and, as a result, there were fewer cases in the village. This could have conferred some protection to those who took none of their INH PT. As noted in the text, taking 50% of one's INH PT over 12 months is not equivalent to simply taking 6 months of consecutive INH PT. Indeed, if the presumed model of protection is accurate (the INH PT only works during random, sporadic spurts of replication by the mycobacteria), the longer-duration regimen would be expected to be more efficacious. This and other concerns have led to reconsideration for the optimal duration of INH PT, perhaps extending the recommended period to 9 months.

at the later date. Thus, those who had received placebo in the first trial eventually received INH, while those who had taken INH in the early study received all or part of a second course of INH. Nonetheless, analyses of these cohorts in 1974 (18) and 1979 (19) revealed that, among those who took little or no INH in the later community program there still was a residual 3.1-fold reduction or 68% reduced morbidity from the INH taken 19 years previously. Notably, most of the demonstrated protection occurred among those persons who entered the early trial with an abnormal x-ray consistent with inactive disease, such as fibrotic lesions. Regarding the extent of protection in relationship to the number of INH doses taken, Fig. 12.7 indicates no significant differences between those who took 50% (6 months) to 170% (20%) of preventive chemotherapy (the latter representing persons who received INH in both Alaskan programs, 1957 and 1964).

Inactive Lesions

Between 1960 and 1964, the USPHS enrolled 4,575 persons from 27 health departments in an effort to ascertain the protective effect of INH on chronic, established infections (11). This was prompted by the observation that, among inmates of mental institutions, tuberculin reactors with x-ray abnormalities were at very high risk of reactivation. Curiously, this series of inactive-lesion patients was never formally reported in a peer-reviewed journal. Details of the study from Ferebee's 1970 review included the following: (a) Criteria for admission were inactive lesions compatible with healed tuberculosis. (b) Approximately two-thirds of the patients were known to have previously active disease; most of these patients had been treated previously. (c) Age, sex, race, and other demographic features were not provided. (d) Results were broken down according to patient category. The highest attack rates in the placebo group and greatest INH protection were demonstrated in the never-previously-active group: 6.86% of those on placebo developed active disease within 5 years, with over half of the cases appearing in the first 2 years, and only 2.57% of those receiving INH developed tuberculosis. Those patients known to have had previously active tuberculosis but who had become inactive without medical treatment had attack rates of 4.5% and 2.41% in the placebo and INH groups, respectively. The lowest attack rates in the placebo group and, consequently, the least protection from INH were seen among the previously treated patients: only 3.30% disease in the placebo group and 2.73% among those assigned INH. Although the attack and protection rates varied modestly, overall the protection from INH averaged 63% over the 5 years.

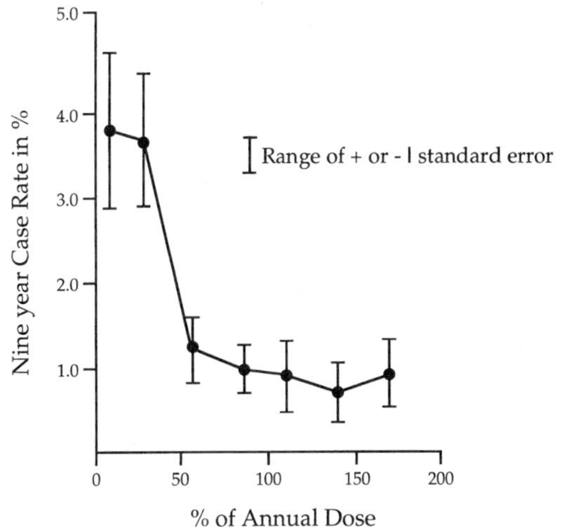

FIG. 12.7. In the USPHS Alaskan study, once INH had been shown to be highly protective, authorities returned to the communities to assure that everyone in the region received INH PT. As a consequence, some persons were prescribed a second course of INH. Through 9 years of observation, no advantage could be seen from roughly 620 doses (70% of annual course) over 180 doses (50% of annual course). Data compiled from Comstock et al. (18).

Other Studies

Preventive chemotherapy studies other than those conducted by the USPHS were generally performed on a small scale or less systematically. Three studies that offer useful data are described below.

Hudson River Hospital Trial

Contrasting strongly with the USPHS trial for patients with inactive lesions reviewed above are the findings of a study in a New York State Mental Institution, Hudson River Hospital, reported in 1964–1965 (20,21). In this study, 513 patients with chest x-rays compatible with inactive tuberculosis were randomly allocated to 2 years of INH 300 mg daily or placebo. Among these patients, 225 had not had active disease, and 288 had previously been found active, many of them having received chemotherapy. Unlike the USPHS findings, in the Hudson River Hospital Trial the incidence of new tuberculosis was considerably higher among these persons with previously active tuberculosis than among those never known to be active: 24.53% of the previously active group assigned to placebo developed active disease within 6 years, whereas only 9.35% of the never-active group on placebo did so. The INH reduced the incidence of tuberculosis among the previously active group by 46% over 6 years but did not alter case rates among those never active.

Veterans Administration Trial

Subsequent to Ferebee's review, Falk and Fuchs reported in 1978 on the effect of INH in Veterans Administration patients with inactive tuberculosis (22). In the study 7,036 patients were randomly assigned to 2 years of INH, 2 years of placebo, or 1 year of INH followed by a year of placebo. In this study, the incidence of reactivation was very low, probably because of extensive and prolonged preenrollment screening to preclude disease activity and because many high-risk persons (alcoholic, homeless, otherwise unreliable) were excluded from the trial. Among those patients who had been previously treated, no benefit from INH could be shown. However, among those never treated, INH reduced the risk of disease by 60%. Consonant with the findings from the Alaskan Trials discussed above, 1 year of INH was equally effective as 2 years.

International Union Against Tuberculosis Trial

Outside the collective USPHS Trials, the largest and most important study of the effectiveness of INH preventive therapy was conducted by the International Union Against Tuberculosis (IUAT) in Eastern Europe (23). In this study, nearly 28,000 tuberculin reactors with chest x-rays consistent with healed tuberculosis were allocated to placebo or INH. Unique to this study were varying durations of INH treatment—12, 24, or 52 weeks—and quantification of the radiographic abnormalities. Compliance with treatment was estimated on the basis of pill counts and urine testing. Results of this study include the following. (a) As shown in Fig. 12.8, the risk of reactivation increased with the extent of radiographic parenchymal abnormalities: pleural changes without parenchymal shadows were very low risk. (b) For those patients with larger abnormalities, the 52-week regimen was significantly more effective than the 24-week regimen, 89% protection versus 67% ($p < .05$); (c) For patients with lesser parenchymal shadows, 24 weeks of INH was comparable in protection to 52 weeks, 66% protection versus 64%. (d) In total, the 6-month regimen reduced tuberculosis morbidity by 65%, the 12-month regimen by 75% (Fig. 12.9). For persons regarded as compliant with these regimens, there was 69% and 93% protection, respectively; see Table 12.2 for summary of IUAT results. (e) The 3-month regimen resulted in an overall reduction over 5 years of 22%; for patients identified as compliant with therapy, this duration yielded a 31% reduction in tuberculosis. (f) There was a modest risk for INH-related hepatitis, with 95 cases (0.46%) occurring

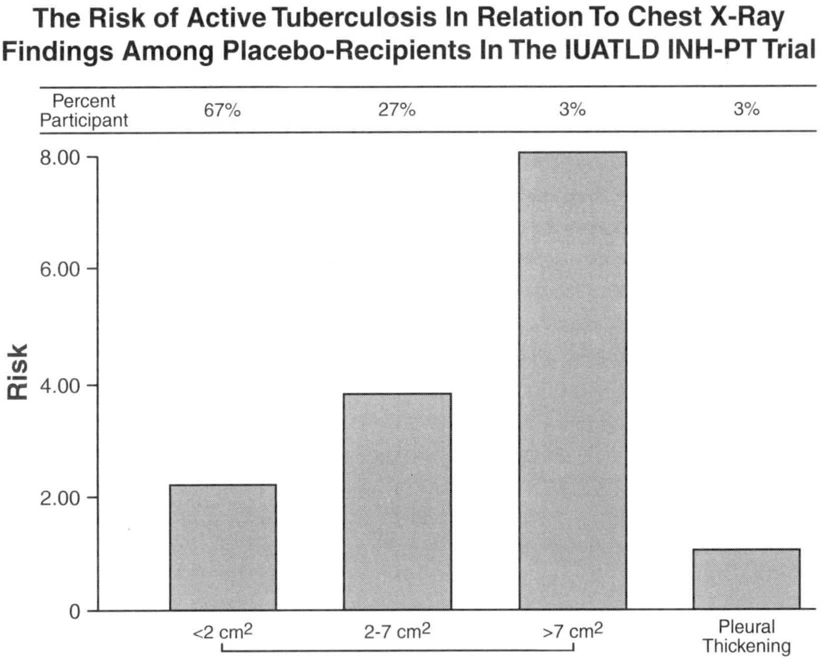

FIG. 12.8. In the International Union Against Tuberculosis (IUAT) trial of isoniazid preventive therapy (INH PT), the extent of chest x-ray abnormality was quantified. The upper-zone fibronodular opacities were assigned by surface area to three groups: <2 cm^2, 2–7 cm^2, or >7 cm^2. The patients were carefully assessed to be sure they did not have active disease before going on the INH PT. Nonetheless, the risk was considerably greater among placebo-recipient patients with larger lesions. Patients with clear lung fields but apical pleural thickening were at very low risk.

among the 20,840 persons receiving INH, with hepatitis noted in only 0.10% of those on placebo (see below).

A BRIEF HISTORY OF PREVENTIVE THERAPY GUIDELINES

Based on the results of the USPHS Trials, the American Thoracic Society, working in concert with the tuberculosis program of the Centers for Disease Control, has issued an evolving set of guidelines to indicate preventive therapy practices. These guidelines have been authored by ad hoc committees of the Scientific Assembly on Tuberculosis of the American Thoracic Society with CDC representation. Before publication as official statements of the ATS and CDC, the documents were reviewed and approved by the parent agencies.

1965 American Thoracic Society Guidelines

As noted, the first formal recommendations in the United States were published by the American Thoracic Society in 1965 (4). The documents advocated treatment of persons with latent infection to prevent emergence of active disease; high-risk groups targeted included those with inactive lesions on chest x-ray, recent tuberculin converters with particular emphasis on children and adolescents, and selected special conditions. Treatment with 12 to 18 months of INH was recommended, noting that for persons with previously untreated/inadequately managed active disease, INH and PAS might be used initially.

1967 ATS/CDC

By 1967, the earlier statement had been amended to recommend just 12 months of INH

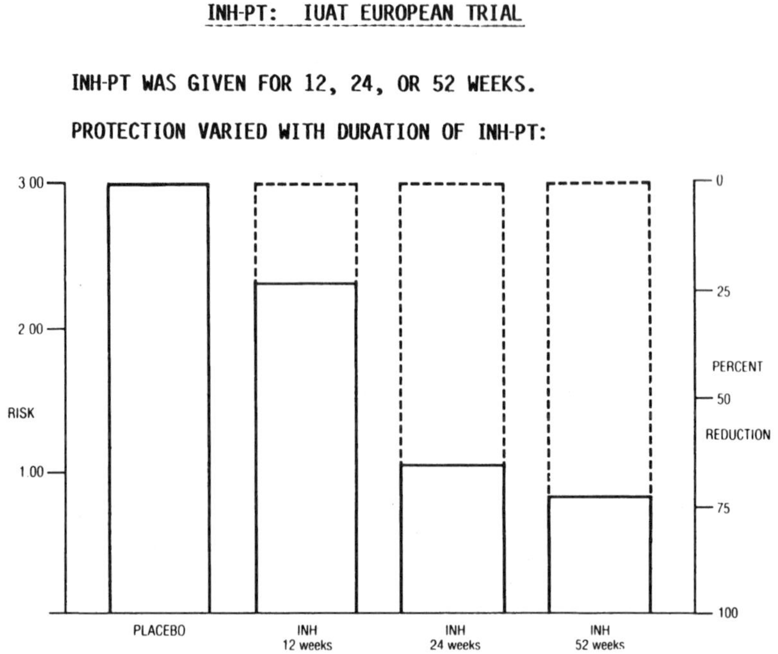

FIG. 12.9. As noted in the text, the duration of INH PT was randomized in this trial. Overall, there was only minimally more protection seen with the 52- versus the 24-week regimen. However, among those patients who were more compliant (≥80% of doses), there was statistically greater protection with 52 than 24 weeks (Table 12.2). Among the patients with the larger parenchymal shadows, the longer duration was again significantly more efficacious. From Krebs et al. *Bull IUAT* 1979; 34:65–69, with permission.

TABLE 12.2. *Effects on efficacy of INH preventive therapy: effects of treatment duration and compliance, IUAT trial*

Regimen	Subjects	5-yr incidence of TB		Reduction vs. placebo	
All subjects					
Placebo	6,990	97 cases	(1.43%)	—	(RR = 4.0)
3-INH	6,956	76 cases	(1.13%)	21% ↓	(RR = 3.1)
6-INH	6,965	34 cases	(0.50%)	65% ↓	(RR = 1.4)
12-INH	6,919	24 cases	(0.36%)	75% ↓	(RR = 1.0)
Compliant subjects (≥80% INH)					
Placebo	5,616	83 cases	(1.50%)	—	(RR = 13.6)
3-INH	6,039	61 cases	(1.04%)	31% ↓	(RR = 9.4)
6-INH	5,437	25 cases	(0.47%)	69% ↓	(RR = 4.3)
12-INH	4,543	5 cases	(0.11%)	93% ↓	(RR = 1.0)

Overall, there was a modest benefit to extending the duration of INH PT to 12 months among these patients with suspicious fibrotic lesions. However among persons with smaller radiographic abnormalities (measuring < 2 cm^2), there was no benefit: 6-INH yields 64% protection, 12-INH only 62% protection. Thus, it has been reasoned that among subjects with "normal" chest x-rays, 6 months should be adequate and equivalent (except for persons with HIV infection).

for preventive therapy (24). Targeted groups remained similar, although there was specific identification of contacts as a primary focus group.

1974 ATS/CDC

The guidelines were modified minimally in 1974, giving more weight to the potential hazards of INH-related hepatitis (25). Recommendations still entailed 12 months of INH for, in order of priority, household or other close contacts, tuberculin reactors with chest roentgenograms consistent with inactive tuberculosis, newly infected persons, tuberculin reactors with special clinical situations, and other tuberculin reactors up to age 35, even without risk factors.

1986 ATS/CDC

In 1986 (26), there were several significant modifications of the guidelines including the following. (a) Based on the IUAT Trial, the recommended duration for treatment was reduced from 12 to 6 months except for those persons with inactive lesions on chest film and persons with HIV infection. (b) The special risk factors category was expanded to include AIDS or positive tests for antibody to AIDS virus, end-stage renal disease, and clinical conditions associated with rapid weight loss or chronic undernutrition. (c) For persons 35 or older, monthly biochemical monitoring was advocated. (d) For high-risk contacts of index cases with INH-resistant disease or high-risk individuals intolerant of INH, rifampin preventive treatment was identified as a suitable option.

1985 American College of Chest Physicians

In 1985, the American College of Chest Physicians (ACCP) held a conference that addressed, among other things, tuberculosis preventive chemotherapy (27). The particular purpose of this conference was to address, by consensus, current problems for which there were not good scientific bases for resolution. Among the unique aspects of these recommendations were the standard use of 9 months of INH PT, except for inactive lesions cases, and for the use of twice-weekly, high-dose (900 mg) directly observed INH for high-risk, likely-to-be-noncompliant individuals such as prison inmates (28).

CONTEMPORARY ISSUES IN PREVENTIVE THERAPY: THE TUBERCULIN SKIN TEST AND INH-RELATED HEPATITIS

Updated guidelines for preventive therapy in the United States were issued in 1990. These recommendations were issued under the aegis of the Advisory Council for Elimination of Tuberculosis (ACET), a group composed of academic physicians and public health practitioners as well as representatives of the CDC (29). A central element of this statement is the attempt to reconcile two confounding factors in tuberculosis prevention: the diminishing utility of the tuberculin skin test in identifying persons infected with *M. tuberculosis* and the relative hazards of INH-related hepatitis versus the benefits of tuberculosis prevented. Because of their great relevance, both of these issues will be reviewed below.

The Tuberculin Skin Test (TST) and Preventive Therapy

False-negative TSTs occasionally occur in patients because the infection has occurred so recently that delayed hypersensitivity has not yet evolved or because there is anergy from coexisting conditions such as HIV infection. However, the major confounding factor of the TST in regard to preventive chemotherapy is the false-positive test. These false positives are engendered mainly from cross-reactivity from infection with *Mycobacteria*, other than tuberculosis, or prior BCG vaccination (30,31). They typically appear as spurious conversions: initial TSTs are negative due to waned hypersensitivity, but exposure to tuberculin antigen boosts reactivity so that on subsequent TSTs the individuals become reactive (so-called "boosting") (32). These phenomena mean that some persons who are not infected at all with *M. tuberculosis* or that others who are mistakenly believed to have been recently infected with the tubercle bacillus will be given INH preventive therapy. The central issues here are exposing persons who are at very low risk of tuberculosis to the potential dangers of INH and of consuming vital health resources in a nonproductive endeavor.

The performance of the TST is strongly influenced by the prevalence of infection by *M. tuberculosis* in the population to be tested. Thus, the TST performed quite adequately in times (early 20th century) or communities (Bethel, Alaska in the 1950s) wherein a majority of those tested had been exposed to and infected with tubercle bacilli early in their lives and repeatedly thereafter; see below for details. In this setting, false-positive tests constitute a small fraction of reactive TSTs. However, as the prevalence of tuberculosis has receded in the United States, these spurious results have become increasingly problematic.

Functionally, the vital aspects of the TST (or any test, for that matter) are its *sensitivity, specificity,* and *predictive values.* The *sensitivity* of the test indicates the percentage of those with the disease/condition in question who have a positive test; false positives do NOT influence the sensitivity because all that matters is that those with the disease/condition react positively to the test. Those with the disease/condition who do not have a positive test are said to have false-negative results. We know that among persons with active tuberculous disease there are substantial numbers who have false-negative responses to the TST. In HIV-negative populations, 15% to 25% of newly diagnosed cases do not have positive TSTs (32–34), and considerably higher rates of anergy exist among HIV-infected or AIDS patients (see Chapter 8). What we do *not* know is the proportion of individuals with latent tuberculosis infection who have false-negative tests because it is by tuberculin reactivity that we usually define latent infection. The presumption is that the percentage of false-negative tests is lower in those with latent infection than with active disease because debilitating tuberculosis has been shown to transiently suppress tuberculin hypersensitivity.

Specificity of a test is related to the number or proportion of individuals without the disease/condition who have a reactive test; in the case of tuberculosis, if none other than those infected with *M. tuberculosis* reacted significantly to the TST, the test would be 100% specific. However, as noted, cross-reactions among those infected with *M. avium* complex or other environmental mycobacteria may result in considerable induration to the TST; also, prior vaccination with BCG may result in tuberculin hypersensitivity (30,31). These would be considered classic false-positive responses.

Skin testing in a population that has been infected with *M. tuberculosis* generates a range of reactivity that is arrayed along the normal bell-shaped curve of distribution; typically, the mean reaction size is 15 to 18 mm of induration (Fig, 12.10A). On the left shoulder of this curve are persons with reactions between 5 and 10 mm of induration; this range has been referred to as indeterminate because of the potential for confusion with cross-reactions. Because of antigenic heterogeneity, the other mycobacterial infections typically result in negligible or small reactions to the 5-tuberculin unit (TU) TST; these might be seen arrayed in a curve of distribution with the peak in the range of 5 mm (Fig. 12.10B). Unfortunately, when these curves are superimposed, as they would be in a population with infections caused by both the tubercle bacillus and other mycobacteria, it becomes very difficult to distinguish between certain members of those groups (Fig. 12.10C). The prevalence of the tuberculous infection strongly influences the performance or predictive value of the TST. If the TST is only 95% specific (that is, 5% of the population has a positive test caused not by *M. tuberculosis* but by other mycobacterial infection), it is possible to calculate the predictive value of the TST in relation to various prevalences of true infection with tubercle bacilli.

The numbers of true-positive and false-positive reactions to tuberculin (PPD-S or PPD-T) vary greatly according to the prevalences of latent infection with *M. tuberculosis.* This concept is vital in appreciating the utility and limitations of the TST in a tuberculosis screening program. Because infections with the other mycobacteria, most notably *M. avium* complex, are widely prevalent in the United States population today (35), it seems appropriate to me to anticipate that

Tuberculin Skin Test Reactivity Among Hypothetical Population Infected Only With *M. tuberculin*, Only With MOTT, or Both

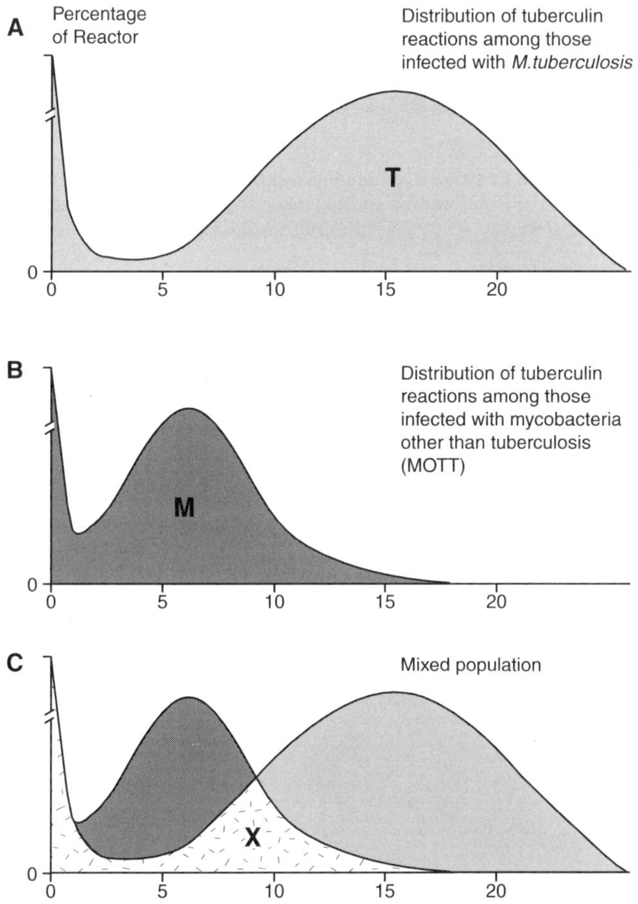

FIG. 12.10. A: Among persons infected with *M. tuberculosis,* this would be a typical distribution of tuberculin skin test reactions to PPD-T. Even without the influence of HIV infection, a modest but consistent proportion of persons presenting with active tuberculosis are anergic (see text). However, no data are available for anergy among those with latent infection because the tuberculin reaction is used to define this state. **B:** By contrast, among persons deemed to be infected with mycobacteria other than tuberculosis (MOTT), such as *M. avium* complex, the distribution of skin test reactions to PPD-T might be as represented here. In contrast to those infected with *M. tuberculosis,* wherein the mode is about 16 mm and the majority react with more than 10 mm induration, the mode and the majority of reactions are less than 10 mm. **C:** When we superimpose these two distributions, as might occur in a population with significant rates of both tuberculosis and MOTT infections, there is considerable overlap. A modest number of those infected with *M. tuberculosis* yield tuberculin reactions less than 10 mm, and a small but vexing fraction of those with MOTT infections yield reactions greater than 10 mm. By increasing the size of reaction that is deemed significant (indicative of tuberculosis infection), the test has a greater positive predictive value, but it loses sensitivity.

a small but functionally meaningful number of persons in most populations will have tuberculin cross-reactivity. Thus, if we are to obtain useful data from TST programs, we must employ this tool in populations with a high prior probability of being infected with *M. tuberculosis.* This can be demonstrated graphically in Fig. 12.11. From this model, we see that in a population with 90% to 95% prevalence of tuberculosis infection (Situation 1 or the United States early in the 20th Century or Alaskan natives in the 1950s), the small number of infections caused by mycobacteria other than tuberculosis (MOTT) was almost inapparent (Fig. 12.11A). However, in a

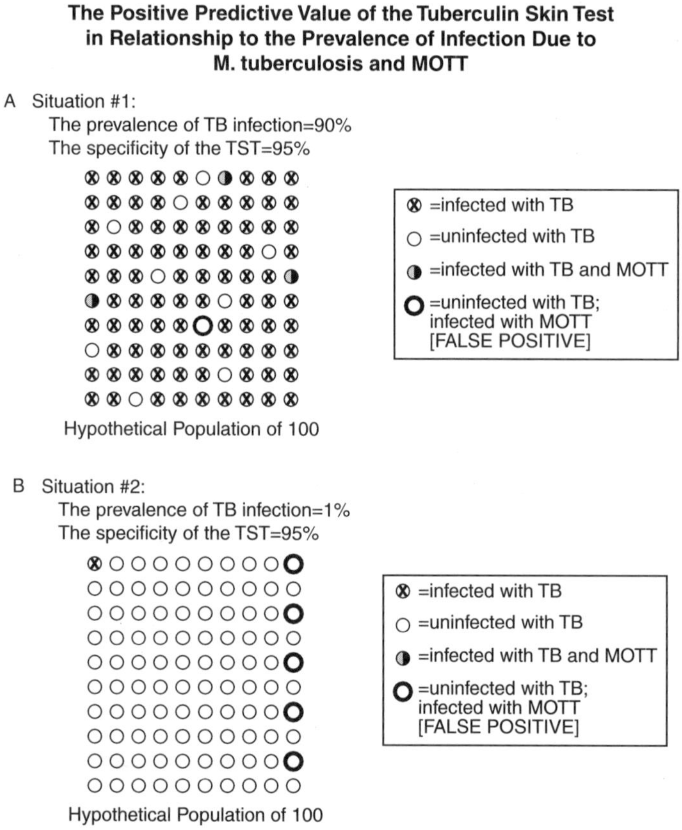

FIG. 12.11. The positive predictive value of the tuberculin skin test (TST) in relation to the prevalence of infection with *M. tuberculosis* and MOTT. **A: Situation 1:** Assume that 90 of 100 persons are truly infected with *M. tuberculosis* and have a positive TST (TB^+). Assume that the prevalence of infection with mycobacteria other than tuberculosis (MOTT) is such that 5 of 100 persons would have a significant reaction to the TST (specificity 95%). Then, because 90 are truly infected with *M. tuberculosis* and only ten are not (TB^-), the odds are that four of the MOTT infections will occur in persons already infected with TB (meaning the positive skin test will be a *true* positive) and that only one of the MOTT infections would occur in a person not infected with TB (resulting in a *false*-positive tuberculin reaction). Total results of TST of these 100 subjects are: 90 true positive (TP), 9 true negative (TN), and one false positive (FP). The positive predictive value is thus TP/(TP + FP) = 90/91 = 98.9%. **B: Situation 2:** Assume that only one of 100 is truly infected with TB (TB^+), resulting in a positive TST. Assume that 25 of 100 are infected with MOTT (TB^-) and that, of these, five have positive TSTs (Fig 12.10B). Then, the probability of MOTT infections occurring in the *one* person infected with TB is **(1/100)** × **5** = 0.05; consequently, the likelihood of the MOTT infection occurring in someone uninfected with TB is **(99/100)** × **5** = 4.95. The total results of the TST on these 100 are: one true positive, 94 true negative, and 5 false positive. The positive predictive value is then TP/(TP + FP) = 1/(1 + 5) = 16.7%.

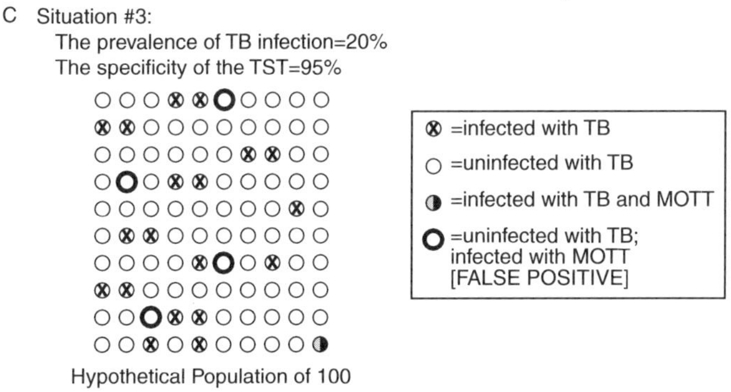

FIG. 12.11. *Continued.* **C: Situation 3:** Assume only 20 of 100 persons are truly infected with *M. tuberculosis* and have a positive TST (TB^+). Assume the prevalence of infection with the MOTT is such that 5 of 100 persons would have a significant reaction to the TST (specificity 95%). Then, the number of people with MOTT infections who are also infected with TB is $(20/100) \times 5 = 1$; conversely, the number of cases of MOTT occurring in people uninfected with TB is $(80/100) \times 5 = 4$. The total results of the TST on these 100 subjects are: 20 true positive, 76 true negative, and 4 false positive. The positive predictive value is thus TP/(TP + FP) = 20/(20 + 4) = 83%.

modern middle-class population (Situation 2), where the prevalence of tuberculosis infection is only 1% and MOTT infection prevalence is sufficient to yield 5% tuberculin reactivity, the number of false positives would greatly exceed the true positives (Fig. 12.11B). In this situation, a reactive TST would have a positive predictive value of only 16.7%. In an intermediate population, Situation 3, a tuberculosis infection prevalence of 20%, the TST would have a positive predictive value of 83% (Fig. 12.11C).

Although there are no sound data on the prevalence of tuberculin reactivity from infection with MOTT, there are considerable inferential data to indicate that these other mycobacteria can result in large tuberculin reactions ranging up to and above 15 mm induration (35–37). Skin-testing surveys done among U.S. Navy recruits indicated a strong predilection for *Mycobacterium avium* complex (MAC) infections in the Southeastern states; at that time, 1958 to 1965, clinical disease from MAC seemed largely sequestered in this region as well. However, recent clinical experience has demonstrated that MOTT disease, including MAC, is found widely throughout the United States (38). These and other data change in the ecology of these mycobacteria and indicate that no region or population may be presumed to be free of background MOTT infection.

Isoniazid-Associated Hepatitis

It is truly remarkable that in the early years of INH usage reports of hepatitis were extremely rare. As noted previously, thousands of patients initially received the drug without clinical recognition of liver injury. Among the approximately 36,000 persons assigned to INH during the major USPHS prevention trials, there were only four notifications of hepatitis (11). The incidence of hepatitis in these and other studies are displayed in Table 12.3. Because the USPHS study organizers did not expect liver injury, the INH PT trials were not designed to detect it. As noted by Ferebee, patients were not encouraged to register complaints about the treatment lest it reduce adherence. Although it is only circumstantial evidence, the fact that complaints related to INH increased with the ages of persons in the USPHS Trials is potentially reflective of the age-related risk of hepatitis recognized in later studies. Liver chemistries were not routinely monitored and may not have been performed despite complaints that, in retrospect, may have been hepatic in origin. For instance, in the house contact studies (14,15), more persons stopped INH than placebo bcause of gastrointestinal problems (146 vs. 110) and because they "felt sick" (35 vs. 23). Similarly, in the inactive lesions trial there were excessive numbers of pa-

TABLE 12.3. *Isoniazid-associated hepatitis[a]: incidence in large series, 1957–1978*

Series	Dates	Patients	Incidence	Nature	Comments
USPHS Trials (11)	1957–1964	36,000	4 cases (0.011%)	All with jaundice	No deaths; very likely underreported; LFTs done rarely
Inactive lesions, Veterans Administration (22)	1964–1968	7,030	None reported	NA	INH stopped in some because of nausea or rash, but LFTs not reported
Inactive lesions, Europe, IUAT (40)	1969–1972	27,840	95 cases (0.46%)	75 with jaundice	3 deaths; LFTs monitored *ad lib*
Capitol Hill Employees (41)	1970–1971	2,321	19 cases (0.82%)	13 with jaundice	12 with acute onset; 47.4% in first 2 months; two deaths, both male
Hospital Employees, Louisiana (42)	1970–1971	427	5 cases (1.17%)	1 with jaundice	No deaths; others stopped INH without symptoms, only abnormal LFTs; LFTs monitored in all patients
Maryland Health Department (43)	1973–1977	5,300	140 cases (2.64%)	15 with jaundice	Increased risk with age; 1 death; most cases in first 2 months; LFTs monitored *ad lib*
USAF personnel (44)	Before 1979	1,000	17 cases (1.7%)	NA	Most cases among whites, age 40–49; no deaths; LFTs monitored regularly

These large, generally consecutive-patient series of INH PT recipients suggest that serious hepatitis was relatively rare in the late 1950s to early 1960s when the USPHS trials were conducted. By the late 1960s to early 1970s, it was either moderately more common, or growing awareness of the problem led to more frequent ascertainment. If there was a trend toward a higher incidence of INH-related hepatitis, plausible hypotheses might include cofactors such as emerging viral hepatitis and/or medication such as acetaminophen; see text for further discussion.

[a] Abnormal liver chemistries in association with symptoms leading to INH discontinuation.

tients receiving INH who discontinued their medication because of gastrointestinal complaints (53 vs. 37) and "hypersensitivity" reactions (39 vs. 21); notably, among the 39 INH patients with hypersensitivity reactions, there were three cases with jaundice while none of the placebo group experienced jaundice (11). Ferebee, in her 1970 review, identified only one other person in the formal trials who developed jaundice; however, she did note that when INH preventive therapy subsequently was given to 300-odd Public Health Service employees, four cases of jaundice developed within 3 months. This led to reexamination of the four cases seen in the formal trials, ultimately determining that all eight cases had been seen among patients receiving INH from two lots prepared specially for the trials. Toxicological studies were done to determine if there were impurities in these lots, but apparently none were found.

Sporadic reports of liver injury associated with INH appeared during the 1960s (39–41); in virtually all of these cases, jaundice was part of the clinical presentation. However, Scharer and Smith first described asymptomatic elevations of serum transaminase levels without jaundice among persons taking INH (42); in this report, both patients receiving multidrug treatment for active disease and hospital employees receiving INH preventive monotherapy experienced significant disturbances of liver chemistry values, 10.4% and 10.0%, respectively. Although none of these patients became clinically ill, liver biopsies indicated hepatocellular damage in five of eight persons tested. INH was stopped in two of nine employees; however, liver chemistries normalized in the other seven despite continuation of the drug.

The first large-scale recognition of INH-related hepatitis occurred in 1972 in association with an outbreak of tuberculosis on Capitol Hill in Washington, D.C. (43). Following seven cases of tuberculosis with two deaths among federal employees on Capitol Hill between 1968 and 1970, contact investigations indicated a high prevalence of tuberculin reactivity. Thus, 2,321 persons were begun on INH in February 1970. In the first 3 months, 250 stopped the drug because of side effects, including 143 with vague gastrointestinal complaints, 32 with fever and chills, and five with "symptoms or signs of hepatic dysfunction." During the eighth month of the program, two men receiving INH developed fatal hepatitis, leading to discontinuation of the program. Intensive study of the population receiving INH revealed that 19 of the 2,321 (0.82%) developed hepatitis; ten were female and nine male, with a mean age of 49.4 years; nine of the cases occurred in the first 2 months, the other ten over the ensuing 6 months. Most patients, 12 of 19, experienced an abrupt illness marked by nausea, vomiting, chills, and fever as high as 103–104°F; 13 of the 19 developed jaundice. Only one case of hepatitis was identified in a matched control group of 2,154 other employees (0.05%); therefore, the risk of hepatitis in association with INH was highly significant. An additional fascinating aspect of this report was the notation in the report that, following the early reports of the Capitol Hill outbreak, the Centers for Disease Control (CDC) received more than 100 additional notifications of patients who had developed hepatitis while taking INH.

Thus, there emerged a growing awareness of the risk of INH-associated hepatitis. In the 1965 American Thoracic Society statement, there was no mention of toxicity, and the initial 1967 American Thoracic Society statement said, "There are virtually no side effects." Curiously, there was a revised version of the 1967 statement that was published subsequently under the aegises of both the American Thoracic Society and the CDC, which acknowledged that "hepatic dysfunction in persons receiving isoniazid for preventive therapy is reported more frequently than it was in previous years" (unable to identify when this was published). With the 1972 Capitol Hill outbreak noted above, however, there remained no ambiguity regarding the risk of hepatitis.

Following the Capitol Hill episode, the CDC conducted a large-scale surveillance study in 21 cities across the United States in 1971–1972 (44). The study examined various risk factors in relation to the likelihood of developing hepatitis while receiving INH. Notably, liver function tests were not routinely monitored but rather obtained when the patients developed symptoms suggestive of hepatitis. There were 12,838 enrollees; 53% were female; 44% were black, 37% white, and 19% other (mostly Asian). By age, 18% were under 20 years, 23% were 20 to 34 years, 30% were 35 to 49 years, 23.6% were 50 to 64 years, and 5.0% were 65 years or older.

Criteria for hepatitis were developed by an expert panel and include the following. Probable case: SGOT $\geq$ 250 Karmen units (KU) or SGOT $<$ 250 KU but SGPT $>$ SGOT and HbsAg negative (if done) and other causes of hepatitis not apparent. Possible case: SGOT $<$ 250 KU or SGOT $\geq$ 250 KU in the presence of other causes of liver disease or SGOT $\geq$ 250 KU but lacking other tests. All potential cases reported were reviewed and categorized by this panel. A detailed analysis of the criteria and of these, plus other cases of putative INH-related hepatitis, was published in 1975 (45). "Probable" INH-related hepatitis occurred in 92 patients (0.66%), and "possible" cases in 82 (0.59%); the total risk represented by these 174 cases was 1.26%. Among the probable cases, roughly two-thirds had occurred by the third month, and over 80% had occurred by the end of the sixth month; however, sporadic cases occurred throughout the entire year of treatment. In terms of liver chemistries, 86 of the patients had SGOT elevations to greater than 250 KU, and 87 had bilirubin levels of 2.5 μg/100 ml or greater. Notable findings in terms of specific risk factors included the following: (a) there was wide diversity in case rates among the participating cities; (b) there were distinct differences by age group; (c) overall, there were no differences in rates between men and women, 1.02% and 1.05%, respectively; (d) there were modest differences according to race, with case rates among Asians 1.80%, whites 1.39%, and blacks 0.94%; notably, these differences derived from high rates among Asian men and low rates among black men; (e) there was an alleged relationship between the amount of alcohol consumed and the risk of INH-related hepatitis—among nondrinkers the risk of probable/possible hepatitis was 0.81%, among occasional drinkers 1.30%, and among daily drinkers 2.63%; and (f) there were no differences in case rates in regard to the source of the raw INH chemicals from West Germany or the United States.

As noted above, in the IUAT European INH PT Trial, 95 cases (0.46%) of hepatitis occurred among the 20,840 persons on INH; 75 of the patients developed jaundice. There were seven cases of hepatitis of the 6,990 on placebo (0.10%). Salient features of this study included: (a) the cumulative risk of hepatitis increased, as expected, with the duration of INH therapy: the incidence in the 12-week regimen was 0.28%, the 24-week regimen 0.36%, and the 52-week regimen 0.52%; (b) the risk of INH-related hepatitis increased significantly in those with either of two underlying disorders, previous cholelithiasis/cystitis or ongoing alcohol abuse, the incidence being 0.31% in patients with one of these conditions and 0.21% in those without; (c) although the overall risk of hepatitis increased with age, it did so only because of striking increases among elderly persons with previous liver disorders; the incidence actually fell slightly among older individuals without predisposing hepatobiliary disorders (Fig. 12.12); (d) notably, the temporal appearance of INH-related

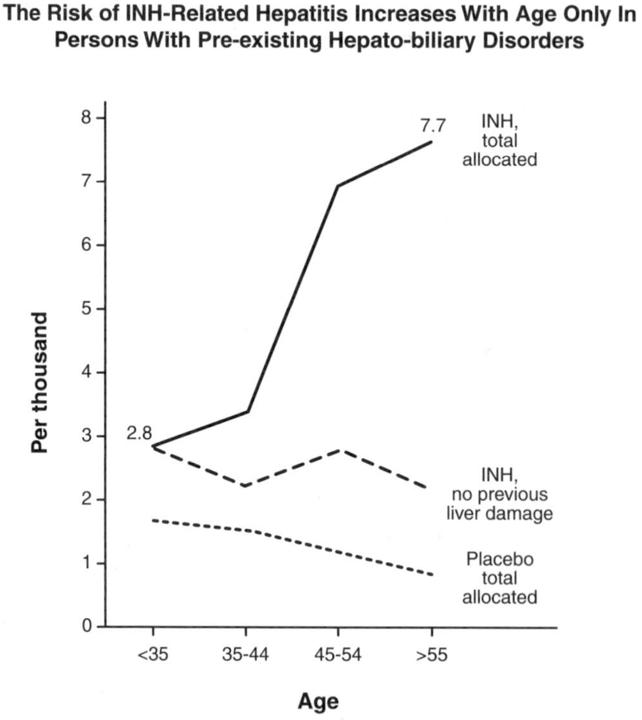

FIG. 12.12. Among persons in the IUAT Trial with preexisting hepatobiliary disorders, the risk of INH-associated hepatitis increased with age. Among the others, however, there was a gradual reduction with increasing age. This raises the issue of cofactors in the pathogenesis of liver injury caused by INH (see text).

hepatitis among those with and without previous liver damage was modestly different, the cases among persons with no liver disease occurring predominately in the first 20 weeks, with a sharp spike between 4 and 8 weeks, and those among patients with preexisting conditions occurred more uniformly throughout the year. Remarkably, these two disorders were uncommon in the placebo group, cholelithiasis in 1.9% and regular intake of alcohol in 3.2%, yet they appeared in 15.8% and 12.8% of the 95 INH-related hepatitis cases, eightfold and fourfold overrepresentation, respectively; and (e) also remarkable was the fact that regular intake of other drugs, unfortunately not specified, was recorded in 16.8% of persons with INH-associated hepatitis, mindful perhaps of the observation by Moulding and colleagues from California of use of drugs associated with fatty degeneration of the liver in 12 of 19 persons with fatal INH-related hepatitis (see below). Because 9.7% of those on placebo also reported use of other drugs, there was not a significant difference between the INH and placebo groups. However, this leaves open the possibility that some of those other drugs may have acted as cofactors in producing hepatitis.

Several other studies in this era reported on liver function test abnormalities among patients receiving INH. Bailey and colleagues in New Orleans followed 178 hospital employees receiving INH PT, comparing them with 93 controls (46); 12% of INH recipients but no controls experienced increased SGOT to over 100 mU/ml. Mitchell and associates observed 358 men in a psychiatric hospital who were receiving INH PT following a tuberculosis outbreak (47). To avoid the dilemma of coping with elevated transaminase levels, bloods were drawn, frozen, and analyzed after treatment was completed; only symptomatic individuals were assessed during the study. Because blood samples were not obtained consistently, actual percentages of elevated transaminase or bilirubin levels were not reported. However, similar to New Orleans health care workers (HCWs), 13.3% had at least one SGOT value $\geq$ 60. Also, three of these patients developed mild icterus with bilirubin levels between 2.5 and 5.3. The risk of hepatitis increased with age. None of the patients with hepatic derangements went on to serious hepatitis despite continuation of the drug.

Despite the trend toward increased risk of INH-related hepatitis with advancing age in the above reports, studies from New York City among adolescents aged 12 to 16 years (48), from Greece among children aged 9 to 14 years (49), and from Montreal among children and adolescents aged 1 to 18 years (50) showed elevated transaminase levels in the range of 7% to 10% of patients. Hepatitis severe enough to discontinue treatment occurred in only 2 of 239 (0.8%) in the Greek children, in 4 of 369 (1.1%) of the Montreal cohort, in 1 of 534 pediatric patients from New York City (51), and in none of other groups from New York City (48) and Virginia (52).

In several of these studies it was clear that, even if transaminase values did not fall outside the normal ranges, the mean SGOT and/or SGPT values of those on INH rose above the baseline values and were substantially higher than the controls (46–49). From these data, one may conclude that INH does have a predictable effect on the liver in a considerable portion of those receiving the drug. However, in the great majority of cases, as long as the patients were asymptomatic, jaundice was not noted, and transaminase elevations were moderate, continued use of the drug was safe. Moreover, in all of these studies, there was no evidence to suggest that even late, delayed, or chronic effects related to this use of INH.

The possible contributions of cofactors such as other medications or viral hepatitis are discussed subsequently.

Fatalities Related to Isoniazid Hepatitis

Eight of the 174 patients with probable/possible INH-related hepatitis died during the 1971–1972 multicenter USPHS study; this represented a 4.6% risk of fatality for persons with INH hepatitis or a 0.058% risk of fatality among all persons started on INH preventive therapy (44). The fatal cases occurred among persons ages 38 to 65 years with the average age of 54. Peculiar aspects of the fatalities were that six of the eight were among women, five of the six were black, and that seven of the eight deaths occurred in Baltimore. Thus, in Baltimore the apparent risk for fatal liver damage was 0.22% among those receiving INH PT, whereas in the remainder of the country it was 0.009%, a 24-fold difference. These findings suggested a possible confounding factor, and, indeed, a subsequent analysis revealed an increase in deaths from liver disease in that region during this period among persons not taking INH (53).

As noted, in the IUAT Preventive Therapy Trial, the risk of hepatitis was 0.46% among those on INH and 0.10% of those receiving placebo (54). There were three deaths among the 95 cases of INH-associated hepatitis for a case fatality risk of 3.16%, or an overall fatality rate of 0.014% among persons in the trial receiving INH. Clinically noteworthy, all persons who died had continued to take INH despite being overtly symptomatic.

In a report that included the probable/possible cases from the USPHS Trial cited above plus other patients seen by these authors, the hepatologists involved with this study described isoniazid-associated hepatitis in a total of 114 patients, among whom there were 13 deaths with an ostensible fatality rate of 11.4% (45). This rate clearly reflects strong bias in terms of case referral because these severely ill patients were sent to specialty centers wherein they came to the attention of the authors. Because of the skewed data, I believe it is grossly inappropriate to use this artificially high fatality rate in calculating risk–benefit ratios for INH preventive therapy.

Similarly, a series of patients who died while being treated with INH was reported from California in 1989 (55). The article, which reflected an intensive inquiry by one of the authors, identified 20 persons who died of hepatic failure between 1973 and 1986. Although I am sure that many of these deaths truly were related to INH, it is difficult to translate this report into a quantitative assessment of risk because there were no denominator data; that is, the authors had no reasonable estimate of the number of persons receiving INH during this era. In addition, there were various other shortcomings to the document (56). Nonetheless, several aspects of this report merit professional notice: (a) most of these patients had not been monitored regularly during treatment; (b) in the majority of cases, the patients continued to take INH at least a week after the appearance of symptoms; (c) 16 of the 20 deaths occurred in women; (d) four of these cases developed during the postpartum period; (e) eight of the deaths occurred among persons 35 years of age or younger, including one 5-year-old and two 15-year-olds; (f) despite substantial use of INH among Asian patients during this period, there were no deaths in Asians in this (or previous) series; and (g) in 12 of the 19 cases for which data were available, the patients had conditions or drug use that have been associated with fatty changes in the liver.

More recently, Snider and Caras undertook a comprehensive review of INH-related hepatitis deaths (57). Through a very intensive review of the literature, FDA records, and a national network of tuberculosis clinicians and public health officers, they identified 177 cases including the above-described series. Among the most pertinent aspects of their report are these: (a) 69% of the patients were female, (b) 21.6% of the deaths occurred in persons 34 years or younger, (c) among 21 women aged 15 to 44 years for whom history was available, eight (38%) of the deaths occurred within one year of parturition, (d) deaths were highest between 1972 and 1982; whether the declining numbers thereafter reflect improved surveillance techniques, fewer patients taking preventive therapy, shorter courses of INH, other covariables, or all of the above is moot, and (e) based on the number of patients given INH preventive therapy by state and local health departments between 1972 and 1988, the authors calculated the risks for fatal hepatitis to be 14 per 100,000 or 0.014% for those beginning therapy and 23 per 100,000 or 0.023% for those completing a course of INH. Because this calculation predictably underestimated the number of patients receiving INH preventive therapy (by excluding patients being treated by private practitioners), it is I believe a high-range estimate for INH-hepatitis lethality.

In 1993, the CDC reported eight patients who had developed severe hepatitis while receiving INH PT; progressive liver damage had led to referral for liver transplantation (58). These cases were culled from three transplant centers in New York and one in Pennsylvania between January 1991 and May 1993. No information was available regarding the numbers of persons receiving INH PT nor of the cases of INH-associated hepatitis from which these patients were derived. Notable aspects of this report included: (a) 75%, six of eight, of the patients were female; (b) the median age was 33 years, with three patients under 20 years; (c) hepatitis became manifest between 21 and 142 days of therapy, the median being 57 days; (d) four patients died, three before and one after transplantation; (e) as in other series, all patients had continued to take the INH after the onset of symptoms typical of hepatitis, with seven of the eight taking the drug more than 10 days while clinically ill, (f) other drugs with potential hepatotoxocity were being taken by these patients: one on phenytoin and estropipate, another on prednisone, methimazole, and nadolol, and the third on metaclopromide; one of these patients and two others had also taken acetominophen concurrently with INH; and (g) serological markers for antecedent viral hepatitis were positive in four patients, hepatitis A and B in two each; one other patient had indeterminate serological markers for hepatitis C. The potential role of viral agents in the copathogenesis of INH-related hepatitis is discussed more fully below.

In view of the powerful influence that INH-related hepatitis deaths have on risk–benefit analyses and clinical decision making, Salpeter reviewed published and unpublished data on this topic in 1993 (59). This report focused particularly on the experience after the 1983 revised guidelines and/or among patients who had been monitored for drug toxicity. Data in this analysis included previously unpublished information on over 180,000 patients begun on INH PT from 26 metropolitan areas and four counties across the United States as reported to the CDC. In this group, 1.2% developed hepatitis requiring termination of INH, and two deaths were recorded. Also, among published reports, data were available on 16,705 patients begun on INH PT and an additional 3,507 patients begun on INH plus another drug(s) for preventive treatment. In these two groups, hepatitis requiring discontinuation of therapy occurred in 1.8% and 0.6% of patients, respectively; no deaths were recorded in either group. In the aggregate, the death rate from hepatitis related to INH was 0.001% or 1 per 100,000 patients.

This ratio is an order of magnitude less than that reported among patients on INH PT without monitoring, 0.01%. Notable also in the Salpeter analysis was the inclusion of substantial numbers of persons older than 35 years: one death occurred among 43,334, a rate of approximately 0.002%. The upper limit of the confidence interval for the overall true incidence of death, calculated by the Poisson distribution, was 0.003% or 3 per 100,000.

These data have been used for a decision analysis regarding the risk–benefit profile of INH PT (60). Although one may quarrel with some of the data in this recent article (61), the analysis appears robust. See Recent Recommendations for discussion.

Viral Infections and INH-Related Hepatitis

Given the paucity of serious hepatitis among early recipients of INH for prevention or disease treatment, the escalating numbers of cases beginning in the 1970s raised that possibility of copathogenic factors. The Capitol Hill experience (43) and subsequent USPHS survey (44) indicated increased risk for death from INH-related hepatitis in the Chesapeake Bay area, posing the question of an infectious agent, perhaps borne by shellfish or other local agents. However, fragmentary serological studies in these and other studies failed to demonstrate consistent evidence of viral hepatitis A or B (43–47,55,57), while one series from Philadelphia failed to show an increased risk for hepatitis among southeast Asian chronic carriers of hepatitis B who received INH PT (62).

However, four of eight young individuals in the Northeast United States with acute liver failure following INH PT were seropositive for hepatitis A or B, and one had equivocal serological evidence for hepatitis C (58).

Formerly referred to as non-A, non-B viral hepatitis, hepatitis C appears to be an emerging pathogen (63–65) that plays a surreptitious role in chronic hepatitis (66) and helps cause fulminant hepatic failure (67). Until recently, though, a relationship between hepatitis C and drug-induced hepatitis was only speculative. However, a recent study from Florida showed a clear and dramatic risk for hepatitis from either INH or rifampin (68). Among 134 consecutive patients admitted to the A.G. Holley Tuberculosis Hospital, 22 developed drug-related hepatitis; 12 (55%) of them were HCV seropositive. Curiously, 12 were also HIV seropositive, involving overlapping but not identical groups. The authors calculated that persons with hepatitis C were at fivefold risk, those with HIV were at fourfold risk, and those with both viruses were at 14.4-fold greater risk of drug-induced hepatitis.

Additional evidence that suggested a causal role of hepatitis C in predisposing to drug-induced hepatitis in these Florida patients included the treatment of four of the hepatitis C patients with α-interferon. With their viral hepatitis in remission, all four tolerated reintroduction of the offending drug(s). Notable in this group of patients, also, was the fact that neither hepatitis A nor B appeared associated with this phenomenon.

Although it is not possible to definitely ascribe all or any of the previously described INH-related hepatitis to hepatitis C, this is a highly plausible hypothesis that merits careful clinical and research attention. Obtaining viral hepatitis serologies among candidates for preventive or disease chemotherapy is probably most suitable for persons with baseline abnormal LFTs, history of prior hepatitis, or risk factors for hepatitis C including injection drug use or multiple transfusions. And, such serologies might be drawn for persons manifesting significant hepatitis with chemotherapy. We should also keep in mind the potential for other viral agents in the copathogenesis of drug-induced hepatitis (69–71).

CURRENT RECOMMENDATIONS FOR THE PREVENTIVE CHEMOTHERAPY OF TUBERCULOSIS

Recent guidelines for prevention include the 1990 recommendations of the Advisory Committee for Elimination of Tuberculosis or ACET (72). Subsequently, this document was supplanted in 1994 by the latest of the ATS/CDC Guidelines (73). The basic recommendations are outlined in Table 12.4.

The clear focus of the guidelines lies with identification of persons harboring latent infection with *M. tuberculosis* who are at particularly high risk of experiencing reactivation. Because of the variable performance of the tuberculin skin test, dependent on the populations in which it is employed, the new guidelines apply new cut points for significance in interpreting skin-testing results. Although epidemiologically sound, these floating values have, in my experience, engendered considerable confusion, particularly among health professionals who do not do such testing frequently. Therefore, these policies will be examined in considerable detail.

Basically, the variable cut points for the tuberculin skin test have been derived in order to lower the sensitivity and increase the specificity of the test in order to assure physicians and the public that the indications for treatment have been maximized. Because of the potential risks of INH-hepatitis and the inhibiting effect this has had on prescribing practices (74), efforts have been made to identify persons or groups for whom the risk–benefit ratios unassailably favor INH therapy.

HIV/AIDS

Persons who are HIV infected (or by history are reasonably presumed to be so) or suffer AIDS are currently regarded as the highest priority because of their relatively greater risk of developing active disease within the near future. Various studies indicate that the annual risk for reactivation for those coinfected with HIV and *M. tuberculosis* to be in the range of 5% to 10%; see Chapter 8 for a more thorough discussion.

Because of the potential for suppressed delayed-type hypersensitivity, I believe it is appropriate to consider such persons for preventive therapy independently of their tuberculin reactivity. Early articles demonstrated that persons with advancing HIV infection were at risk for cutaneous anergy (75,76). In that setting, the CDC recommended anergy panel testing for HIV-infected persons with unreactive PPD tests

TABLE 12.4. *Isoniazid PT: 1994 ATS/CDC guidelines*

Condition	Treatment duration	PPD status	Comments
1. HIV-positive or suspect	12 mo	≥5 mm induration or regardless of PPD	May give PT to those at high risk of TB by epidemiological features
2. Close contact to newly diagnosed, infectious case	6 mo	≥5 mm induration or regardless of PPD	PT for infants/young children exposed; may stop if still PPD-negative at 3 months
3. Recent tuberculin conversion (in past 2 years)	6 mo	≥10 mm increased induration, <35 years old; ≥15 mm increased induration, ≥35 years old	PT for all PPD reactors <4 years old; note difference in increased induration related to age
4. Fibronodular scarring in lung apex	12 mo	≥5 mm induration	Any age group; consider multidrug prevention therapy; rule out active disease
5. Medical conditions with increased TB risk	6 mo	≥10 mm induration	IDDM, prolonged steroids, other immunosuppressive Rx, silicosis, cancers, ESRD, rapid loss of weight or malnutrition, IDU, crack cocaine
6. PPD reactor <35 years old at risk of TB with varied social and/or economic risk factors	6 mo	≥10 mm induration	Foreign–born, high-risk area; disadvantaged poor/minority; residents of at-risk facilities (NHs, correctional, or psych)
7. PPD reactor <35 years old without special risk factors	6 mo	≥15 mm induration	Consider risk-benefit on *ad hoc* basis.

These are the broad current recommendations regarding candidates for INH PT. Important variables in this system include the suggested duration of INH therapy. Missing in this table are the recommendations for infants and children, for whom the American Academy of Pediatrics advised 9 months of INH PT (see Chapter 9 for details of this policy). As indicated in the text, 12 months is recommended for persons with HIV infection because of fear that progressively compromised immunity will put them at risk for reactivation tuberculosis. Please see Chapter 8 for an extended review of the issues around INH PT in such persons.

IDDM, insulin-dependent diabetes millitus; Rx, therapy; IDM, injection drug use; NHs, nursing homes.

(77). However, various factors have combined to persuade the CDC to withdraw the recommendations for anergy panel testing (78), including the following: anergy panels were not reliable in discerning latent tuberculosis infection (79), anergy was not strongly associated with the risk for subsequent tuberculosis in a U.S. population (80), and, in an anergic Ugandan population, INH PT was not significantly helpful in averting tuberculosis (81).

This is a confusing picture for these reasons: (a) in the U.S. anergy study cited above, INH PT did result in a 56% reduction compared to placebo (0.4% risk vs. 0.9%), but this did not reach statistical significance; (b) the INH PT did not protect anergic Ugandans, but a simultaneous group of PPD-positive Ugandans whose risk of tuberculosis was almost identical to anergic patients did profit significantly from INH PT. Thus, in the U.S. patients, INH PT appeared protective, but anergy was not a powerful risk factor for TB; in Uganda, anergy was predictive of TB, but INH PT was not protective!

Despite evidence in a Spanish population that anergy among an HIV-infected population was associated with increased risk for tuberculosis (82), a recent study from San Francisco failed to demonstrate such a risk (83). The cause of this disparity is unclear, although it may be that the risk of TB in Spain was related to a higher risk of exogenous infection than in San Francisco.

On balance, the evidence indicates that tuberculin reactivity in HIV-infected persons predicts a high risk for tuberculosis and merits strong consideration for preventive therapy. Anergy is much more difficult to define (84) and is considerably less clear in implication. I would still feel justified in recommending INH PT for an HIV-infected tuberculin nonreactor at high risk for tuberculosis by epidemiological parameters but do not believe that population screening for anergy in a U.S. group is a justifiable practice (85).

As noted in Table 12.4, 12 months of INH is currently recommended, even if the HIV-infected person has a normal chest x-ray. This extended treatment is based on the premise that antituberculosis chemotherapy is less effective in sterilizing hosts with impaired immunity. As a generalization, patients with HIV infection or AIDS with active tuberculosis respond well to conventional chemotherapy with conversion of sputum cultures to negative in about the same period as normal hosts; see Chapter 8 for details. However, authorities are concerned that deficient cellular immunity might result in microbial persistence with a higher risk of recrudescence in these persons. These concerns, as well as problems with the extended treatment leading to noncompliance, have led to interest in short-course, multidrug preventive therapy (see Decision Analyses below).

Contacts

Close contacts to newly diagnosed, infectious tuberculosis cases have been found to be at considerable risk for the development of tuberculosis over a 2- to 3-year period. In the USPHS Trial noted above, INH PT reduced the 10-year risk by 60%. The highest case rates among the placebo recipients occurred in the first year, with 86 of the total 215 cases (40%) found then; INH PT resulted in a 78% reduction in morbidity in that year. This emphasizes the importance of performing prompt and thorough contact investigations. The cut point of 5 mm tuberculin reactivity is based largely on data from this study. Rates of tuberculosis among placebo recipients during observation and extent of protection by INH PT are as follows:

Patients with a 10-mm induration have 1-year and 10-year TB risks of 1.22% and 2.94%; their INH protection is 60.2%. Those with induration of 5 to 9 mm have 1-year and 10-year risks of 0.50% and 1.92% and INH protection of 45.3%. Conversion during year 1 in the 10-year study is 3.69%, and protection is 61.0%. Placebo recipients in the age group 15 to 34 years were the highest-risk group, tuberculosis developing in 4.23% of that population.

Stead recently analyzed risks for a distinctive group of high-risk contacts, health care workers exposed nosocomially (86). In this review he contrasted the very high risk for developing active tuberculosis among previously tuberculin-negative HCWs who convert their tuberculin skin test following known exposure. This topic is discussed in the next section.

Recent Convertors

Persons found to have newly reactive TSTs are another very high-risk group. As noted above, contacts whose tuberculin reactivity increased significantly in the past year were particularly prone to the development of tuberculosis in the near future. The most likely explanation for this phenomenon is simple selection of biologically vulnerable hosts. Let us imagine a hypothetical group of 100 tuberculin-negative, previously uninfected persons without specific, identifiable risk factors who are similar in age, sex, and race. They are put in a chamber and exposed to an aerosol of fine particles containing virulent *M. tuberculosis.* Each person is infected with an equal number of mycobacteria sufficient to cause all 100 persons to develop significant tuberculin reactivity—to convert. A number of these individuals, varying according to factors intrinsic to their group, will develop active disease, pulmonary or extrapulmonary, within the ensuing 2 years. We presume that those who become ill are identified ipso facto as the most vulnerable of their group. Because we cannot readily identify those at highest risk prospectively, the recommended practice is to administer INH PT to all of them.

Although this is a logical model and surely involves favorable risk–benefit performance, it has been compromised by shortcomings of the tuberculin skin test, including imprecision of reading and boosting through serial testing. Early guidelines relating to INH PT for convertors called for nearly a 6-mm increase in induration, increasing from less than 10 mm to greater than 10 mm induration in 2 years or less (25). However, substantial reader-to-reader and even intrareader variation in measuring induration means that there is great risk for error working with such a small interval of change. Hence, recent guidelines have called for larger increases to designate conversion. In the 1990 ACET recommendations, distinction was made also on the basis of the age of the individual: for persons under 35 years, an increase of 10 mm or more, but for those 35 years or older, increases of 15 mm or more were advocated. This age discrimination reflects two considerations: older persons are more likely to experience spurious conversion from boosting and are at greater risk for INH-related hepatitis. Hence, these modifications were made to make the criteria less sensitive but more specific among persons 35 and older. For a Spanish population, among whom BCG was a common factor, March-Ayuela concluded that only increases of 12 to 18 mm were compatible with known risks for infection (87); however, he conceded that these criteria would miss some newly infected persons.

The above analysis of recent convertors basically applies to persons who are being followed routinely with serial tuberculin skin tests. However, we should be aware of a variation of this situation with significantly different implications. Stead's recent analysis of the risks for health care workers whose tuberculin skin tests become positive following exposure to an infectious case (88) indicates a substantially higher risk than the 5% to 10% 2-year figure given routinely (73). Indeed, in a series of reported nosocomial outbreaks, Stead calculated that 19% of recent convertors developed active tuberculosis before preventive therapy could be given. The cause of this inordinately great risk is not clear. In some respects, it may reflect reporting bias, such as, the manuscript was prepared and published because of the extreme morbidity. It could also reflect the possibility that in such large outbreaks the infecting inocula were greater and/or the particular strains were more virulent. In any case, when deciding about the risk–benefit ratio for INH PT for HCWs so exposed and infected, this apparently greater risk should be considered.

Fibrotic Lesions

Upper lung zone fibronodular shadows on the chest x-rays of tuberculin reactors increase their risk of tuberulosis very significantly. As noted in Chapter 5, surveys indicate that these "fibrotic" or "inactive" lesions are associated with a 30-fold higher risk of reactivation than matched individuals with normal chest films. Factors relating to the radiographic abnormalities that influence the probability of tuberculosis include these: (a) Essentially all of the studies indicate that classical, upper-zone fibronodular shadowing known by the eponym "Simon focus" are the lesions that mark persons at risk, not the isolated granulomatous focus or Ghon lesion (Fig. 12.13) (6). (b) The greater the extent of such lesions, the higher the risk (23). (c) The newer these lesions, the more the likelihood of reactivation (23). For instance, among patients who were known to have active disease in the prechemotherapy era and to have undergone spontaneous remission, reactivation rates are relatively low despite extensive residual chest x-ray abnormalities (11,22). (d) Prior antituberculosis therapy dramatically reduces the risk of active disease.

Current guidelines have called for either 12 months of INH PT or shorter-duration, multidrug preventive therapy for persons with upper-zone fibronodular abnormalities thought to be tuberculous (73). The latter tactic is particularly applicable to the patient in whom it is unclear whether these findings are old and stable or new and evolving. In these cases, multidrug treatment is begun on the possibility of active disease. If all cultures return negative and the patient experiences no radiographic or symptomatic improvement, preventive therapy may be terminated at 3 months, and the patient deemed to have received PT. If there is symptomatic or radiographic improvement, despite negative cultures, the patient is regarded to have smear- and culture-negative disease and is treated for 4 months.

Medical Risk Factors

Certain illnesses or disorders have been identified because they are associated epidemiologically with increased risks for tuberculosis. How-

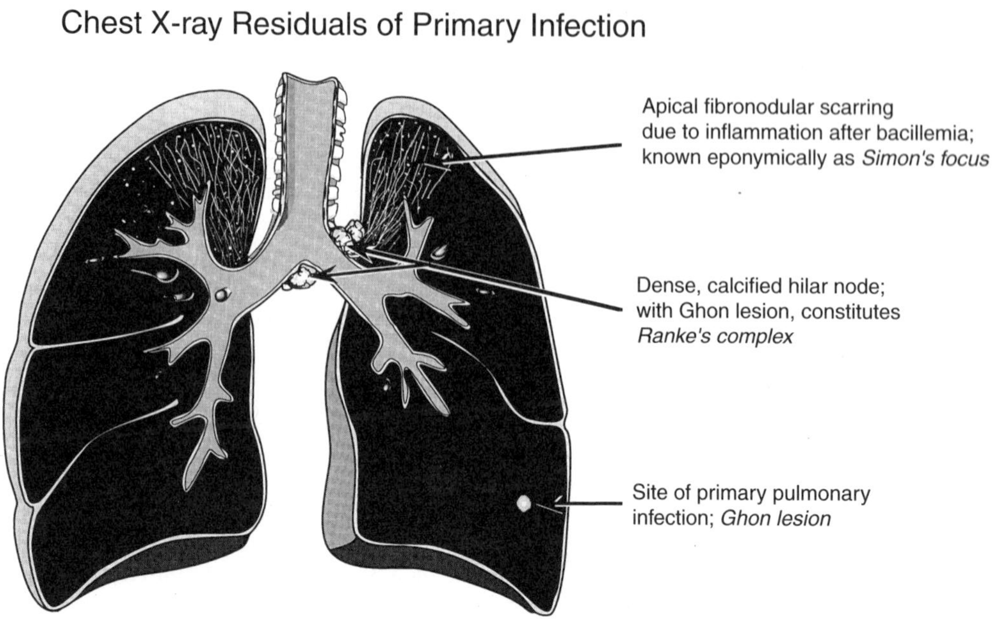

FIG. 12.13. Schematic of chest x-ray residuals of primary infection. Following the primary infection with *M. tuberculosis,* a minority of subjects apparently experience an asymptomatic or minimally symptomatic period with disease in the lung apex(ices). Although it does not bring them to medical attention, it does leave distinctive fibrotic and nodular shadowing in the upper zones (this is known eponymically as a "Simon focus"). Such shadows mark persons at considerable risk for reactivation disease.

ever, I personally find this topic to be one of the murkiest areas in the practical application of preventive therapy for the reasons noted below.

Although reports certainly do indicate that injection drug users (83) as well as those who use crack cocaine by inhalation (88,89) appear at substantial risk of tuberculosis, presumably because of social congregation factors as well as biological disturbances, experience tells us that such individuals in the community are unlikely to comply with an INH PT program.

Persons with silicosis are assuredly at higher risk for both tuberculosis and infection with other mycobacteria (see Chapter 5); however, the limited data on INH PT in this setting indicate marginal efficacy (90). A recent report from Hong Kong suggests that intensive, short-course preventive treatment with INH, rifampin, and pyrazinamide may be a more effective means of prevention than regular INH PT (91). However, another series involving gold miners from South Africa given a similar three-drug preventive regimen failed to demonstrate significant benefits (92). See "Decision Analyses," below, for a more extensive discussion of multidrug preventive therapy.

Diabetes mellitus was shown to be a very powerful predisposition in the era before insulin, but in the modern era the risk appears to be rather modest, with the incidence of tuberculosis in insulin-dependent diabetes ranging from two- to fourfold higher than that in the general population (see Chapter 5 for a more thorough discussion). There are no good data available to suggest that there is an association between type II obesity-related diabetes and tuberculosis.

Therapy with corticosteroids has been designated as a risk factor justifying INH PT since the first ATS Guidelines in 1965; this recommendation was based primarily on animal model work with only anecdotal human reports. Indeed, the 1965 recommendations emphasized that the risk from steroids was particularly noteworthy in persons with large tuberculin reactions and radiographic abnormalities. Modern retrospective surveys show only a vague relationship between steroids and the risk of tuberculosis. However, there is no real information regarding the critical dose per day and/or the duration of such dosage required to raise the danger of reactivation significantly. The 1986 ATS/CDC Statement identifies the equivalence of prednisone, 15 mg per day for 2 to 3 weeks, because this schedule has been shown to suppress cutaneous delayed-type hypersensitivity to tuberculin (26). Certainly, veteran clinicians have all seen patients who experienced active tuberculosis, often disseminated or multifocal, while receiving corticosteroids. However, in most of these cases, there were variable combinations of very high steroid dosage extended over many months, often associated with other immunosuppressive drugs and/or diseases that themselves were immunocompromising. Thus, it is highly problematic for me to determine along a simple dosage–time continuum the point at which steroids alone pose a sufficiently great risk for tuberculosis to justify INH PT.

Similarly, the inclusion of such conditions as immunosuppressive therapy and hematological and reticuloendothelial diseases such as leukemia or Hodgkin's disease are without quantification or sound epidemiological support. They broadly reflect the experiential or intuitive sense of risk and probably were more valid in earlier decades in the United States, when the prevalence of latent tuberculosis infection was high among virtually all sectors of the population.

End-stage renal disease was identified as an indication for INH PT for the first time in ATS Guidelines in 1986. Again, there are limited data that indicate that renal insufficiency does impair tuberculoimmunity but that the actual risk of reactivation tuberculosis is significant only in persons who are at high risk for other reasons, such as minority or immigrant status. Two practical and compelling reasons to be alert to the issue of tuberculosis in this group are the risk for nosocomial transmission to others with renal disease in congregate settings such as dialysis centers or hospitals and the potential risk for reactivation if the patient were to undergo kidney transplantation with the immunosuppression attendant thereto.

Substantial, rapid weight loss and chronic undernutrition were listed as explicit risk factors initially in 1986; previously, they had been linked solely to gastrectomy surgery. The demonstrated significant risk for reactivation tuberculosis among individuals with the premorbid slender, asthenic habitus noted in U.S. Navy recruits, inmates of mental institutions, and the general population of Norway was not mentioned in these guidelines despite the fact that the positive predictive value for this phenotype was as great as that of other, less-well documented, risk factors (see Chapter 5 for details). Chronic undernutrition may be seen as secondary to dietary inadequacies or malabsorption or debilitating illnesses.

Racial, Social, and Economic Risk Factors

Additional candidates for INH PT identified in the 1994 Guidelines are persons less than 35 years of age with 10 mm or more tuberculin reactivity who belong to epidemiological high-risk groups, including (a) foreign-born from high-prevalence countries, (b) low-income minority populations such as blacks, Hispanics, and Native Americans, who suffer much higher rates of tuberculosis than whites (see Chapter 5 for detailed discussion), and (c) residents of long-term care facilities such as prisons and mental institutions—facilities where tuberculosis has historically been both endemic and epidemic. The document also identifies nursing homes in this grouping, but it seems unlikely that there would be many residents under 35 years of age in such facilities. Note that neither the special risk factors listed in Table 12.3 nor an abnormal chest x-ray nor recent tuberculin conversion is required for this group. The rationale for this strategy is simply that although the annual risk of tuberculosis for such persons is relatively low, because they are young and have long life expectancy, their cumulative risk is substantial. Also, because they are young, their risk of significant hepatitis is relatively low.

There is little controversy about the relatively high risks for tuberculosis for the above enumerated groups, but a practical consideration is how realistic is delivery of INH PT for them.

The Seattle Public Health Tuberculosis Clinic reported low compliance with an INH PT program for Southeast Asian refugees (93). As a result, case rates ranged between 200 and 300 per 100,000 per year for their first 4 years in the United States. They calculated that noncompliance with INH PT resulted in a sixfold increased risk for tuberculosis. By contrast, the Denver Public Health Clinic reported considerable success with a screening and INH PT program for foreign-born persons (94). There were several major differences in these populations, however. The group in Denver were largely Mexican nationals who had been living in the United States and were applying for legalization of their status and for citizenship. In this report, 716 of 1,029 applicants (70%) completed at least 6 months of INH PT.

Homeless persons have also proven problematic. Again, the group from Seattle has provided useful information (95). Following an outbreak in a shelter, they demonstrated that twice-weekly, high-dose INH PT could be delivered with reasonable efficiency to a group of men, the majority of whom were alcoholic. The Public Health Tuberculosis Clinic in San Francisco compared these tactics for getting PPD-positive subjects to report to clinic (96). In order, financial incentives (84%), peer health advisors (75%), and usual care consisting of referral slips and bus tokens (53%) were diminishingly effective in promoting an initial clinic visit. Predictors of failure included injection drug use and age under 49 years. The article reported only on initiation, not completion, of INH PT.

Finally, regarding INH PT for persons released from jails, the Seattle group reported discouraging results (97). After screening for infection in the jail, both directly observed PT (DO-PT) and self-administered INH PT were offered postrelease. Of 262 infected inmates, 40% were lost immediately on release; 63 of 105 (60%) on DO-PT completed therapy; but only 15 of 52 (29%) completed self-administered PT (SA-PT). Based on its low return, Nolan and colleagues terminated this program and did not recommend it to others.

Others

The final category of patient to be considered for INH PT includes persons less than 35 years of age with 15 mm or more induration to the TST but no other medical, racial, social, or economic risk factors for tuberculosis. This construct is a clear effort to make the tuberculin skin test less sensitive but more specific by increasing the induration required to be considered positive. Once again, the logic is that although the annual risk is low, the cumulative lifetime risk is not trivial, and the risk of serious hepatitis is extremely modest.

DECISION ANALYSES AND INH PT

To aid with the selection of treatment or policy options, decision analysis (DA) has been employed with increasing frequency over the past two decades. DA consists of constructing a branching tree describing various choices, the probable results for those choices, and the aggregate results or implications of the alternative pathways. The outcomes may be described in terms of morbidity, mortality, economic, or other markers. Obviously, the quality or predictability of the data fed into the DA plays a dominant role in the reliability or accuracy of the outcomes. By varying the data employed at the different nodes or branch points, one can calculate the impact of these factors on the results.

Although DA has played a prominent role in the discussions surrounding INH PT in the United States, it is vital to emphasize that virtually all of the controversy has surrounded the least important component of an INH PT program in America, namely, the relatively low-risk group described in the preceding section, "Others."

The suggestion that INH PT should be recommended or offered to low-risk persons marked only by positive tuberculin skin tests and no other risk factors evolved from early USPHS/CDC analyses; this practice was incorporated in early ATS guidelines specifically for persons up to age 35 years (25). Moulding first challenged the practice in 1971 on the basis of cost-ineffectiveness (98). However, the battle was joined seriously in 1981 when a group from Harvard challenged the ATS/CDC Guidelines with a DA that suggested that INH PT for low-risk persons would result in more cases of hepatitis than cases of tuberculosis prevented (99); thus, INH

PT would result in a net loss of life for this group. An editorial by Comstock that accompanied the DA criticized the data fed into the model, stating that the authors had underestimated the risk of tuberculosis, overestimated the risk of hepatitis, and grossly exaggerated the likelihood of death from INH-related hepatitis (100).

From this point, debate always ardent, occasionally acrimonious has surrounded this issue. Multiple DAs have since been performed regarding INH PT for low-risk young adults (60, 101–105). Based on variations on the data input, subtle differences in outcomes resulted. Most DAs found in favor of the practice of INH PT, but the benefits were usually subtle or marginal. The powerful influence of death rates from INH-related hepatitis came prominently into play with the report by Salpeter of extremely low death rates with monitored INH PT (59) and the subsequent DA using the low mortality to calculate the utility of INH PT for low-risk tuberculin reactors of all ages (60). In this model, INH PT performed favorably in terms of both risk–benefit and cost-effectiveness for all ages, one year through 70 years. Although Moulding challenged some of the assumptions employed in this DA (61), no other major criticisms have surfaced.

Other DAs have been employed to calculate the utility of INH PT in HIV-infected persons (85), the use of INH PT in areas with various levels of INH resistance (106), the applicability of INH PT in the elderly (107), the cost-effectiveness of INH PT (108), the optimal duration of INH PT (109), the utility of INH PT for patients with fibrotic lesions and other health and age variables (110), or the effectiveness of INH PT or a hypothetical vaccine in protecting physicians from tuberculosis (111). Broadly speaking, these DAs usually found in favor of INH PT, but, in all such modeling, the data put into the calculations determine the outcomes. Furthermore, although I largely agree with the results, we should continue to recalculate these decisions in terms of newly revised data and evolving trends. As Snider commented in an editorial accompanying one of the DAs noted above, "The results of this particular analysis are not useful for influencing individual (or public policy) decisions on this subject because some of the input data were inappropriate and several of the assumptions were incorrect" (112).

A CHECKLIST FOR INITIATING AND MONITORING INH PREVENTIVE THERAPY

Assessment Before PT

Before INH PT is initiated, certain precautions should be taken to assure that the therapy is appropriate and optimally safe. Table 12.5 represents a modified version of ATS/CDC recommendations for evaluating these candidates.

Monitoring for Hepatitis

Current guidelines advocate monthly symptom review for persons less than 35 years of age but baseline and periodic monitoring of hepatic enzymes as well as monthly symptom review for those 35 years and older. There are significant programmatic/financial implications surrounding the recommendations to monitor liver function tests (LFTs). (a) Because of the increased costs entailed in such testing, it is important that individuals at particularly high risk for tuberculosis be enrolled in INH PT programs in order that favorable cost-effectiveness returns be preserved. (b) Confusion will be generated by such monitoring because, predictably, 10% to 20% of persons receiving INH PT will experience elevation of transaminase values above the normal range (see above). Although most of these persons will not experience clinically significant hepatitis despite continued use of the INH, there is concern that these elevated LFTs may be premonitory for severe liver damage. Arbitrarily, but reasonably I believe, the following conditions are offered as criteria to discontinue INH:

1. Significant elevations of any LFTs in the presence of any symptomatology suggestive of hepatitis without other apparent causes.
2. Elevations of the SGOT value fivefold above baseline or threefold above the upper range of normal.
3. Significant elevations of the bilirubin (along with transaminases) without other apparent causes.

TABLE 12.5. *Assessment before initiating INH preventive chemotherapy*

To assure appropriateness	
Exclude active pulmonary disease	For patients with "fibrotic lesions," especially when serial x-rays are not available, obtain sputum before INH PT. If suspicious of activity, may begin multidrug therapy while awaiting cultures.
Exclude active extrapulmonary disease	Even with a normal chest x-ray, do careful review of systems to exclude active disease at common sites (see Chapter 7); special precautions with HIV-infected persons who are at high risk of extrapulmonary tuberculosis should be taken.
Is patient infected with an INH-resistant strain?	If there is a high likelihood of INH resistance, consideration must be given to alternative agents such as rifampin or other drugs based on the resistance pattern of the source case; see Chapter 11
Probability of adherence with therapy	If the person is at high risk of tuberculosis, and there are potentially severe adverse consequences of its reactivation, consideration should be given to twice-weekly, high-dose, directly observed INH PT.
To assure safety	
Prior history of major toxicity from INH	Symptomatic or biochemically severe hepatitis; lupus-like reaction; fever, rash, hypersensitivity; psychosis; seizures
Adequacy of communications or contact	Able to converse well and/or availability of skilled translators; appropriate translations of precautionary information; available for monthly interview; face-to-face preferred; telephonic contact is minimal acceptable standard; accessible for periodic monitoring of liver chemistries when indicated.
Preexisting factors that increase the risk or possible implications of INH hepatitis	Preexisting virus-, alcoholic-, or drug-induced liver damage that reduces reserve hepatocellular capacity
	Chronic alcohol use, which may increase risk of INH hepatitis (see text for details)
	Recent use of medications associated with fatty degeneration of liver, general anesthetic agents, or acetaminophen (see text for details)
	The use of INH during pregnancy may be associated with increased risk for postpartum liver failure; hence, use INH PT after delivery (see text for details); if a woman is thought to be newly/primarily infected during pregnancy, prompt preventive therapy is indicated to lessen the risk of bacillemic infection of the placenta/fetus.
Predisposition for or existing peripheral neuritis	INH is rarely associated with peripheral neuritis at ≤300 mg/day dosing, but for persons at risk for vitamin depletion (malnutrition/alcoholism/pregnancy) or primary neuritis (diabetes mellitus/alcoholism), may include pyridoxine/B at 10 to 30 mg/day

These recommendations are largely derived from the 1994 ATS/CDC guidelines (77). However, I regard preexisting liver damage as a more powerful contraindication than the guidelines suggest. Although the likelihood of INH-related hepatitis may not be greater with preexisting or chronic liver disease, the clinical implications of drug-induced hepatocellular injury for such a patient may be profound or life-threatening, including hepatic encephalopathy, bleeding, or rapid-onset liver failure. Regarding chronic alcohol use, the CDC survey in the 1970s concluded that daily use of ethanol increased the risk of INH-induced hepatitis (49). However, I believe that the methodology of the study resulted in erroneously ascribing LFT derangements to INH rather than alcohol ingestion; because of the high risk for tuberculosis among urban alcoholics, I am disposed to offer INH PT despite ongoing regular alcohol use if the patient is motivated and monitoring is feasible. Finally, regarding pregnancy, the practice of treating newly infected pregnant women is not identified in the ATS/CDC guidelines, but, given the plausible risk for congenital tuberculosis (see Chapter 9), I believe this to be an appropriate practice.

Although I am sure that this scheme will result in the unnecessary termination of INH in some cases, I believe it is critical that a conservative stance be taken in order to reassure both clinicians and the public of the safety of this prevention strategy. If 80% or more of the planned INH PT has been delivered at this point, one might conclude at this point. If less therapy has been delivered and the patient is deemed at high risk for tuberculosis, PT may be completed with rifampin (see below).

What to Do when PT Is Interrupted

The most common question asked at the Tuberculosis Course offered at National Jewish is what do we do when a patient receiving INH PT elopes after 3 months, then reappears 6 months later (or some variation thereof)? No ideal data are available to inform the reply, but by extrapolating from the Alaskan and IUAT Trials, I believe that, if 6 months of INH PT can be delivered within a 12-month bloc of time, this should perform reasonably well. However, if too long a period has elapsed, the possibility that the bacillary population involved with the latent infection has regrown to its original size suggests to me that an entire new course of INH PT should be resumed.

ALTERNATIVES TO INH PT

Whether because of the likelihood of nonadherence among persons at very high risk for tuberculosis, disease caused by strains of tubercle bacilli highly resistant to INH, hepatitis or other causes of intolerance to INH, or the impracticality or unfeasibility of delivering 6 to 12 months of PT, there recently has been greatly increased interest in other methods of conducting preventive chemotherapy.

Twice-Weekly High-Dose INH PT

Based on therapeutic success and freedom from toxicity with INH given at 15 mg/kg twice weekly for 18 months to patients with active tuberculosis, a group from Denver proposed twice-weekly high-dose INH PT (TW/HD INH PT) in the early 1970s (113). The 1985 ACCP Consensus Conference endorsed this approach for selected situations (114). Nolan and colleagues reported on the deliverability of TW/HD IPT among a group of homeless alcoholics in Seattle (95). In addition, I have received personal accounts of this strategy being employed fairly extensively in prison systems.

The efficacy of TW/HD IPT will probably never be shown in a rigorous controlled trial. However, extrapolating from disease treatment reports, animal, and in vitro studies, a sophisticated group of students of tuberculosis thought it worthy of endorsement by consensus (114).

The two obvious circumstances in which TW/HD IPT might be employed are prisons, where the likelihood of nonadherence makes direct observation desirable, and in homes where outreach workers are treating a household member twice weekly for active disease. In the latter situation, contacts might be seen simultaneously for directly observed PT.

Rifamycin Preventive Therapy

Rifampin or other rifamycin agents might be superior agents for PT than INH. Evidence in support of this concept include the performance of rifampin in reducing the duration of chemotherapy required for use (see Chapter 10), the activity of rifamycins in animal studies (115–118), and sophisticated pulsed-exposure in vitro studies in which rifampin was much more effective in killing tubercle bacilli (119,120). Isoniazid, however, has been proven efficacious in large clinical trials that will never be recapitulated with a rifamycin; and INH is and will remain far cheaper than any rifamycin because of its simplicity of production. Hence, INH will probably remain the standard for usual PT.

Nonetheless rifampin or other agents such as rifapentine or rifabutine may find expanded future use in special settings: (a) close, high-risk contacts exposed to an INH-resistant source case. Anecdotal experience suggests efficacy (50,121,122), (b) high-risk candidates for PT with hepatitis ascribed to INH or other significant toxic reactions (unproven, but logic suggests probable efficacy, or (c) other. For some PT candidates, directly observed treatment is clearly desirable. High-dose INH may suffice, but it is probable that an intermittent rifamycin may be more efficacious in a shorter period of time. Because of its extremely long half-life, rifapentine may make once-weekly PT feasible (116,117).

Multidrug Short-Course PT

Animal studies indicate that rifamycin-containing multidrug regimens are considerably more effective in sterilizing chronic, nonprogressive infections than INH alone (115–118). Despite obviously increased costs for medications, the possibility of delivering highly effective preventive therapy in a few months of intermittent treatment has generated considerable interest (123). Among the obvious advantages are that reduced duration lessens noncompliance, intermittency facilitates directly observed therapy, and multiple drugs provide coverage despite INH resistance.

The efficacy of 3- to 4-month multidrug regimens in the treatment of patients in Hong Kong

TABLE 12.6. *Multidrug, short-course prevention therapy in humans*

Study	Population	Regimens	Completion	Results: Case (%)	Results: R/R	Comments
I. Halsey (124)	Haitian adults, HIV-positive and PPD-positive	(a) 6 I_7	55%	3.8	1.0	Follow-up 4 years
		(b) 2 R_2R_2	74%	5.0	1.32	
II. Whalen (81)	Ugandan adults, HIV-positive and PPD-positive	(a) 6 I_7	88%	1.08	0.33	Follow-up 2+ years
		(b) 3 $I_7R_7R_7$	86%	1.32	0.40	
		(c) 3 $I_7R_7R_7$	80%	1.73	0.51	
		(d) Placebo	89%	3.41	1.00	
III. Gordin (125)	Multinational, adults HIV-positive and PPD-positive	(a) 12 I_7	68%	1.2	1.0	Follow-up 3 years
		(b) 2 R_7P_7	80%	1.2	1.0	
IV. Hong Kong[a]	Silicotics with abnl CXRs and PPD-positive	(a) 3 R_7	NA	5.0	0.19	Follow-up 5 years
		(b) 3 I_7R_7	NA	8.0	0.30	
		(c) 6 I_7	NA	10.0	0.37	
		(d) 6 placebo	NA	27.0	1.00	
V. South Africa (92)	Silicotics with abnl CXRs and PPD-positive	(a) 3 $I_5R_5P_5$	"100%"	5.7	0.73	Follow-up 4 years; PT was "observed" but not enforced
		(b) 3 $placebo_5$	"100%"	7.8	1.0	

The regimens are represented in this manner: The first number is duration in months; I, INH; R, rifampin; P, pyrazinamide; the subscript number is the days per week the medication was given; NA, not available. For data relating to normal hosts, one can extrapolate from the efficacy of treatment for smear and culture negative cases in Hong Kong (Chapter 10).

[a] Hong Kong Chest Service/Tuberculosis Research Centre/British Medical Research Council. A controlled clinical comparison of 6 and 8 months of antituberculosis chemotherapy in the treatment of patients with silicotuberculosis in Hong Kong. *Am Rev Respir Dis* 1991;143:262–267.

deemed to have active pulmonary disease despite multiple negative sputum smears gives strong support to the supposition that similar regimens should be highly effective preventive therapy for other patients with normal or minimally abnormal chest x-rays; see Chapter 10 for extensive discussion of treatment of smear-negative disease.

Table 12.6 is a compilation of multidrug short-course (MD/SC) PT regimens in humans. HIV-infected persons were the subjects of therapy in three of the five studies; silicotic men were the subjects in the other two reports (124,125). Overall, the results suggest that shorter-duration, multidrug regimens are reasonably effective; however, it is not clear how much the drugs other than rifampin contribute to the efficacy of these regimens. Pyrazinamide (PZA) daily clearly resulted in increased intolerance in the Ugandan trial (Table 12.6). If, as suggested by Mitchison, PZA plays a specific limited role in the treatment of active pulmonary disease—attaching bacilli in the acidic debris lining the acutely inflamed cavity—it may not contribute substantially in PT in humans, where such an environment does not exist (see Chapter 10 for more discussion) (126).

At this time, the data regarding MD/SC PT are interesting and encouraging, but future studies should attempt to clarify the relative contributions of the components of these regimens. If the primary effect is derived from the rifamycin, cheaper and less toxic regimens can be concocted.

SUMMARY

There is no question that the current epidemiology of tuberculosis in the industrialized nations favors the utility of preventive chemotherapy given to those with latent infection over mass vaccination of the uninfected. Isoniazid monotherapy has been the treatment of choice because of its proven efficacy, general tolerability, and safety. However, the current acceptability of this strategic weapon has been compromised considerably by concerns for safety, difficulty identifying optimal populations, largely because of inadequacies of the tuberculin skin test, noncompliance, and the risk of prevalence of INH-resistant strains of *M. tuberculosis.* Existing guidelines for INH PT, although generally well founded in epidemiology, have not been consistently employed by clinicians. The number of persons started on INH PT has drifted downward over the 1980s. Hence, I believe it is time to reconsider our existing policies and attitudes toward this potentially useful but controversial tool.

In order to allay professional and public concerns about the relative balance of risk to benefit of INH PT, it is appropriate that we direct the bulk of our attention and resources toward those patients for whom the most recent and robust data exist documenting the risks for tuberculosis. These persons should be actively pursued and screened for INH PT. For others, who include older and less compelling risk profiles, clinicians encountering these persons in the course of other medical care should evaluate them for possible INH PT, factoring in not only risk for tuberculosis but the patient's willingness and capacity to participate in the treatment. Arbitrarily, I would designate these categories as *active* or *passive* screening targets for preventive therapy. By screening, I mean clinician/public health officer-initiated survey programs in which tuberculin skin testing and, when appropriate, chest x-rays are performed on groups of asymptomatic persons for the express purpose of identifying candidates for INH PT. Passive screening would refer to individual cases in which a specific finding, come upon in the course of rendering other care services, leads to the recognition of a person with risk factors sufficient to merit consideration. Some of such cases, notably individuals with chest x-ray findings suggestive of inactive tuberculosis, may be at relatively high risk of TB. Although there is no reasonable way to routinely screen for such radiographic risk factors, when inactive lesions are identified on chest x-rays done for other purposes, INH PT should be vigorously encouraged. Based on assessments of the risks for tuberculosis, the proven efficacy of INH PT in such groups, the practicality of conducting treatment, and the potential benefit to both the patient and society, reasonable decisions about INH PT can be reached. Categories of patients with proven or presumed tuberculous infection for whom preventive therapy unquestionably should be considered include: HIV-infected; high-risk contacts to recent, infectious cases; persons with upper-lobe fibronodular scarring; and recent immigrants from regions endemic for tuberculosis.

The role of alternative regimens for preventive therapy should be explored with ongoing trials.

The first and foremost priorities of tuberculosis control programs must be effective case detection and treatment to cure; focused preventive therapy may significantly help curtail tuberculosis rates in appropriate populations.

REFERENCES

1. Comstock G. Prevention of tuberculosis among tuberculin reactors: maximizing benefits, minimizing risks (editorial). *JAMA* 1986;256:2729–2730.
2. Centers for Disease Control. A strategic plan for the elimination of tuberculosis in the United States. *MMWR* 1989;38:1–25.
3. Ferebee SH. An epidemiological model of tuberculosis in the United States. TB control: with present methods? with BCG vaccination? or with isoniazid prophylaxis? *NTA Bull* 1967;53:4–7.
4. American Thoracic Society. Preventive treatment in tuberculosis. A statement by the Committee on Therapy. *Am Rev Respir Dis* 1965;91:297–298.
5. Small PM, Hopewell PC, Singh SP, et al. The epidemiology of tuberculosis in San Francisco. A population-based study using conventional and molecular methods. *N Engl J Med* 1994;330:1703–1709.
6. Alland D, Kalkut GE, Moss AR, et al. Transmission of tuberculosis in New York City. An analysis by DNA fingerprinting and conventional epidemiologic methods. *N Engl J Med* 1994;330:1710–1716.
7. Frieden TR, Woodley CL, Crawford JT, Lew D, Dooley SM. The molecular epidemiology of tuberculosis in New York City: the importance of nosocomial transmission and laboratory error. *Tubercle Lung Dis* 1996;77:407–413.
8. Zorini AO. Recent developments in the chemoprophylaxis of tuberculosis with isoniazid (historical vignette). *Cardiopul Med* 1978:15–16.
9. Lincoln EM. The effect of antimicrobial therapy on the prognosis of primary tuberculosis in children. *Am Rev Tuberc* 1954;69:682–689.
10. United States Public Health Service. United States Public Health Service tuberculosis prophylaxis trial. Prophylactic effects of isoniazid on primary tuberculo-

sis in children: preliminary report. *Am Rev Tuberc* 1957;76:942.
11. Ferebee SH. Controlled chemoprophylaxis trials in tuberculosis. A general review. *Adv Tuberc Res* 1970;17: 28–106.
12. Mount FW, Ferebee SH. Preventive effects of isoniazid in the treatment of primary tuberculosis in children. *N Engl J Med* 1961;265:713–721.
13. Wallgren A. The time-table of tuberculosis. *Tubercle* 1948;29:245–251.
14. Mount FW, Ferebee SH. The effect of isoniazid prophylaxis on tuberculosis morbidity among household contacts of previously known cases of tuberculosis. *Am Rev Respir Dis* 1962;85:821–827.
15. Ferebee SH, Mount FW. Tuberculosis morbidity in a controlled trial of the prophylactic use of isoniazid among household contacts. *Am Rev Respir Dis* 1962; 85:490–510.
16. Ferebee SH, Mount FW, Murray FJ, Livesay VT. A controlled trial of isoniazid prophylaxis in mental institutions. *Am Rev Respir Dis* 1963;88:161–175.
17. Comstock GW, Ferebee SH, Hammes LM. A controlled trial of community-wide isoniazid prophylaxis in Alaska. *Am Rev Respir Dis* 1969;95:935–943.
18. Comstock GW, Ferebee-Woolpert S, Baum C. Isoniazid prophylaxis among Alaskan Eskimos: a progress report. *Am Rev Respir Dis* 1974;110:195–197.
19. Comstock GW, Baum C, Snider DE Jr. Isoniazid prophylaxis among Alaskan Eskimos: a final report of the Bethel studies. *Am Rev Respir Dis* 1979;119:827–830.
20. Katz J, Kunofsky S, Damijonaitis V, LaFleur A, Caron T. Effect of isoniazid upon the reactivation of inactive tuberculosis. Preliminary report. *Am Rev Respir Dis* 1962;86:8–15.
21. Katz J, Kunofsky S, Damijonaitis V, LaFleur A, Caron T. Effect of isoniazid upon the reactivation of inactive tuberculosis. Final report. *Am Rev Respir Dis* 1965; 91:345–350.
22. Falk A, Fuchs GF. Prophylaxis with isoniazid in inactive tuberculosis. A Veterans Administration Cooperative Study XII. *Chest* 1978;73:44–48.
23. IUAT Committee on Prophylaxis. The efficacy of varying durations of isoniazid preventive therapy for tuberculosis: five years of follow-up in the IUAT trial. *Bull WHO* 1965;60:555–564.
24. American Thoracic Society. Chemoprophylaxis for the prevention of tuberculosis. *Am Rev Respir Dis* 1967; 96:558–560.
25. American Thoracic Society. Preventive therapy of tuberculous infection. *Am Rev Respir Dis* 1974;110: 371–374.
26. American Thoracic Society. Treatment of tuberculosis and tuberculosis infection in adults and children. *Am Rev Respir Dis* 1986;134:355–363.
27. American College of Chest Physicians Consensus Conference on Tuberculosis. Preventive Chemotherapy of Tuberculosis. *Chest* 1985;87(2 Suppl):115s–149s.
28. Bailey WC, Byrd RB, Glassroth JL, Hopewell PC, Reichman LB. Preventive treatment of tuberculosis. *Chest* 1985;87(Suppl):128s–132s.
29. Centers for Disease Control. Screening for tuberculosis and tuberculosis infection in high-risk populations, and the use of preventive therapy infection in the United States. *MMWR* 1990;39:1–12.
30. Menzies R, Vissandjee B, Amyot D. Factors associated with tuberculin reactivity among the foreign-born in Montreal. *Am Rev Respir Dis* 1992;146:752–756.
31. Menzies R, Vissandjee B, Rocher I, St Germain Y. The booster effect in two-step tuberculin testing among young adults in Montreal. *Ann Intern Med* 1994;120: 190–198.
32. Holden M, Dubin MR, Diamond PH. Frequency of negative intermediate-strength tuberculin sensitivity in patients with active tuberculosis. *N Engl J Med* 1971; 285:1506–1509.
33. Rooney JJ, Crocco JA, Lyons HA. Tuberculous pericarditis. *Ann Intern Med* 1970;72:73–78.
34. Nash DK, Douglass JE. A comparison between positive and negative reactors and an evaluation of 5-TU and 250-TU skin test doses. *Chest* 1980;77:32–37.
35. von Reyn CF, Green PA, McCormick D, et al. Dual skin testing with Mycobacterium avium sensitive and purified protein derivative: an open study of patients with *M. avium* complex infection or tuberculosis. *Clin Infect Dis* 1994;19:15–20.
36. Judson FN, Feldman RA. Mycobacterial skin tests in humans 12 years after infection with *M. marinum. Am Rev Respir Dis* 1974;109:544–547.
37. Wolinsky E. Nontuberculous mycobacteria and associated diseases. *Am Rev Respir Dis* 1979;119:107–159.
38. Chan ED, Iseman MD. Hypothesis: prior infection with *Histoplasma capsulatum* predisposes to pulmonary *Mycobacterium avium* complex infection? *Am J Respir Crit Care Med* 1996;153:A329.
39. Davies D, Glowinski JJ. Jaundice due to isoniazid. *Tubercle* 1961;42:504–506.
40. Cohen R, Kaiser MH, Thompson RV. Fatal hepatic necrosis secondary to isoniazid therapy. *JAMA* 1961; 176:877–879.
41. Reynolds E. Isoniazid jaundice and its relationship to iponiazid jaundice. *Tubercle* 1962;43:375–381.
42. Scharer L, Smith JP. Serum transaminase elevations and other hepatic abnormalities in patients receiving isoniazid. *Ann Intern Med* 1969;71:1113–1120.
43. Garibaldi RA, Drusin RE, Ferebee SH, Gregg MB. Isoniazid associated hepatitis. Report of an outbreak. *Am Rev Respir Dis* 1972;106:357–365.
44. Kopanoff DE, Snider DE Jr, Caras GJ. Isoniazid-related hepatitis. A US Public Health Service Cooperative Surveillance Study. *Am Rev Respir Dis* 1978;117: 991–1001.
45. Black M, Mitchell JR, Zimmerman HJ, Ishak KG, Epler GR. Isoniazid-associated hepatitis in 114 patients. *Gastroenterology* 1975;69:289–302.
46. Bailey WC, Weill H, DeRouen TA, Ziskind MM, Jackson HA, Greenberg HB. The effect of isoniazid on transaminase levels. *Ann Intern Med* 1974;81:200–202.
47. Mitchell JR, Long MW, Thorgeirsson UP, Jollow DJ. Acetylation rates and monthly liver function tests during one year of isoniazid preventive therapy. *Chest* 1975;68:181–190.
48. Litt IF, Cohen MI, McNamara H. Isoniazid hepatitis in adolescents. *J Pediatr* 1976;89:133–135.
49. Spyridis P, Sinaniotis C, Papadea I, Oreopoulos L, Hadjiyiannis S, Papadatos C. Isoniazid liver injury during chemoprophylaxis in children. *Arch Dis Child* 1979;54:65–67.
50. Beaudry PH, Brickman HF, Wise MB, MacDougall D. Liver enzyme disturbances during isoniazid chemo-

prophylaxis in children. *Am Rev Respir Dis* 1974;110: 581–584.
51. Nakajo MM, Rao M, Steiner P. Incidence of hepatotoxicity in children receiving isoniazid chemoprophylaxis. *Pediatr Infect Dis J* 1989;8:649–650.
52. Rapp RS, Campbell RW, Howell JC, Kendig EL Jr. Isoniazid hepatotoxicity in children. *Am Rev Respir Dis* 1978;118:794–796.
53. Levin ML, Moodie AS. Isoniazid prophylaxis and deaths in Baltimore, 1972. *Md Med J* 1974;24:64–67.
54. Riska N. Hepatitis cases in isoniazid treated groups and in a control group. *Bull Int Union Tuberc* 1976;51: 203–208.
55. Moulding TS, Redeker AG, Kanel GC. Twenty isoniazid-associated deaths in one state. *Am Rev Respir Dis* 1989;140:700–705.
56. Iseman MD, Miller B. If a tree falls in the middle of the forest. Isoniazid and hepatitis (editorial). *Am Rev Respir Dis* 1989;140:575–576.
57. Snider DE Jr, Caras GJ. Isoniazid-associated hepatitis deaths: a review of available information. *Am Rev Respir Dis* 1992;145:494–497.
58. Centers for Disease Control. Severe isoniazid-associated hepatitis—New York, 1991–1993. *MMWR* 1993; 42:545–547.
59. Salpeter SR. Fatal isoniazid-induced heptatis. Its risk during chemoprophylaxis. *West J Med* 1993;159: 560–564.
60. Salpeter SR, Sanders GD, Salpeter EE, Owens DK. Monitored isoniazid prophylaxis for low-risk tuberculin reactors older than 35 years of age: a risk-benefit and cost-effectiveness analysis. *Ann Intern Med* 1997;127:1051–1061.
61. Moulding T. Monitored isoniazid prophylaxis for low-risk tuberculin reactors (letter). *Ann Intern Med* 1998;128:1048.
62. McGlynn KA, Lustbader ED, Sharrar RG, Murphy EC, London WT. Isoniazid prophylaxis in hepatitis B carriers. *Am Rev Respir Dis* 1986;134:666–668.
63. Iwarson S, Norkrans G, Wejstal R. Hepatitis C: natural history of a unique infection. *Clin Infect Dis* 1995;20:1361–1370.
64. Zein NN, Rakela J, Krawitt EL, et al. Hepatitis C virus genotypes in the United States: epidemiology, pathogenicity, and response to interferon therapy. *Ann Intern Med* 1996;125:634–639.
65. Lau JYN, Davis GL, Prescott LE, et al. Distribution of hepatitis C virus genotypes determined by line probe assay in patients with chronic hepatitis C seen at tertiary referral centers in the United States. *Ann Intern Med* 1996;124:868–876.
66. Schmidt WN, Wu P, Cederna J, Mitros FA, LaBrecque DR, Stapleton JT. Surreptitious hepatitis C virus (HCV) infection detected in the majority of patients with cryptogenic chronic hepatitis and negative HCV antibody tests. *J Infect Dis* 1997;176:27–33.
67. Farci P, Alter HJ, Shimoda A, et al. Hepatitis C virus-associated fulminant hepatic failure. *N Engl J Med* 1996;335:631–634.
68. Ungo JR, Jones D, Ashkin D, et al. Antituberculosis drug-induced hepatotoxicity. The role of hepatitis C virus and the human immunodeficiency virus. *Am J Respir Crit Care Med* 1998;157:1871–1876.
69. Yoto Y, Kudoh T, Haseyama K, Suzuki N, Chiba S. Human parvovirus B19 infection associated with acute hepatitis. *Lancet* 1996;347:868–869.
70. Heringlake S, Osterkamp S, Trautwein C, et al. Association between fulminant hepatic failure and a strain of GBV virus C. *Lancet* 1996;348:1626–1629.
71. Mas A, Rodés J. Fulminant hepatic failure. *Lancet* 1997;349:1081–1085.
72. Centers for Disease Control. The use of preventive therapy for tuberculous infection in the United States: recommendations of the Advisory Committee for Elimination of Tuberculosis. *MMWR* 1990;39:9–12.
73. American Thoracic Society. Treatment of tuberculosis and tuberculosis infection in adults and children. *Am J Respir Crit Care Med* 1994;149:1359–1374.
74. Mehta JB, Dutt AK, Harvill L, Henry W. Isoniazid preventive therapy for tuberculosis. Are we losing our enthusiasm? *Chest* 1988;94:138–141.
75. Graham NMH, Nelson KE, Solomon L, et al. Prevalence of tuberculin positivity and skin test anergy in HIV-1-seropositive and -seronegative intravenous drug users. *JAMA* 1992;267:369–373.
76. Markowitz N, Hansen NI, Wilcosky TC, et al. Tuberculin and anergy testing in HIV-seropositive and HIV-seronegative persons. *Ann Intern Med* 1993;119: 185–193.
77. Centers for Disease Control. Purified protein derivative (PPD)-tuberculin anergy and HIV infection: guidelines for anergy testing and management of anergic persons at risk of tuberculosis. *MMWR* 1991; 40:27–33.
78. Centers for Disease Control and Prevention. Anergy skin testing and preventive therapy for HIV-infected persons: revised recommendations. *MMWR* 1997;46: 1–10.
79. Chin DP, Osmond D, Page-Shafer K, et al. Reliability of anergy skin testing in persons with HIV infection. *Am J Respir Crit Care Med* 1996;153:1982–1984.
80. Gordin FM, Matts JP, Miller C, et al. A controlled trial of isoniazid in persons with anergy and human immunodeficiency virus infection who are at high risk for tuberculosis. *N Engl J Med* 1997;37:315–320.
81. Whalen CC, Johnson JL, Okwera A, et al. A trial of three regimens to prevent tuberculosis in Ugandan adults infected with the human immunodeficiency virus. *N Engl J Med* 1997;337:801–808.
82. Moreno S, Bavaia-Etxabury J, Bouza E, et al. Risk for developing tuberculosis among anergic patients infected with HIV. *Ann Intern Med* 1993;119:194–198.
83. Daley CL, Hahn JA, Moss AR, Hopewell PC, Schecter GF. Incidence of tuberculosis in injection drug users in San Francisco. Impact of anergy. *Am J Respir Crit Care Med* 1998;157:19–22.
84. Pesanti EL. The negative tuberculin test. Tuberculin, HIV, and anergy panels. *Am J Respir Crit Care Med* 1994;149:1699–1709.
85. Jordan TJ, Levit EM, Montgomery EL, Reichman LB. Isoniazid as preventive therapy in HIV-infected intravenous drug abusers: a decision analysis. *JAMA* 1991; 265:2987–2991.
86. Stead WW. Management of health care workers after inadvertent exposure to tuberculosis: a guide for the use of preventive therapy. *Ann Intern Med* 1995;122: 906–912.
87. de March-Ayuela P. Choosing an appropriate criterion for true or false conversion in serial tuberculin testing. *Am Rev Respir Dis* 1990;141:815–820.
88. Centers for Disease Control and Prevention. Crack cocaine use among persons with tuberculosis—Contra

Costa County, California, 1987–1990. *MMWR* 1991; 40:485–488.
89. O'Donnell AE, Selig J, Aravamuthan M, Richardson MSA. Pulmonary complications associated with illicit drug abuse—an update. *Chest* 1995;108:460–463.
90. Snider D. The relationship between tuberculosis and silicosis. *Am Rev Respir Dis* 1978;118:455–460.
91. Hong Kong Chest Service/Tuberculosis Research Center MBMRC. A double-blind placebo-controlled clinical trial of three antituberculosis chemoprophylaxis regimens in patients with silicosis in Hong Kong. *Am Rev Respir Dis* 1992;145:36–41.
92. Cowie RL. Short course chemoprophylaxis with rifampicin, isoniazid and pyrazinamide for tuberculosis evaluated in gold miners with chronic silicosis: a double-blind placebo controlled trial. *Tuberc Lung Dis* 1996;77:239–243.
93. Nolan CM, Aitken ML, Elarth AM, Anderson KM, Miller WT. Active tuberculosis after isoniazid chemoprophylaxis of Southeast Asian refugees. *Am Rev Respir Dis* 1986;133:431–436.
94. Blum RN, Polish LB, Tapy JM, Catlin BJ, Cohn DL. Results of screening for tuberculosis in foreign-born persons applying for adjustment of immigration status. *Chest* 1993;103:1670–1674.
95. Nazar-Stewart V, Nolan CM. Results of a directly observed intermittent isoniazid preventive therapy program in a shelter for homeless men. *Am Rev Respir Dis* 1992;146:57–60.
96. Pilote L, Tulsky JP, Zolopa AR, Hahn JA, Schecter GF, Moss AR. Tuberculosis prophylaxis in the homeless. A trial to improve adherence to referral. *Arch Intern Med* 1996;156:161–165.
97. Nolan CM, Roll L, Goldberg SV, Elarth AM. Directly observed isoniazid preventive therapy for released jail inmates. *Am J Respir Crit Care Med* 1997;155: 583–586.
98. Moulding T. Chemoprophylaxis of tuberculosis: when is the benefit worth the risk and cost? *Ann Intern Med* 1971;74:761–770.
99. Taylor WC, Aronson MD, Delbanco TL. Should young adults with a positive tuberculin test take isoniazid? *Ann Intern Med* 1981;94:808–813.
100. Comstock GW. Evaluating isoniazid preventive therapy: the need for more data (editorial). *Ann Intern Med* 1981;94:817–819.
101. Rose DN, Schecter CB, Silver AL. The age threshold for isoniazid chemoprophylaxis. A decision analysis for low-risk tuberculin reactors. *JAMA* 1986;256: 2709–2713.
102. Rose DN, Schechter CB, Fahs MC, Silver AL. Tuberculosis prevention: cost effectiveness analysis of isoniazid chemoprophylaxis. *Am J Prev Med* 1988;4: 102–109.
103. Tsevat J, Taylor WC, Wong JB, Pauker SG. Isoniazid for the tuberculin reactor: take it or leave it. *Am Rev Respir Dis* 1988;137:215–220.
104. Colice GL. Decision analysis. Public health policy and isoniazid chemoprophylaxis for young adult tuberculin skin reactors. *Arch Intern Med* 1990; 150:2517–2522.
105. Jordan TJ, Lewit EM, Reichman LB. Isoniazid preventive therapy for tuberculosis. Decision analysis considering ethnicity and gender. *Am Rev Respir Dis* 1991; 144:1357–1360.
106. Sterling TR, Brehm WT, Frieden TR. Isoniazid preventive therapy in areas of high isoniazid resistance. *Arch Intern Med* 1995;155:1622–1628.
107. Stead WW, To T, Harrison RW, Abraham JH 3rd. Benefit-risk considerations in preventive treatment for tuberculosis in elderly persons. *Ann Intern Med* 1987; 107:843–845.
108. Fitzgerald JM, Gafni A. A cost-effectiveness analysis of the routine use of isoniazid prophylaxis in patients with a positive Mantoux skin test. *Am Rev Respir Dis* 1990;142:828–853.
109. Snider D, Caras G, Kaplan J. Preventive therapy with isoniazid. Cost-effectiveness of different durations of therapy. *JAMA* 1986;255:1579–1583.
110. Sarasin FP, Perrier A, Rochat T. Isoniazid preventive therapy for pulmonary tuberculosis sequelae: which patients up to which age? *Tuberc Lung Dis* 1995;76: 394–400.
111. Nettleman MD, Geerdes H, Roy M-C. The cost-effectiveness of preventing tuberculosis in physicians using tuberculin skin testing or a hypothetical vaccine. *Arch Intern Med* 1997;157:1121–1127.
112. Snider DE Jr. Decision analysis for isoniazid preventive therapy: take it or leave it? *Am Rev Respir Dis* 1988;137:2–4.
113. Moulding T, Iseman MD, Sbarbaro J. Preventing isoniazid heptotoxicity (letter to editor). *Ann Intern Med* 1976;85:398.
114. American College of Chest Physicians. American College of Chest Physicians Consensus Conference on Tuberculosis. *Chest* 1985;87:1152–1158.
115. Lecoeur HF, Truffot-Pernot C, Grosset JH. Experimental short-course preventive therapy of tuberculosis with rifampin and pyrazinamide. *Am Rev Respir Dis* 1989;140:1189–1193.
116. Ji B, Truffot-Pernot C, Lacroix C. Effectiveness of rifampin, rifabutin, and rifapentine for preventive therapy of tuberculosis in mice. *Am Rev Respir Dis* 1993; 148:1541–1546.
117. Chapuis L, Ji B, Truffot-Pernot C, O'Brien RJ, Raviglione MC, Grosset JH. Preventive therapy of tuberculosis with rifapentine in immunocompetent and nude mice. *Am J Respir Crit Care Med* 1994;150:1355–1362.
118. Dhillon J, Dickinson JM, Sole K, Mitchison DA. Preventive chemotherapy of tuberculosis in Cornell model mice with combinations of rifampin, isoniazid, and pyrazinamide. *Antimicrob Agents Chemother* 1996;40: 552–555.
119. Dickinson JM, Mitchison DA. Experimental models to explain the high sterilizing activity of rifampin in the chemotherapy of tuberculosis. *Am Rev Respir Dis* 1981;123:367–371.
120. Gangadharam PR, Pratt PF, Perumal VK, Iseman MD. The effects of exposure time, drug concentration, and temperature on the activity of ethambutol versus *Mycobacterium tuberculosis*. *Am Rev Respir Dis* 1990; 141:1478–1482.
121. Villarino ME, Ridzon R, Weismuller PC. Rifampin preventive therapy for tuberculosis infection. Experience with 157 adolescents. *Am J Respir Crit Care Med* 1997;155:1735–1738.
122. Polesky A, Farber HW, Gottlieb DJ, et al. Rifampin preventive therapy for tuberculosis in Boston's home-

less. *Am J Respir Crit Care Med* 1996;154: 1473–1477.
123. Iseman MD. Less is more: short-course preventive therapy of tuberculosis (editorial). *Am Rev Respir Dis* 1989;140:1187.
124. Halsey NA, Coberly JS, Desormeaux J, et al. Randomised trial of isoniazid versus rifampicin and pyrazinamide for prevention of tuberculosis in HIV-1 patients. *Lancet* 1998;351:786–792.
125. Gordin F, Chaisson R, Matts J, et al. *A randomized trial of 2 months of rifampin (RIF) and pyrazinamide (PZA) versus 12 months of isoniazid (INH) for the prevention of tuberculosis (TB) in HIV-positive (+), PPD+ patients.* Paper presented at the Fifth Conference on Retroviruses, Chicago, IL, 1998.
126. Mitchison DA. Pyrazinamide in the chemoprophylaxis of tuberculosis (letter). *Am Rev Respir Dis* 1990; 142:1467.

13

Vaccination to Prevent Tuberculosis and Immunomodulatory Therapy for Persons with Active Disease

Stimulate the phagocytes. Drugs are a delusion.
"The Doctor's Dilemma," Act I

G. B. Shaw, 1902

These words were uttered by Dr. Bloomfield Bonnington, a bombastic physician in Shaw's play, which dealt with a young artist who was dying of consumption. Shaw, through Bonnington, vented his spleen about contemporary efforts to cure tuberculosis with drugs or chemicals ("a huge commercial system of quackery and poison") and endorsed efforts to enhance the body's intrinsic immunologic defenses ("Nature's remedy"). How did the Irish playwright come to this persuasion? Shaw was a personal friend of Thomas Almroth-Wright, a physician who was subsequently to win a Nobel Prize for his pioneering work in immunology and to be knighted for his labors. Evidently, Sir Thomas shared his views with Shaw during what must have been some highly entertaining fireside conversations.

Although modern drug therapy has come great distances from the turn-of-the-century remedies that left many sicker and all poorer than before treatment, tuberculosis control still begs for an effective vaccine to complement the other tools of prevention. Indeed, as one anticipates the future of tuberculosis augmented by the effects of HIV infection in the early twenty-first century, the need for an effective vaccine will be virtually as compelling as it was in 1902. Although modern chemotherapy is highly effective, the limited resources of the poorer nations, where much of the tuberculosis is found, preclude consistent early diagnosis of disease and make it improbable that even very short-course therapy (3 to 6 months) for treatment or prevention can be delivered predictably.

Hence, new energy has been directed at clarifying the effectiveness and limitations of current preventive vaccines, virtually all of which have been derived from Calmette and Guérin's modification of *M. bovis* (BCG). In addition, recent interest has developed in developing novel vaccines and in using defense-modifying biological products or vaccines to treat persons with active disease to reduce morbidity, mortality, and the duration of chemotherapy required to effect enduring cures.

A HISTORY OF BCG, THE BACILLUS OF CALMETTE AND GUERIN

Based on the prior favorable experience with such vaccines as Jenner's cowpox to prevent smallpox and Kitasako's diphtheria agent, efforts to develop an immunization product for tuberculosis commenced shortly after Koch's description of the bacillus in 1882. Indeed, Koch himself announced at the World Congress of Medicine in 1890 that he had created a substance that both cured and prevented the dreaded disease (1). Koch's lymph, as it was first known, was a glycerin-extracted filtrate of cultures of the tubercle bacillus. Subsequently, it became known as "old tuberculin," a predecessor of today's various protein-based agents used in diagnostic skin testing. Koch's original veiled hints of success were soon confounded by profoundly morbid, even lethal, complications from local and remote hypersensitivity reactions when the agent was administered. This reaction became known as "the Koch phenomenon." Shaw referred to this in "The Doctor's Dilemma" when a group of physicians were discussing a young woman who had been "treated with Koch's tuberculin. . . . instead of curing her, it rotted her arm right off. Yes, I remember. Poor Jane! However, she makes a good living out of that arm now by showing it at medical lectures" (Act I).

Calmette, a physician, and Guérin, a veterinarian, chose instead the organism associated with tuberculosis in cattle, *M. bovis* (2). To lessen bacillary clumping in their culture medium, they added ox bile; serendipitiously they found that the bile also reduced the virulence of the *M. bovis* strain, making it a more attractive vaccine candidate. After 231 serial passages, these attenuated organisms were shown to offer significant protection in animal models and were introduced as a human vaccine in the early 1920s (3). Enthusiasm for its use was dampened by an unfortunate accident in which a laboratory technician comingled a virulent strain of *M. tuberculosis* with BCG. Tragically, 207 of the 251 German infants who received the vaccine developed active tuberculosis, 72 dying within one year in "the Lubeck Disaster" (4).

Two reports from the 1930 to 1946 era strongly suggested the utility of BCG in protecting young persons against tuberculosis. Heimbeck in Norway noted that tuberculin-negative nursing students were at much higher risk of developing active TB during the early years of their professional experience than were their colleagues who were already reactors at the onset of their training. Thus, he began offering BCG to nonreactive nurse trainees. There was no pattern of allocation other than acceptance or refusal of the vaccine by these individuals. Nonetheless, the differences observed over two decades and with nearly 1,500 student nurses were quite impressive: case rates for tuberculin-negative, not-vaccinated nurses were 141 per 1,000 person-years contrasted to 24 for the tuberculin-negative individuals who were vaccinated; the case rate for the group of nurses who were already tuberculin reactors (and did not get BCG) was 12 (5).

Similarly, among a group of 305 Danish children who were exposed to a tuberculous teacher during World War II, widely disparate rates of active TB were seen depending on tuberculin and BCG status: 14 of 94 (15%) tuberculin-negative not-vaccinated children developed disease in comparison to 2 of 106 (2%) tuberculin-negative children who had been vaccinated before their exposure (6). Curiously, the tuberculin-positive children who had not been given BCG developed active TB at a very high rate, 9 of 105 (9%).

Based on the recognition that tuberculosis case rates had soared during and following prior wars, BCG vaccination was widely applied following World War II (7). Authorities estimate that it is the most extensively used immunization in the world, with several billion doses having been given.

It should be noted that Koch and others have attempted to use vaccines not only to prevent infection but also to treat persons with active disease. It appears superficially implausible that vaccination given to an individual experiencing active disease could be beneficial. However, as indicated below, there is a theoretical basis for attempting to redirect the host's immune responses, which, as a function of the pathogenic properties of the microbe, may have been diverted into pathways that serve the parasite better than the host. Recently, efforts have been directed also to the use of various biological compounds involved with cell–cell interaction in the effort also to favorably affect the immune response.

MECHANISMS OF BCG ACTIVITY

In the simplest manner, BCG vaccination represents an analogue to Jenner's use of inoculation with the benign cowpox virus to protect against the more virulent infections with the related organism smallpox. BCG is a living vaccine prepared from *M. bovis* (BCG), an organism that is so closely related to *M. tuberculosis* that it is deemed taxonomically a subspecies within the "tuberculosis complex" (see Chapter 2 for details). It typically is administered by subcutaneous or intradermal inoculation, usually in the left deltoid region; peroral or aerosol use is extremely uncommon. The bacilli cause a localized infection, occasionally associated with regional lymphadenitis. Because of the slow growth rates of these bacilli, this process typically takes 6 to 8 weeks. Delayed-type hypersensitivity (DTH) to tuberculoprotein commonly evolves during this period, with most but not all recipients developing a reactive tuberculin skin test. Curiously, the protective effects of a vaccine are not consistently associated with its potency in inducing DTH (8).

Smith, based on extensive experience with animal models for BCG, believes that such vaccination serves primarily to help limit the bacillemia associated with the primary pulmonary infection (9). Such hematogenous spread is believed to be a central component of the pathogenesis of human tuberculosis (see Chapter 4). In animals studied by Smith, even those in which BCG had induced significant capacity for intracellular inhibition of bacillary growth, there was no ability to prevent pulmonary implantation or early intrapulmonary replication. After 14 days, however, the number of bacilli recovered from the lungs of BCG-vaccinated mice was significantly less than that in the nonvaccinated animals.

Corresponding to these animal studies, autopsy reports from persons having been vaccinated in an early Finnish BCG program indicated that there was evidence of primary-type tuberculous lesions in the expected frequency; however, there was little evidence of postprimary disease elsewhere (10).

In spite of an inability to prevent local lung implantation, BCG should theoretically be able to reduce both pulmonary and extrapulmonary tuberculosis because classical apical pulmonary disease is thought to be produced by bacillemic seeding of the upper lung zones, not airborne implantation of these regions (see Chapter 4).

Extrapulmonary tuberculosis is believed to reflect implantation of these organs by bacillemic seeding from intrathoracic sites. In most instances, such seeding is thought to occur during the primary infection; hence, BCG or other vaccines that confer preexisting immunity could and very likely do reduce the frequency of extrapulmonary disease. This has been demonstrated most readily in infants and young children, in whom extrapulmonary disease constitutes a large component of their tuberculous morbidity.

ANALYSES AND LARGE BCG TRIALS

Among the first controlled vaccination studies was a trial begun in 1935, using a strain of BCG (Phipps) among Native Americans in Arizona, North and South Dakota, and Alaska (10); a 75% protective effect against disease was seen. Subsequently, many studies of various descriptions have been conducted, involving numerous variables including vaccine strains, routes of administration, dosage, age at vaccination, race and ethnicity of vaccinees, geographical location of study populations, as well as other factors discussed below. Effects of BCG vaccination ranged up to 80% protection and down to negative 56% effect, i.e. more tuberculosis seen among those receiving the vaccine than among the controls (Fig. 13.1). Numerous scholars have reviewed the phenomenon of the extraordinary variability of BCG protection, none offering a universally accepted explanation. These analyses are delineated below.

Clemens, Chuong, and Feinstein (1983)

The authors reviewed in detail eight large-scale community trials of BCG (11). They paid particular attention to the methodological aspects of the studies, focusing on four possible sources of outcome distortion:

1. Susceptibility bias: Were the subjects, when allocated to BCG or control, comparable in terms of their risks for tuberculosis?

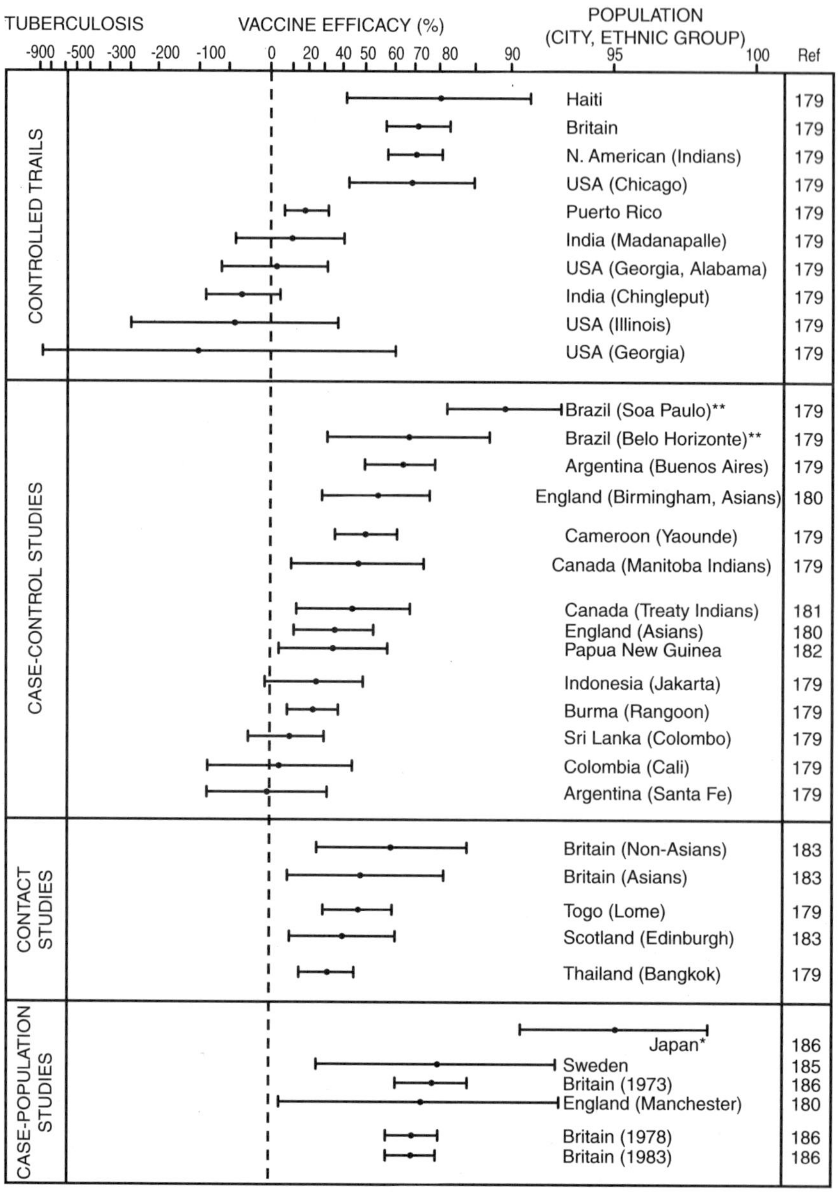

FIG. 13.1. Range of efficacy of various BCG trials. These trials were described in a 1990 review by Rodrigues and Smith (178). They were broken down according to trial format. Three of the studies *(asterisks)* (179,184) describe protection against meningitis only. The sources of the data are contained in these eight articles (179–186). This analysis did not include the recent disappointing results from Malawi (26,27). Fine later analyzed these and other BCG trials with regard to their geographical relationship to the equator and the mixture of urban and rural populations (22) (see Fig. 14.2). Modified from Rodrigues and Smith (178).

2. Surveillance bias: Was the ongoing observation of the study participants controlled to provide comparable attention (symptom monitoring, laboratory testing) to each group?
3. Diagnostic testing bias: If sputa, chest x-rays, or other tests were ordered, were they performed with similar frequency in both groups?
4. Diagnostic interpretation bias: Were the results of symptom monitoring and test interpretation comparable between the two groups?

Among the eight trials so analyzed, these authors noted that adequate assurance of unbiased detection of tuberculosis was demonstrated only in the three trials that reported high levels of protection.

Furthermore, the authors observed that among the trials demonstrating negative or low levels of BCG efficacy, there were wide confidence intervals that could not exclude significant protective effect. By contrast, however, the studies demonstrating high levels of protection had narrow confidence intervals that excluded low efficacy.

Although their analysis may be correct in ascribing methodological variables as the cause for the poor performance of BCG in these selected studies, it is quite important to note that there were geographical variables as well. The three trials in which BCG performed best were conducted either in relatively northern Chicago (12), England (13), or arid climes (Native Americans) (14). By contrast, the studies showing low levels of efficacy were done in more southern, humid climates where "atypical mycobacteria" or other variables may compromise the vaccine's performance—Georgia (15), Puerto Rico (16), Georgia–Alabama (17), or South India (18,19). (See below for further development of this hypothesis.)

Comstock (1994)

Similar to the above analysis, Comstock, arguably the most experienced and astute contemporary student of tuberculosis in the United States, recently published his review of 19 controlled trials of vaccination (8). This article provides a rich lode of information regarding these studies done between 1927 and 1968 including the BCG strains employed, routes of administration, characteristics of the study populations, and protective efficacy. Salient aspects of this analysis include careful scrutiny of the implications of vaccinating persons who are already infected with *M. tuberculosis* and who presumably would not profit from BCG. As Comstock demonstrates, if there were a high prevalence of latent tuberculosis infection among the vaccinees, the endogenous reactivation of these cases would substantially reduce the apparent effect of that vaccine. He points out that many trials did not perform prevaccination tuberculin testing, and thus, this effect cannot be calculated. However, among trials in which such data were available, he contrasts the British Medical Research Council trial (13) with the Chingleput WHO Study (19). In the former, there were relatively few initial tuberculin reactors to provide a pool for subsequent tuberculosis, the vaccine proved highly efficacious among the nonreactive/uninfected, and the overall effect of BCG on tuberculosis case rates was substantial. By contrast, in the Chingleput Study, there were substantial numbers of initial tuberculin reactors who were responsible for the great preponderance of cases, the vaccine appeared to have no measurable protective effect, and the net result of massive BCG programs involving over 200,000 vaccinations was nil.

An additional unique element of Comstock's report is his graphic demonstration of the lack of predictable association between post-BCG tuberculin reactivity and protection, as seen in Fig. 13.2. Although there was a general trend toward concordance, some vaccines that resulted in high rates of postvaccination reactivity were ineffective; and, conversely, some vaccine trials resulted in very low rates of tuberculin reactivity but high levels of protection. This is a demonstration, I believe, of a human equivalent to animal models in which DTH can be dissociated from CMI (see Chapter 4).

Springett and Sutherland (1994)

In examining the results of the Chingleput BCG Trial, these authors were struck by the unavoidable conclusion that, not only did the vac-

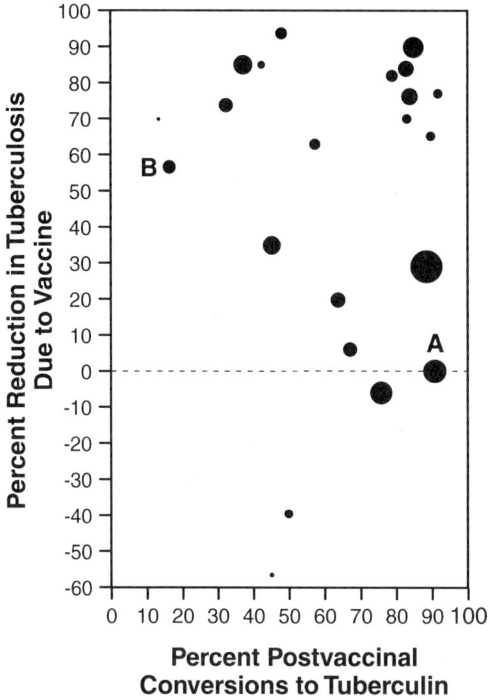

FIG. 13.2. Postvaccinal conversion rates and corresponding reduction in tuberculosis attributable to vaccination in 10 controlled trials. Comstock analyzed a number of BCG trials to assess the relationship between vaccine-conferred tuberculin reactivity and demonstrated protection against tuberculosis. The areas of the *circles* are proportional to the square roots of the combined numbers of vaccinated and control subjects. As may be seen, there was no ready correlation between these variables. Indeed, in some studies, nearly all vaccinated subjects became tuberculin-reactive, yet no protection was seen *(circle A),* whereas in other studies, fewer than 20% of vaccinees became tuberculin-positive, yet nearly 60% protection was seen *(circle B).* (Please see original article to identify these studies.).

cines not provide protection, but there was more tuberculosis in all age groups of vaccinees during the first 5 years postvaccination, overall a 32% excess ($p < .01$). Their retrospective analysis was directed at providing possible explanations for what they deemed to be a true paradoxical effect of the vaccination, not merely an "extreme chance" result as was posited in the original trial report.

The vaccines employed in the Chingleput study were considered the best strains available on the basis of proven records of efficacy: Institute Pasteur (Paris) and Tokyo (derived from the Copenhagen vaccine, which descended from the original Paris strain). Candidates for the study in India were screened by pretesting with both PPD-S, 3 or 5 TU, and PPD-B. The assessment of vaccine efficacy was based solely, however, on protection of these with initial reactions of 0 to 7 mm induration to PPD-S.

The essential hypothesis of Springett and Sutherland was that vaccines employed were effective, "75% protective," in suitable candidates, but the Chingleput paradoxical negative protection resulted from a combination of two adverse factors: (a) inclusion of a group of patients, presumably in the control arm, that already had some cross-protection as a result of infection with environmental mycobacteria such as *Mycobacterium avium* complex, and (b) inclusion in the vaccination arm of a group of patients for whom BCG would result in more detectable cases of tuberculosis. In this model, factor (a) would result in fewer cases of tuberculosis among the control subjects, thus obscuring the potential benefit of BCG in the vaccines, while factor (b) would raise the number of tuberculosis cases in the vaccinees, thus further disguising any beneficial effects of the vaccine.

Factor (a) has been long considered a possible confounder of BCG trials and is reviewed at length by Fine (see below). Animal studies as well as other data substantially validate the potential for mycobacteria other than tuberculosis to vitiate BCG's protective effects. However, as the authors point out, this phenomenon cannot readily explain surplus cases among vacinees.

Factor (b) is rather less intuitively grasped. Springett and Sutherland argue that, by including persons with low-level tuberculin reactivity in the BCG arm, complicated immunological events ensue that result in more patients manifesting active tuberculosis. They suggest that the vaccination results in heightened delayed-type hypersensitivity. Rather than true protection, this amplified DTH results in enhanced inflammation with increased symptoms and/or radiographic abnormalities. They offer as a model for this process the concept of "focal reactions," a phenomenon that dates back to the era of Koch.

In this construct, inflammation (such as that provoked by BCG) initiated at one site in the body results in a generalized increase in inflammation including flares of tuberculosis localized in other organs. This was believed to occur in patients whom Koch treated with his tuberculin who experienced acute deterioration, "Koch's phenomenon."

In support of their thesis, the authors offer the following data. (a) Children aged 1 to 14 whose initial response to PPD-S ranged from 0 to 7 mm boosted to an average reaction of 16.7 mm 2 1/2 months after getting a 0.1-mg dose of BCG. (b) Other BCG trials, even those in which good protective efficacy was ultimately shown, commonly show an early paradoxical increase in tuberculosis among vaccinees to be followed by demonstrated protection (as was ultimately the case in Chingleput: after a (−)32% effect at 7.5 years, a net (+)2% effect was ultimately recorded at 15 years). (c) BCG trials that screened enrollees with high doses of tuberculin tend to result in higher vaccine efficacy, whereas those such as Chingleput that screened with lower doses of tuberculin tend to show lower levels of protection. They reason that the higher-dose tuberculin screening was more likely to identify persons with prior infection with *M. tuberculosis* or mycobacteria other than tuberculosis.

They conclude by indicating that, if their analysis is fundamentally sound, the application of BCG most likely to be efficacious would be to vaccinate, "early in life, before infection with any form of mycobacterium is likely to have occurred."

Colditz et al. (1994)

Because of the confusion surrounding the efficacy of the vaccine(s), the U.S. Centers for Disease Control recently commissioned the Harvard School of Public Health to perform a meta-analysis of the published BCG experience. A concise review of these findings was published in 1994 (20). This was a highly sophisticated study that commenced with 1,264 references relating to BCG. Based on descriptions of methodology, 26 reports were eventually deemed to be of sufficient quality to include in the final assessment. The group divided these reports into two types, trials and case-controlled studies. The trials, which were prospective in orientation, variously employed random, alternate, or systematic allocation. Case-control studies, which are retrospective means of assessing the utility of the intervention, compared BCG vaccination rates among cases of tuberculosis with rates among "controls" without tuberculosis, inferring levels of protection.

Among the trials analyzed in the Harvard report, the overall protective effect of BCG in preventing tuberculosis disease or morbidity was 51%, and, in the seven trials that reported death rates, BCG had a 71% protective effect versus death.

The case-control studies indicated similar levels of benefit, 55% overall protection against tuberculosis, including pulmonary disease. Protection in these case-control studies against meningitis among newborns receiving BCG was 64%, and, versus disseminated disease, it was 78%.

In this meta-analysis, considerable attention was given to understanding or reconciling the apparent, gross disparities in the utility of BCG. Two variables were significantly associated with the reported differences, explaining 66% of the heterogeneity in a random-effects regression model: (a) the efficacy of the vaccination increased with increasing distance from the equator, and (b) the better the study methodology ("data validity scoring"), the more likely the trial was to show protection.

Although the authors examined reports of BCG vaccination given to health care workers, none of these met methodological criteria for inclusion in the meta-analysis. The potential utility of BCG for physicians is discussed below.

In their original article, the authors state that mean age at vaccination did not change the results of their random-effects regression model. However, in an extended report of their study, they showed that there was, in the aggregate, lower efficacy when BCG was given at a later age: estimated protective effect if vaccinated at birth was 85%; at 10 years, 73%; and at 20 years, 50% (20). Although this phenomenon did not explain interstudy variability, it is still of clinical interest.

Regarding individual strains of BCG, the authors traced the pedigrees of five of the major contemporary vaccines. They observed that within each of four arms of this pedigree there were studies that demonstrated significant protection and others that showed no benefit. Because of these considerations, the authors did not use strains as a covariant in the meta-analysis (21).

In consideration of the applicability of the results of this meta-analysis, Fine suggests that, "it is invalid to combine existing data into a single overall estimate. Not only does the enormous heterogeneity ($p < .00001$) make an average inappropriate, but the available efficacy data do not represent the geographic pattern of actual BCG use" (22). See the following section for a more thorough discussion.

Fine (1995)

Fine argued in this analysis that exposure to environmental mycobacteria with resultant cross-immunity is the major factor responsible for variation in vaccine efficacy (22,23). He notes that Palmer and Long in the U.S. Tuberculosis Research Program first proposed that explanation in 1966 (24). Updating information first compiled by these investigators, Fine provides graphic evidence of the relationship between BCG efficacy in relationship to latitude or distance from the equator. According to his calculation, the trend is highly significant ($p <$ .00001). Similarly, Colditz and colleagues involved with the Harvard meta-analysis estimated that latitude could explain 41% of the variance among the studies they analyzed (25).

In addition to latitude, Fine examines another component of geography that might influence exposure to environmental mycobacteria, namely, urban or rural environments. He observes that the efficacy of BCG in the USPHS Puerto Rico Trial was lower in the rural vaccinees, 18%, than urban, 42% (16). Moreover, as also indicated in Fig. 13.3, most of the trials showing poor efficacy were done among rural populations in tropical or subtropical countries. The implication of these observations is that persons living in rural environments are more likely to be exposed to/infected with environmental mycobacteria (Fig. 13.4).

In further support of his thesis, Fine cites both animal studies and human observations indicating the capacity for mycobacteria other than tuberculosis to confer protection against *M. tuberculosis.* Of particular relevance are the data he offers in support of protection in humans: (a) cohort natural history studies that show that persons with low-level or "indeterminate" tuberculin reactivity are at lower risk of developing tuberculosis than those with negative (or strongly positive) tuberculin skin tests. He infers that this reflects prior immunological experience with environmental mycobacteria, citing the highest levels of protection against tuberculosis found in U.S. Navy recruits with indeterminate reactions to PPD-S and larger reactions to PPD-B, the antigen of *M. avium* complex (MAC); (b) like Springett and Sutherland, Fine notes that BCG trials that excluded persons with reactivity to high doses of tuberculin were more likely to demonstrate protective efficacy; (c) he reasons that declining protection seen over extended periods of postvaccine observation up to 20 years may be explained by accumulated protection by infection with environmental mycobacteria, (d) studies of peripheral blood monocytes (PBM) from unvaccinated teenagers from South India were more competent at inhibiting intracellular proliferation of *M. microti* than were the PBMs from unvaccinated teens in England; from this he infers that more exposure to the environmental mycobacteria in India provided heterologous immunity; and (e) demonstration of protection from BCG against other mycobacterial infections including MAC, *M. ulcerans,* and *M. leprae.*

Like Springett and Sutherland, Fine develops a quantitative model to calculate the capacity for cross-immunity from environmental mycobacteria to nullify BCG protection. Fine estimates but does not prove that such heterologous immunity may, in fact, be fully equal to that afforded by BCG vaccine.

Implications of the Malawi (Karonga) Trial

The most recent large-scale study of BCG was conducted too recently to be included in the anal-

STUDY	Lat	U/R	Type	OR and 99% CI	VE
NORWAY, gen popn[42]	65	U+R	COH		81%
SWEDEN, gen popn[43]	62	U+R	COH		80%
SWEDEN, military[44]	62	U+R	COH		55%
DENMARK, school[45]	56	U	O/B		94%
IRELAND, school[46]	55	R	O/B		82%
CANADA Indians[47*]	55	R	T		81%
CANADA ALBERTA, Indians[48*]	55	R	C.C		57%
CANADA MANITOBA, Indians[49*]	55	R	C.C		70%
UK, schoolchildren[50*]	53	U+R	T		77%
UK, gen popn 1973[51]	53	U+R	COH		79%
UK, gen popn 1978[52]	53	U+R	COH		74%
UK, gen popn 1983[7]	53	U+R	COH		75%
UK, Asians[53*]	53	U	C.C		49%
UK, BIRMINGHAM Asians[54*]	52	U	C.C		64%
UK, BIRMINGHAM[55]	52	U	COH		88%
USA, indians[25*]	52	R	T		79%
USA, CHICAGO infants[56*]	42	U	T		72%
USA, NEW YORK infants[57]	41	U	T		7% →
KOREA, SEOUL[58]	38	U	H/H		74%
ARGENTINA, BUENOS AIRES[59*]	35	U	C.C		73%
USA, GEORGIA school[26*]	33	U+R	T		-56% →
USA, GEORGIA ALABAMA, gen popn[60*]	33	U+R	T		16%
ISRAEL, children[61]	31	U+R	COH		38%
SOUTH AFRICA, miners[62*]	27	U+R	T		62%
AUSTRALIA, QUEENSLAND[63*]	20	U+R	C.C		41%
PUERTO RICO[15*]	18	R+U	T		29%
HAITI[64*]	18	R+U	T		80%
BURMA, RANGOON[65*]	17	U	C.C		38%
THAILAND, BANGKOK[66]	14	U	C.C		74%
THAILAND, BANGKOK[67]	14	U	C.C		83%
THAILAND, BANGKOK[68]	14	U	H/H		47%
INDIA, MADANAPALLE[27*]	13	R	T		20%
INDIA, CHINGLEPUT[10*]	13	R	T		-19%
PAPUA NEW GUINEA[69]	10	U+R	C.C		41%
MALAWI, KARONGA[8]	10	R	COH		-11%
INDONESIA, JAKARTA[70*]	6	U	C.C		37%
TOGO, LOME[71]	6	U	H/H		66%
COLUMBIA, CALI[72*]	4	U	C.C		16%
CAMEROON, YAOUNDE[73]	4	U	C.C		66%
KENYA, KISUMU[17]	0	R	C.C		22%

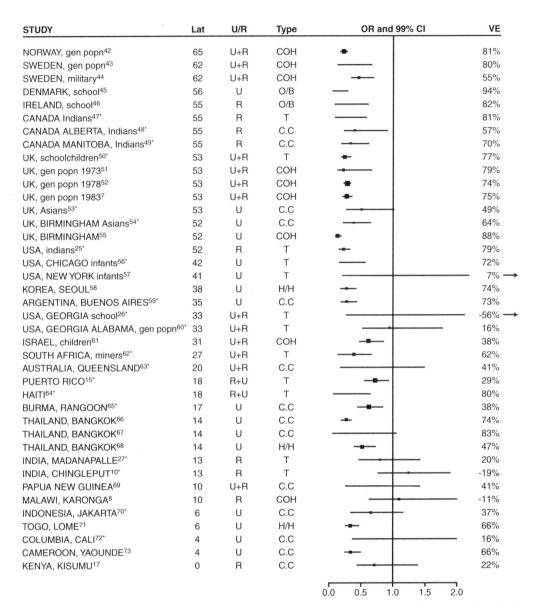

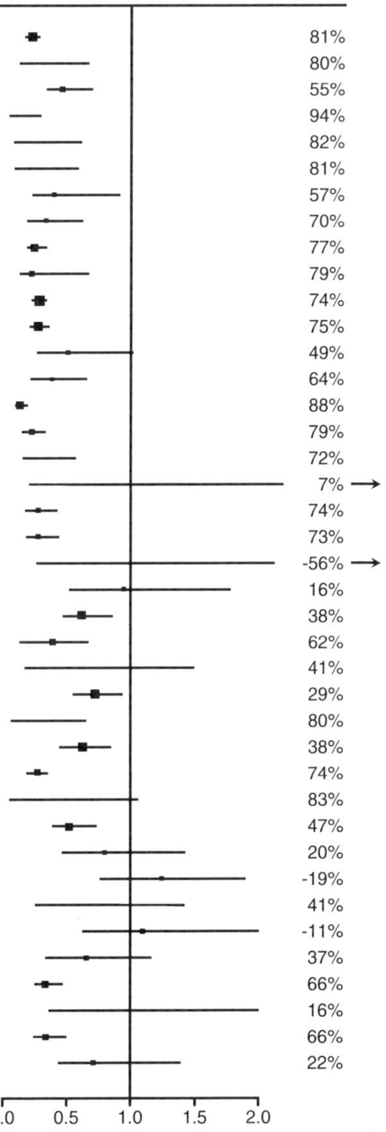

FIG. 13.3. Efficacy of BCG in relation to distance from equator and mixture of urban and rural subjects. Fine's recent reanalysis of the influence of latitude on the varying efficacy of BCG showed a clear, statistically significant trend for diminishing efficacy among equatorial populations (179). There also appeared to be a tendency toward less protection in rural areas, where presumably there would be greater exposure to the environmental mycobacteria. The total series analyzed by Fine showed a highly significant trend in relation to latitude, ($p < .00001$). Lat, latitude in degrees north or south from equator; U/R, urban or rural; type, study type (T, trial; COH, cohort; C-C, case control; O/B, outbreak; H/H, household contact study); OR, odds ratio; VE, vaccine efficacy (1 − OR). Reproduced with permission from Fine (22). Study references in this table are from Fine's bibliography.

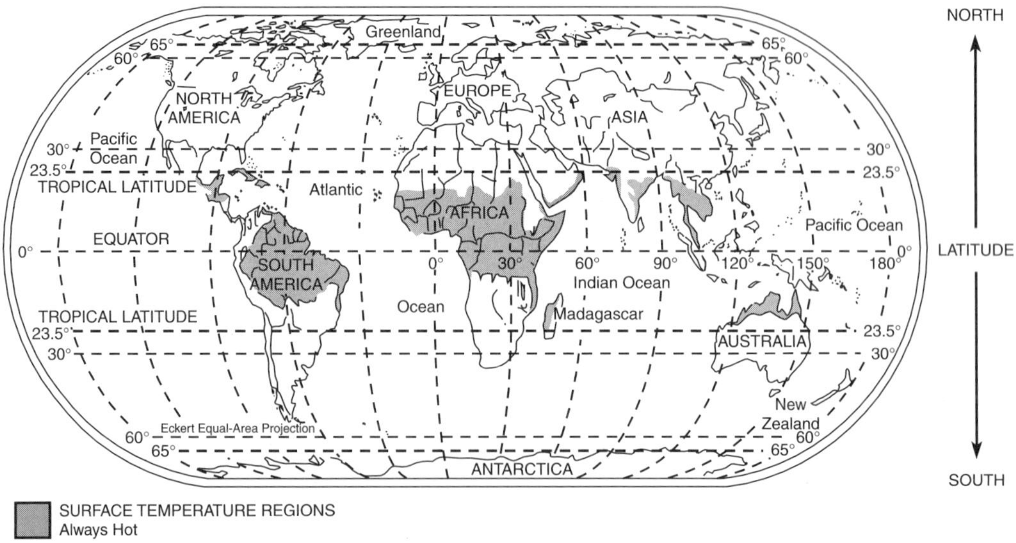

FIG. 13.4. In the tropical and subtropical regions, the year-round warmth promotes lush vegetation and, presumably, a wide prevalence of environmental nontuberculous mycobacteria. This observation is consistent with the hypothesis of Fine and others that community exposure to these microbes nullifies any demonstrable protection by BCG.

yses above. A mass program of vaccination using the Glaxo strain of BCG was introduced in 1974 into the Karonga District of Malawi, a small nation in south central Africa lying to the west of Lake Malawi (26). Nearly 84,000 individuals were followed between 1979 and 1989 in the first Malawi trial with the following results. In the aggregate, there was a −11% efficacy versus tuberculosis; among persons born after 1954, this was −9%; among those born after 1974, −65%. By contrast, the vaccine was highly effective against leprosy, an overall protective effect of +49%. Notably, the incidence rates for tuberculosis were substantially higher in vaccine recipients in the 45-55 years age range.

A second component of this BCG program was reported in 1996, a follow-up program of vaccination between 1986 and 1989 for persons in the Kawonga District (27). In this study, those without a BCG scar were randomly allocated to vaccination with BCG or BCG plus killed *M. leprae,* whereas those with a scar were given placebo, BCG, or BCG with *M. leprae.* Again, the results were disappointing with regard to tuberculosis. There were significantly higher rates of pulmonary tuberculosis among scar-positive persons who had received a second dose of BCG with or without killed *M. leprae.* Curiously, there were reduced numbers of lymph node tuberculosis among recipients of BCG. As before, the vaccinations did afford significant protection versus leprosy, +50% over a first BCG vaccination.

As noted in this report, and amplified by Rieder in an accompanying editorial (28), the surplus of pulmonary cases among vaccine recipients was largely found, 14 of 15, among HIV-positive persons. Although inconclusive, the data raised the possibility that BCG had perhaps had a paradoxical effect in this group, conceivably through the mechanism of chronic BCG-related infection inducing HIV replication.

There are subtle issues to be resolved in this interpretation of these data, but it is impossible not to conclude that BCG in this population did not protect against tuberculosis.

Overview

Examining the confusing array of findings and opinions enumerated above, one must struggle to derive a quantitative sense of the potential benefits from BCG and to identify the most appropriate applications of such vaccination programs.

The Harvard meta-analysis suggests an overall 50% level of protection from BCG in the generic. However, as noted by Fine, examining aggregate data for a modality that ranges from 80% protective to a negative 11% effect may not be a suitable way to consider such an agent (22). Others have recently shown that meta-analyses are not infallible; comparing the predictions of meta-analyses with the largest trial results, the authors found a 40% probability of disparity between the trial results and the predictions of the aggregate analysis (29).

As a component of a national control program, BCG appears to remain a desirable element for nations in which there are high rates of tuberculosis among young adults and their children. Virtually all of the case-controlled pediatric studies indicate highly significant reductions in tuberculous morbidity including miliary and meningeal disease among young vaccinees. These observations are consonant with the above-described models in which it is believed that prior infection with *M. tuberculosis* may result in more clinical tuberculosis following BCG vaccination or that prior infection with environmental mycobacteria confers comparable protection to BCG, thereby making such intervention superfluous. If the vaccine is given before such corrupting events occur, it may well reduce potentially lethal tuberculosis in children. Colditz and colleagues' meta-analysis demonstrated aggregate protective effects of 0.74 among randomized, controlled trials and 0.52 in case-control studies of BCG in infants and newborns (30). However, in countries with low prevalences of tuberculosis, discontinuation of BCG programs has not had a discernible effect on pediatric tuberculosis case rates (31–34). Thus, in 1994, the IUATLD issued a statement regarding discontinuation of BCG in low-prevalence countries (35); basic criteria included (a) annual rates of sputum smear-positive pulmonary disease $\leq$5/100,000/year for 3 years, or (b) annual rates of tuberculous meningitis in children under 5 years age $<$1 per 10 million population for 5 years, or (c) the annual risk of infection is $\leq$0.1%.

BCG has failed sorely to reduce rates of pulmonary tuberculosis in adults. Therefore, it has had no significant effect on the overall patterns of transmission and morbidity, even in countries with extensive vaccination programs. Should national BCG programs continue? In light of the large numbers of cases of communicable pulmonary cases that are either belatedly found or not detected, infants and children in developing nations remain at high risk for infection with *M. tuberculosis*. As HIV makes it way through sexually active young adults (who, not coincidentally, are parents), this risk will escalate. And, given the unaffordability/unachievability of large-scale contact investigation/preventive chemotherapy for these pediatric contacts, BCG may be the only means of reducing tuberculous morbibity/mortality in these populations. Nonetheless, the ongoing havoc of tuberculosis may lead to reconsideration of the feasibility in preventive chemotherapy in the near future.

However, the use of BCG for adults either in the general population or in high-risk groups such as health care workers remains a dubious proposition in my eye. If, as the Chingleput or Malawi studies suggest, BCG has no measurable benefit in general populations, programs to vaccinate (or revaccinate) adults may be seen as merely ineffective, expensive diversions from the primary priorities of a national tuberculosis program. Early and efficient case finding and treatment to cure must remain the central objectives. As Ian Sutherland noted, one man's cure is many men's prevention (36).

Issue: Should BCG Be Used for HCWs?

Should BCG be used for health care workers (HCWs) exposed to tuberculosis? As a component of the Harvard meta-analysis project, the possible utility of BCG for HCWs was assessed from the available literature (37). The analysis indicated that none of the trials of BCG in nursing or medical students employed methodological designs adequate to allow meaningful conclusions. However, the authors concluded that the studies "suggest that vaccination with BCG is effective in reducing the incidence of tuberculosis among health care workers." Similar data have been used in "decision analyses" to support the use of BCG for American HCWs either exposed routinely (38,39) or to MDR TB cases (40).

Because of the inadequacies of the existing BCG studies in HCWs and the extraordinary number of potential variables in such contemporary decision analysis, I am highly concerned that greater mischief than benefit might derive from wholesale use of BCG. As detailed in Chapter 12, potentially deleterious aspects of BCG vaccination for HCWs include: (a) obscuring tuberculin skin test surveillance with the attendant option of predictably effective INH preventive therapy, (b) creating a false sense of security among HCWs and those administratively responsible for creating safe working environments, (c) local or systemic complication of BCG, and (d) paradoxical increases in tuberculosis case rates. Anyone contemplating BCG in these circumstances should consider the possibility of 0% benefit from the vaccine. Perhaps if an individual had absolutely no reactivity whatsoever to PPD-S or T and none to PPD-B (without other evidence of anergy), they might be a theoretically better candidate for BCG, but PPD-B is not available, and this is an unproved hypothesis. See below for a more extensive critique of this rationale.

Special concern also has been given as well to HCWs who are infected with the human immunodeficiency virus, particularly in light of the extensive morbidity and mortality experienced by HIV-infected HCWs exposed in the MDR TB outbreaks in the United States (see Chapters 5 and 11). However, giving BCG to persons already HIV-infected poses significant risks of infectious complications from the vaccine, including the possibility that a live-bacterial vaccine that sets up a long-standing chronic infection might quicken progress to CD4 depletion and AIDS and might possibly result in an excess of TB and other OIs among vaccine recipients. This is, I believe, an unmitigated bad idea.

The 1997 publication of the CDC's Advisory Committee on Immunization Practices and Hospital Infection Control Practices Advisory Committee recommended that BCG for HCWs should be considered on an individual basis in health-care settings where all of the following conditions are met: a high percentage of TB patients are infected with *M. tuberculosis* strains that are resistant to both isoniazid and rifampin; and, transmission of such drug-resistant *M. tuberculosis* strains to HCWs is likely; and, comprehensive TB infection-control precautions have been implemented and have not been successful (41). Like Santa Claus's workshop, such a location is frequently mentioned but never found. They also delineate a number of conditions and disclaimers to be reviewed with the HCW before BCG is given. They also recommend that BCG not be given to HIV-infected or otherwise immunocompromised HCWs. However, for HCWs in countries with fewer resources, the practice of BCG vaccination might be justified.

ADVERSE CONSEQUENCES OF THE USE OF BCG

As with all preventive modalities, BCG vaccination has potentially undesirable results. Although some of the trials discussed above indicated that BCG vaccinees appeared to be at slightly higher risk of tuberculosis, this does not appear with sufficient frequency or magnitude to constitute a generalized drawback. Rather, the more significant issues are those delineated below.

Loss of Utility of the Tuberculin Skin Test and Isoniazid Preventive Therapy

By confounding the tuberculin skin test (TST), BCG nullifies the only practical tool to indicate recent infection and, thus, candidacy for preventive chemotherapy. As described in Chapter 12, isoniazid preventive therapy offers 60% to 90% protection against tuberculosis. Unless there is exogenous reinfection, this protection probably is lifelong. New infection is traditionally identified by conversion from tuberculin nonreactivity to various levels of indurated response. However, among recipients of BCG, 15% to 90% initially become tuberculin reactive (8). Although the percentage of reactors ebbs with time following vaccination, 8% to 25% of young adults react to the TST following vaccination in infancy or after 5 years of age, respectively (42). Also, BCG recipients who do not react to an initial TST are found to be at substantial risk for "boosting" of reactivity to subsequent TSTs by the initial test; 10% of young adults with a history of childhood BCG converted their TSTs on repeat testing in a recent report from Canada (43). Similar findings were described in a series of young adults in Chile, in whom the likelihood of tuberculin reactivity on initial TST in adulthood was proportional to the number of BCG vaccinations in childhood (44). Comparable data were seen in a large series from Spain (45). Furthermore, among both groups, boosting with serial tuberculin testing was relatively common; this likelihood of boosting effectively precludes monitoring these individuals with sequential tuberculin skin testing were they to be employed in high-risk settings or otherwise exposed.

It has been argued that BCG vaccination is tactically superior to tuberculin skin testing and isoniazid preventive therapy (TST/IPT) for health care workers such as house staff trainees and medical students (38). In this logic, loss of TST validity from BCG use would not constitute a drawback. The authors of this decision analysis concluded that, if the BCG vaccine were only 13.1% effective in preventing tuberculosis, it would be of superior overall utility. Elements in their analysis that militated against the utility of TST/IPT included historical noncompliance with skin-testing programs, refusal to take or nonadherence to prescribed isoniazid, and the morbidity including loss of work time secondary to isoniazid-induced hepatitis.

Although the authors claimed to have taken into their analysis a variety of parameters for and against both BCG and TST/IPT, it should be pointed out that some of the data they employed were inaccurate, reflecting detrimentally on the potential efficiency of TST/IPT. I will not recapitulate their entire analysis here. For those with an in-depth interest in this issue, I suggest reading the analysis, keeping in mind these questionable assumptions or data: (a) Only "63%" of at-risk house staff or medical students will participate in the TST program. Certainly, in the past students and residents have been notorious for failure to comply with such mandated testing (46,47). However, this probably reflects more on the lack of commitment on the part of those conducting TST programs than anything else. With reasonable institutional resolve, such tests can be completed at close to 100%, which then compels higher performance from BCG to favor this tactic (see below). (b) Among those who "convert" their TST, only "45%" will commence IPT. Certainly, inertia and denial, amplified by fears of isoniazid hepatotoxicity, must be addressed. However, such a low performance largely speaks to a lack of enthusiasm on the part of those running the TST/IPT surveillance program and a failure to educate potential recipients of the risks and benefits involved (48). Again, if there were higher acceptance of IPT, BCG protection would have to be substantially better than 13.1% to be the preferred tactic (see below). (c) By using an index termed the "Quality Adjusted Life Years," the authors calculated that 2.68 cases of isoniazid-induced hepatitis were the morbidity equivalent of one case of tuberculosis. The derivation of this index is somewhat obscure and dubious, and it is my strong impression from 25 years of work in the field that this is a gross misrepresentation. Among well-informed persons taking isoniazid, medications are withheld promptly with the onset of hepatitis symptoms or significant perturbations of liver function tests, and there are no "28 days confined to home" or "6.8 days in the hospital and 21 days confined to home." Nearly all persons who are appropriately monitored experience little more than transient, mild distress, fleeting abnormalities of liver chemistries, and no residual or ongoing hepatic dysfunction. Deaths or liver failure requiring transplantation, although of potentially immense import, are exceedingly rare among individuals who are alert to early symptoms and signs of hepatitis and who have suitable surveillance of liver chemistries. Tuberculosis, on the other hand, even when successfully treated, leaves residual scarring and nonfunctional tissue in the lungs or other involved organs; thus, we should not equate "curing" a case of tuberculosis with a return to the normal, premorbid state. (d) The authors estimated the benefit of IPT given for one year to be "60%," with a range of 50% to 70% protective. This probably is a significant underestimation of the potential protection of IPT. In Eastern European studies conducted by the International Union Against Tuberculosis (IUAT), 12 months of IPT among compliant patients with fibrotic lesions on their chest x-rays yielded 93% protection; 6 months of IPT in such patients offered approximately 70% protection (see Chapter 12 for details) (49). The IUAT studies indicated that patients with smaller x-ray fibrotic abnormalities were at progressively lower risk of reactivation tuberculosis and that for such patients 6 months of therapy was equal in protection to 12. Hence, it is reasonable to infer that newly infected persons who have normal chest x-rays, the most common scenario, should enjoy protection in the range of 70% to 90%. Similarly, the authors of the analysis calculated the efficacy of partial treatment (persons who prematurely terminate or are erratically adherent to IPT) to be only "12% to 21%" protection. In the IUAT trials, patients with fibrotic lesions who were compliant with just 12 weeks of IPT had 30% protection at 5 years follow-up. (e) The protective efficacy of BCG ranges between "25%" and "80%." The authors did not consider the possibility of a paradoxical early effect as seen in the initial phase of the Chingleput trial (see above), a factor of which potential recipients of the vaccine should be aware.

Even within the parameters noted above, which underestimate the potential utility of IPT, the authors of the decision analysis concluded that, if all complied with tuberculin skin testing and every convertor commenced IPT, BCG efficacy would have to be 46% to be the preferred tactic. Furthermore, if all completed IPT, the vaccine would have to be 58% effective. And, as noted, the authors ignored both the possibility of a nil or negative impact of BCG on the vaccinees and the modest but not inconsequential morbidity associated with giving BCG (see below).

The most compelling case for BCG for health care workers lies with exposure to patients with multidrug-resistant tuberculosis (defined currently as resistance to isoniazid and rifampin with or without resistance to other drugs; see Chapter 11). Because these two drugs are by far the most active bactericidal agents, their presumable lack of utility for preventive therapy makes treatment of individuals newly infected with an MDR-TB strain highly problematic. Thus, one might very appropriately consider BCG for persons so exposed. Indeed, a well-reasoned recent decision analysis suggested BCG for health care workers exposed to MDR-TB patients (40). However, at the National Jewish Medical and Research Center, where we treat almost exclusively MDR TB, we have not chosen BCG but have relied instead on aggressive environmental controls featuring in-room ultraviolet germicidal irradiation to reduce the risk of transmission (see Chapter 14). Clearly, we have the advantage that virtually all of our tuberculosis patients are previously identified and can be placed in suitable isolation. However, other institutions can (and should, in my estimation) be more aggressive in employing UVGI routinely in areas where tuberculosis patients, especially MDR cases, are likely to be encountered.

Inflammatory Complications of BCG Vaccination

Inoculation with BCG typically results in a local inflammatory response that persists for several months (50). This may be tender, erythematous, and weeping and commonly leaves a depressed scar with mottled pigmentation on healing. Infrequent complications include the following (51). Deep, sloughing abscesses at the inoculation site have been noted. Regional lymph nodes may be inflamed as well, presenting with tender, swollen adenitis or actually breaking down with fistulous tracts. In addition, various forms of remote complications occur, including disseminated mycobacterial infections, focal osteitis or osteomyelitis, diffuse lymphadenitis, hepatosplenomegaly, and genitourinary lesions. Responses that appear to be mediated by hypersensitivity reactions, rather than direct infection, are also recorded, including diffuse erythrodermic rashes, erythema nodosum, phlyctenular keratoconjunctivitis, and vasculitis with pyoderma gangrenosum. Anaphylactoid reactions seen in association with BCG vaccination appear most likely to be caused by response to dextran, which is used for vaccine suspension, and not by the mycobacteria themselves (52,53).

The frequency with which these complications have been reported varies immensely. In an effort to calculate more accurately the dimensions of the problem, the International Union Against Tuberculosis conducted a comprehensive analysis (51). Although the authors invested a heroic effort in this project, it was very difficult to truly estimate the complication rates because of the large number of variables involved, including vaccine strains, doses, routes of administration, skill of staff administering vaccine, reporting/nonreporting systems, race and demographic factors, and definitions of adverse events. They concluded that the most reliable estimates were for the dramatic events, disseminated infection, and hypersensitivity; also, because of superior surveillance systems, studies from Europe afforded the most reliable data. Included in this report were data from both intradermal and peroral routes of BCG administration.

Osteitis is the most commonly described complication of BCG in normal hosts. A very interesting report from Finland found that the role of osteitis varied in relation to the vaccine employed, ranging overall between 7 and 30 cases/100,000 vaccinations (54). Another report from the Finnish group described diagnostic criteria for this condition and noted the anatomical predilection for the metaphyses of the long bones, the lower extremities, sternum, and ribs (55). A recent report from Chile noted an incidence of osteitis of 3/100,000 vaccinations and also noted the preponderance of cases to involve the lower extremities (56).

Prolonged regional lymphadenitis was noted to occur in <1% of Japanese children receiving Tokyo BCG (57). In their discussion, the Japanese group noted that the frequency of lymphadenitis in two recent reports from Taiwan and Korea involved higher rates of lymphadenitis with Pasteur BCG than with the Japan vaccine, but these articles were not available in English.

The most serious inflammatory complication of BCG is disseminated infection. Talbot and colleagues from Duke recently described such a case and identified 27 other published, well-documented cases in their literature review (58). Salient aspects of their report included the notation that 24 of the 28 had various immune-deficiency statuses including nine with AIDS, five with SCID, and three with chronic granulomatous disease; 68% were male; and treatment outcome was unfavorable, with 71% mortality.

Potential for Adverse Events or Paradoxical Increases of Tuberculosis Cases Among HIV-Infected Persons Receiving BCG

The global resurgence of tuberculosis is being propelled in part by the effects of HIV infection, particularly in sub-Saharan Africa, some Pacific Rim nations, South Asia, India, and parts of Latin America. BCG has been employed previously in these regions, and consideration has been given to intensifying vaccination in an effort to help control the scale of the epidemic.

No data exist that clearly characterize the protective effects of BCG given before acquisition of HIV infection. However, cases of disseminated "BCG-osis" among persons with AIDS have been reported (59–69); in these cases, it appears as though the disrupted immunity has facilitated either progressive primary infection or recrudescence of quiescient foci of BCG infection. Hence, considerable concern exists regarding the wisdom of giving BCG vaccine to persons with known HIV infection.

An additional potential hazard of BCG in persons/populations with HIV infection has been previously noted. In a recent (1986–1989) trial of BCG in Malawi, one component of the study was to examine the impact of a second BCG vaccination on the risks for tuberculosis and leprosy (27) (see above). The second dose of BCG resulted in a significantly *higher* case rate of pulmonary tuberculosis than the placebo-treated controls (risk ratio 1.74, $p = .05$). This higher rate resulted from excess cases among HIV-infected persons who received the second BCG dose (risk ratio 13.98, $p = .0009$). Note that all cases were confirmed to be *M. tuberculosis,* not

BCG disease. The authors of this Karonga trial felt that this was not likely to be a true causal relationship, but Rieder, an epidemiologist, argued that we cannot be assured of this (28). Based on a demonstrated increase in HIV-viral load following administration of other vaccines as well as accelerated depletion of CD4 counts with progression to AIDS in HIV-infected persons who develop active tuberculosis (see Chapter 8), it is a plausible thesis that BCG vaccination, through chronic inflammatory stimulation, may make HIV-infected persons more vulnerable to both endogenous reactivation and exogenous new infections with tuberculosis.

Sequelae of Intravesical BCG for Bladder Cancer

During the past 25 years, BCG has been given as an immune adjuvant for a wide assortment of neoplastic conditions. The greatest therapeutic utility has been described in superficial cancer of the bladder (59). Although it does not fit the immediate context of this chapter, the inflammatory complications of this procedure are sufficiently common to merit attention.

Sporadic reports have described a variety of sequelae, including febrile reactions and local infections of the bladder, prostate, and epididymis (60). Also, systemic febrile illnesses including diffuse, miliary shadowing on chest x-rays have been reported. In some cases, cultures were positive for BCG, confirming disseminated infection (61,62); in others, smears and cultures were negative, and the authors concluded that the illness was a hypersensitivity reaction (63). Recently, there have been two reported cases of BCG vertebral osteomyelitis following intravesical instillation (64,65). We have also treated another patient who developed highly destructive BCG spondylitis. In this case, following intravesical BCG, the patient experienced a motor vehicle accident and a compression fracture of the T-12 vertebra; this injury appeared to facilitate the osteomyelitis through the principle of *locus minoris resistentiae* (66). Also, granulomatous hepatitis has been described in relation to intravesical BCG (67–69).

Management of these various complications has not been well described because of their sporadic nature. For local or focal infections, multidrug chemotherapy has been prescribed, generally with good outcome. For most patients with acute or subacute miliary illness with respiratory embarrassment, simultaneous administration of chemotherapy plus steroids to suppress hypersensitivity has been employed (62,70); in other cases, only chemotherapy has been used (70,71). In another case, steroid treatment alone was given when intensive studies failed to demonstrate mycobacteria in numerous sites, presuming a noninfectious hypersensitivity phenomenon (72). Although successful in this instance, this strategy is highly problematic because of the potential implications of immunosuppressing an individual with cryptic disseminated mycobacterial disease. Because *M. bovis* BCG is predictably resistant to pyrazinamide, empirical therapy should consist of isoniazid, rifampin, and probably ethambutol (the necessity for this agent is unproven, but during early therapy it should afford protection against acquired resistance).

EPIDEMIOLOGICAL AND PUBLIC HEALTH ISSUES IN DETERMINING THE POTENTIAL UTILITY OF BCG VACCINATION

The decision regarding use of preventive chemotherapy or BCG vaccination as the central tactical component of a tuberculosis control program is substantially determined by the dynamics of the disease in the community and the availability of various assets.

Reactivation Versus Recent Transmission

Ferebee's model of tuberculosis in the United States in 1964 was the historical justification for the choice of tuberculin skin testing and isoniazid preventive therapy over BCG vaccination in the United States. This model is discussed in detail in Chapter 11. It is similar to the observations of Comstock (above) that, in addition to the efficacy of the vaccine used, the portion of the total tuberculosis morbidity derived by reactivation of remote tuberculosis infection strongly determines the overall impact of BCG.

Thus, for public health policy makers, the actual patterns of tuberculosis in a population are vital elements in selecting a prevention strategy. For the industrialized, more affluent nations, the dominant pattern has been congruent with the Ferebee model described above. This consideration has led to discontinuation of universal BCG vaccination programs in many of the Western nations over the last decade. In some countries, vaccination has been employed only for infants and children from high-risk minority or immigrant families.

Recently, however, the validity of this model has been called to question in some communities. Surveys based on DNA fingerprinting (restriction fragment length polymorphism [RFLP]) have indicated that approximately 40% of the new cases in San Francisco (73), parts of New York City (74), and Amsterdam, the Netherlands (75) were clustered by RFLP, strongly suggesting new transmission rather than late reactivation. These clusters were in some cases traced to point-source, common exposures and risk factors: shelters, clinics, hospitals, specific homes, or substance abuse (76–78). Often, though, conventional epidemiological tracing could not link the cases. Conventional epidemiological contact tracing failed to identify the site or time of apparent transmission in over 90% of the cases in which RFLP suggested clustering in two of these reports (73,75). These observations have led some to reason that the strategy/tactics of contact investigation/INH-preventive therapy would not be efficient and that BCG for a group such as the homeless might be more effective (79). By contrast, Burman in Denver was able to identify linkage in 40 of 51 cases (78%) in which RFLP indicated recent transmission (80).

Overall, these data indicate that in selected communities, a relatively greater proportion of new cases of tuberculosis can be ascribed to new infection than earlier models would have indicated. And, because a considerable proportion of these cases occurred in individuals who would not have been identified by contact investigations of new cases, the tuberculin skin test/preventive chemotherapy strategy would not have proven useful. In view of these recent findings, reconsideration of tuberculosis control programs in the United States and other industrialized nations has occurred. A major issue in these deliberations is the fact that, for many of the populations at high risk of acquiring new tuberculous infections and proceeding quickly to overt disease, ready access to and willingness to employ conventional health facilities are highly problematic (see below).

Availability of Diagnostic Services, Treatment Programs, Contact Investigation, and Preventive Chemotherapy

Choice of prevention strategy must also take into account the availability and feasibility of the services enumerated above. In a resource-rich community with a motivated population, programs to screen at-risk groups and to provide preventive treatment are practical. However, even in such communities, it is sorely unrealistic to expect a mobile population of disadvantaged, disaffected, and/or disconnected persons to regularly participate in skin-testing programs or if tested to return for reading, to have chest x-rays done if indicated, and, if recommended, to take 6 months of chemotherapy. Although directly observed therapy of active cases of tuberculosis is an appropriate goal for such individuals, wholesale programs of directly observed preventive therapy for cases of latent infection are neither feasible nor cost-effective. Hence, we are compelled to contemplate the other strategy, vaccination. Unfortunately, as described above, one cannot readily identify a vaccine that will predictably provide significant protection for the populations in question.

In developing nations, BCG vaccination, with all of the shortcomings described, remains the bulwark of prevention. Certainly in countries with a high prevalence of tuberculosis, vaccinating infants to protect them against more hazardous forms of extrapulmonary disease including miliary, meningeal, and vertebral tuberculosis is clearly indicated. The major issue to be addressed in such populations is what can be done to impact adult-type pulmonary disease that results in continued transmission of infection. As conceded by Farga, BCG programs have largely failed to contain the continued spread of infection (81).

Overall, the epidemiology of tuberculosis in industrialized nations continues to represent three distinct elements: (a) low-level reactivation of remote latent infection among the indigenous population, largely among persons ages 60 and above; (b) more recent transmission ("epidemics") among younger minorities and socioeconomically disadvantaged; and, (c) a relatively high prevalence ("endemic") among immigrants from high-risk countries. There is some spillover from group (b) to group (a) (82,83), but for the most part, these processes tend to run in parallel (84–90).

Although it may be tempting to employ BCG in some situations, I believe that a clearly preferable option is to improve case finding, introduce DOT to assure rapid cures and thereby to halt transmission, and practice aggressive but focused contact investigation and preventive chemotherapy for high-risk contacts. If, however, vaccines of greater efficacy can be developed, the role of this strategy should be reevaluated. Efforts to develop mathematical models to weigh the relative contributions of the preventive chemotherapy strategy or vaccination, although desirable, are very sensitive to the assumptions fed into these analyses. A 1996 report by the Harvard group, associated with the earlier BCG meta-analysis, calculated that a BCG program that reached 10% of eligible children and 1% of eligible adults each year would produce a 17% reduction in cases and an 11% decline in deaths over 10 years (91). They also concluded that preventive chemotherapy among the general population would have little effect on the number of tuberculosis cases. However, as indicated by Castro and Miller in an editorial that accompanied this article, the analysis did not realistically acknowledge the shortcomings of vaccination and, it seemed, willfully to underestimate the potential of preventive chemotherapy except for HIV-infected persons (92). I will not pretend to be unbiased on this issue. I do not feel BCG should be used in the manner described by this distinguished group because their assessment overestimates the efficacy of BCG and underestimates the programmatic and biological difficulties with the vaccine; they also underestimate the efficacy and overestimate the morbidity, mortality, and complexity of a focused program of preventive chemotherapy.

VACCINE CANDIDATES OTHER THAN BCG

Because of the demonstrated shortcomings of BCG, considerable effort has recently been directed toward the development of novel agents that might confer higher levels of protective immunity. Orme recently reviewed various candidates for such vaccines (93). Using his schema, I attempt to briefly analyze the theoretical bases and current experience with them.

Mycobacterial DNA

To most immunologists' surprise, DNA from a number of bacteria, viruses, and parasites has been shown to be effective in animal vaccine models (94). For tuberculosis, one group showed murine protection following vaccination with the mycobacterial gene (derived from *M. leprae,* incidentally) for the 60-kDa heat-shock protein (95). Another group employed the gene for another secreted mycobacterial product, vaccinating with a plasmid that was encoded for a 30- to 32-kDa protein, antigen 85A (96). Yet another group vaccinated with the genes encoding for two secreted protein antigens, hsp60 and a 36-kDa protein (97).

All of these efforts demonstrated significant levels of protection from experimental challenge with virulent *M. tuberculosis.* In some cases, the protection appeared to persist, perhaps related to the residual presence of the genetic antigen at the vaccination site. However, as indicated by Orme, given the association with hsp60 as an autoimmunity-inducing substance, issues of safety will surround this approach.

Culture Filtrate Proteins/Secreted Antigens

As noted in Chapter 4, Orme and others have reasoned that early immunity against invading tubercle bacilli might be directed against proteins elaborated by the viable bacilli held within macrophages that were incompetent to kill the mycobacteria. If such immunity were engendered, the earlier host response might help limit the bacillary dissemination.

Thus, there have been multiple studies attempting to delineate which of these protein antigens might confer protection. Orme's group has published a series of articles on this topic (98–101). Others have also shown variable levels of immune responses or protection following vaccination with such products, including Andersen and colleagues in Denmark (102–104) and Horwitz's group in California (105,106). The California group has also recently reported a method to express large quantitites of four of the candidate proteins by use of a rapid-growing mycobacterial vector, *M. smegmatis* (107).

However, as summarized by Orme, there remain substantive issues regarding the potency and long-term effectiveness of such vaccines.

"Auxotrophic" BCG Vaccines

Auxotrophic microbes are mutants that have different nutrient requirements than their parent strains. Research has been performed attempting to produce living vaccines of lessened virulence or durability by this phenomenon. Recent reports have described an auxotroph of *M. bovis* BCG (108), have noted this organism to have restricted growth in macrophages (109), and have shown the auxotroph to confer comparable protection to native BCG in a normal laboratory murine strain, BALB/c mice (110). Because of concern over the possibility of producing progressive or disseminated infection with conventional BCG among persons with AIDS, regular BCG and the auxotrophic strains were given to mice with severe combined immune deficiency syndrome or SCIDS (110). BCG killed all of the SCIDS mice within 8 weeks, but the auxotroph did not appear lethal for these mice and, in fact, was not recovered from their tissues after 16 to 32 weeks.

These observations suggest that this attenuation of an already attenuated vaccine may prove of utility among persons with HIV infection or other immunosuppressed states.

New Recombinant BCG Vaccines

Considerable investigation has been directed toward the use of BCG as a living vaccine vector to present various antigens from other pathogens including Lyme disease (111), *Leishmania* (112), and even HIV (113).

In view of the capacity to modify the antigens presented by the BCG bacillus, we should consider the possibility of custom tailoring to prominently present tuberculosis antigens, which are found to be protective, and perhaps delete those antigens that promote pathogenesis or confound immunity.

In summary, promising work is being conducted seeking improved vaccines for tuberculosis. However, unless there is a vaccine with such extraordinary efficacy that it clearly distinguishes itself from the pack, we are unlikely to see such novel agents widely employed within a decade. The costs of vaccine development, the expenses of organizing human trials, and the time required to confirm effectiveness and safety in humans are daunting obstacles.

IMMUNOTHERAPY OF PATIENTS WITH ACTIVE TUBERCULOSIS

Robert Koch was the first to attempt specific immunotherapy of tuberculosis; his intuition as well as fragmentary successes in animals and humans have continued to inspire interest in this approach.

Early investigators working with animal models and with patients recognized broadly that there were two types of responses after sensitization to tuberculosis antigens. On the one hand, there were intensely inflammatory, necrotizing reactions including, at the extreme, Koch's phenomenon. On the other hand, there were less intensely inflammatory reactions that were nonetheless associated with apparent inhibition of mycobacterial replication and survival. In an ill-defined way, these patterns came to be called delayed-type hypersensitivity (DTH) and cell-mediated immunity (CMI).

Based on these dichotomous observations, clinicians and scientists have attempted throughout the twentieth century to modify the immune responses to tuberculosis to both facilitate cures and ameliorate symptoms and tissue injury. Hence, this section is divided into two segments, one related to enhancing immune capacity, the other to downregulation of immune-mediated inflammation.

Immunity-Enhancing Therapy

Efforts to reinforce the host's protective immunity may be seen in several broad, albeit arbitrary, arenas: (a) adding substances, usually cytokines, that are seen to drive proimmune processes, (b) inhibiting substances that result in downregulation of immunity, as with TGF-β inhibitors, (c) shifting the T-lymphocyte maturation away from the Th2 to the Th1 pathway, as with *M. vaccae,* or (d) using exogenous serum to promote cellular immune pathways, as with transfer factor, or humoral immunity, with passive antibody or serum therapy.

Interferon-γ

Produced by CD4 and CD8 lymphocytes, natural killer cells, and δ/γ-lymphocytes, IFN-γ stimulates both production of TNF-α and antigen presentation by macrophages. Based on its apparent centrality in cellular immunity, IFN-γ has been used in leprosy (114–116), other nontuberculous mycobacterial infections (117,118), and tuberculosis (119,120).

Among leprosy patients, local injections of IFN-γ were given into lepromatous leprosy lesions (a very permissive form of advanced disease in which the bacilli proliferate massively and the host appears incapable of mounting an effective immune response); the cytokine appeared to promote considerable local immune response (114). A subsequent trial of systemic IFN-γ for patients with lepromatous leprosy resulted in the transformation in six of ten patients to a condition called erythema nodosum leprosum (ENL, a highly inflammatory, febrile state with exhuberant, tender nodules, high fever, and histologic features of vasculitis); this was believed to be associated with the induction of very high levels of TNF-α production (115). A third trial of IFN-γ also employed interleukin-2 (IL-2) therapy; both of these cytokines elicited substantial inflammation believed related to TNF-α (116). In all of these studies, the IFN-γ appeared to result in diminished burdens of mycobacteria in the tissues but at the cost of severe inflammation. Thalidomide was helpful in controlling the inflammatory complications (see below).

Holland and colleagues from the National Institutes of Health (NIH) described seven patients with refractory, disseminated nontuberculous mycobacteria (NTM) infections who were successfully treated with systemic IFN-γ (117). However, all of these patients were found to have substantial underlying abnormalities of their cellular immune systems (see Chapter 4 for details). Perhaps more applicable to the usual patient would be a single case report of a patient from France with refractory, localized pulmonary disease caused by *M. avium* complex (118). Treated with three courses of inhaled IFN-γ, the patient enjoyed modest bacteriological response to this therapy.

There are two reports of the use of IFN-γ for tuberculosis. One was a case report of the treatment of a patient with lymphocytic leukemia and a refractory, multidrug-resistant tuberculoma of the CNS (119); simultaneous therapy with subcutaneous IFN-γ and GM-CSF resulted in striking improvement. At autopsy, from a leukemic death, there was no residual evidence of tuberculosis. The other report involved a group of five patients from Bellevue Hospital in New York with refractory multidrug-resistant (MDR) pulmonary tuberculosis (120). By contrast, these patients received inhaled IFN-γ thrice-weekly for 1 month. The inhaled therapy was well tolerated and resulted in transient sputum smear negativity in all patients, delays in time until cultures became positive, and modest radiographic improvement.

Unpublished data from one institution include the use of IFN-γ by subcutaneous injection (Holland's NIH protocol) for five patients with refractory MDR pulmonary tuberculosis. In this unblinded study, we were not able to discern any significant improvement among these patients with long-standing, chronic disease.

On balance, it appears as though IFN-γ may modestly enhance immunity among normal hosts with refractory mycobacterial infections. The limited experience raises the possibility that inhaled therapy may be more effective than systemic for pulmonary disease. However, at best, it remains a form of rescue therapy rather than an affordable, practical modality that might be employed widely to accelerate the curative response among large numbers of patients (see below under "*Mycobacterium vaccae*").

Interferon-α/Imiquod

Most studies of antimycobacterial immunity have focused upon IFN-γ; however, a recent report from Italy described a series of patients with drug-susceptible pulmonary tuberculosis who were treated with aerosolized IFN-α (121). In this trial, 20 HIV-negative adult patients were randomized to conventional chemotherapy or chemotherapy plus aerosolized IFN-α, 3 MU thrice-weekly for 2 months. In addition to conventional laboratory studies, bronchoscopy with BAL was done on entry and at completion of the IFN-α therapy. In this unblinded trial, the authors indicated that the cytokine therapy resulted in more rapid reduction in fever, sputum mycobacterial burden, and radiographic abnormalities. Also, they described reduced levels of BAL inflammatory cytokines IL-1β, IL-6, and TNF-α during the 2 months of IFN-α treatment. Although the observed changes were modest, the trends were consistently favorable for the treated group.

The authors concluded that IFN-α had similar effects to IFN-γ in stimulating T-cell function, particularly in the Th1 mode, without as many systemic side effects.

These observations have suggested the possibility of using Imiquod, an oral agent that has been shown to induce the production and release of IFN-α (122). Although not used yet in the therapy of patients with mycobacterial disease, Imiquod has been used in a Phase I trial for 12 patients with early HIV infection (123). Given once weekly, the Imiquod appeared to have potent effects in increasing IFN-α levels along with surrogate markers of IFN activity, β_2-microglobulin, and neopterin. However, there were dose-limiting side effects. Nonetheless, oral administration and infrequent dosing schedules make this a potential candidate for immune-enhancing therapy in view of the findings of the Italian group above.

Interleukin-12

A proimmune cytokine produced primarily by mononuclear phagocytes, interleukin-12 (IL-12) stimulates production of IFN-γ by Th1 lymphocytes and NK cells and promotes maturation of Th1 phenotypic lymphocytes. Recent studies of several children with extreme genetically determined vulnerability to disseminated mycobacterial infections have shown a central role for this cytokine in protective immunity (see Chapter 4).

Used in the immune-deficient beige mouse model, IL-12 has shown significant activity in reducing burdens of *M. avium* complex (MAC) in various tissues; however, it had considerable toxicity (124). Young and colleagues have shown that the simultaneous use of IL-12 and clarithromycin, a potent anti-MAC antibiotic, resulted in less toxicity and enhanced antimycobacterial effects.

Although it has been given parenterally and clearly has considerable toxicity, the potency of its antimycobacterial activities makes IL-12 an ongoing candidate for immunotherapy.

Granulocyte–Macrophage Colony-Stimulating Factor

Colony-stimulating factors have been shown to drive the proliferation and maturation of a variety of hematopoietic cell lines (125). GM-CSF, while having a variety of stimulating effects, has been shown to drive the monocyte–macrophage series.

GM-CSF was employed by Deresinski and colleagues in California in the treatment of a young woman with a highly refractory, perplexing disseminated infection with *M. kansasii* (126). Despite receiving many months of very aggressive antimycobacterial therapy with agents to which her organisms were susceptible, she experienced protracted high fevers, persistence of massive retroperitoneal lymphadenitis, and relative neutropenia with total white cell counts around 3,000. In vitro studies showed that peripheral blood monocytes, when infected with *M. kansasii* or MAC, were extremely permissive for their replication; these findings were partially corrected after exposure to GM-CSF. Treatment with this colony-stimulating factor eventually led to clinical and radiological resolution of the disseminated mycobacteriosis and, despite discontinuation of the GM-CSF, long-term freedom from recurrence.

As noted above, a patient with refractory CNS infection with MDR TB was treated simultaneously with IFN-γ and GM-CSF, resulting ultimately in control of the tuberculosis (119). The authors inferred, though, that the IFN-γ had played no prominent beneficial role.

More recently, Devesinski's group reported on the effects of GM-CSF in bacteremic MAC infection in four patients with AIDS (127). Although the drug did not influence the extent of bacteremia, it did result in increased production of reactive oxygen intermediates (ROIs) and improved antimycobacterial activity by peripheral blood monocytes in vitro.

Once again, this agent does not appear to be a strong candidate as a general agent to improve host defenses against tuberculosis. Rather, its utility probably resides in the care of patients with clear-cut deficiencies in mononuclear phagocyte maturation or function. Its profound, acute side effects mandate that it be used with caution.

Levamisole

Developed as a veterinary antihelminthic agent, this compound was described to promote cellular immunity (128). In a 1980 report, levamisole was reported to have resulted in more rapid sputum conversion and radiographic improvement in a series of pulmonary tuberculosis from India (129); and a 1981 report, also from India, described accelerated radiographic clearing (130). However, a 1989 report from East Africa done with the British Medical Research Council failed to demonstrate either bacteriological or radiographic advantage from 4 or 8 weeks of levamisole (131). The earlier studies had reported higher lymphocyte counts and restoration of skin-test sensitization to DNCB following levamisole, but such assays were not done in the East African trial because of technical problems.

Unfortunately, the putative value of levamisole was not confirmed, and, to my knowledge, no further studies have been performed with this agent in patients with tuberculosis.

Transfer Factor

Originally described by Lawrence as a serum factor that would convey DTH reactivity to a recipient from a skin-test–positive donor (132), Transfer factor (TF) was shown in early reports to improve or normalize cellular immune responses in small numbers of patients with Wiskott-Aldrich syndrome (133,134), patients with chronic mucocutaneous candidiasis (135–137), or patients with lepromatous leprosy (138) or coccidioidomycosis (139). Whitcomb and Rocklin in 1973 described dramatic clinical improvement following TF therapy of a young woman with refractory pulmonary and disseminated drug-susceptible tuberculosis (140). Like the young woman with disseminated *M. kansasii* infection described above, this patient had unexplained pancytopenia and some type of cellular immune deficit.

Although used subsequently in patients with MAC disease (141), refractory *M. xenopi* infection (142), *M. fortuitum* (143), and tuberculous osteomyelitis (144), little work has been reported.

In perspective, TF appears to be potentially useful in reconstituting cellular immune function among patients with various deficits. Ongoing research is being conducted into the structure, function, and clinical applications of TF (C. H. Kirkpatrick, *personal communication*).

Inhibitors of Transforming Growth Factor-β

Ellner and colleagues in Cleveland have studied extensively the factors associated with the normal downregulation of tuberculosis immune-mediated inflammation. Among the substances that appear prominently involved with this process is TGF-β (see Chapter 4 for a more detailed exposition). In 1997, they reported on the capacity of two naturally occurring substances, decorin and latency-associated peptide, to reverse the suppression of T-cell function seen in patients with advanced pulmonary tuberculosis (145). In vitro assays showed that these substances corrected depressed T-cell proliferation and increased IFN-γ production twofold; these effects were seen both with PBMs from diseased hosts and from mononuclear phagocytes infected in vitro with *M. tuberculosis*.

Although this approach is far from clinical application, the concept of inhibiting inhibitors of immunity merits future considerations.

Mycobacterium vaccae

The most explicit proposal for the potential avenues of immune enhancement has been delineated by Grange, Stanford, Rook, and colleagues and has culminated in their extensive studies of *M. vaccae* as an immune-enhancing vaccine for patients with active tuberculosis (146). This model is based on studies that have identified two subpopulations of T helper cells, Th1 and Th2, with distinctive patterns of cytokine production and functional activity (147). In various chronic parasitic infestations and viral infections, hosts may alternately mount an immune response characterized by predominance of either Th1 or Th2 pathways (148). In general, the Th1-dominant responses are characterized by more effective inhibition of the microbe, controlled inflammation, limited tissue injury, and favorable outcome for the host. However, among effective pathogens there is a propensity for switching the host response to the Th2 variety that is associated with extensive tissue necrosis and a worsened prognosis.

Regarding tuberculosis, Grange, Stanford, Rook, and colleagues have hypothesized that experience of the immune system with various mycobacteria including *M. tuberculosis* and other "environmental" strains would influence the dominance of Th1 or Th2 pathways (149,150).

Indeed, their hypothesis was originally driven by the observation that BCG vaccination appeared to be particularly effective in Uganda, where a common environmental mycobacteria was a rapid grower, *M. vaccae* (151). Their research had shown that certain mycobacteria were prone to elicit a "*Listeria*"-type response rather than the classic Koch response. In contrast to the Koch type, the "*Listeria*" reaction evolved in days rather than weeks following infection and, on subsequent skin testing, resulted in somewhat earlier indurated responses that were softer, less tender, earlier to resolve, and not necrotizing or ulcerating (152). In an animal model, they demonstrated that immunization that induced one type of response, Koch or Listerial, tended to block the other and speculated that this could explain some of the diversity seen in BCG trials.

Their current assumption is that these responses are elicited by groups of antigens that are represented variously in the different mycobacterial species. In particular, they believe that the antigens common to all mycobacterial species (group 1) and those unique to species (group 4) are central to the phenomenon. Group 1 epitopes, which are found to be predominant antigens in *M. vaccae,* appear to direct initial immune responses to Th1 or to switch responses away from the Th2 into Th1 patterns. By contrast, group 4 species-specific epitopes, which are prominently represented in *M. tuberculosis,* tend to elicit Th2-pathway responses, downregulating or suppressing Th1 activity.

In one recent iteration of their model, so-called "Koch's phenomenon" is seen to be of utility in helping the human host establish local control of a small tuberculous lesion (necrosis → fibrosis → walling-off of bacilli). However, in advanced, progressive disease, it is maladaptive, causing cavitation that facilitates mycobacterial replication, downregulation of effective cellular immunity, and diminished vulnerability of the bacilli to drugs within necrotic lesions (because of slowed metabolism induced by the acidic milieu). The pathogenesis of this caseating necrosis of Koch's phenomenon is believed to be caused by a complex cascade of cytokines (153).

A study by this group has shown that in the mouse model TNF-α could either help induce protective immunity or worsen tissue injury with necrosis (154). This experiment involved priming the murine immune systems into low (107) or high (109) doses of heat-killed *M. vaccae.* After the low-dose immunization, the mice responded with a Th1 cytokine profile; and, when challenged later with TNF-α, there was no tissue necrosis, and the response was similar to that previously noted to provide effective immunity. By contrast, following the high-dose immunization, there was a mixed cytokine response with features of Th1 and Th2 (and Th0) patterns. When these animals were challenged with TNF-α, there were exaggerated local inflammation and injury, patterns seen with failing host protection.

To summarize this group's theory of immunopathogenesis and immunomodulation: as tuberculosis advances in a vulnerable subject, there is a shift away from the Th1 cytokine pathway (that produces effective bacteriostasis without extensive tissue damage) to the mixed Th1/Th2/Th0 pattern (that is associated with intense, necrotizing inflammation that adversely affects host survival). Because *M. vaccae* predominantly presents group 1 antigens that allegedly promote dominance of the Th1 pathway, vaccination of a patient experiencing active, destructive tuberculosis could/should redirect the errant Th2 response into the preferred pathway.

Indirect evidence from human disease status that is offered in support of the theory includes these indicators of Th2 pathway activity: (a) elevated levels of IgE antibodies to *M. tuberculosis,* release of IL-4 from peripheral T cells in response to mycobacterial antigens, and relief of constitutional symptoms by thalidomide, a TNF-α inhibitor, in patients with active tuberculosis, (b) other chronic infections including AIDS, downgrading leprosy, schistosomiasis, leishmaniasis, and syphilis in which shifts from Th1 to Th2 dominant responses in association with clinical and microbiological worsening have been documented.

The British group has participated in a variety of studies employing *M. vaccae* immunotherapy, and their 1993 review indicated that it resulted in significantly improved cure rates for newly diagnosed pulmonary tuberculosis (155).

The authors point out that the immunomodulatory activity in this setting is primarily effective in the elimination of "persistor" tubercle bacilli. In their putative model, there are three populations of tubercle bacilli in the untreated patient: a large population of rapidly proliferating organisms that are very susceptible to and rapidly killed by chemotherapy, a less rapidly metabolizing population that lives within and is inhibited by acidic inflammatory debris and is killed less rapidly by chemotherapy, and the semidormant persistors, which are only sporadically sufficiently active metabolically to be killed by medication. The latter two populations, and particularly the persistors, are the reason that antituberculosis treatment must be extended so long. The advocates of *M. vaccae* immunotherapy contend that by switching the host to a more efficient mode of cellular response, Th1 pathway, the duration of chemotherapy required to effect enduring cure can be substantially shortened.

In addition, they believe that *M. vaccae* immunotherapy can aid in the management of patients with multidrug-resistant tuberculosis. In one report from Iran, an uncontrolled experience, *M. vaccae* was given up to four times for patients with chronic MDR TB (156). Although the study design and patient attrition did not allow firm conclusions, the authors noted that 11 of the original 41 patients entered into the study became sputum negative whereas their prior experience with such patients would have predicted only 1 in 100 responders.

In a 1991 essay, which now seems unfortunate, three of this group suggested that the future of tuberculosis control in Africa was lost and proposed that *M. vaccae* might prove so effective that chemotherapeutic regimens as short as 1 to 8 weeks coupled with immunotherapy could provide substantial rates of cure (157).

An adage learned in my youth warned that, "if something seems too good to be true, it probably is [too good to be true]." This model appeared to be one of the most intriguing, potentially useful issues currently under clinical study in tuberculosis. However, more recent trials of *M. vaccae* that were randomized and controlled have failed to show clinical utility of such vaccine therapy (158). It is not clear now whether this reflects inadequacy of previous study design, variations in vaccine strain efficacy, or differences in study populations. Given the scientific accomplishments of this group, I am disposed to take a wait-and-see attitude rather than totally dismiss this approach.

Humoral (Antibody) Therapy

Conventional wisdom of this era indicates that antibody or humoral immunity does not participate significantly in the human defense against tuberculosis, and certainly, the preponderance of clinical and experimental evidence supports this model. However, it is counterintuitive to believe that this major component of defense against other bacterial infections has been wholly excluded from involvement with this disease.

Glatman-Freedman and Casadevall have recently performed an extraordinary review of the history of serum therapy for tuberculosis (159). Worth reading for its historical interest alone, this article traces the theory and practice of treatment with immune serum from various animal sources, performed mostly from the late 1890s through 1920. Given the predictable issues with study design, there is little evidence, favorable or negative, that stands up to rigorous scrutiny. However, the authors note that some investigators reported fairly dramatic improvements. They also describe plausible mechanisms by which antibodies might influence the pathogenesis or immune defenses against tuberculosis, including adhesion, phagosome–lysosome fusion, neutralization of inflammatory moieties, or opsonization. Also, they remind us of evidence that humoral immunity has been shown to be of importance in defense against an intracellular fungal infection, *Cryptococcus neoformans.*

On balance, this review should provoke contemporary scientists to reexamine some of the ongoing riddles of tuberculosis with a more open mind to humoral phenomena.

Suppression of Immune-Mediated Inflammation

As noted in Chapter 4, tubercle bacilli do not elaborate classical endotoxins, exotoxins, or destructive enzymes associated with other notorious bacterial pathogens. Rather, the vast preponderance of tissue injury results from the body's urgent efforts to rid itself of this tenacious intracellular invasion. In the previous sections of this chapter, we have reviewed methods that (a) stimulate immunity to prevent disease via enhanced defense against spread from the primary infection site in the lungs and (b) to control refractory disease by improving the quality of the cellular immune response.

However, in the modern era of chemotherapy we are presented with an additional therapeutic option. Multidrug regimens that include isoniazid and a rifamycin are so potent that we may be able to effect cures while suppressing some components of the immune response, preferably those that are responsible for injury to important tissues or organs and cause miserable or disabling symptoms including high fevers, drenching sweats, prostration, anorexia, and weight loss. Some of the potential modalities for such interventions are reviewed below.

Thalidomide

Made forever infamous by its association with phocomelia or short-limb deformities in infants of mothers who received this drug to control morning sickness, thalidomide has been revisited because of its ability to inhibit TNF-α.

The group from Rockefeller University in New York City began using IFN-γ to enhance cellular immunity in patients with lepromatous leprosy. In doing so, some patients developed a profoundly inflammatory condition, erythema nodosum leprosum. Based on in vitro evidence that thalidomide inhibited TNF-α from stimulated monocytes (160), the group gave the drug to patients with ENL (115). They observed that thalidomide resulted in considerable reductions in IFN-γ–stimulated production of TNF-α and amelioration of clinical toxicity. Subsequently, they showed that a mechanism of thalidomide action was causing accelerated degradation of mRNA for TNF-α production (161). Kaplan in 1993 noted that thalidomide downregulated TNF-α without interfering with other monocyte cytokines necessary for normal immune function (116). However, another group in 1997 noted that thalidomide also inhibited production by peripheral blood monocytes of IL-12, a critical proimmune cytokine described above and in Chapter 4 (162).

Nonetheless, in 1995 thalidomide was given to 15 patients with pulmonary tuberculosis, with or without coexisting HIV infection (163). Given for single or multiple 2-week cycles, the drug was reportedly well tolerated and resulted in enhanced weight gain. Other observations included diminished TNF-α production, increased IFN-γ levels, and no impairment of in vitro DTH reaction to PPD with thalidomide.

Recently, the Rockefeller group described a rabbit model of mycobacterial meningitis in which thalidomide plus chemotherapy appeared more effective in preventing death than chemotherapy alone (164).

Thalidomide has also been employed in a variety of other human diseases including aphthous ulcers in HIV-infected persons (165), AIDS-related wasting syndrome (166), refractory adult-onset Still's disease (167), and the mucocutaneous lesions of the Behçet syndrome (168). These reports generally describe some degree of therapeutic efficacy but were notable also for side effects, toxicity, and unanticipated results such as the appearance of erythema nodosum and peripheral neuropathy in Behçet syndrome patients.

In 1998, an unusual case of pulmonary MAC disease, associated with idiopathic CD4 lymphocytopenia and unresponsive to conventional antimicrobial therapy but that responded favorably to thalidomide, was reported from Italy (169). Receiving thalidomide as well as conventional anti-MAC therapy, this patient experienced defervescence, weight gain, clearance of mycobacteria from her blood and sputum, restoration of cellular DTH functions, and increases in CD4 lymphocyte counts. This case clearly is anomalous; MAC bacteremia is exceedingly rare outside of persons with AIDS, and thalidomide should not be attempted in other patients simply for refractory pulmonary MAC. However, the clinical response and improvements of lymphocyte function suggest that thalidomide may have an expanded role in the therapy of various defects of cellular immunity.

Thalidomide's role in controlling inflammation in tuberculosis and other disorders is not yet clearly defined. Perhaps the side effects such as sedation and toxicity including peripheral neuropathy will limit its widespread use; 24 of 56 (43%) of HIV-infected persons stopped the drug because of adverse effects in a recent trial (170). Furthermore, thalidomide's potential for birth defects will surely preclude its use in women at risk of pregnancy. However, the general mechanism of inhibiting TNF-α appears a potentially fruitful avenue of exploration (see pentoxifylline below).

Pentoxifylline

A phosphodisesterase inhibitor, this xanthine derivative has been used in the United States primarily for the management of claudication in peripheral vascular disease. However, studies have also demonstrated inhibition of TNF-α production in vitro (171) and in vivo (172); in addition to TNF-α inhibition, pentoxifylline inhibits inducible nitric oxide synthase in murine macrophages (173).

Clinically, pentoxifylline has been used recently in persons with HIV infections to lower TNF-α levels with two objectives: limit HIV replication and control the AIDS wasting syndrome (174,175). The first trial employed 400 mg thrice daily, the second, 800 mg twice daily. Both studies demonstrated reduced production of TNF-α from peripheral blood monocytes stimulated with lipopolysaccharide; gastrointestinal side effects made the higher dose less acceptable.

At this point, the clinical efficacy of pentoxifylline for management of tuberculosis-related inflammation has not been studied. However, a trial focusing on patients with more extensive signs, symptoms, and evidence of tissue damage might be appropriate.

Corticosteroids

The one category of anti-inflammatory agents that has been employed widely in tuberculosis is glucocorticoids. There is a vast literature relating to the effects of these steroids on various forms of pulmonary and extrapulmonary tuberculosis; these reports were well summarized in a 1997 review (176). Most clinicians are familiar with usage in tuberculous meningitis and pericarditis, but there have also been large trials in pulmonary, pleural, and other forms of disease. The specific utility of steroids for these types of tuberculosis is reviewed in Chapters 6 and 7. Briefly, though, the most readily demonstrated advantages have been shown with meningitis and pericarditis, but rapid reductions in constitutional symptoms, cough, pulmonary radiographic abnormalities, and local inflammatory phenomena have been shown consistently.

On balance, the side effects and potential complications of doses of glucocorticoids sufficient to reduce inflammation are such that wholesale use of these agents is not justified. However, for individual cases, clinical utility is possible.

Cyclosporine A and Other Agents

Derived from a fungus, cyclosporine A (CsA) is a cyclic polypeptide with a very selective inhibitory effect on T lymphocytes. It may be given parenterally or orally. Used almost exclusively to suppress cell-mediated rejection of transplanted organs, it was shown to be highly effective in a murine model in reducing granulomatous lung inflammation following intravenous injection of *M. bovis* BCG (177). It has not been studied systematically as an agent to control tuberculosis-associated inflammation, and, because of the potential of profound immunosuppression, it clearly would not be appropriate for wide usage. However, for highly selected cases in which there are potentially life-threatening complications of tuberculosis, if corticosteroids do not prove adequate, one might consider this agent. In particular, I would have in mind advanced meningitis. Note that, if used with rifampin, the dosage of CsA should be increased because of accelerated elimination by the hepatic system cytochrome P450.

Other agents such as tacrolimus or mycopherolic acid are potential candidates, although clinical experience with these agents is far less than with CsA.

SUMMARY

As medical science advances, our understanding of the pathogenesis and immune defenses against tuberculosis should allow us to prevent and modify disease caused by this and other mycobacteria. BCG vaccine given to infants and children in high-prevalence countries offers significant protection against some of the more destructive forms of tuberculosis; however, it has failed to significantly alter the prevalence of disease among the general population. New vaccines and/or vaccine strategies must be developed if we are to have measurable impact on the ongoing epidemic in the developing nations.

For patients with active tuberculosis, we find ourselves in the paradoxical situation of contemplating means to strengthen the immune responses (to either cure refractory cases or lessen the time required to effect cures with chemotherapy) or to suppress immune-mediated inflammation to attenuate the clinical illness or lessen damage to vital organs. Regarding the latter issue, we must appreciate that curing a patient of tuberculosis rarely returns him or her to the premorbid health. Lung function, susceptibility to subsequent pulmonary infections, skeletal integrity and work capacity, renal function, and intellectual capacity may all be adversely impacted despite successful chemotherapy. The future management of tuberculosis should focus on minimizing such morbid sequelae.

REFERENCES

1. Koch R. Weitere Mitteilungen über ein Heilmittel gegen Tuberculose. *Dtsch Med Wochenschr* 1890;16: 1029–1032.
2. Sakula A. BCG: who were Calmette and Guérin? *Thorax* 1983;38:806–812.
3. Guérin C. The history of BCG. In: Rosenthal S, ed. *BCG vaccination against tuberculosis.* Boston: Little, Brown, 1957:48–53.
4. Anonymous (Berlin correspondent). The Lübeck trial. *Lancet* 1931;2:1038.
5. Heimbeck J. BCG vaccination of nurses. *Tubercle* 1948;29:84–88.
6. Hyge TV. The efficacy of BCG vaccination. Tuberculosis epidemic in a state school with an observation period of 12 years. *Dan Med Bull* 1957;4:13–15.
7. Comstock GW. The International Tuberculosis Campaign: a pioneering venture in mass vaccination and research. *Clin Infect Dis* 1994;19:528–540.
8. Comstock GW. Field trials of tuberculosis vaccines: how could we have done them better? *Control Clin Trials* 1994;15:247–276.
9. Smith DW. Protective effect of BCG in experimental tuberculosis. In: Fox W, Grosset J, Styblo K, eds. *Advances in tuberculosis research.* Basel: Karger, 1985: 1–97.
10. Townsend J, Aronson J, Saylor R. Tuberculosis control among North American Indians. *Am Rev Tuberc* 1942; 45:41–52.
11. Clemens JD, Chuong JJH, Feinstein AR. The BCG controversy. A methodological and statistical reappraisal. *JAMA* 1983;249:2362–2369.
12. Rosenthal SR, Loewinsohn E, Graham ML, Liveright D, Thorne MG, Johnson V. BCG vaccination against

tuberculosis in Chicago. A twenty-year study statistically analyzed. *Pediatrics* 1961;28:622–641.

13. Hart PD, Sutherland I. BCG and vole bacillus vaccines in the prevention of tuberculosis in adolescence and early adult life. Final report to the Medical Research Council. *BMJ* 1977;2:293–295.
14. Aronson JD, Aronson CF, Taylor HC. A twenty-year appraisal of BCG vaccination in the control of tuberculosis. *Arch Intern Med* 1958;101:881–893.
15. Comstock GW, Webster RG. Tuberculosis studies in Muscogee County, Georgia. VII. A twenty-year evaluation of BCG vaccination in a school population. *Am Rev Respir Dis* 1969;100:839–845.
16. Comstock G, Livesay V, Woolpert S. Evaluation of BCG vaccination among Puerto Rican children. *Am J Public Health* 1974;64:283–291.
17. Palmer C, Shaw L, Comstock G. Community trials of BCG vaccination. *Am Rev Respir Dis* 1958;77:877–907.
18. Frimodt-Møller J, Acharyulu GS, Kesava Pillai K. Observations on the protective effect of BCG vaccination in a South Indian rural population: fourth report. *Bull Int Union Tuberc* 1973;48:40–50.
19. Tripathy SP. Fifteen-year follow-up of the Indian BCG prevention trial. *Bull Int Union Tuberc Lung Dis* 1987; 62:69–72.
20. Colditz GA, Brewer TF, Berkey CS, et al. Efficacy of BCG vaccine in the prevention of tuberculosis. Meta-analysis of the published literature. *JAMA* 1994;271: 298–702.
21. Brewer TF, Colditz GA. Relationship between Bacille Calmette-Guérin (BCG) strains and the efficacy of BCG vaccine in the prevention of tuberculosis. *Clin Infect Dis* 1995;20:126–135.
22. Fine PEM. Variation in protection by BCG: implications of and for heterologous immunity. *Lancet* 1995; 346:1339–1345.
23. Fine PEM, Sterne JAC, Pönnighaus JM, Rees RJW. Delayed-type hypersensitivity, mycobacterial vaccines and protective immunity. *Lancet* 1994;344:1245–1249.
24. Palmer CE, Long MW. Effects of infection with atypical mycobacteria on BCG vaccination and tuberculosis. *Am Rev Respir Dis* 1966;94:553–568.
25. Wilson ME, Fineberg HV, Colditz GA. Geographic latitude and the efficacy of bacillus Calmette-Guérin vaccine. *Clin Infect Dis* 1995;20:982–991.
26. Pönninghaus JM, Fine PEM, Sterne JAC, et al. Efficacy of BCG vaccine against leprosy and tuberculosis in northern Malawi. *Lancet* 1992;339:636–639.
27. Karonga Prevention Trial Group. Randomised controlled trial of single BCG, repeated BCG, or combined BCG, and killed *Mycobacterium leprae* vaccine for prevention of leprosy and tuberculosis in Malawi. *Lancet* 1996;348:17–24.
28. Rieder HL. Repercussions of the Karonga prevention trial for tuberculosis control. *Lancet* 1996;348:4.
29. Villar J, Carroli G, Belizán JM. Predictive ability of meta-analyses of randomised controlled trials. *Lancet* 1995;345:772–776.
30. Colditz GA, Berkey CS, Mosteller F, et al. The efficacy of Bacillus Calmette-Guérin vaccination of newborns and infants in the prevention of tuberculosis: meta-analyses of the published literature. *Pediatrics* 1995;96:29–35.
31. Romanus V. Childhood tuberculosis in Sweden: an epidemiological study made six years after the cessation of general BCG vaccination of the newborn. *Tubercle* 1983;64:101–110.
32. Romanus V, Svensson A, Hallander HO. The impact of changing BCG coverage on tuberculosis incidence in Swedish-born children between 1969 and 1989. *Tuberc Lung Dis* 1992;73:150–161.
33. Trnka L, Dankova D, Svandova E. Six years' experience with the discontinuation of BCG vaccination: risk of tuberculosis infection and disease. *Tuberc Lung Dis* 1993;74:167–172.
34. Tala-Heikkilä MM, Tuominen JE, Tala EOJ. Bacillus Calmette-Guérin revaccination questionable with low tuberculosis incidence. *Am J Respir Crit Care Med* 1998;157:1324–1327.
35. International Union Against Tuberculosis and Lung Disease. Criteria for discontinuation of vaccination programmes using Bacille Calmette-Guérin (BCG) in countries with a low prevalence of tuberculosis. *Tuber Lung Dis* 1994;75:179–181.
36. Sutherland I. Epidemiology of tuberculosis. Is preventing better than treating? (French). *Bull Int Union Tuberc* 1981;56:127–128.
37. Brewer TF, Colditz GA. Bacille Calmette–Guérin vaccination for the prevention of tuberculosis in health care workers. *Clin Infect Dis* 1995;20:136–142.
38. Greenberg PD, Lax KG, Schechter CB. Tuberculosis in house staff: a decision analysis comparing the tuberculin screening strategy with the BCG vaccination. *Am Rev Respir Dis* 1980;143:490–495.
39. Marcus AM, Rose DN, Sacks HS, Schechter CB. BCG vaccination to prevent tuberculosis in health care workers: a decision analysis. *Prevent Med* 1997;26: 201–207.
40. Stevens JP, Daniel TM. Bacille Calmette Guérin immunization of health care workers exposed to multidrug-resistant tuberculosis: a decision analysis. *Tuber Lung Dis* 1996;77:315–321.
41. Centers for Disease Control and Prevention. Immunization of health-care workers. *MMWR* 1997;46:1– 42.
42. Menzies R, Vissandjee B. Effect of Bacille Calmette-Guérin vaccination on tuberculin reactivity. *Am Rev Respir Dis* 1992;145:621–625.
43. Menzies R, Vissandjee B, Rocher I, St Germain Y. The booster effect in two-step tuberculin testing among young adults in Montreal. *Ann Intern Med* 1994; 120:190–198.
44. Sepulveda RL, Ferrer X, Latrach C, Sorensen RU. The influence of Calmette-Guérin bacillus immunization on the booster effect of tuberculin testing in healthy young adults. *Am Rev Respir Dis* 1990;142:24–28.
45. Miret-Cuadras P, Pina-Gutierrez JM, Juncosa S. Tuberculin reactivity in Bacillus Calmette-Guérin vaccinated subjects. *Tuberc Lung Dis* 1996;77:52–58.
46. Barrett-Connor E. The epidemiology of tuberculosis in physicians. *JAMA* 1979;241:33–38.
47. Geisler PJ, Nelson KE, Crispen RG. Tuberculosis in physicians. Compliance with preventive measures. *Am Rev Respir Dis* 1987;135:3–9.
48. Miller B, Snider DE Jr. Physician noncompliance with tuberculosis preventive measures. *Am Rev Respir Dis* 1987;135:1–2.
49. Krebs A, Farer LS, Snider WE, Thompson NJ. Five years of follow-up of the IUAT trial of isoniazid pro-

phylaxis in fibrotic lesions. *Bull Int Union Against Tuberc* 1979;54:65–69.
50. Brewer MA, Edwards KM, Palmer PS, Hinson HP. Bacille Calmette-Guérin immunization in normal healthy adults. *J Infect Dis* 1994;170:476–479.
51. Lotte A, Wasz-Hockert O, Poisson N, Dumitrescu N, Verron M, Couvet E. BCG complications. Estimates of the risks among vaccinated subjects and statistical analysis of their main characteristics. In: Fox W, Grosset J, Styblo K, eds. *Advances in tuberculosis research.* Basel: Karger, 1984:107–193.
52. Rudin CH, Amacher A, Berglund A. Anaphylactoid reaction to BCG vaccination. *Lancet* 1991;337:377.
53. van Assendelft AHW. BCG anaphylaxis. *Tubercle* 1986;67:233–235.
54. Kröger L, Brander E, Korppi M, et al. Osteitis after newborn vaccination with three different Bacillus Calmette-Guérin vaccines: twenty-nine years of experience. *Pediatr Infect Dis J* 1994;12:113–116.
55. Kröger L, Korppi M, Brander E, et al. Osteitis caused by Bacille Calmette-Guérin vaccination: a retrospective analysis of 222 cases. *J Infect Dis* 1995;172: 574–576.
56. Castro-Rodriguez JA, González R, Girardi G. Osteitis caused by Bacille Calmette-Guérin vaccination: an emergent problem in Chile? *Int J Tuberc Lung Dis* 1997;1:417–421.
57. Mori T, Yamauchi Y, Shiozawa K. Lymph node swelling due to bacille Calmette-Guérin vaccination with multipuncture method. *Tuberc Lung Dis* 1996;77: 269–273.
58. Talbot EA, Perkins MD, Silva SFM, Frothingham R. Disseminated Bacille Calmette-Guérin disease after vaccination: case report and review. *Clin Infect Dis* 1997;24:1139–1146.
59. Lamm DL, Blumenstein BA, Crawford ED, et al. A randomized trial of intravesical doxorubicin and immunotherapy with Bacille Calmette-Guérin for transitional-cell carcinoma of the bladder. *N Engl J Med* 1991;325:1205–1209.
60. Lamm DL. Complications of bacillus Calmette-Guerin immunotherapy. *Urol Clin North Am* 1992;19:565–572.
61. McParland C, Cotton DJ, Gowda KS, Hoeppner VH, Martin WT, Weckworth PF. Miliary *Mycobacterium bovis* induced by intravesical Bacille Calmette-Guérin immunotherapy. *Am Rev Respir Dis* 1992;146:1330–1333.
62. Palayew M, Briedis D, Libman M, Michel RP, Levy RD. Disseminated infection after intravesical BCG immunotherapy. Detection of organisms in pulmonary tissue. *Chest* 1993;104:307–309.
63. Israel-Biet D, Venet A, Sandron D, Ziza JM, Chretien J. Pulmonary complications of intravesical Bacille Calmette-Guérin immunotherapy. *Am Rev Respir Dis* 1987;135:763–765.
64. Civen R, Berlin G, Panosian C. Vertebral osteomyelitis after intravesical administration of bacille Calmette-Guérin. *Clin Infect Dis* 1994;18:1013–1014.
65. Fishman JR, Walton DT, Flynn NM, Benson DR, deVere White RW. Tuberculosis spondylitis as a complication of intravesical Bacillus Calmette-Guérin therapy. *J Urol* 1993;149:584–587.
66. Morgan MB, Iseman MD. *Mycobacterium bovis* vertebral osteomyelitis as a complication of intravesical administration of Bacille Calmette-Guérin. *Am J Med* 1996;100:372–373.
67. Marans HY, Bekirov HM. Granulomatous hepatitis following intravesical bacillus Calmette-Guerin therapy for bladder carcinoma. *J Urol* 1987;137:111–112.
68. Proctor DD, Chopra S, Rubenstein SC, Jokela JA, Uhl L. Mycobacteremia and granulomatous hepatitis following initial intravesical bacillus Calmette-Guerin instillation for bladder carcinoma. *Am J Gastroenterol* 1993;88:1112–1115.
69. Leebeek FWG, Ouwendijk RJT, Kolk AHJ, et al. Granulomatous hepatitis caused by bacillus Calmette-Guerin (BCG) infection after BCG bladder instillation. *Gut* 1996;38:616–618.
70. Kesten S, Title L, Mullen B, Grossman R. Pulmonary disease following intravesical BCG treatment. *Thorax* 1990;45:709–710.
71. Gupta RC, Lavengood R Jr, Smith JP. Miliary tuberculosis due to intravesical Bacillus Calmette-Guérin therapy. *Chest* 1988;94:1296–1298.
72. LeMense GP, Strange C. Granulomatous pneumonitis following intravesical BCG. What therapy is needed? *Chest* 1994;106:1624–1626.
73. Small PM. *Molecular epidemiology of TB cases in San Francisco.* Paper presented at the World Congress on Tuberculosis, Bethesda, MD, 1992.
74. Alland D, Kalkut GE, Moss AR, et al. Transmission of tuberculosis in New York City. An analysis by DNA fingerprinting and conventional epidemiologic methods. *N Engl J Med* 1994;330:1710–1716.
75. van Deutekom H, Gerritsen JJJ, van Soolingen D, van Ameijden EJC, van Embden JDA, Coutinho RA. A molecular epidemiological approach to studying the transmission of tuberculosis in Amsterdam. *Clin Infect Dis* 1997;25:1071–1077.
76. Friedman CR, Quinn GC, Kreiswirth BN, et al. Widespread dissemination of a drug-susceptible strain of *Mycobacterium tuberculosis. J Infect Dis* 1997;176: 478–484.
77. Frieden TR, Woodley CL, Crawford JT, Lew D, Dooley SM. The molecular epidemiology of tuberculosis in New York City: the importance of nosocomial transmission and laboratory error. *Tubercle Lung Dis* 1996;77:407–413.
78. Barnes PF, El-Hajj H, Preston-Martin S, et al. Transmission of tuberculosis among the urban homeless. *JAMA* 1996;275:305–307.
79. Nettleman MD. Use of BCG vaccine in shelters for the homeless. A decision analysis. *Chest* 1993;103:1087–1090.
80. Burman WJ, Reves RR, Hawkes AP, et al. DNA fingerprinting with two probes decreases clustering of *Mycobacterium tuberculosis. Am J Respir Crit Care Med* 1997;155:1140–1146.
81. Farga V. A turning point in the fight against tuberculosis. *Bull Int Union Against Tuberc* 1979;54:228–229.
82. Genewein A, Telenti A, Bernasconi C, et al. Molecular approach to identifying route of transmission of tuberculosis in the community. *Lancet* 1993;342:841–844.
83. Pfyffer GE, Strässle A, Rose N, Wirth R, Brändli O, Shang H. Transmission of tuberculosis in the metropolitan area of Zurich: a 3 year survey based on DNA fingerprinting. *Eur Respir J* 1998;11:804–808.
84. Bradford WZ, Koehler J, El-Hajj H, et al. Dissemination of *Mycobacterium tuberculosis* across the San

Francisco Bay area. *J Infect Dis* 1998;177:1104–1107.

85. Kimerling ME, Benjamin WH, Lok KH, Curtis G, Dunlap NE. Restriction fragment length polymorphism screening of *Mycobacterium tuberculosis* isolates: population surveillance for targeting disease transmission in a community. *Int J Tuberc Lung Dis* 1998;2:655–662.
86. Braden CR, Templeton GL, Cave MD, et al. Interpretation of restriction fragment length polymorphism analysis of *Mycobacterium tuberculosis* isolates from a state with a large rural population. *J Infect Dis* 1997;175:1446–1452.
87. Van Soolingen D. *Use of DNA fingerprinting in the epidemiology of tuberculosis.* Dissertation, University of Utrecht, The Netherlands, 1996.
88. Yang ZH, de Haas PEW, Wachman CH, van Soolingen D, van Embden JDA, Anderson AB. Molecular epidemiology of tuberculosis in Denmark in 1992. *J Clin Microbiol* 1995;33:2077–2081.
89. Hermans PWM, Messadi F, Guebrexabher H, et al. Analysis of the population structure of *Mycobacterium tuberculosis* in Ethiopia, Tunisia, and the Netherlands: usefulness of DNA typing for global tuberculosis epidemiology. *J Infect Dis* 1995;171:1504–1513.
90. Dwyer B, Jackson K, Raios K, Sievers A, Wilshire E, Ross B. DNA restriction fragment analysis to define an extended cluster of tuberculosis in homeless men and their associates. *J Infect Dis* 1993;167:490–494.
91. Brewer TF, Heymann SJ, Colditz GA, et al. Evaluation of tuberculosis control policies using computer simulation. *JAMA* 1996;276:1898–1903.
92. Miller B, Castro KG. Sharpen available tools for tuberculosis control, but new tools needed for elimination. *JAMA* 1996;276:1916–1917.
93. Orme IM. Progress in the development of new vaccines against tuberculosis. *Int J Tuberc Lung Dis* 1997;1:95–100.
94. Donnelly JJ, Ulmer JB, Lui MA. Immunization with DNA. *J Immunol Methods* 1994;176:145–152.
95. Silva SL, Lowrie DB. A single mycobacterial protein (hsp60) expressed by a transgenic antigen-presenting cell vaccinates mice against tuberculosis. *Immunology* 1994;82:244–248.
96. Huygen K, Content J, Denis O, et al. Immunogenicity and protective efficacy of a tuberculosis DNA vaccine. *Nat Med* 1996;8:893–898.
97. Tascon RE, Colston MJ, Ragno S, Stavropoulos E, Gregory D, Lowrie DB. Vaccination against tuberculosis by DNA injection. *Nature Med* 1996;2:888–892.
98. Orme IM, Collins FM. Crossprotection against nontuberculous mycobacterial infections by *Mycobacterium tuberculosis* memory immune T lymphocytes. *J Exp Med* 1986;163:203–208.
99. Orme IM. Characteristics and specificity of acquired immunologic memory to *Mycobacterium tuberculosis* infection. *J Immunol* 1988;140:3589–3593.
100. Orme IM. Induction of nonspecific acquired resistance and delayed-type hypersensistivity, but not specific acquired resistance, in mice inoculated with nonliving mycobacterial vaccines. *Infect Immun* 1988;56:3310–3312.
101. Roberts AD, Sonnenberg MG, Ordway DJ, et al. Characteristics of protective immunity engendered by vaccination of mice with purified culture filtrate protein antigens of *Mycobacterium tuberculosis. Immunology* 1995;85:502–508.
102. Andersen P, Askgaard D, Gottschau A, Bennedsen J, Nagai S, Heron I. Identification of immunodominant antigens during infection with *Mycobacterium tuberculosis. Scand J Immunol* 1992;36:823–831.
103. Andersen P, Askgaard D, Ljungqvist L, Weis Bentzon M, Heron I. T-cell proliferative response to antigens secreted by *Mycobacterium tuberculosis. Infect Immun* 1991;59:1558–1563.
104. Andersen P. Effective vaccination of mice against *Mycobacterium tuberculosis* infection with a soluble mixture of secreted mycobacterial proteins. *Infect Immun* 1994;62:2536–2544.
105. Pal PG, Horwitz MA. Immunization with extracellular proteins of *Mycobacterium tuberculosis* induces cell-mediated immune responses and substantial protective immunity in a guinea pig model of pulmonary tuberculosis. *Infect Immun* 1992;60:4781–4792.
106. Horwitz M, Lee B, Dillon B, Harth G. Protective immunity against tuberculosis induced by vaccination with major extracellular proteins of *Mycobacterium tuberculosis. Proc Natl Acad Sci USA* 1995;92:1530–1534.
107. Harth G, Lee B-Y, Horwitz MA. High-level heterologous expression and secretion in rapidly growing non-pathogenic mycobacteria of four major *Mycobacterium tuberculosis* extracellular proteins considered to be leading vaccine candidates and drug targets. *Infect Immun* 1997;65:2321–2328.
108. McAdam RA, Weisbrod TR, Martin J, et al. In vivo growth characteristics of leucine and methionine auxotrophic mutants of *Mycobacterium bovis* BCG generated by transposon mutagenesis. *Infect Immun* 1995;63:1004–1012.
109. Bange FC, Brown AM, Jacobs WR. Leucine auxotrophy restricts growth of *Mycobacterium bovis* BCG in macrophages. *Infect Immun* 1996;64:1794–1799.
110. Guleria I, Teitelbaum R, McAdam RA, Kalpana G, Jacobs WR Jr, Bloom BR. Auxotrophic vaccines for tuberculosis. *Nature Med* 1996;2:334–337.
111. Stover CK, Bansal GP, Hanson MS, et al. Protective immunity elicited by recombinant bacille Calmette-Guerin (BCG) expressing outer surface protein A (OspA) lipoprotein: a candidate Lyme disease vaccine. *J Exp Med* 1993;178:197–209.
112. Abdelhak S, Louzir H, Timm J, et al. Recombinant BCG expressing the *Leishmania* surface antigen Gp63 indices protective immunity against *Leishmania* major infection in Balb/c mice. *Microbiology* 1995;141:1585–1592.
113. Winter N, Lagranderie M, Gangloff S, Leclerc C, Gheorghiu M, Gicquel B. Recombinant BCG strains expressing the SIVmac251 *nef* gene induce proliferative and CTL responses against *nef* synthetic peptides in mice. *Vaccine* 1995;13:471–478.
114. Nathan CF, Kaplan G, Levis WR, et al. Local and systemic effects of intradermal recombinant interferon-γ in patients with lepromatous leprosy. *N Engl J Med* 1986;315:6–15.
115. Sampaio EP, Moreira AL, Sarno EN, Malta AM, Kaplan G. Prolonged treatment with recombinant interferon γ induces erythema nodusum leprosum in lepromatous leprosy patients. *J Exp Med* 1992;175:1729–1737.

116. Kaplan G. Recent advances in cytokine therapy in leprosy. *J Infect Dis* 1993;167:S18–S22.
117. Holland SN, Eisenstein EM, Kuhns DB, et al. Treatment of refractory disseminated nontuberculous mycobacterial infection with interferon gamma. *N Engl J Med* 1994;330:1348–1355.
118. Chatte G, Panteix G, Perrin-Fayolle M, Pacheco Y. Aerosolized interferon gamma for *Mycobacterium avium* complex lung disease. *Am J Respir Crit Care Med* 1995;152:1094–1096.
119. Raad I, Hachem R, Leeds N, Sawaya R, Salem Z, Atweh S. Use of adjunctive treatment with interferon-γ in an immunocompromised patient who had refractory multidrug-resistant tuberculosis of the brain. *Clin Infect Dis* 1996;22:572–574.
120. Condos R, Rom WM, Schluger NW. Treatment of multidrug-resistant pulmonary tuberculosis with interferon-γ via aerosol. *Lancet* 1997;349:1513–1515.
121. Giosué S, Casarini M, Alemanno L, et al. Effects of aerosolized interferon-α in patients with pulmonary tuberculosis. *Am J Respir Crit Care Med* 1998;158:1156–1162.
122. Miller R, Birmachu W, Gerster J, et al. Imiquimod: cytokine induction and antiviral activity. *Int Antiviral News* 1995;3:111–113.
123. Goldstein D, Hertzog P, Tomkinson E, et al. Administration of Imiquimod, an interferon inducer, in asymptomatic human immunodeficiency virus-infected persons to determine safety and biologic response modification. *J Infect Dis* 1998;178:858–861.
124. Bermudez LE, Petrofsky M, Wu M, Young LS. Clarithromycin significantly improves interleukin-12–mediated anti-*Mycobacterium avium* activity and abolishes toxicity in mice. *J Infect Dis* 1998;178:896–899.
125. Steward WP. Granulocyte and granulocyte–macrophage colony-stimulating factors. *Lancet* 1993;342:153–157.
126. Bermudez LE, Kemper CA, Deresinski SC. Dysfunctional monocytes from a patient with disseminated *Mycobacterium kansasii* infection are activated in vitro and in vivo by GM-CSF. *Biotherapy* 1995;8:135–142.
127. Kemper CA, Bermudez LE, Deresinski SC. Immunomodulatory treatment of *Mycobacterium avium* complex bacteremia in patients with AIDS by use of recombinant granulocyte–macrophage colony-stimulating factor. *J Infect Dis* 1998;177:914–920.
128. Willoughby DA, Wood C, eds. Forum on immunotherapy. The history and development of levamisole. *R Soc Med* 1977;1:3–11.
129. Yaseen NY, Thewaini AJ, Al-Tawil NG, Jazrawi FY. Trial of immunopotentiation by levamisole in patients with pulmonary tuberculosis. *J Infect* 1980;2:125–136.
130. Singh MM, Kumar P, Malaviya AN, Kumar R. Levamisole as an adjunct in the treatment of pulmonary tuberculosis. *Am Rev Respir Dis* 1981;123:277–279.
131. A Kenyan/Zambia/British Medical Research Council Collaborative Study. Controlled clinical trial of levamisole in short-course chemotherapy for pulmonary tuberculosis. *Am Rev Respir Dis* 1989;140:990–995.
132. Lawrence HS. Transfer factor. *Adv Immunol* 1969;11:195–266.
133. Levin AS, Spitler LE, Stites DP, Fudenberg HH. Wiskott-Aldrich syndrome, a genetically determined cellular immunologic deficiency: clinical and laboratory responses to therapy with transfer factor. *Proc Natl Acad Sci USA* 1970;67:821–828.
134. Spitler LE, Levin AS, Stites DP, et al. The Wiskott-Aldrich syndrome. Results of transfer factor therapy. *J Clin Invest* 1972;51:3216–3224.
135. Schulking MD, Adler WH III, Altemeier WA III, Ayoub EM. Transfer factor in the treatment of a case of chronic mucocutaneous candidiasis. *Cell Immunol* 1972;3:606–615.
136. Pabst HF, Swanson R. Successful treatment of candidiasis with transfer factor. *Br Med J* 1972;2:442–443.
137. Kirkpatrick CH, Rich RR, Bennett JE. Chronic mucocutaneous candidiasis: model-building in cellular immunity. *Ann Intern Med* 1971;74:955–978.
138. Bullock WE, Fields JP, Brandriss MW. An evaluation of transfer factor as immunotherapy for patients with lepromatous leprosy. *N Engl J Med* 1972;287:1053–1059.
139. Graybill JR, Silva J Jr, Alford RH, Thor DE. Immunologic and clinical improvement of progressive coccidioidomycosis following adminstration of transfer factor. *Cell Immunol* 1973;8:120–135.
140. Whitcomb ME, Rocklin RE. Transfer factor therapy in a patient with progressive primary tuberculosis. *Ann Intern Med* 1973;79:161–166.
141. Thestrup-Pedersen K, Thulin H, Zachariae H. Transfer factor applied to intensify the cell-mediated immunological reactions against *Mycobacterium avium. Acta Allergol* 1974;29:101–116.
142. Dwyer JM, Gerstenhaber BJ, Dobuler KJ. Clinical and immunologic response to antigen-specific transfer factor drug-resistant infection with *Mycobacterium xenopi. Am J Med* 1983;74:161–168.
143. Fudenberg HH, Wilson GB, Smith CL. Immunotherapy with dialyzable leukocyte extracts and studies of their antigen-specifc (transfer factor) activity. *Proc Virchow-Pirquet Med Soc* 1980;34:3–87.
144. Rubinstein A, Melamed J, Rodescu D. Transfer factor treatment in a patient with progressive tuberculosis. *Clin Immunol Immunopathol* 1977;8:39–50.
145. Hirsch CS, Ellner JJ, Blinkhorn R, Toossi Z. In vitro restoration of T cell responses in tuberculosis and augmentation of monocyte effector function against *Mycobacterium tuberculosis* by natural inhibitors of transforming growth factor β. *Proc Natl Acad Sci USA* 1997;94:3926–3931.
146. Grange JM, Stanford JL, Rook GAH, Onyebujoh P, Bretscher PA. Tuberculosis and HIV: light after darkness. *Thorax* 1994;49:537–539.
147. Mosmann TR. Regulation of immune responses by T-cells with different cytokine secretor phenotypes. Role of new cytokines: cytokine synthesis inhibitor factors (IL-10). *Int Arch Allergy Appl Immunol* 1991;94:110–115.
148. Sher A, Gazzinelli RT, Oswald IP, et al. Role of T-cell derived cytokines in the down regulation of immune responses in parasitic and retroviral infection. *Immunol Rev* 1992;127:183–204.
149. Grange JM. Immunotherapy of tuberculosis. *Tubercle* 1990;71:237–239.
150. Bahr GM, Shaaban MA, Gabriel M, et al. Improved immunotherapy for pulmonary tuberculosis with *Mycobacterium vaccae. Tubercle* 1990;71:259–266.
151. Stanford JL, Shield MJ, Rook GAW. Hypothesis 1. How environmental mycobacteria may predetermine the protective efficacy of BCG. *Tubercle* 1981;62:55–62.

152. Rook GAW, Bahr GM, Stanford JL. Hypothesis 2. The effect of two distinct forms of cell-mediated response to mycobacteria on the protective efficacy of BCG. *Tubercle* 1981;62:63–68.
153. Stanford JL. Koch's phenomenon: can it be corrected? *Tubercle* 1991;72:241–249.
154. Hernandez-Pando R, Rook GAW. The role of TNF-α in T-cell mediated inflammation depends on the Th1/Th2 cytokine balance. *Immunology* 1994;82:591–595.
155. Stanford JL, Grange JM. New concepts for the control of tuberculosis in the twenty-first century. *J Coll Physicians Lond* 1993;27:218–223.
156. Etemadi A, Farid R, Stanford JL. Immunotherapy for drug-resistant tuberculosis (letter). *Lancet* 1992;340: 1360–1361.
157. Stanford JL, Grange JM, Pozniak A. Is Africa lost? *Lancet* 1991;338:557–558.
158. Stanford JL. *Recent experience with M. vaccae immunotherapy for tuberculosis.* Paper presented at the Frontiers in Mycobacteriology Symposium, Vail, Colorado, 1997.
159. Glatman-Freedman A, Casadevall A. Serum therapy for tuberculosis revisited: reappraisal of the role of antibody-mediated immunity against *Mycobacterium tuberculosis. Clin Microbiol Rev* 1998;11:514–532.
160. Sampaio EP, Sarno EN, Galilly R, Cohn ZA, Kaplan G. Thalidomide selectively inhibits tumor necrosis factor a production by stimulated human monocytes. *J Exp Med* 1991;173:699–703.
161. Moreira AL, Sampaio EP, Zmuidzinas A, Frindt P, Smith KA, Kaplan G. Thalidomide exerts its inhibitory action on tumor necrosis factor α by enhancing mRNA degradation. *J Exp Med* 1993;177:1675–1680.
162. Moller DR, Wysocka M, Greenlee BM. Inhibition of IL-12 production by thalidomide. *J Immunol* 1997; 159:5157–5161.
163. Tramontana JM, Utaipat U, Molloy A, et al. Thalidomide treatment reduces tumor necrosis factor α production and enhances weight gain in patients with pulmonary tuberculosis. *Mol Med* 1995;1:384–397.
164. Tsenova L, Sokol K, Freedman VH, Kaplan G. A combination of thalidomide plus antibiotics protects rabbits from mycobacterial meningitis-associated death. *J Infect Dis* 1998;177:1563–1572.
165. Paterson DL, Georghiou PR, Allworth AM, Kemp RJ. Thalidomide as treatment of refractory aphthous ulceration related to human immunodeficiency virus infection. *Clin Infect Dis* 1995;20:250–254.
166. Reyes-Teran G, Sierra-Madero JG, Martinez del Cerro V. Effects of thalidomide on HIV-associated wasting syndrome: a randomized, double-blind, placebo-controlled clinical trial. *AIDS* 1996;10:1501–1507.
167. Stambe C, Wicks IP. TNFα and response of treatment-resistant adult-onset Still's disease to thalidomide. *Lancet* 1998;352:544–545.
168. Hamuryudan V, Mat C, Saip S, et al. Thalidomide in the treatment of mucocutaneous lesions of the Behçet syndrome. A randomized, double-blind, placebo-controlled trial. *Ann Intern Med* 1998;128:443–450.
169. Gori A, Franzetti F, Marchetti G, et al. Clinical and immunological improvement in a patient who received thalidomide treatment for refractory *Mycobacterium avium* complex infection. *Clin Infect Dis* 1998;26: 184–185.
170. Haslett P, Tramontana J, Burroughs M, Hempstead M, Kaplan G. Adverse reactions to thalidomide in patients infected with human immunodeficiency virus. *Clin Infect Dis* 1997;24:1223–1227.
171. Strieter RM, Remick DG, Ward PA, et al. Cellular and molecular regulation of tumor necrosis factor-alpha production by pentoxifylline. *Biochem Biophys Res Commun* 1988;155:1230–1236.
172. Zeni F, Pain P, Vindimian M, et al. Effects of pentoxifylline on circulating cytokine concentrations and hemodynamics in patients with septic shock: results from a double-blind, randomized, placebo-controlled study. *Crit Care Med* 1996;24:207–214.
173. Loftis LL, Meals EA, English BK. Differential effects of pentoxifylline and interleukin-10 on production of tumor necrosis factor and inducible nitric oxide synthase by murine macrophages. *J Infect Dis* 1997; 175:1008–1011.
174. Dezube BJ. Pentoxifylline for the treatment of infection with human immunodeficiency virus. *Clin Infect Dis* 1994;18:285–287.
175. Dezube BJ, Lederman MM, Spritzler JG, et al. High-dose pentoxifylline in patients with AIDS: inhibition of tumor necrosis factor production. *J Infect Dis* 1995;171:1628–1632.
176. Dooley DP, Carpenter JL, Rademacher S. Adjunctive corticosteroid therapy for tuberculosis: a critical reappraisal of the literature. *Clin Infect Dis* 1997;25: 872–887.
177. Takizawa H, Suko M, Shoji S, et al. Granulomatous pneumonitis induced by bacille Calmette-Guérin in the mouse and its treatment with cyclosporin A. *Am Rev Respir Dis* 1986;134:296–299.
178. Rodrigues LC, Smith PG. Tuberculosis in developing countries and methods for its control. *Trans R Soc Trop Med Hyg* 1990;84:739–744.
179. Fine PEM. BCG vaccination against tuberculosis and leprosy. *Br Med Bull* 1988;44:691–703.
180. Rodrigues LC, Gill ON, Smith PG. BCG vaccination in the first year of life protects children of Indian subcontinent ethnic origin against tuberculosis in England. *J Epidemiol Comm Health* 1990;45:78–80.
181. Houston S, Fanning A, Soskolne C, Fraser N. The effectiveness of Bacillus Calmette-Guerin (BCG) vaccination against tuberculosis. A case-controlled study in Treaty Indians, Alberta, Canada. *Am J Epidemiol* 1990;131:340–348.
182. Murthag K. Efficacy of BCG. *Lancet* 1980;i:423.
183. Capewell S, Leitch AG. The value of contact procedures for tuberculosis in Edinburgh. *Br J Dis Chest* 1984;78:317–329.
184. Mori T, Takizawa H, Aoki M, Shimao T. Tuberculous meningitis in Japan. *Bull Int Un Tuberc* 1984;59: 201.
185. Romanus V. Childhood tuberculosis in Sweden. *Bull Int Union Against Tuberc* 1984;59:193.
186. Sutherland I, Springett VH. Effectiveness of BCG vaccination in England and Wales in 1983. *Tubercle* 1987;68:81–92.

14

Preventing Transmission of Tuberculosis within Institutions

Tuberculosis is transmitted typically by aerial dissemination of small particles, which are inhaled by individuals who share the air in a closed environment with persons with active disease (see Chapter 3). In most cases, such transmission occurs within homes or other private settings. However, large outbreaks with high rates of infection and extensive disease have occurred recently in institutional or congregate settings including hospitals, clinics, residential facilities for persons with AIDS, nursing homes, homeless shelters, drug treatment centers, and prisons. Although outbreaks of TB have occurred in schools, they are not addressed in this chapter because they are so uncommon that systematic measures to prevent their occurrence are not appropriate. Similarly, although there has been some evidence of transmission of infection during prolonged airplane flights, because of the infrequency of this occurrence and the absence of resultant disease in these studies, this topic too is not addressed.

Tuberculosis has been transmitted to other patients or clients in these facilities as well as to health care professionals, lay staff, and visitors. Recently, attention has been given to these phenomena because of two particularly adverse elements—the rising prevalence of multidrug-resistant tuberculosis involved in such outbreaks and high rates of morbidity and mortality among immunocompromised persons, particularly those with AIDS, so infected.

Although there are numerous factors involved in these recent microepidemics, common features have included the following: delayed or failed diagnosis of tuberculosis in the source case(s); closed, recirculating air systems with minimal fresh air ventilation employed (to conserve energy devoted to heating or air conditioning); highly vulnerable persons exposed including those with HIV infection, AIDS, organ transplantation, oncologic chemotherapy, substance abuse, malnutrition, and elderly persons with immunosenescence; and greatly reduced efficacy or failure of chemotherapy as a result of extensive drug resistance among source cases.

In this chapter, information regarding recent, well-studied outbreaks in a variety of facilities is reviewed, potentially useful components of institutional control programs are analyzed, recent guidelines and policies advocated by the Centers for Disease Control and Prevention (CDC), Occupational Safety and Health Administration (OSHA), and American Thoracic Society (ATS) are discussed, and various strategies regarding this problem are delineated.

RECENT INSTITUTIONAL OUTBREAKS

Throughout the twentieth century there has been a growing understanding of the means and the likelihood of transmission; these sentinel studies are reviewed in Chapter 3. Table 14.1 contains reports on more recent outbreaks in the United States that represent the modern era of institutional transmission (1–27). In addition to these specific reports, there have been other community-based surveys that, through molecular biology techniques and/or drug-resistance patterns, indicate clustering of cases in patterns suggesting some components of institutional transmission (28–32). In the New York State

TABLE 14.1. *Recent reports of institutional transmission of tuberculosis, United States*

Report	Site	HIV involved	MDR TB	Infections and/or disease	Comments
CDC, 1980 (1)	Substance abuse rehab center	No	No	40/65 (62%) infected, 7/8 children (88%) exposed had abnl CXRs	Source case ran day-care program
CDC, 1991 (2)	Substance abuse residency	Yes	MDR TB	15/69 (22%) of clients/staff converted	Failure to isolate primary case
Nardell, 1986 (3)	Men's shelter	No	Yes	22 cases clustered	INH and SM (R) strain marked spread
King, 1977 (4)	Jail	No	No	10/14 exposed (71%) converted	Probably underestimated number of infections
Stead, 1990 (5)	Prisons	Possibly	NR	17.5% conversions overall (see comments)	Conversion rates higher for blacks (27%) than whites (14%)
Nolan, 1991 (6)	Men's shelter	NR	No	20 cases clustered	Poor ventilation; higher risk for Amerinds
Daley, 1992 (7)	AIDS residency	Yes	No	11/30 (37%) of exposed developed active disease; 4 others of the 30 exposed (13%) converted	Short incubation from exposure to disease
Stead, 1981 (8)	Nursing home	No	No	49/161 (30%) residents, 21/138 (15%) employees converted; 9 cases of disease	Source case symptomatic for 1 year; delayed diagnosis
CDC, 1980 (9)	Nursing home	No	No	60/135 (44%) of residents, 30/91 (33%) of staff converted; 6 cases of disease	Delayed diagnosis and failure to use INH PT
CDC, 1983 (10)	Nursing home	No	No	56/91 (65%) residents, 38/87 (44%) of employees converted; 11 cases of disease	Delayed diagnosis and failure to use INH PT
Stead, 1990 (5)	Nursing homes	No	No	11.5% conversions overall (see comments)	Higher conversion rates among blacks (15%) than whites (10%)
Ehrenkranz, 1972 (11)	Hospital	No	No	21/60 (35%) and 2/19 (11%) of HCWs on separate wards converted	Possible spread through ventilation system
Catanzaro, 1982 (12)	Hospital (ICU)	No	No	10/13 (77%) at bronchoscopy, 4/32 (13%) elsewhere, HCWs converted	Smear-neg. case, but at bronch, calculated 1 infectious quantum/69 cu ft of air
Kantor, 1988 (13)	Hospital	No	No	9/56 (16%) HCWs infected; 3/9 developed disease	Poor ventilation noted

Hutton, 1990 (14)	Hospital OR/wards	No	No	14% to 85% of HCWs infected, dependent on time/circumstances; 9 active cases	Soft-tissue abscess; aerosols secondary to dressing changes and debridement (see Chapter 3)
Frampton, 1992 (15)	Hospital OR/wards	No	No	11/59 (19%) of exposed HCWs converted; 2 cases of disease	Convertors present at dressing change or debridement
Edlin, 1991 (16)	Hospital	Yes	Yes	14 cases clustered	Inadequate ventilation
Dooley, 1992 (17)	Hospital (Puerto Rico)	Yes	NS	8/48 (17%) of exposed HIV-positive persons developed active TB; high rates of PPD reactivity among exposed HCWs	Short incubation period from exposure to disease
Pearson, 1992 (18)	Hospital	Yes	Yes	11/32 (34%) of exposed HCWs converted; 23 clustered cases	Failure to isolate cases; inadequate ventilation
Fischl, 1992 (19)	Clinic/hospital	Yes	Yes	44 cases assoc. with clinic; 22 cases were contacts to one patient	Higher rates of MDR TB in gay, white males suggest recent transmission
Beck-Sagué, 1992 (20)	Clinic/hospital	Yes	Yes	13/39 (33%) of exposed HCWs converted	Conversion rate related to exposure to smear-positive cases
Jereb, 1995 (21)	Hospital	Yes	Yes	20–23% of exposed HCWs converted; 6 cases of disease	Inadequate isolation practices and ventilation
Ikeda, 1995 (22)	Hospital (prison)	Yes	Yes	20–29% of HCWs on two wards infected; several cases of disease	Prisoner with MDR TB infected guard at prison and HCWs at hospital
Haley, 1989 (23)	ER hospital	No	No	15/44 (34%) of exposed HCWs converted; 5 other HCWs developed active disease	HCWs knew of exposure; infections occurred despite use of surgical masks
Griffith, 1995 (24)	ER/ward hospital	No	No	13/17 (76%) of exposed HCWs converted; 3 of these developed active disease	High risk associated with endotracheal intubation
Templeton, 1995 (25)	Hospital/morgue	No	No	0/40 (0%) of HCWs exposed on ward converted; 5/5 (100%) of those exposed at autopsy converted	Sputum negative antemortem; dissem TB found at autopsy; aerosol ascribed to bone saw; 1 infectious quantum/3.5 cu ft
Frieden, 1996 (26)	Hospitals	Yes	Yes	267 cases of MDR TB (strain W) traced in NYC; 67% of these were probably acquired in 11 hospitals	86% or more of cases associated with AIDS; all cause mortality, 83% within 43 months
Kenyon, 1997 (27)	Hospital	Yes	Yes	11/74 (15%) of exposed HCWs converted [1 HCW with AIDS developed disease]; 5 patients also acquired MDR TB	Room's positive pressure appeared to cause spread to HCWs; the most infectious case had a "normal" CXR

prisons, the annual incidence of tuberculosis rose from 15.4 per 100,000 in 1976–1978 to 105.5 cases in 1986; the risk for tuberculosis was significantly associated with AIDS in this setting (33). Although institutional spread of infections was not documented in this report, recent transmission within such facilities must have been responsible for a substantial component of this increase.

Outside the United States, recent studies of institutional transmission and nosocomial tuberculosis among patients and HCWs have been reported from Italy (34,35) and France (36,37). Indeed, a recent report from Buenos Aires, Argentina was an institutionally spread outbreak of MDR TB second in morbidity and mortality only to New York City (38). In a large referral hospital that served both complicated HIV and tuberculosis cases, 101 patients with MDR TB were seen over 18 months from 1994 to 1995; 68 cases were proven to reflect on-site exposure. This five-drug-resistant organism, termed strain M, was associated with a median survival of only 33 days from date of diagnosis. In 1998 an extensive prison-based outbreak in The General Penetentiary of Madrid, Spain was described (39). Using genetic fingerprinting techniques, it was shown that 74% of cases studied were clustered and that 62% of these cases reflected recent transmission, presumably within the prison. During this outbreak, which occurred in 1993–1994, case rates in the prison doubled within 2 years, reaching the phenomenal level of 2,283 cases/100,000/year. Notable features of this epidemic included nearly comparable risks for those with or without HIV infection, the apparent contribution of noncompliance with treatment to the propagation of transmission, and relatively low levels of drug-resistant strains involved. The authors concluded that, "Perhaps no other form of congregate living carries the risk for *M. tuberculosis* transmission found in today's prisons."

In summary, considerable evidence exists to document transmission of tuberculosis in congregate settings to patients, clients, and staff. Because of the accelerated progression to active disease in immunocompromised persons, routine prevention methods that rely on surveillance by tuberculin skin testing and preventive chemotherapy, although essential, are not sufficient. Also, with the apparent predilection of HIV/AIDS patients for MDR TB (40), preventive chemotherapy may not be feasible for either patients or HCWs exposed in these settings. Thus, improved programs to limit transmission are imperative.

PREVENTING TRANSMISSION

In the broad sense, prevention may be viewed in the following components: early suspicion leading to aggressive efforts at diagnosis, prompt initiation of effective chemotherapy, physical isolation, dilution of the air to limit the concentration of potentially infectious particles, germicidal ultraviolet irradiation of the air to reduce the number of viable bacilli, physical filtration to remove bacilli from the air, and respiratory protective devices to filter out infectious particles from inhaled air. Depending on circumstances, resources, and the scale of the local problem, variable combinations of these tactics may be appropriate for institutions in which tuberculosis transmission is potentially problematic.

Principles of Transmission

In Chapter 3, the general scientific understanding of airborne transmission is reviewed in detail. In brief, animal model studies as well as empirical clinical observations indicate that most new infections occur when an individual inhales microscopic aerosolized particles containing tubercle bacilli. In the vast majority of instances, these particles presumably are elaborated by expiratory maneuvers (such as coughing, sneezing, or singing) by a patient with respiratory tract tuberculosis. However, aerosols may be generated by any physical agitation of tissue or fluids containing the mycobacteria—soft tissue debridement, wound irrigation, or autopsy (see Chapter 3 for details).

Because of the slow replication time and limited tissue-invading capacity of tubercle bacilli, these particles are *much* more likely to infect if they are deposited in the alveoli at the end of the complex respiratory tree. It is sometimes said that the particles *must* reach the alveoli. This derives in part from the belief that the bacilli must be engulfed by a mononuclear phagocyte in order to commence multiplication. Although this is more likely to occur with alveolar deposition, it has not been excluded that invasion might occur with deposition in inflamed airways in which there is macrophage traffic. In order to traverse the ramifying bronchial tree, these particles must be so tiny that they drift with the inspired air rather than impact on the mucous membranes of the proximal airways. Particles less than 10 μm in diameter are capable of behaving in this manner, and it is generally believed that it is the dehydrated residuals of aerosolized particles, droplet nuclei of roughly 0.5 to 5 μm, that are the usual vectors of infection.

The size of particles liberated from a gas–liquid interface is related to the velocity of the air current moving over the liquid surface: the faster the current, the smaller the particle size. However, because of evaporation, particles in the air rapidly lose volume; thus, even larger particles, which are relatively more common in respiratory aerosols, may shrink to the size requisite for transmission if they remain suspended. When larger droplets fall on a surface, they are likely to be physically complexed by miscellaneous debris, forming particles so large that, even if propelled into the air again, they seem very unlikely to be deposited in the distal air spaces.

Potential Means to Control Transmission

The 1990 (41) and 1994 CDC documents (42) on the prevention of transmission in health-care settings enumerate various recommendations or programs to help achieve this end. (Incidentally, the controversies and complexity surrounding the issue are reflected in the relative lengths of these documents: the 1990 version was 29 pages, the 1994 document 132 pages!) Administering preventive chemotherapy to persons with latent tuberculosis infection is included in these documents. Although this tactic potentially would reduce the ultimate number of tuberculosis patients admitted to various facilities, it is not relevant to immediate institutional control methods and is not discussed in this chapter.

The literature and discussions regarding this issue have been oft-times confusing and frequently rancorous. In good measure, the widely diverse attitudes, approaches, and recommendations reflect the disparate groups that have been involved (43). Historically, limiting the transmission of tuberculosis in hospitals has been the bailiwick of practitioners of tuberculosis, who based their practices on the model of Riley (see above); theirs was an empirical approach, wrapped in lore. A more recent participant in the process was the hospital-based infection control specialist. Then, with the appreciation of institutional risks to employees, the Occupational Safety and Health Administration (OSHA), a regulatory agency within the Department of Labor, and the National Institute of Occupational Safety and Health (NIOSH), a research institute within the CDC, joined the fray. Not only did the latter groups bring with them the paradigms of occupational medicine and industrial hygiene, but they came from the model of regulatory compulsion with citations and fines. To many workers in the field, this author included, the creation of rigid, mandated practices, typically in the absence of supporting data, felt like an arbitrary, even arrogant, exercise in power. Based on the anticipated expenses, perceived impracticality, and arguable lack of efficacy of some of these regulations, there was a predictable backlash. The evolution toward more appropriate, mutually agreed-on recommendations is traced below.

Early Diagnosis

Programs are advocated to aid staff in the prompt recognition of patients who, through historical, epidemiological, clinical, laboratory, or radiological features, might be deemed at particular risk of tuberculosis. Personnel involved with triage or emergency visits as well as routine hospital and clinic intake systems should have ongoing education regarding persons or groups who are most likely to present with potentially communicable tuberculosis. Relevant data might include risk profiles based on race, ethnicity, national origin, age, occupations, social history, institutional experience, substance abuse, HIV exposure, as well as clinical features suggestive of tuberculosis. Personnel should also be instructed on steps to be taken to minimize immediate risk of transmission, e.g., early isolation, covering coughs, prompt acquisition of diagnostic studies, and initiation of chemotherapy.

For selected high-risk settings with particularly high prevalences of active disease, chest x-ray screening may be appropriate. Most tuberculosis screening programs rely primarily on tuberculin skin testing. However, this technique has significant drawbacks: difficulty inducing patients/clients to return at 72 hours to read tests; delayed availability of results; diminished sensitivity (persons with advanced HIV infection or inanition from other causes are likely to be falsely nonreactive (even normal hosts with active pulmonary tuberculosis have a 20% to 25% risk of false-negative tuberculin testing); and lack of specificity (depending on the region and the group screened, a considerable portion of reactors may not be infected with *M. tuberculosis* but with other mycobacteria). Thus, tuberculin testing has diminishing credibility as a screening tool in such settings. Chest radiography has the advantages of being prompt, one-step, and generally sensitive for patients most likely to have transmissible tuberculosis (assuming timely, competent reading of x-rays). Obviously, the expense is substantial and must be weighed carefully. For instance, in jails where inmates are held for brief periods but typically there is crowding and a relatively high proportion of vulnerable exposees (including HIV-infected and injecting drug abusers), prompt identification of persons with pulmonary tuberculosis could substantially reduce institutional transmission and favorably impact the community at large as well. A similar argument could be made for selected homeless shelters. Wholesale use of these tactics would not be responsible, but for high-prevalence communities, chest radiographic screening should be carefully considered.

Prompt Isolation

The cardinal reason for early identification of patients with tuberculosis is to place them in areas where the risk of transmission may be minimized. Potential elements of isolation include negative-pressure rooms, dilution by frequent air changes, sterilization by ultraviolet germicidal irradiation, and/or filtration by devices capable of removing infectious particles. The decision to place suspected persons in isolation usually will be made on the basis of the epidemiological-historical features noted above, supplemented, when practical, by laboratory studies. However, it must be appreciated that obtaining such studies as sputum smears and chest x-rays may result in delays and entail transportation to high-risk areas. For example, sputum microscopy is relatively insensitive; smears made directly from raw sputum can only detect very large numbers of bacilli. To be optimal, microscopy should be done on sputum that has been digested, decontaminated, and concentrated by centrifugation; this process typically requires one day in current laboratories. To send a patient to the radiology department for chest films may involve an extended period of time in an area crowded with vulnerable persons. In facilities where significant numbers of tuberculosis patients are seen annually, it might therefore be prudent to have radiological facilities within the triage/emergency intake areas with negative pressure waiting and examination rooms abetted by ultraviolet germicidal irradiation systems or other engineering controls.

For patients being admitted to the hospital, current CDC or OSHA guidelines indicate that those with suspected or proven communicable tuberculosis should be housed in isolation rooms. However, because of the high ratio of suspects to actually proven cases, this means that many persons would be sent needlessly to isolation.

Administratively, a critical suspect of this process is defining a "tuberculosis suspect." A senior OSHA physician indicated in 1994 that, if a clinician considered the risk of tuberculosis to be great enough to merit ordering sputum for mycobacterial smears and culture, this patient should be deemed a suspect (44). The potential implications of this policy could be staggering. In a community with relatively low risk for tuberculosis, candidates for isolation on the basis of CDC risk factors and admission chest x-rays would have exceeded actual tuberculosis cases by 92:1 (45). The group from Grady Memorial Hospital in Atlanta reported on the evaluation of their empirical isolation practices. In their initial analysis, they described in 1995 the impact of their control program, which consisted primarily of administrative measures, on two markers of risk, (a) exposure episodes wherein a patient with potentially communicable tuberculosis comes in contact with HCWs in unsafe environments, and (b) tuberculin skin test conversion rates among HCWs (46). They noted that their measures reduced the exposure episodes from 4.4 to 0.6 per month; commensurately, TST conversions fell sequentially from 3.3% to 0.4%. Subsequently, they reported on the efficiency of their administrative measures, an expanded respiratory isolation policy (47). The initial program had resulted in empirical isolation of over 95% of patients with eventual diagnoses of tuberculosis but did so by the isolation of eight non-TB patients for each TB case. To refine their selection, they identified five criteria: (a) chest x-ray with an upper lobe infiltrate, (b) chest x-ray with a cavity, (c) a history of knowing someone with tuberculosis, (d) a reported history of TST reactivity, and (e) a reported history of INH-preventive therapy. Applying these criteria would have reduced unnecessary isolations from 253 to 95 but would have missed 19%, 8 of 42 cases, with tuberculosis. Thus, the actual practice of early isolation needs refinement with careful consideration of local historical patterns and resources. This function should fall to hospital infection control committees or specially designated tuberculosis task forces.

For the high-risk facilities other than hospitals enumerated above, policies and procedures should be developed with community or public health advisors to help identify, isolate, and expedite evaluation of persons with potentially communicable tuberculosis.

Early Initiation of Chemotherapy

The impact that initiation of chemotherapy has on the infectiousness of pulmonary tuberculosis cases was demonstrated in community studies from Madras, India (48) and Little Rock, Arkansas (49). In these similar projects, some patients were hospitalized for treatment until sputum cultures were negative, while others were never hospitalized or were treated briefly within institutions; investigation of disease (India) or infection rates (Arkansas) among their household contacts demonstrated comparable rates of morbidity in both groups of contacts. Other studies from Cincinnati (50) and Baltimore (51) confirmed that treatment prevented or rapidly blunted household transmission. The Cincinnati study involved two weeks of hospital treatment before discharge. In the Baltimore report, patients with tuberculosis were assigned to hospital or home treatment in a non-random manner. Surveillance of 25 tuberculin-negative household contacts of patients who were treated entirely at home did not indicate ongoing infectiousness. Data from the Baltimore VAH studies where guinea pigs were exposed to effluent air from the rooms of patients receiving chemotherapy also confirmed that infectiousness rapidly diminished in most cases (see Chapter 3 for details of this study).

Quantification of the numbers of viable bacilli in sputum from patients receiving modern regimens has confirmed a prompt and dramatic early reduction in counts. The first report of quantitative culture reports for patients with drug-susceptible tuberculosis receiving regimens containing isoniazid and rifampin came from New York in 1973 (52). Pretreatment cultures ranged from 1.2 million to 240 million bacilli per milliliter of sputum; following approximately 2 weeks of therapy, the number of cultivable bacilli had fallen to the range of 0 to 700,000 with reduction by 2 to 6 logs, the mean reduction being 3 $\log_{10}$ colony-forming units/ml. Similarly, a 1980 report from Africa revealed dramatic reductions in the numbers of bacilli in the sputa of patients receiving various drugs and drug combinations (53). Indeed, among those patients who received the regimen of isoniazid, rifampin, pyrazinamide, and streptomycin, the number of bacilli fell from a mean of 7.2 $\log_{10}$ CFU/ml pretreatment to roughly 4.0 logs by day 14. Notably, during the first 2 days of therapy, the mean fall in bacillary numbers was 0.44

log_{10} CFU/ day. This obviously would have immense impact on the infectivity of pulmonary tuberculosis cases. Data approximating the bacillary decline in the four patients on a four-drug regimen (isoniazid, rifampin, pyrazinamide, and streptomycin) in the African study above are displayed in Fig. 14.1. Superimposed on these numbers is another factor that alters the likelihood of transmission, the diminishing frequency of cough for patients (from another series) started on treatment (54). The data on cough frequency came from an earlier era of chemotherapy when isoniazid, streptomycin, and PAS were employed. As seen, the number of coughs per 8-hour period fell steadily, presumably exerting an additional favorable effect (above the bacillary reductions from medication), lessening the probability of generating infectious particles.

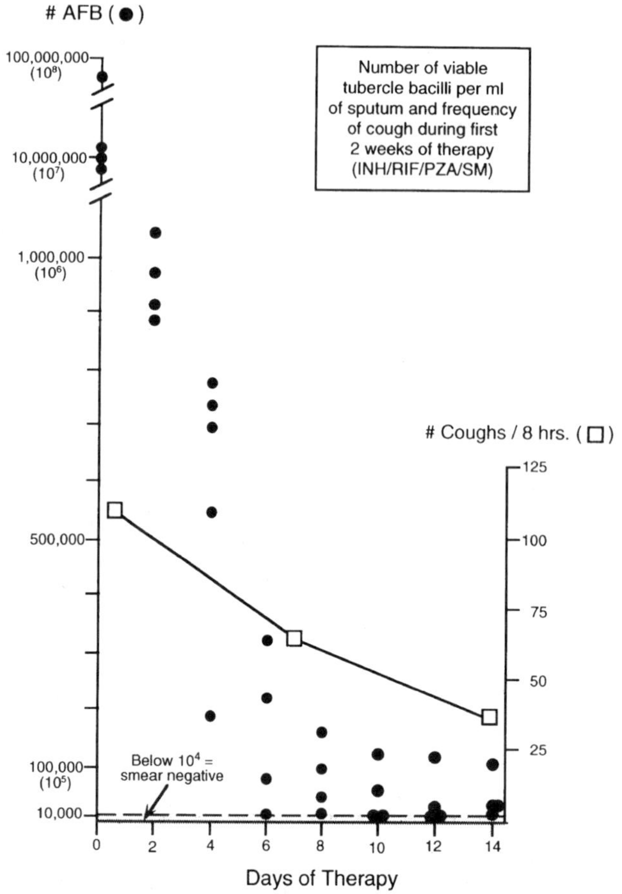

FIG. 14.1. Bacillary counts are rapidly reduced by modern chemotherapy; also, the frequency of coughing is quickly suppressed by treatment. Quantitative sputum cultures were performed on four patients receiving isoniazid, rifampin, pyrazinamide, and streptomycin for pulmonary tuberculosis (53). Before therapy, there were approximately 1 to 10 million bacilli per milliliter of sputum. Within 7 days, viable bacilli had fallen two or more logs, and by 14 days, counts were less than 10,000 in all four patients. Superimposed on this graph are data from a prior study in which patients with pulmonary tuberculosis were monitored by cough frequency during the initial 2 weeks of treatment (54). As may be seen, the introduction of chemotherapy may have two powerful effects in lessening the likelihood of transmitting tuberculosis. Hence, the likelihood of infecting contacts should diminish quickly. However, this is a generalization, not a predictable principle. Factors that might confound this model include extremely high bacillary burdens, extraordinary aerosol generation as in laryngeal tuberculosis, drug-resistant strains, nonadherence with therapy, or—possibly—exquisitely susceptible contacts.

Ventilation

Introducing fresh air into spaces inhabited by confirmed or suspected cases of tuberculosis will dilute the concentration of potential infective particles, thereby lowering the likelihood of transmission. In general, contact investigation experience as well as outbreak analyses suggest a significant impact by the volume of shared area on infectivity. The CDC currently recommends that there be 6 or more air changes per hour in isolation facilities. Industrial hygienists generally concur that introduction of fresh air creates a more comfortable environment and should be encouraged for that reason alone. As calculated by industrial hygienists, 6 air changes per hour would remove 90% of airborne contaminants in 23 minutes. However, if infectious droplets were being elaborated continuously, such a level of ventilation might still entail significant risk of exposure/infection. This principle was demonstrated in an analysis of an outbreak of office-based transmission in which a patient with cavitary, smear-positive pulmonary tuberculosis with a 4-week work exposure had resulted in new infections in 27 of 67 (40%) of tuberculin-negative fellow-workers (55). The building in which transmission occurred was ventilated at the lower range of acceptable levels, 15 cubic feet per minute (cfm) per occupant. In the model adapted by the authors to analyze this particular outbreak, increasing the ventilation to 25 cfm would have reduced infections among co-workers to 27%, while 35 cfm fresh ventilation (currently regarded as optimal) would have still resulted in 22% of the employees being infected. Thus, the utility of exogenous ventilation is limited in cases such as this wherein the source case was a particularly prolific generator of infectious aerosols.

Overall, for reasons of comfort as well as sanitation, maintaining appropriate levels of fresh ventilation is a laudable goal, 25 to 35 cubic feet per minute *per person* being an acceptable range. Certainly, for facilities where there is a predictable risk of exposure to airborne infectious diseases including tuberculosis, institutions should be encouraged to strive for fresh air introduction within the high range of that which is recommended, feasible, and affordable. However, the impracticality, both engineering and financial, of compelling all existing facilities to achieve and sustain 6 or more air changes per hour should be considered in a realistic, responsible program to limit nosocomial transmission. For some older structures in which engineering revisions might be highly complicated and expensive, widespread deployment of UVGI or air filtration systems might well provide comparable or greater levels of protection at much lower expense (56).

Ultraviolet Germicidal Irradiation

As discussed in detail in Chapter 3, UVGI has demonstrated utility in killing tubercle bacilli suspended in fine particles in the air. Indeed, it is because the particles are so tiny that there is such efficient killing: in the droplet nuclei (which are most likely to traverse to airways to initiate alveolar infection), the mycobacteria are readily exposed to the irradiation in contrast to other bacteria imbedded in dense collections of proteinaceous debris.

In the ultraviolet spectrum, there are three subtypes of UV irradiation: UV-A, wavelength band 320–400 nm; UV-B, wavelength band 290–320 nm; and UV-C, wavelength band 100–290 nm (56). UV-C embraces the wavelengths that are deemed to be germicidal, 254–260 nm. UV-A and UV-B, which are prominently represented in sunlight, have been demonstrated to cause actinic damage, skin cancer, and cataracts. By contrast, UV-C is capable of only superficial penetration of human tissue and is not believed likely to produce either cancer or cataracts. However, extended or intensive exposure can produce keratoconjunctivitis or cutaneous irritation, but these effects can be avoided with proper design (56). Current UVGI devices typically employ mercury vapor lamps with a peak wavelength of 253.7 nm and are representative of the units employed in Riley's room disinfection studies.

Riley and colleagues demonstrated substantial protection for guinea pigs (animals exquisitely vulnerable to tuberculosis) exposed to effluent air from a 6-bed unit housing patients with active tuberculosis *if* the air underwent UVGI before passage through the guinea pig cages (57). Subsequently, experiments were conducted using a nonvirulent strain of *M. bovis* BCG as a surrogate for *M. tuberculosis* to demonstrate rapid killing by UVGI of aerosolized mycobacteria in a typical patient room (58). In this study, comparable killing of BCG and virulent *M. tuberculosis* was first demonstrated in an aerosol chamber. Then, BCG was aerosolized into a room where there was seen to be a slow reduction in the number of bacilli in the air, dependent on the frequency of air changes. When upper room fixtures with UVGI were activated, there was rapid reduction in the number of viable bacilli in the air, equivalent to 12 to 37 air changes per hour.

The UVGI has been employed extensively over the past 25 years in tuberculosis clinical facilities and laboratories with the widely held perception that it was both safe and effective. Stead commented on its apparent efficacy in a tuberculosis ward in Milwaukee and homeless shelter in Arkansas (59). We also have employed an improvised UVGI system at National Jewish in Denver on our ward where large numbers of MDR TB patients have been hospitalized for extended periods (60). Following tuberculin skin test conversions in three staff persons in 1982–1983, we found that the ventilation on the ward had become unbalanced—there was less negative pressure and fewer air changes within the rooms than originally designed. Rather than perform extensive revisions of the ventilation system and windows (which leaked, causing the rooms to occasionally become positive pressure with respect to hallways), we installed UVGI active ventilation devices in each room and in common areas or lounges where the MDR TB patients congregated. In contrast to the method employed by Riley et al. in the 1976 study noted above (which employed a UV fixture in the upper room and relied on convection or movement to create air currents to bring the infectious particles into the zones that were irradiated), the National Jewish system placed the UVGI fixtures within a galvanized air duct in the false ceiling above the rooms; a fan drew the air from the room through a coarse filter (to remove dust to prevent deposition on the UV bulbs) and passed the air through roughly 8 to 10 feet of duct, wherein (because of reflectance) it was intensely irradiated during its entire travel time. The air was returned to the patient's room, presumably sterilized, but without loss of the energy previously invested in heating or cooling. In addition, there was no significant UVGI within the rooms and no reports of irritation of skin or eyes. In the now 13 years following installation of these units, there have been only three other skin test conversions among nursing and ward clerk staff who were systematically tested (we believe that two of these three conversions occurred from failure to enforce isolation policies) and none among physicians, who were less regularly surveyed (60). It should be noted, also, that during this time, personal respiratory protection was used only infrequently and optionally by the staff and that the devices employed were disposable surgical masks, which subsequently have been shown to be totally ineffective in filtering out particles of the size believed to cause tuberculosis infection (61).

Nardell and Riley have described a passive (no special efforts to move air) upper-room UVGI system that would be less costly to install, operate, and maintain than the National Jewish active-ventilation system (62). In such a system, UV-C units are placed on walls or suspended from ceilings using baffles to assure that there is minimal UV-exposure in the lower room where patients and staff would be found. A requirement for such an arrangement is that the ceiling height be at least 8 feet. Certainly, the data from Riley's 1976 study indicate that a similar system is potentially effective (58). However, to assure better air mixing within rooms housing these units, it might be desirable to augment such a system with some fans.

Although there are no controlled studies that document or quantify the protection of HCWs and other patients by UVGI, I believe that these or similar systems would be highly effective and relatively very economical in the prevention or abatement of transmission (63). As suggested previously, UVGI might well be employed within patient isolation rooms, in congregate settings where potentially infectious tuberculosis patients may be anticipated (hospital visiting rooms, triage areas, AIDS clinics, tuberculosis clinics, high-risk men's shelters, and jails), in corridors of high-risk hospital areas, in recirculation air ducts leading out of hospital areas where infectious patients are most likely to be housed, and in other special settings such as mycobacteriology laboratories or autopsy suites (56).

High-Efficiency Filtration

The CDC and OSHA previously endorsed the use of high-efficiency particulate aerosol (HEPA) filtration units for removal of infectious matter both within patient rooms and in recirculation ductwork leading out of rooms that house confirmed or suspected infectious patients (42). HEPA units, by definition, remove 99.97% of particles down to 0.3 μm in diameter. Thus, such systems might reasonably be assumed to substantially sterilize air. However, there are very significant practical impediments to the employment of HEPA units. High-efficiency filters inherently have increased resistive load. Therefore, they must be precisely installed lest air flow around and not through them. Also, they require more powerful ventilation units to pull/push air through them. In addition, because mycobacteria can survive in the environment for many weeks in a viable, potentially virulent state, these filters must be treated as high-grade biohazards when they are repaired, replaced, or disposed of.

No direct comparisons of the efficacy, efficiency, and costs of HEPA-filtered systems and UVGI systems have been conducted. Earlier OSHA regulations appeared to favor filtration, indicating that HEPA-filtered air may be recirculated but UVGI-treated air may not be. However, assessment of the relevant literature and my professional experience suggest that UVGI systems would be more effective, affordable, and practical to install and maintain than HEPA systems. A more efficient and sustainable air filtration system using devices with less resistive load than HEPA filters may prove to be an acceptable compromise.

Personal Respiratory Protective Devices

Over the past 6 years, CDC guidelines and OSHA or NIOSH policies have called for variable levels of use of personal respirators to protect HCWs from tuberculosis transmission. These published documents have followed a highly convoluted pathway marked by confusing semantics, uncertainty, and vacillation, resulting in wholesale distress among health professionals.

Before 1990, surgical masks, usually one-piece disposable units, were used on a sporadic basis. The usual indications were unavoidable exposure to a newly diagnosed case with forms of tuberculosis deemed highly infectious, such as laryngeal disease, extensive cavitation, strongly smear-positive, or highly productive cough. Masks were typically used by HCWs when involved with cough-inducing procedures as well. Beginning with the 1990 CDC Guidelines, however, there was a rapid escalation in respirator requirements.

The 1990 CDC document advocated the use of personal respirators when HCWs were likely to be exposed to infectious aerosols, recommending use at least of a dust/mist-level device (41).

However, in October 1992, OSHA in Region II (including, most notably, New York City) issued a policy requiring a higher-level respirator, the dust/mist/fume devices. At roughly the same time, NIOSH recommended the use of powered air-purifying respirators (PAPRs) to assuredly prevent infection of HCWs.

By October 1993, the CDC published *draft* guidelines on this topic, eliciting nearly 3,000 letters of comment. Based on these suggestions as well as further investigation, the 1994 CDC Guidelines included for the first time performance criteria for respirators. They also called for all health-care facilities in the United States to develop comprehensive plans to limit transmission not only to HCWs and other patients but to visitors, volunteers, and other persons within these facilities. Primarily intended for hospitals, medical wards at correctional facilities, nursing homes, and hospices, the guidelines also provided recommendations for ambulatory care facilities, emergency departments, home health-care settings, medical and dental offices, and various other ill-defined settings. Although it contained generally useful information, this bureaucratic leviathan spawned widespread frustration and uncertainty, particularly with regard to personal respirators.

In 1996, NIOSH released revised criteria for the evaluation and classification of personal respirators (64). This represented a shift away from the traditional nomenclature and testing of particulate respirators. In this system, NIOSH identified three types of respirators, N, P, and R. The N class respirators are intended for use against *non*-oil-based aerosols such as aqueous aerosols including secretions or fluids bearing tubercle bacilli. Within each of these three classes, respirators are rated on their efficiency at excluding particles of 0.3 μm mass median aerodynamic diameter. The levels identified are 99.97%, 99%, and 95%.

From this hierarchy has come the recent recommendations that, based on relative consideration of effectiveness, cost, comfort, and acceptability, HCWs use N-95 personal respirators as the devices of choice. Currently, there are numerous devices meeting these criteria on the market.

Now, having reached this plateau in the struggle to provide suitable protection for HCWs and others exposed to communicable forms of tuberculosis, we must still address the issue of *when* to employ personal respirators. This is a controversial, even inflammatory, question with many unresolved issues of science. In my estimation, the most balanced, informative delineation of the subject was recently authored by Fennelly (65). This essay not only reviews the physical nature and function of the various respirators but addresses the equally or more important issues of the relationship between levels of ventilation and the utility of personal respirators, fit-testing, and acceptance/compliance on the part of HCWs. In addition, the reviews detail the nature of the potentially infectious aerosols and create practical scenarios for tactics to interrupt transmission.

Fennelly and Nardell have developed a mathematical model that describes the relationships among three critical variables in the transmission of tuberculosis: the concentration of infectious particles, the ventilation, and the efficacy of various personal respiratory protection devices (66). These interrelationships can be displayed on a three-dimensional graph (Fig. 14.2). By this modeling, the likelihood of an HCW contracting infection can be calculated at varying levels of ventilation or while wearing personal respirators with different *assigned protection factors* (APF). As readily seen, in rooms with 6 to 12 ACs/hr, little benefit can be anticipated by wearing high-efficiency respirators in the setting of a relatively low level of infectious particle generation, 1.25 quanta per hour. However, in the case of a patient generating more infectious particles (Fig. 14.3), a respirator with a higher APF may be anticipated to confer significant benefit. This model provides a rational framework for decision making. Health care workers involved with high-risk situations (bronchoscopy, intubation, autopsy, etc.) might reasonably wear a fit-tested, high-APF device or a powered air-purifying respirator. However, other HCWs attending patients without extraordinary risk factors in a well-ventilated room with/without UVGI might well wear no personal respiratory protective device.

Why, if there is even a remote risk of infection, might a HCW choose *not* to use personal respiratory protection? There are numerous issues, some subtle or subjective, that influence that decision. From the perspective of the relationship to the patient, many HCWs, including me, feel that a respirator or PAPR constitutes a major barrier to emotional and verbal contact with the patient. Humans read one another's faces to form bonds of trust and affection, and this is denied by these devices. Words of informational or supportive content are obscured by these barriers. Many persons with tuberculosis are minorities or foreign-born for whom English is a second language; verbal contact is significantly impaired by the muffling of the HCW's voice and the inability to watch the HCW's mouth for additional cues. Finally and inevitably, the patient must feel stigmatized and isolated when all of the HCWs they encounter are masked.

From the perspective of the HCW, these devices are often perceived to be uncomfortable, to interfere with visual fields, to cause fogging of glasses, to disturb one's grooming while donning or removing, or to be a heavy-handed man-

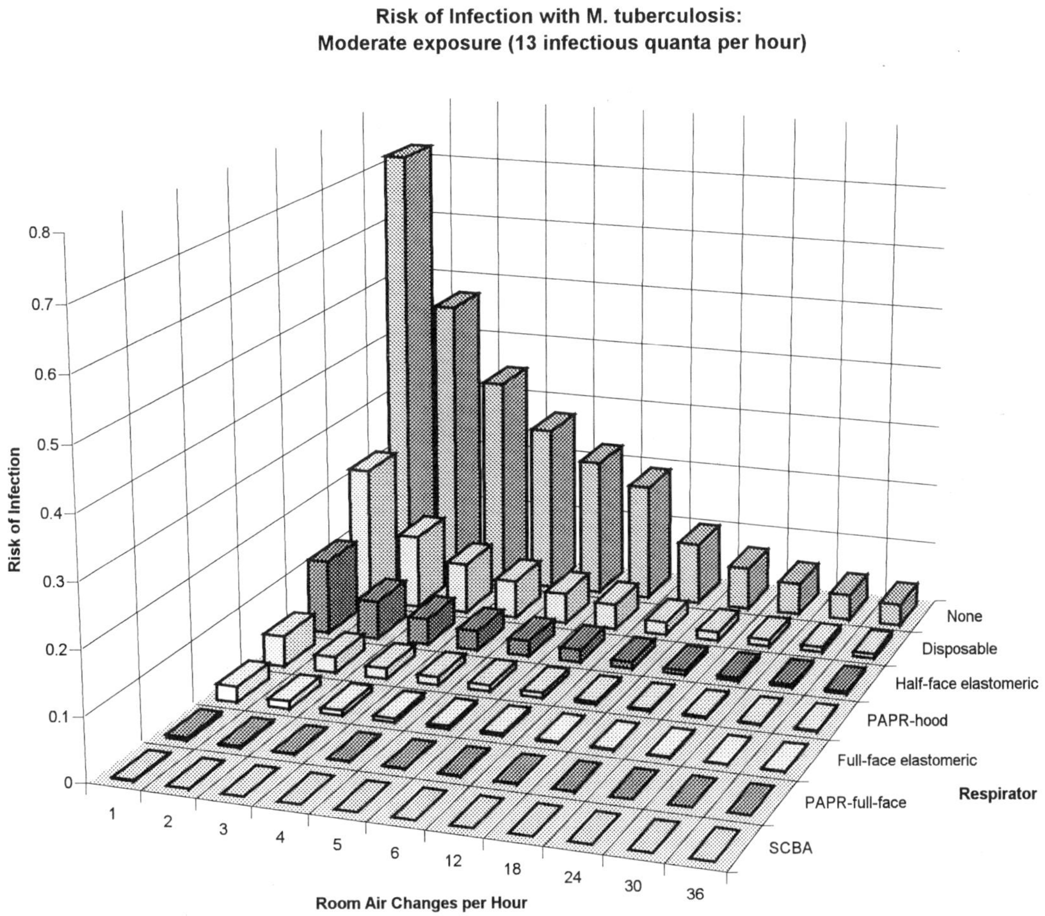

FIG. 14.2. In this mathematical analysis, Fennelly and Nardell demonstrate the relationships among the risk of infection, the number of air changes (ACs) per hour, and the use of various personal respiratory protective methods; they calculate these variables under the situation of moderate exposure, for example, a patient who produces 13 infectious quanta per hour. As may be seen, the risk of infection varies in nearly direct relationship to the number of ACs in which no respiratory protection is employed, but, even with 12 ACs per hour there is nearly a 10% risk of infection. However, with six or more ACs per hour, all of the personal respirators substantially lessened the risk. The likelihood of infection with different levels of infectious quanta generation is displayed in Fig. 14.3. From ref. 66, with permission.

ifestation of a remote authority that does not understand the subtleties of patient care. If the use of these devices were limited to situations in which there is an obvious, definite rationale, all parties would respond more favorably, programs would have more credibility, and substantial financial savings would result.

Should patients with confirmed or suspected tuberculosis be required to wear respirators? This issue has not been clearly or consistently addressed. Although I am not aware of any data regarding the capacity of masks to control the elaboration of infectious particles, the proposition appears very dubious for the following reasons. If, as indicated by research and empirical findings, it is high velocity exhalational maneuvers such as cough or sneezing which generate the great majority of microscopic particles likely to be infectious (see Chapter 3 for details), an occlusive respiratory mask with high efficiency (and resistive load) would be blown away from the face by the explosive event. Although the

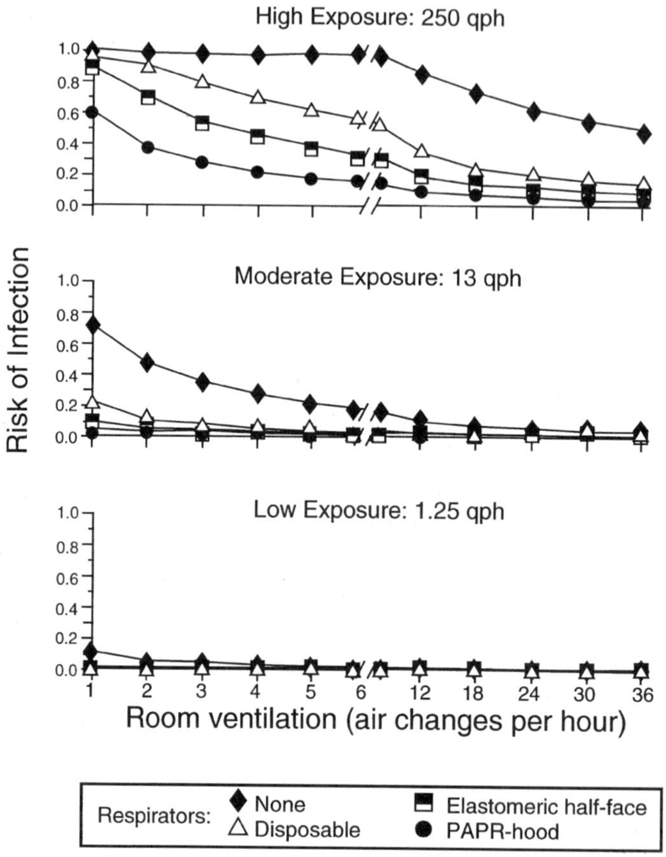

FIG. 14.3. Fennelly and Nardell's mathematical model also allows us to calculate the risk of infection in relation to air changes (ACs) per hour for hyperexcreters, producing 250 quanta per hour, such as seen in bronchoscopy procedures or autopsy suites, down to the low-level excretions that are typical of the usual tuberculosis patient, about 1.25 quanta per hour. As may be readily appreciated, even near-tornadic air movement (36 ACs/hr) is inadequate to protect those in the presence of a hyperexcreter. In this situation, high-level personal respiratory protection is clearly indicated. By contrast, under circumstances of low-level exposure, very little benefit may be demonstrated from respirators in the presence of even minimal air movement. From ref. 66, with permission.

mask might reduce the number of particles released, it seems far more efficient to teach the patients to cover their mouths and noses with tissue during cough or sneeze. Also, many patients early in the course of their illness have considerable dyspnea and may even require supplemental oxygen; in either of these cases, wearing a respirator would likely prove intolerable or impossible for the patients. For patients deemed likely to generate high numbers of infectious particles, wearing some device when they must visit or travel through the general milieu of a facility may seem intuitively appropriate. However, we should not mistake this for a practice of proven efficacy.

Surveillance (Tuberculin Testing) of Employees

The CDC and OSHA clearly place a very high priority on programs to regularly survey HCWs regarding the risk of tuberculosis infection. Such programs do not directly prevent transmission, but, by identifying areas or tasks that are associated with significant risk of occupationally acquired infection, they allow institutions to direct remediation. Current policies call for baseline and periodic tuberculin skin testing for all employees. The frequency with which periodic retesting is to be performed depends on whether the institution itself or units within the institution are shown on survey to be low, intermediate, or high risk for tuberculosis. The criteria for this are spelled out in the 1994 CDC/OSHA Guideline (42).

Other aspects of surveillance for workers include the obligation to perform chest x-rays and clinical assessments on all tuberculosis reactors or convertors to exclude active tuberculosis or to evaluate for preventive chemotherapy.

One of the more controversial aspects of the tuberculin surveillance recommendations is the mandate to perform tuberculin testing every 3 months among persons working in settings deemed high risk. This clearly speaks to the administrative and biological naiveté of the authors. Anyone who has worked in a health facility knows that it is not feasible without Draconian measures to administer and read Mantoux tests every 90 days for employees whose schedules are typical of hospital staff. Moreover this frequent schedule is simply not needed for normal hosts (who take months or years to develop diseases after infection) and is not suitable for persons with AIDS (who may develop tuberculous disease rapidly but are very likely to be anergic).

The mandate that health-care facilities test *all* employees is likewise problematic. For decades, such widespread screening has been discouraged, with the focus instead on persons or groups deemed at higher risk. Compelling all employees to be skin-tested annually has placed substantial burdens on overworked employee health services for negligible returns in most institutions in the United States. And, OSHA has another highly dubious practice in this regard. The current policy is to regard tuberculin skin test conversion of *any* employee of a health facility as an institutionally acquired infection. Particularly for urban facilities, which typically employ large numbers of minorities and immigrants from low-income neighborhoods, there is a predictable level of tuberculin conversion that reflects community-acquired infections. As noted in Chapter 5, in a population with an annual incidence of 48 cases per 100,000, it has been calculated that 1% of those uninfected would be newly infected each year. Thus, in an inner city where annual case rates may exceed 100, one would predict that staff living in these neighborhoods would experience roughly 2% annual rates of infection. If these individuals were employees of a health-care facility, under OSHA criteria they would be classified as institutional infections. Although there are both public and individual health advantages to the detection of these infections, the *appearance* of high rates of nosocomial tuberculosis infections creates immense problems for the institutions. Indeed, in just such a situation, analysis of tuberculin reactivity of the staff of an urban hospital in St. Louis indicated that new infection correlated with increasing age, minority race, and residency in low-income postal zones; over 50% of the convertors had no patient exposure (67). The potential mischief to arise from this situation is related to the institutional risk assessment described by OSHA: by designating all new infections as institutionally acquired, this system compels inappropriate and costly efforts at remediation and excessive frequency of tuberculin testing. Universal employee surveillance is indicated only in regions or institutions with demonstrated burdens of tuberculosis, in my estimation, and, if the initial results of institution-wide testing demonstrate no meaningful transmission in various groups, these facilities should be allowed to terminate routine surveillance of these persons.

Finally, if we are truly committed to preventing nosocomial tuberculosis in health care workers, we must inevitably confront the issue of HIV infection. Clearly, a vastly disproportionate share of tuberculosis morbidity and mortality among health care workers exposed during the well-studied outbreaks on the East Coast fell on those with underlying HIV/AIDS. Although it is an extremely sensitive political issue, educational programs for HCWs, consistent encouragement of HIV serology testing, and strong efforts to discourage HIV-infected persons from working in units with predictable, high-risk exposure to communicable tuberculosis may be the most effective measure to diminish tuberculosis among HCWs.

PRACTICAL CONSIDERATIONS IN LIMITING TRANSMISSION

The current situation regarding efforts to control tuberculosis transmission represents a substantial shift in U.S. public health practices. Until the early 1990s, preventing transmission had been a professional endeavor driven by broad notions of protection for patients and staff as well as general public good. Implicit in the guidelines and practices was a sense of the inherent *im*perfectability of institutions such as the large, heavily burdened urban hospitals that provided care for many tuberculosis patients, imperfect because of the predictable constraints on personnel and material assets.

As noted above in the section on personal respiratory protection, the occupational perspective historically has been that, if a single tubercle bacillus might cause infection, then the permissible exposure level is zero. From this binary system ("all or none") flows, by internal logic, the stringent requirement for very high-level protection measures to *prevent infection.*

By comparison, the infection control paradigm entails the view of a wide continuum of levels of exposure and likelihood of infection. Also, tuberculosis control programs historically have tacitly factored in the *unlikelihood* of infection progressing to disease and the relative benignity of most forms of tuberculosis when promptly treated. Among normal hosts who are infected with *M. tuberculosis,* there is calculated to be 10% or less lifetime risk of developing active tuberculous disease. And, if new infections with drug-susceptible strains of tuberculosis are detected by tuberculin skin test conversion, preventive chemotherapy can reduce the risk of disease from 10% to 1–3%. Finally, among those who develop overt disease with drug-susceptible bacilli, 6 months of therapy offers a 98% lifetime cure rate.

Nonetheless, in view of the extraordinary risks involved with HIV-infected patients or HCWs and multidrug-resistant tuberculosis, there is legitimate cause to reevaluate traditional methods to limit transmission. The OSHA methodology, although apparently useful and feasible in protecting workers in other industrial settings, seems to me to be not well suited to the problem of airborne tuberculosis spread. The impracticality of the occupational paradigm in this model is captured best, perhaps unwittingly, in the words of a physician in an essay explaining and justifying the OSHA position:

> The [correct] observation by the infection control community that there is no proof that TB transmission occurs with the use of dust/mist masks when the 1990 CDC guidelines are properly implemented, is simply irrelevant; the standard of the law is not prevention of transmission but prevention of exposure. (68)

If this is indeed an accurate representation of OSHA's policy and practice, then institutions and practitioners will inevitably be driven to extreme, impractical, and expensive measures that will distract from the mission, divert precious resources, and breed mistrust and disrespect for OSHA. Certainly, no one in the field of tuberculosis or infection control can feel sanguine about seeing a fellow health care worker infected with or diseased by the tubercle bacillus. Rather, the issue is what measures can be applied in a real-life, sustainable, cost-effective system that are compatible with a humane, professional environment for care (69).

REFERENCES

1. Centers for Disease Control. Tuberculosis in a drug rehabilitation center—Colorado. *MMWR* 1980;29:543–544.
2. Centers for Disease Control. Transmission of multidrug-resistant tuberculosis from an HIV-positive client in a residential substance-abuse treatment facility—Michigan. *MMWR* 1991;40:129–131.
3. Nardell E, McInnis B, Thomas B, Weishaas S. Exogenous reinfection with tuberculosis in a shelter for the homeless. *N Engl J Med* 1986;315:1570–1575.
4. King L, Geis G. Tuberculosis transmission in a large urban jail. *JAMA* 1977;237:791–792.
5. Stead W, Senner J, Reddick W, Lofgren J. Racial differences in susceptibility to infection by *Mycobacterium tuberculosis. N Engl J Med* 1990;322:422–427.
6. Nolan CM, Elarth AM, Barr H, Saeed AM, Risser DR. An outbreak of tuberculosis in a shelter for homeless men. A description of its evolution and control. *Am Rev Respir Dis* 1991;143:257–261.
7. Daley CL, Small PM, Schecter GF, et al. An outbreak of tuberculosis with accelerated progression among per-

sons infected with the human immunodeficiency virus. An analysis using restriction-fragment-length polymorphisms. *N Engl J Med* 1992;326:231–235.
8. Stead WW, Dutt AK. Tuberculosis in elderly persons. *Annu Rev Med* 1991;42:267–276.
9. Centers for Disease Control. Tuberculosis in a nursing care facility—Washington. *MMWR* 1983;32:121–129.
10. Centers for Disease Control. Tuberculosis in a nursing home—Oklahoma. *MMWR* 1980;29:465–467.
11. Ehrenkranz NJ, Kicklighter JL. Tuberculosis outbreak in a general hospital: evidence for airborne spread of infection. *Ann Intern Med* 1972;77:377–382.
12. Catanzaro A. Nosocomial tuberculosis. *Am Rev Respir Dis* 1982;125:559–562.
13. Kantor HS, Poblete R, Pusateri SL. Nosocomial transmission of tuberculosis from unsuspected disease. *Am J Med* 1988;84:833–838.
14. Hutton MD, Stead WW, Cauthen GM, Bloch AB, Ewing WM. Nosocomial transmission of tuberculosis associated with a draining abscess. *J Infect Dis* 1990; 161:286–295.
15. Frampton M. An outbreak of tuberculosis among hospital personnel caring for a patient with a skin ulcer. *Ann Intern Med* 1992;117:312–313.
16. Edlin BR, Tokars JI, Grieco MH, et al. An outbreak of multidrug-resistant tuberculosis among hospitalized patients with the acquired immunodeficiency syndrome. *N Engl J Med* 1992;326:1514–1521.
17. Dooley SW, Villarino ME, Lawrence M, et al. Nosocomial transmission of tuberculosis in a hospital unit for HIV-infected patients. *JAMA* 1992;267:2632–2635.
18. Pearson ML, Jereb JA, Frieden TR, et al. Nosocomial transmission of multidrug-resistant *Mycobacterium tuberculosis.* A risk to patients and health care workers. *Ann Intern Med* 1992;117:191–196.
19. Fischl MA, Uttamchandani RB, Daikos GL, et al. An outbreak of tuberculosis caused by multiple-drug-resistant tubercle bacilli among patients with HIV infection. *Ann Intern Med* 1992;117:177–183.
20. Beck-Sagué C, Dooley SW, Hutton MD, et al. Hospital outbreak of multidrug-resistant *Mycobacterium tuberculosis* infections. Factors in transmission to staff and HIV-infected patients. *JAMA* 1992;268:1280–1286.
21. Jereb JA, Klevens M, Privett TD, et al. Tuberculosis in health care workers at a hospital with an outbreak of multidrug-resistant *Mycobacterium tuberculosis. Arch Intern Med* 1995;155:854–859.
22. Ikeda RM, Birkhead GS, DiFerdinando GT Jr, et al. Nosocomial tuberculosis: an outbreak of a strain resistant to seven drugs. *Infect Control Hosp Epidemiol* 1995;16:152–159.
23. Haley CE, McDonald RC, Rossi L. Tuberculosis epidemic among hospital personnel. *Infect Control Hosp Epidemiol* 1989;10:204–210.
24. Griffith DE, Hardeman JL, Zhang Y, Wallace RJ, Mazurek GH. Tuberculosis outbreak among healthcare workers in a community hospital. *Am J Respir Crit Care Med* 1995;152:808–811.
25. Templeton GL, Illing LA, Young L, Cave D, Stead WW, Bates JH. The risk for transmission of *Mycobacterium tuberculosis* at the bedside and during autopsy. *Ann Intern Med* 1995;122:922–925.
26. Frieden TR, Sherman LF, Maw KL, et al. A multi-institutional outbreak of highly drug-resistant tuberculosis. Epidemiology and clinical outcomes. *JAMA* 1996; 276:1229–1235.
27. Kenyon TA, Ridzon R, Luskin-Hawk R, et al. A nosocomial outbreak of multidrug-resistant tuberculosis. *Ann Intern Med* 1997;127:32–36.
28. Small PM, Hopewell PC, Singh SP, et al. The epidemiology of tuberculosis in San Francisco. A population-based study using conventional and molecular methods. *N Engl J Med* 1994;330:1703–1709.
29. Alland D, Kalkut GE, Moss AR, et al. Transmission of tuberculosis in New York City. An analysis by DNA fingerprinting and conventional epidemiologic methods. *N Engl J Med* 1994;330:1710–1716.
30. Friedman CR, Stoeckle MY, Kreiswirth BN, et al. Transmission of multidrug-resistant tuberculosis in a large urban setting. *Am J Respir Crit Care Med* 1995;152:355–359.
31. Bifani PJ, Plikaytis BB, Kapur V, et al. Origin and interstate spread of a New York City multidrug-resistant *Mycobacterium tuberculosis* clone family. *JAMA* 1996;275:452–457.
32. Barnes PF, El-Hajj H, Preston-Martin S, et al. Transmission of tuberculosis among the urban homeless. *JAMA* 1996;275:305–307.
33. Braun MM, Truman BI, Maguire B, et al. Increasing incidence of tuberculosis in a prison inmate population. Association with HIV infection. *JAMA* 1989;261: 393–397.
34. DiPerri G, Cruciani M, Danzi MC, et al. Nosocomial epidemic of active tuberculosis among HIV-infected patients. *Lancet* 1989;2:1502–1504.
35. DiPerri G, Cadeo GP, Castelli F, et al. Transmission of HIV-associated tuberculosis to health-care workers. *Lancet* 1992;340:682.
36. Bader J-M. France: nosocomial multidrug resistant TB. *Lancet* 1992;340:1533.
37. Longuet P, Pierre J, Lacassin F. *A limited multidrug-resistant* Mycobacterium tuberculosis *(MDR TB) outbreak: screening of contact hospitalized patients (pts).* Paper presented at the 35th Interscience Conference on Antimicrobial Agents and Chemotherapy, 1995.
38. Ritacco V, Di Lonardo M, Reniero A, et al. Nosocomial spread of human immunodeficiency virus-related multidrug-resistant tuberculosis in Buenos Aires. *J Infect Dis* 1997;176:637–642.
39. Chaves F, Dronda F, Cave MD, et al. A longitudinal study of transmission of tuberculosis in a large prison population. *Am J Respir Crit Care Med* 1997;155:719–725.
40. Bradford WZ, Martin JN, Reingold AL, Schecter GF, Hopewell PC, Small PM. The changing epidemiology of acquired drug-resistant tuberculosis in San Francisco, USA. *Lancet* 1996;348:928–931.
41. Centers for Disease Control. Guidelines for preventing the transmission of tuberculosis in health-care settings, with special focus on HIV-related issues. *MMWR* 1990;39:1–29.
42. Centers for Disease Control. Guidelines for preventing the transmission of *Mycobacterium tuberculosis* in health-care facilities, 1994. *MMWR* 1994;43:1–132.
43. Gerberding JL. Occupational infectious diseases or infectious occupational diseases? Bridging the issues on tuberculosis control. *Infect Control Hosp Epidemiol* 1993;14:686–688.
44. MacDiarmid M. Comment at conference. In: *TB and the Health Care Environment. A National Seminar on Integrating Infection Control and Engineering Systems, Dallas,* January, 1994.

45. Scott B, Schmid M, Nettleman MD. Early identification and isolation of inpatients at high risk for tuberculosis. *Arch Intern Med* 1994;154:326–330.
46. Blumberg HM, Watkins DL, Berschling JD, et al. Preventing the nosocomial transmission of tuberculosis. *Ann Intern Med* 1995;122:658–663.
47. Bock NN, McGowan JE Jr, Ahn J, Tapia J, Blumberg HM. Clinical predictors of tuberculosis as a guide for a respiratory isolation policy. *Am J Respir Crit Care Med* 1996;154:1468–1472.
48. Kamat SR, Daawson JJY, Devadatta S, et al. A controlled study of the influence of segregation of tuberculous patients for one year on the attack rate of tuberculosis in a 5-year period in close family contacts in South India. *Bull WHO* 1966;34:517–532.
49. Gunnells JJ, Bates JH, Swindoll H. Infectivity of sputum-positive tuberculous patients on chemotherapy. *Am Rev Respir Dis* 1974;109:323–330.
50. Brooks SM, Lassiter NL, Young EC. A pilot study of the infection risk of sputa positive tuberculous patients on chemotherapy. *Am Rev Respir Dis* 1973;108: 799–894.
51. Riley RL, Moodie AS. Infectivity of patients with pulmonary tuberculosis in inner city homes. *Am Rev Respir Dis* 1974;110:810–812.
52. Hobby GL, Holman AP, Iseman MD, Jones J. Enumeration of tubercle bacilli in sputum of patients with pulmonary tuberculosis. *Antimicrob Agents Chemother* 1973;4:94–104.
53. Jindani A, Aber VR, Edwards EA, Mitchison DA. The early bactericidal activity of drugs in patients with pulmonary tuberculosis. *Am Rev Respir Dis* 1980;121: 939–949.
54. Loudon RG, Romans WE. Cough frequency and infectivity in patients with pulmonary tuberculosis. *Am Rev Respir Dis* 1969;99:109–111.
55. Nardell EA, Keegan J, Cheney SA, Etkind SC. Airborne infection. Theoretical limits of protection achievable by building ventilation. *Am Rev Respir Dis* 1991;144: 302–306.
56. Riley R, Nardell E. Cleaning the air: the theory and application of ultraviolet air disinfection. *Am Rev Respir Dis* 1989;139:1286–1294.
57. Riley R, Mills C, O'Grady F, Sultan LU, Wittstadt F, Shivpuri DN. Infectiousness of air from a tuberculosis ward. Ultraviolet irradiation of infected air: comparative infectiousness of different patients. *Am Rev Respir Dis* 1962;85:511–525.
58. Riley RL, Knight M, Middlebrook G. Ultraviolet susceptibility of BCG and virulent tubercle bacilli. *Am Rev Respir Dis* 1976;113:413–418.
59. Stead W. Clearing the air: the theory and application of ultraviolet air disinfection (letter). *Am Rev Respir Dis* 1989;140:1832.
60. Madsen L, Carbajal J, Iseman M. Low incidence of nosocomial infection of health care workers on a tuberculosis ward equipped with ultraviolet germicidal irradiation. *Am J Respir Crit Care Med* 1994;149: A855.
61. Fennelly KP, Martyny JW, Ackerson LM, Mueller KL. The role of disposable particulate respirators in the prevention of occupational tuberculosis: respiratory protection, acceptance, and fit testing in a hospital setting (abstract). *Am J Respir Crit Care Med* 1994;149: A527.
62. Nardell E. Fans, filters or rays? Pros and cons of the current environmental tuberculosis control strategies. *Infect Control Hosp Epidemiol* 1993;14:681–685.
63. Iseman MD. A leap of faith—what can we do to curtail intrainstitutional transmission of tuberculosis? [editorial]. *Ann Intern Med* 1992;117:251.
64. USDHHS. *NIOSH guide to the selection and use of particulate respirators certified under 42 CFR 84.* Washington, DC: USDHHS, 1996.
65. Fennelly KP. Personal respiratory protection against *Mycobacterium tuberculosis.* In: Iseman MD, Huitt GA, eds. *Clinics in chest medicine.* Philadelphia: WB Saunders, 1996:1–17.
66. Fennelly KP, Nardell EA. The relative efficacy of respirators and room ventilation in preventing occupational tuberculosis. *Infect Control Hosp Epidemiol* 1998;19: 754–759.
67. Bailey TC, Fraser VJ, Spitznagel EL, Dunagan WC. Risk factors for a positive tuberculin skin test among employees of an urban, midwestern teaching hospital. *Ann Intern Med* 1995;122:580–585.
68. Decker MD. OSHA enforcement policy for occupational exposure to tuberculosis (special report). *Infect Control Hosp Epidemiol* 1993;14:689–693.
69. Nolan CM. Tuberculosis in health care professionals: assessing and accepting the risk. *Ann Intern Med* 1994; 120:964–965.

Subject Index